Essentials of Orthognathic Surgery

Third Edition

Essentials of
ORTHOGNATHIC SURGERY

THIRD EDITION

Johan Reyneke, BChD, MChD, FCMFOS (SA), PhD

Director
Centre of Orthognathic Surgery
Mediclinic
Cape Town, South Africa

Clinical Professor
Department of Oral and Maxillofacial Surgery
University of Florida College of Dentistry
Gainesville, Florida

Extraordinary Professor
Department of Maxillofacial and Oral Surgery
University of the Western Cape
Cape Town, South Africa

Associate Professor
Division of Oral and Maxillofacial Surgery
Universidad Autónoma de Nuevo León
Monterrey, Mexico

Clinical Professor
Department of Surgical Sciences
Division of Oral and Maxillofacial Surgery
University of Oklahoma College of Dentistry
Oklahoma City, Oklahoma

With contributions from

Steven M. Sullivan, DDS
Professor and Chair
Department of Surgical Sciences
Division of Oral and Maxillofacial Surgery
University of Oklahoma College of Dentistry
Oklahoma City, Oklahoma

QUINTESSENCE PUBLISHING

Berlin | Chicago | Tokyo
Barcelona | London | Milan | Mexico City | Moscow | Paris | Prague | Seoul | Warsaw
Beijing | Istanbul | Sao Paulo | Zagreb

Library of Congress Cataloging-in-Publication Data

Names: Reyneke, Johan P., author.
Title: Essentials of orthognathic surgery / Johan P. Reyneke.
Description: Third edition. | Batavia, IL : Quintessence Publishing Co, Inc, [2021] | Includes bibliographical references and index. | Summary: "Clinical manual for the diagnosis and treatment of different dentofacial deformities with orthognathic surgery, including patient assessment with cephalometric analysis and surgical techniques such as Le Fort I osteotomy, bilateral sagittal split osteotomy, and genioplasty"-- Provided by publisher.
Identifiers: LCCN 2019036472 (print) | LCCN 2019036473 (ebook) | ISBN 9780867159561 (hardcover) | ISBN 9780867159691 (ebook)
Subjects: MESH: Dentofacial Deformities--surgery | Dentofacial Deformities--diagnosis | Malocclusion--surgery | Orthognathic Surgical Procedures--methods | Atlas | Case Reports
Classification: LCC RK521 (print) | LCC RK521 (ebook) | NLM WU 600.7 | DDC 617.6/43059--dc23
LC record available at https://lccn.loc.gov/2019036472
LC ebook record available at https://lccn.loc.gov/2019036473

A CIP record for this book is available from the British Library.
ISBN: 9780867159561

QUINTESSENCE PUBLISHING
USA

Quintessence Publishing Co, Inc
411 N Raddant Road
Batavia, IL 60510
www.quintpub.com

5 4 3 2 1

Editor: Marieke Zaffron
Design: Sue Zubek
Production: Angelina Schmelter

Printed in Croatia

CONTENTS

PREFACE

From the outset, the fundamental purpose of *Essentials of Orthognathic Surgery* was to provide the clinician with basic and "to the point" information regarding the assessment, diagnosis, treatment planning, and treatment of individuals with dentofacial deformities. The general plan of the third edition is unaltered; however, as with most fields in medicine, orthognathic surgery is a dynamic science that is developing exponentially over time. It was therefore exciting to refresh the text by adding new developments and ideas and use clinical cases as demonstration.

This edition is enhanced by extending several chapters and by the addition of several new sections such as the diagnosis and treatment of hemifacial microsomia, the role of total temporomandibular joint replacement in orthognathic surgery, functional and esthetic nasal control with Le Fort I osteotomy, functional tongue reduction for open bite cases, and indications and implementation of a unilateral sagittal split osteotomy for the correction of mandibular asymmetry.

Since Vilray Blair completed a bilateral osteotomy of the mandible under chloroform anesthesia in 1897, the correction of mandibular dentofacial deformities has developed into a routine surgical procedure that is carried out all over the world. We are fortunate to have been able to stand on the shoulders of giants in the field of orthodontics and oral and maxillofacial surgery who lay the foundations of this surgical science. It is, however, our responsibility to develop the science and art of orthodontics and surgery further and to share our experience with our students and colleagues to the benefit of our patients.

There is an old saying: "A pleasure shared is a pleasure doubled." Successful treatment allows the clinician to share the functional and esthetic changes with not only the patient but also the patient's family and friends and the orthognathic treatment team. We don't change faces, we change lives. I have been blessed with the privilege of correcting dentofacial deformities for more than 40 years and honored by sharing experience gained over this time through this book and other contributions. Sharing experience is an essential ingredient of education, and I thank all the postgraduate residents in oral and maxillofacial surgery who honored me by allowing me to participate in their education.

Acknowledgments

I would like to express my sincere appreciation and gratitude to my good friend and colleague Steven Sullivan, who added further value by contributing two new sections: the management of the airway in the orthognathic surgery patient and 3D virtual treatment planning for orthognathic surgery.

1

Principles of Orthognathic Surgery

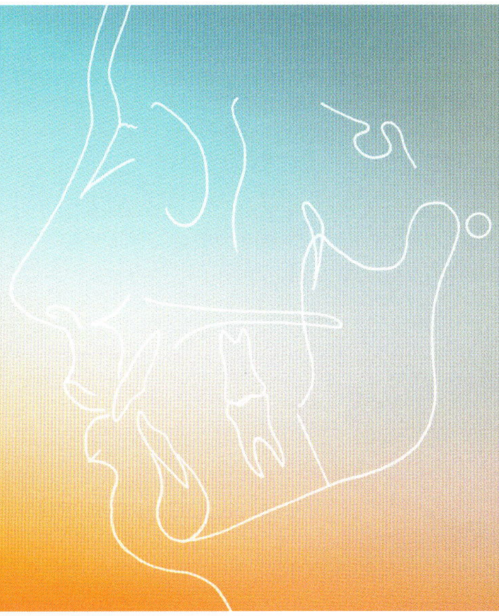

When people recognize malpositioned teeth or obvious jaw deformities, they usually seek treatment from an orthodontist, who can improve tooth alignment, function, and facial esthetics. More severe deformities that require a combination of orthodontics and surgery for correction are called *dentofacial deformities*. These deformities can affect physical orofacial function in several ways. Mastication can be impaired, and—especially in severe cases—this impairment can affect digestion and general nutritional health. Lip incompetence due to excessive vertical growth of the maxilla results in mouth breathing, which eliminates the physiologic effect of the nose on breathing. Speech is often affected by dentofacial deformities despite the body's adaptive capabilities. Malpositioned teeth may have a profound effect on proper oral hygiene maintenance, making teeth more susceptible to dental caries and periodontal disease. The patency of the airway and normal breathing is certainly affected by the position of the jaws, and dentofacial deformities are currently considered an important etiologic factor in the development of obstructive sleep apnea. Several types of dentofacial deformities also affect temporomandibular function. The physical effects of a dentofacial deformity are important, but the psychosocial impact of a dentofacial deformity on an individual is often paramount. This type of deformity can profoundly affect the quality of life and may entail lifelong adjustment.

Treatment Options for Dentofacial Deformities

The combination of surgery and orthodontic treatment makes it possible to treat dentofacial deformities that are not possible to correct with orthodontics alone (eg, vertical maxillary excess and severe anterior open bite malocclusion). Orthognathic surgery has created new and exciting opportunities in the treatment of patients with dentofacial deformities and provided the orthodontist with options other than compromised treatment for patients with skeletal disharmony. Experience in orthognathic surgery, an increased understanding of its biologic basis, and a refinement of its art form now enable us to routinely deliver a stable, esthetic, and functional result to patients. When severe skeletal discrepancies result in malocclusion, three kinds of treatment are available: growth modification, orthodontic camouflage, and orthognathic surgery.

Growth modification

This treatment approach should only be considered for mild skeletal deformities. In growing children, dentofacial orthopedics can alter the expression of growth to some extent. However, the extent of growth alteration varies, and this topic remains controversial. The following facial growth patterns may be influenced by growth modification in adolescents:

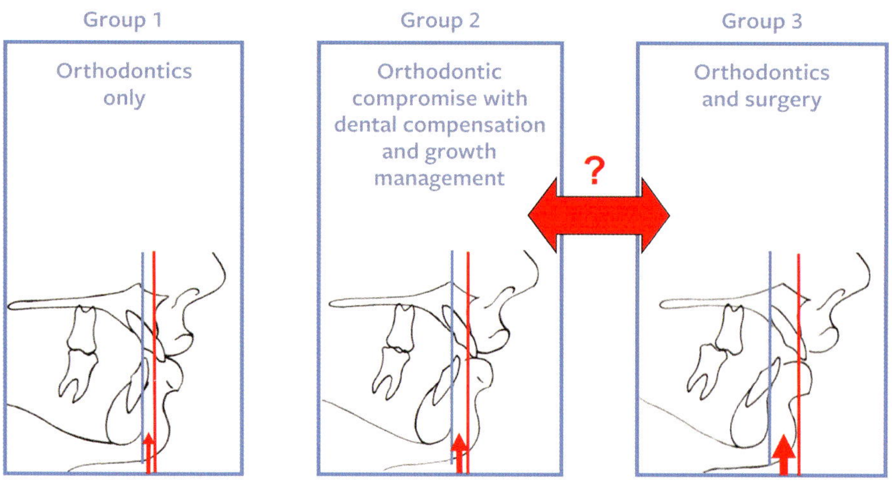

Fig 1-1 Patients who may seek treatment for their malocclusions from an orthodontist can in general be divided into three categories according to the severity of their skeletal deformities. When planning treatment, it can be challenging but is essential to differentiate between groups 2 and 3.

- *Maxillary anteroposterior excess:* Excessive horizontal growth of the maxilla may be impeded by headgear or camouflaged by extraction of the maxillary first premolars and orthodontic retraction of the incisors.
- *Maxillary anteroposterior deficiency:* Moderate improvement can be established by orthodontic protraction.
- *Vertical maxillary excess:* High-pull headgear with temporary anchorage devices can impede the vertical growth of the maxilla and diminish the severity of the deformity.
- *Mandibular anteroposterior deficiency:* Headgear combined with functional appliances may improve mandibular projection.

Skeletal deformities such as mandibular anteroposterior excess, vertical maxillary deficiency, and microgenia cannot be easily influenced by growth modification. In addition, there are some patients who may undergo growth modification for a long period of time with headgear or elastics and end up still requiring a surgical approach. This can be very disappointing and frustrating for the patient as well as their family and health care providers.

Preparing for surgery in these cases would often also require "reverse" orthodontics, decompensating the attempts to compenstate the dentition before orthognathic surgery, prolonging treatment even further.

Orthodontic camouflage

Certain patients with mild skeletal discrepancies would benefit from orthodontic camouflage rather than surgery. Dental compensation for a skeletal deformity, or orthodontic camouflage, may, however, be associated with impaired esthetics, questionable posttreatment stability, and prolonged treatment time (see Figs 1-2 and 1-3). Corrective treatment may require rebanding and a second orthodontic treatment followed by orthognathic surgery.

Orthognathic surgery

Combined orthodontic and surgical correction is considered the best treatment modality for dentoskeletal imbalances once growth has ceased. Although orthognathic surgery is associated with certain risks and challenges, it has become a more refined and less traumatic procedure for patients and therefore is now a reasonable treatment option. Improving skeletal relationships will result in remarkable facial changes, and this is an important goal to consider.

Selecting a treatment

Patients seeking orthodontic treatment have a wide range of functional and esthetic needs and can be divided into three groups (Fig 1-1):

- *Group 1:* Those with a normal skeletal relationship and malocclusions that can be treated using routine orthodontic techniques.
- *Group 2:* Those with mild to moderate skeletal discrepancies. The malocclusions of many of the patients in this group can be corrected by dental compensation and growth management. Both options—pursuing only orthodontic treatment and pursuing combined treatment—will have advantages and disadvantages that must be discussed between the clinicians, the patient, and the patient's parents (if necessary). There are several factors that will determine the treatment decision.

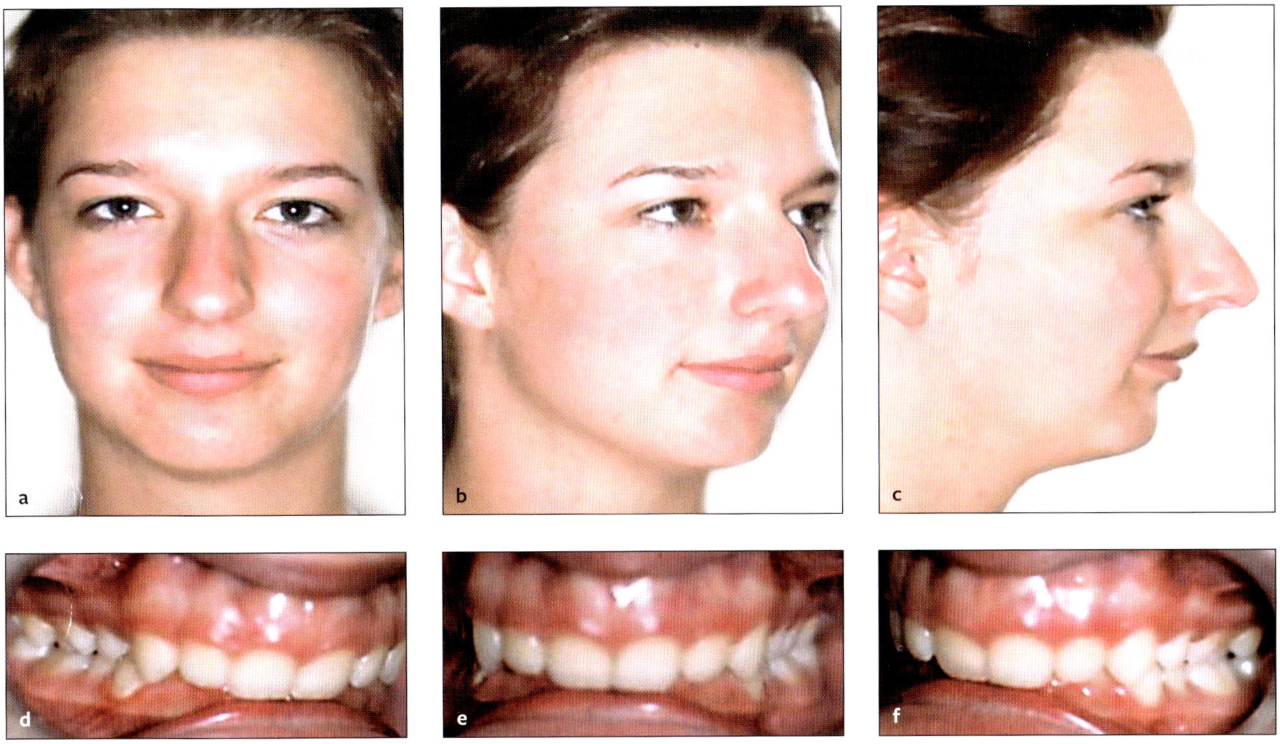

Fig 1-2 (*a to f*) A 19-year-old patient with a skeletal Class II relationship who would be considered to fall into group 3. Her maxillary first premolars were removed and the maxillary incisors retracted in an attempt to correct her occlusion. Unfortunately, the treatment compromised her esthetics and occlusion, resulting in a severe convex profile that accentuated her prominent nose and a Class II deep bite malocclusion.

- *Group 3:* Those with moderate to severe skeletal discrepancy and noticeable facial imbalance. The negative effects of compromised orthodontic treatment for patients in the third group would be unacceptable, making combined surgery and orthodontics the treatment of choice. In cases when the surgical option is not acceptable to the patient, it would be wise for the surgeon not to accept the patient for treatment. Orthodontic treatment alone for patients in this group will certainly worsen the esthetics, have doubtful stability, and possibly have negative long-term periodontic implications (Figs 1-2 and 1-3). On the other hand, only pursuing surgery without orthodontics would also lead to compromise.

An important challenge for the clinician is to differentiate between patients on the borderline between group 2 and group 3. An orthodontic camouflage treatment for patients in group 3 would be a mistake, just as surgical treatment of certain patients in group 2 would be inappropriate. The decision regarding the best treatment for borderline patients is influenced by various factors:

- *The patient's main complaint and preferences.* Some patients are interested only in improving occlusion, whereas esthetic change is a high priority for others. The patient's priority is an important factor in treatment planning: The patient needs to be able to weigh the two treatment options against each other and must therefore be well informed.
  1. Long orthodontic treatment. This often involves headgear, functional appliances, and a different extraction pattern with a compromised treatment outcome. The possibility of worsening esthetics, instability, and long-term periodontal problems should be discussed with the patient (and parents when applicable).
  2. Shorter orthodontic treatment combined with surgery. The surgical implications, possible complications, and improved treatment outcome must be discussed with the patient (and parents when applicable).
- *The orthodontist's preferences and skills.* If the orthodontist has encountered poor surgical results with previous patients, there will be a natural hesitation to continue

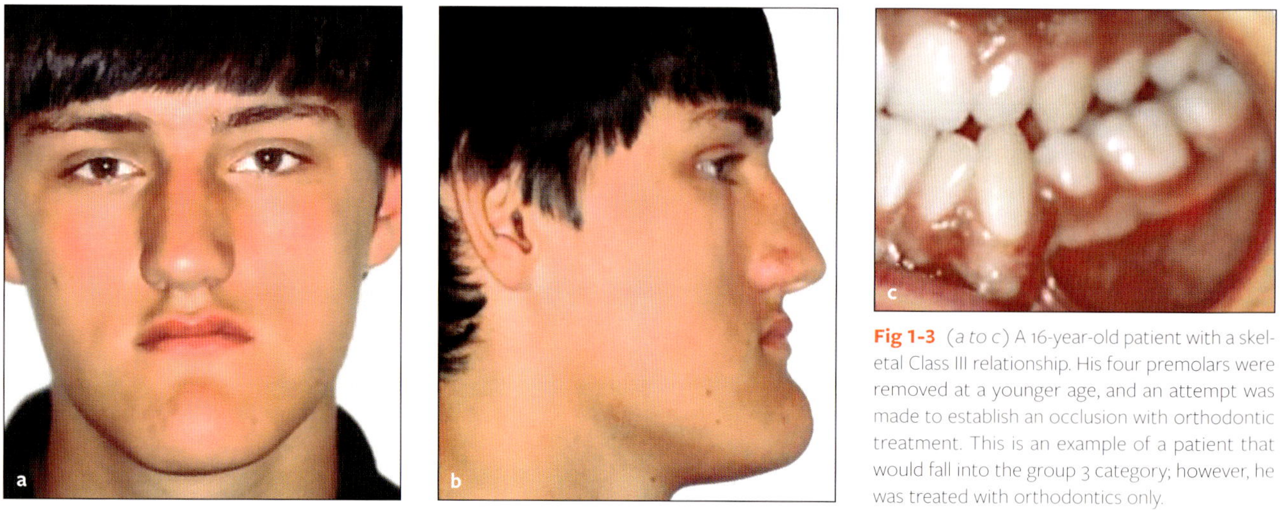

Fig 1-3 (*a to c*) A 16-year-old patient with a skeletal Class III relationship. His four premolars were removed at a younger age, and an attempt was made to establish an occlusion with orthodontic treatment. This is an example of a patient that would fall into the group 3 category; however, he was treated with orthodontics only.

to recommend surgery. The orthodontist's confidence in the success of surgery is an important factor.

- *Available surgical skills.* Orthognathic surgical expertise may not be available in the area, and the patient may be unable to travel.
- *Lack of insurance coverage.* The financial implications of orthodontic treatment with the added burden of surgery and hospitalization can be substantial, and this is a significant factor for patients to consider.

Treating patients in group 3 with orthodontics alone (group 2 treatment) may create additional problems (eg, occlusal relapse, worsening of the profile, obstructive sleep apnea (OSA), periodontal and temporomandibular joint decline) rather than solving the existing problem. Surgical treatment of patients in group 2 is appropriate when camouflage treatment would produce an unacceptable esthetic result or when orthodontics alone cannot achieve the desired facial change. Camouflage treatment also can be considered an alternative treatment method that should render acceptable functional, stable, and esthetic results.

Treatment Objectives in Orthognathic Surgery

Four treatment objectives are fundamental in orthognathic surgery: (*1*) function, (*2*) esthetics, (*3*) airway patency, and (*4*) stability of results. These objectives form the basic goals in treating patients with dentofacial deformities and often go hand in hand.

Function

Functional and esthetic deformities often exist concurrently, so treatment should be designed to correct both. The orofacial functional objectives should not only incorporate the bite and chewing functions but also include normal breathing, speech, swallowing, and temporomandibular joint function. When correcting a functional problem, the clinician should make full use of the opportunity to improve facial esthetics at the same time. It is particularly challenging to treat patients whose function is poor but esthetics are already good. Careful planning is essential to avoid additional esthetic deformity while providing optimal functional relationships.

Esthetics

The patient's main concern is often their facial appearance, and it is paramount to establish what the patient perceives as esthetically wrong. As Leo Tolstoy said in *Childhood*, "I am convinced that nothing has so marked influence on the direction of a man's mind as his appearance, and not his appearance itself so much as his conviction that it is attractive or unattractive."

Esthetic imbalance is often the result of a significant dentoskeletal deformity. Esthetic results can be improved by surgery alone in some patients, although the functional problem will not necessarily be treated. For example, if a patient with mandibular anteroposterior deficiency is treated with surgical advancement of the chin, this may result in a Class II malocclusion. In contrast, for a patient with vertical maxillary excess, it may be possible

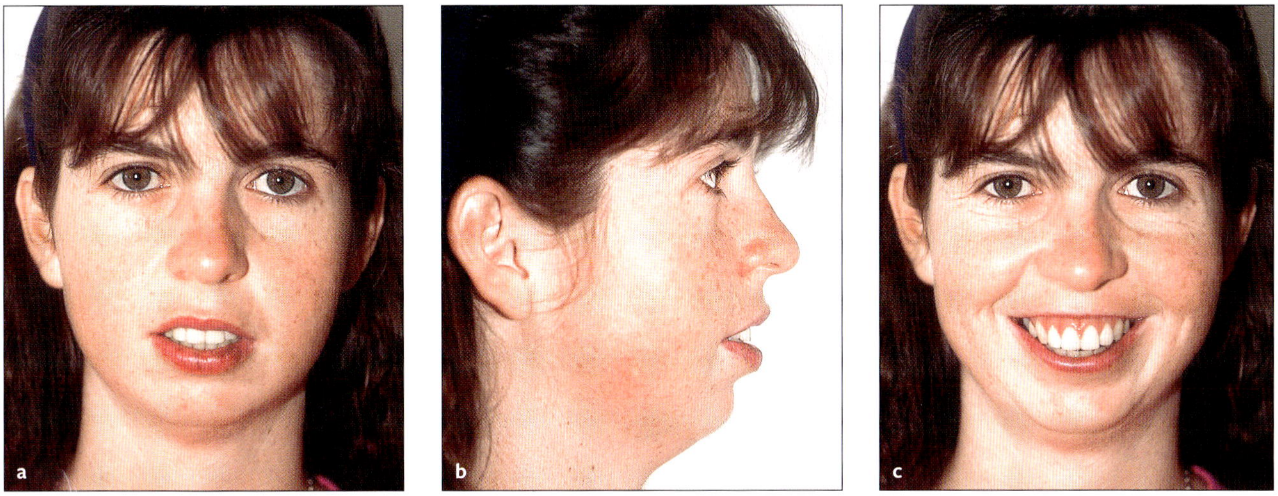

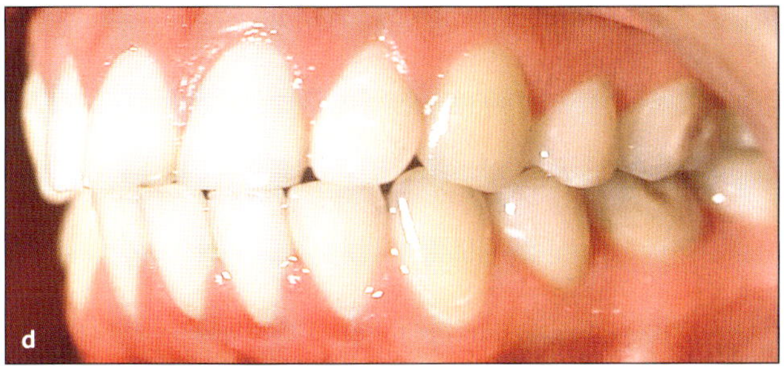

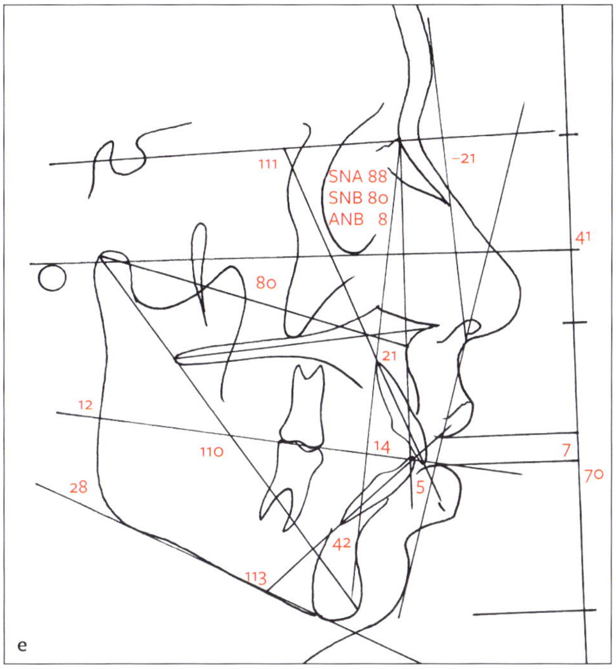

Fig 1-4 This 20-year-old patient was referred to the surgeon with the main complaint that her chin appeared too small and she did not like her "gummy smile." Previous orthodontic treatment lasted 3 years and consisted of extraction of four first premolars, retraction of maxillary incisors, and proclination of mandibular incisors. She was not offered the option of surgical correction of her skeletal problem. (*a*) Frontal view. (*b*) Profile. (*c*) Smile. The dental compromise for the skeletal disharmony is evident in the occlusion (*d*) and the cephalometric analysis (*e*). The ideal treatment for this patient would have been the preoperative orthodontic creation of a Class II malocclusion (possibly with a different extraction pattern), followed by the vertical repositioning of her maxilla and advancement of her mandible. In this case, however, an acceptable, although compromised, esthetic result was achieved by superior repositioning of her maxilla and advancement genioplasty, while the existing occlusion was maintained.

to achieve a Class I occlusion by orthodontic treatment alone; however, an ideal esthetic result is not possible.

Because the orthodontic placement of the teeth dictates surgical movement (and ultimately facial changes), the orthodontist must carefully assess patients with musculoskeletal deformities before orthodontic treatment is begun. Accurate preoperative orthodontic and surgical planning that considers the indicated surgical movement is necessary to ensure not only good functional results but also an optimal esthetic outcome. As seen in the patient in Fig 1-4, the dentition has been compromised for skeletal vertical maxillary excess and mandibular anteroposterior deficiency. Function and questionable stability have been achieved; however, the esthetic result is poor. An acceptable result is achieved after surgical compromise.

The patient in Fig 1-5 decided against surgical correction of her Class II malocclusion and vertical maxillary excess dentofacial problem. The orthodontic compromise treatment plan consisted of extraction of first maxillary premolars, retraction of maxillary incisors, and establishment of an occlusion. Four months after beginning orthodontic treatment, the patient thought her appearance was worsening and realized that this treatment option would not be acceptable to her. It was then decided to decompensate the maxillary incisors to open the extraction spaces in the maxilla. The surgical treatment plan consisted

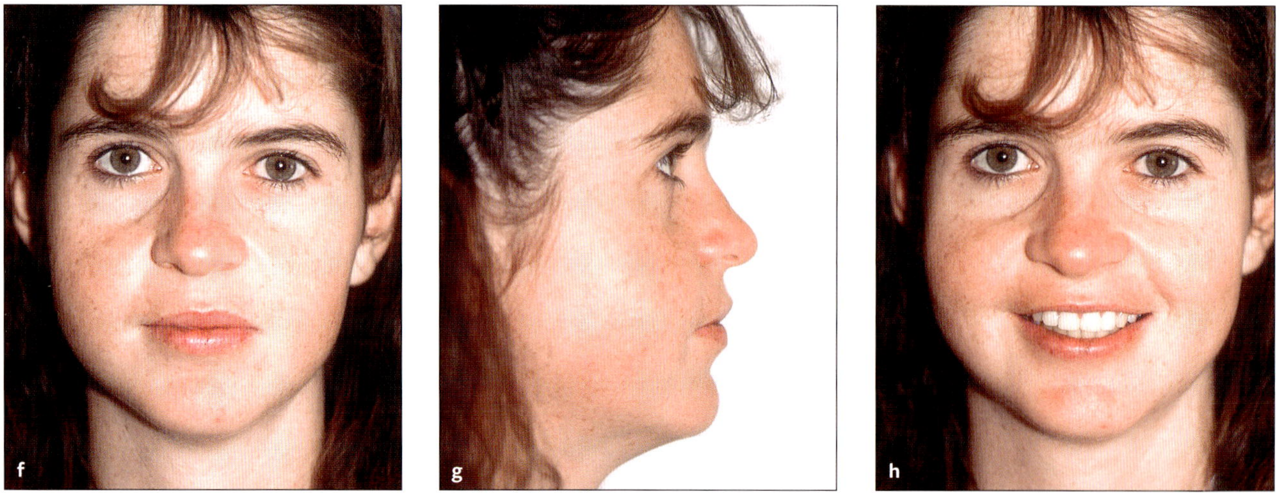

Fig 1-4 *(cont)* (*f*) Postoperative frontal view. (*g*) Postoperative profile. (*h*) Smile.

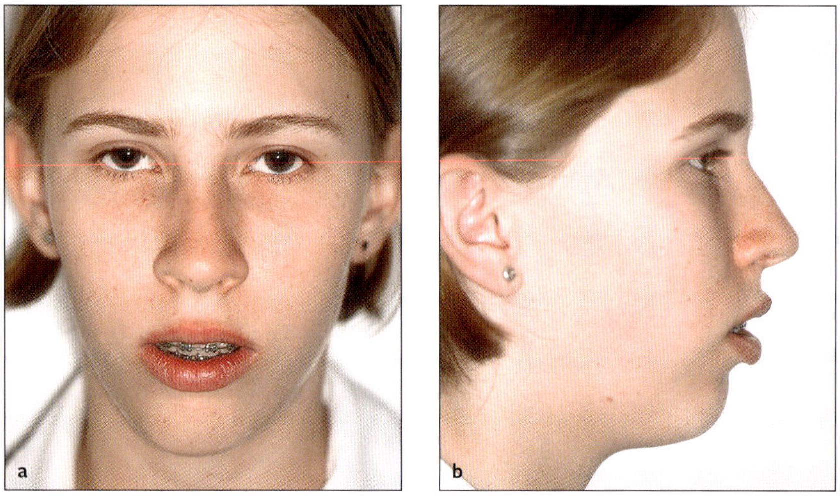

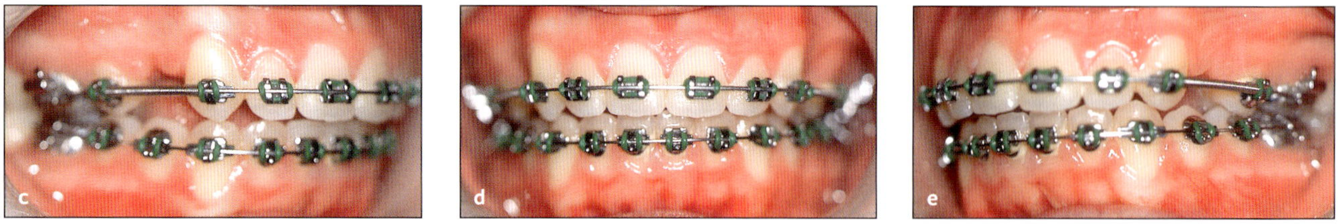

Fig 1-5 Because the patient decided not to have surgery, the compromise orthodontic treatment consisted of extraction of the maxillary first premolars and retraction of the maxillary incisors. The deteriorating esthetic results are evident in the frontal (*a*) and profile (*b*) views. (*c to e*) The diagnosis of vertical maxillary excess and microgenia with a Class II malocclusion is confirmed by the occlusion.

of a two-piece Le Fort I maxillary osteotomy, superior repositioning of the maxilla, and surgical closure of the extraction spaces by advancement of the posterior maxillary segment (see Figs 1-5g and 1-5h). The mandible would autorotate, and the chin would be surgically advanced by means of a sliding genioplasty. In this case, an acceptable surgical solution could be found (see Figs 1-5i to 1-5m); however, in other cases, the surgical compromise for the orthodontic compromise may be limited from either an esthetic, functional, or stability aspect. In some patients with orthodontic compromise, the compromised dentition may cause challenges with solving the dentofacial problems and may even prevent a solution.

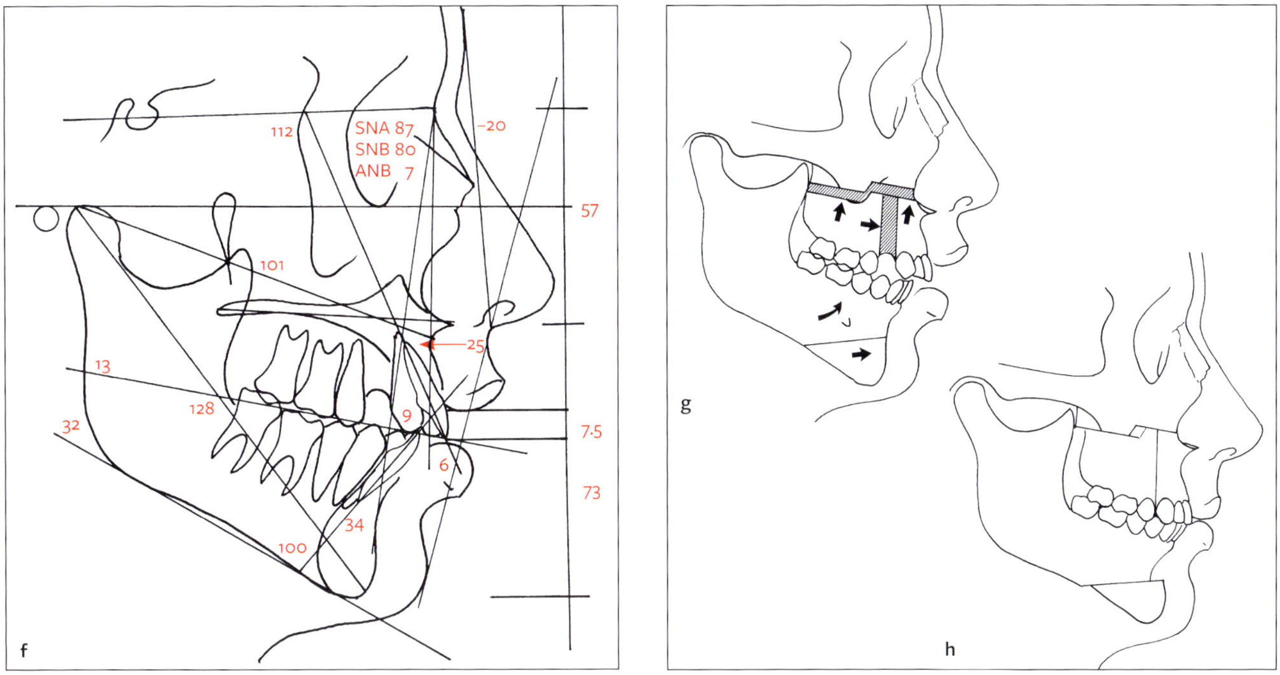

Fig 1-5 *(cont)* (*f*) Cephalometric tracing confirming diagnosis. (*g*) Surgical treatment plan. The maxillary incisors were decompensated, opening the spaces where the first premolars had been extracted. The surgery consisted of a two-piece Le Fort I maxillary osteotomy, superior repositioning of the maxilla, and advancement of the posterior segment to close the spaces. The chin was advanced by means of a sliding genioplasty. (*h*) Postoperative dental, skeletal, and soft tissue positions. (*i*) Postoperative frontal view. (*j*) Postoperative profile. (*k to m*) Postoperative occlusion.

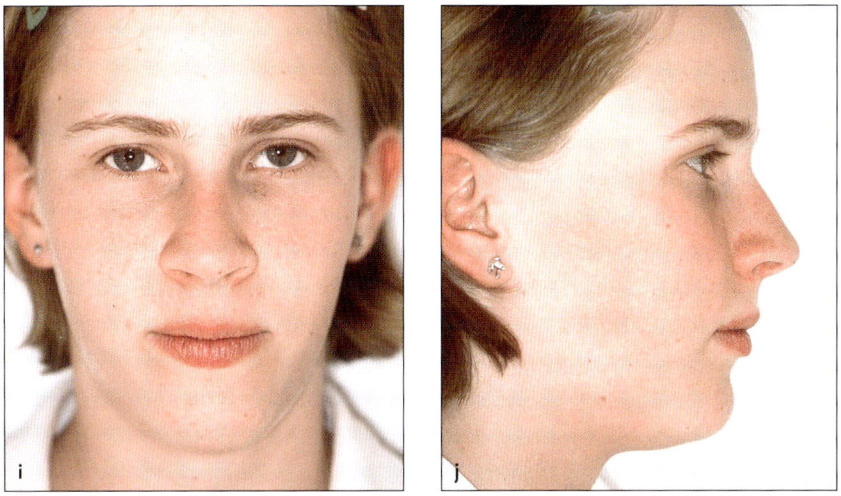

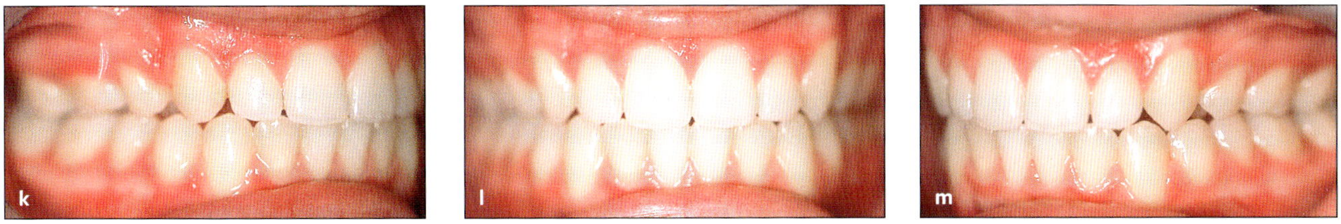

Airway patency

There are several anatomical risk factors that may play a role in causing OSA. These include regional obesity, alteration of the nasal cavity, enlargement of other critical soft tissue structures of the upper airway, inadequate pharyngeal muscle tone, and a retrusive maxillomandibular skeleton. Patients with dentofacial deformities may suffer from OSA or be candidates to develop OSA. Some changes caused by dentoskeletal treatment when the patient is young may result in development of OSA when the patient gets older. A thorough medical and sleep history should be taken and a physical examination completed when indicated. See “Airway Considerations in Orthognathic Surgery” in chapter 2.

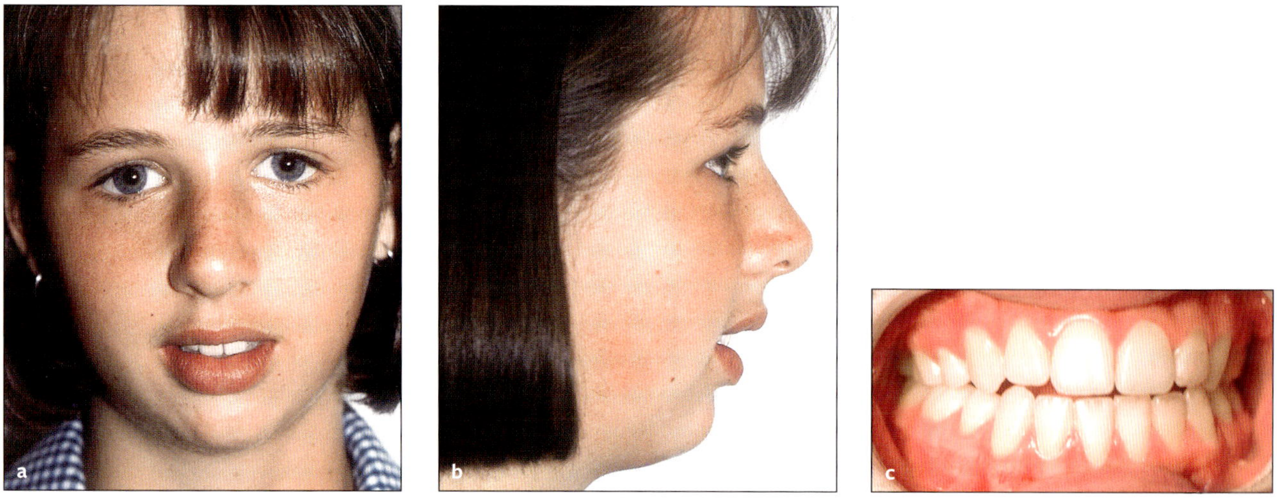

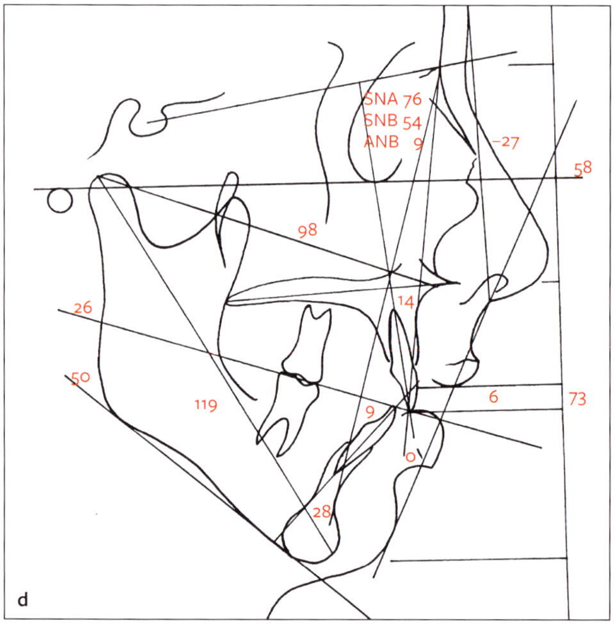

Fig 1-6 A 15-year-old patient reported an inability to bite certain foods with her front teeth. She recalled that she had an open bite before orthodontic treatment. Her four first premolars were removed as part of her orthodontic treatment, which lasted 2 years. Her bite was good at the time of band removal. Her frontal (*a*) and profile (*b*) views revealed a convex profile, maxillary vertical excess, and mandibular anteroposterior deficiency. (*c*) She had a Class II anterior open bite malocclusion. (*d*) The skeletal soft tissue and dental relationship is evident on the cephalometric tracing. The patient was rebanded and the maxillary arch aligned in three segments; the anterior segment contained the incisors, whereas the right and left posterior segments included all the teeth from the canines to the second molars. The surgery consisted of a three-piece Le Fort I maxillary osteotomy with superior repositioning and expanding of the posterior segments, which allowed the mandible to autorotate. The chin was advanced by means of a sliding genioplasty. The acceptable esthetic and functional result is seen in the postoperative frontal view (*e*) and profile (*f*) as well as in the occlusion (*g*).

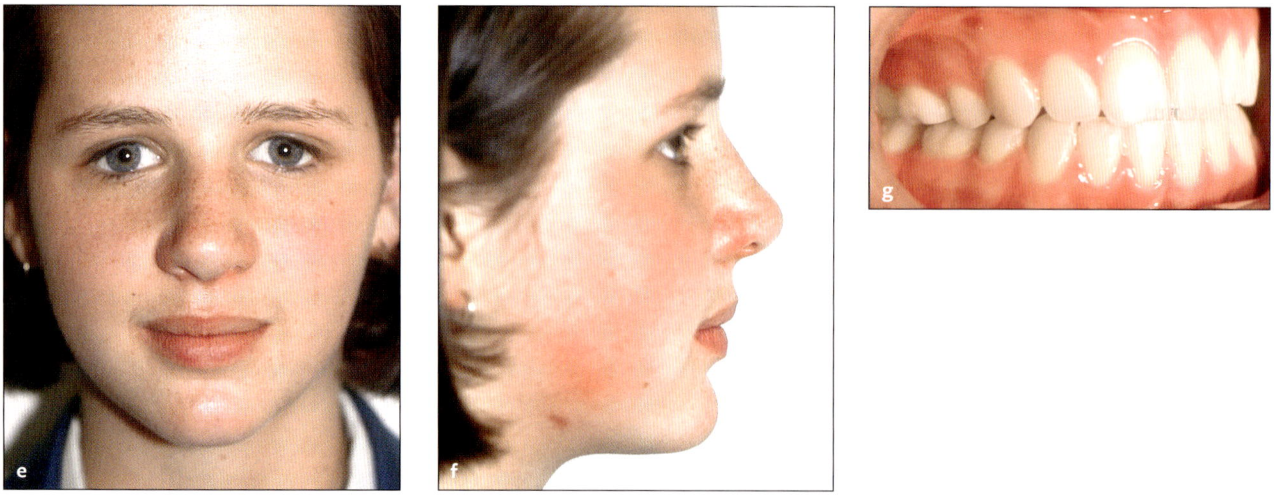

Stability

A treatment outcome of good function of pleasing esthetics is not acceptable without stability. Certain orthodontic tooth movements have questionable stability. An example is the extrusion of teeth to correct a skeletal anterior open bite; any preoperative orthodontic attempt to correct this type of open bite adds significant instability to the overall result. After the jaws are surgically repositioned beyond their biologic parameters, they will relapse into a more harmonious musculoskeletal relationship for the individual. Figure 1-6 demonstrates a case in which the orthodontic treatment of an open bite led to poor stability and unacceptable esthetics. Occlusal stability at any moment is the result of the sum of all the forces acting against the teeth (Enlow, 1990). A good occlusion is often the best retainer. It has been shown that the use of sound orthodontic mechanics and surgical techniques will produce optimal stability, function, airway, and esthetics.

Patient Consultation

There will be separate consultations with the orthodontist and with the surgeon, and each will have both an initial consultation to inform the patient about treatment and a definitive consultation to begin the treatment. Before the final consultation with the patient, the orthodontist and surgeon will formalize and agree on a diagnosis and treatment plan.

First orthodontic consultation

Because people with malpositioned teeth and a jaw deformity usually seek treatment from an orthodontist, the orthodontist must usually discuss the possible need for a surgical procedure at the initial consultation. During the first orthodontic consultation, a clinical examination is performed and the appropriate records obtained. The surgeon will need a copy of these records as well.

Definitive orthodontic consultation

The final pretreatment consultation takes place only after a systematic patient evaluation has been conducted and the orthodontist and surgeon have agreed on a final treatment plan. It is mandatory that the patient (and perhaps the parents or spouse) be well informed. Well-informed patients follow instructions and, as a general rule, are easy to treat.

Orthodontists and surgeons should develop their own methods of informing patients about treatment options and gaining their confidence. It is important to keep explanations simple and to use the patient's radiographs and dental casts to demonstrate the problems. Solutions for the problems should be discussed in general terms, and the need for surgery must be explained. The patient and their family (if applicable) must understand the importance of properly aligning the teeth, and that the bite may not improve or even get worse during the preoperative phase. Word choice is important for the orthodontist in discussing the type of surgery required. Terms such as *reposition*, *lengthen*, or *shorten* should be used when describing the surgical procedures. The final and more detailed explanation of the surgery should be left to the surgeon. Treatment results of patients with similar problems may be used to demonstrate specific treatment objectives.

For most patients, the treatment time is extremely important, but it is preferable not to give a specific length of time. It is important, however, to give the patient a general idea of the length of treatment and a treatment profile explaining various phases of the treatment, the sequence of the stages, and the time each phase could take. The patient should be alerted to factors that might influence the treatment time and surgical precision, such as bone density, periodontal disease, patient cooperation, age, and tooth extractions. It is also important at this stage to inform the patient about the cost of the orthodontic aspect of the treatment.

Explanation of typical treatment profile

A typical treatment profile consists of six phases:

1. *Placement of orthodontic bands on the teeth*. Any necessary extractions of teeth (including third molars) are completed at this time. The orthodontic bands are usually fitted 2 to 3 weeks later.
2. *Preoperative/preparatory orthodontic phase (9 to 18 months, on average)*. The teeth are now aligned in their optimal positions in each arch. When the orthodontist is satisfied that this preparation is complete, the patient is referred back to the surgeon.
3. *Surgical phase and healing time (4 to 6 weeks)*. The surgeon surgically repositions the jaw or jaws into their most favorable relationship to establish a good occlusion (bite) and balanced facial proportions. After a short healing period, the patient returns to the orthodontist for the final correction of the bite. It is very important that the patient see the orthodontist 2 to 3 weeks after surgery for postoperative orthodontic control.

4. *Postoperative orthodontic phase to perfect the bite (3 to 6 months).* The purpose of orthodontics after the surgery is to refine the bite. Minor tooth movement occurs during this phase to finalize the occlusion and achieve a satisfactory result.
5. *Removal of orthodontic bands.*
6. *Retention phase (6 to 12 months).* When orthodontic treatment has been completed, the teeth that have been moved through bone need to be stabilized in their new positions for a time. The orthodontist manufactures and fits a retention appliance, which must be worn by the patient as instructed by the orthodontist.

The duration of the presurgical orthodontic phase will vary as the severity and type of malocclusion varies. For example, mandibular advancement will be performed earlier in the orthodontic phase for Class II deep bite cases than for mandibular setback cases. In fact, in some cases, the orthognathic surgery may be performed before the orthodontic treatment begins. When performing surgery first, it is mandatory that an acceptable, stable occlusion can be established at the time of surgery. This treatment approach requires an experienced and competent orthodontist and surgeon.

First surgical consultation

The initial surgical consultation includes a general discussion of the basic principles of combined orthodontic and surgical treatment and why surgery is necessary. Most patients are apprehensive at this consultation, and the fact that they may need surgery has often come as a surprise to them. The surgeon should therefore use this consultation as an opportunity to inform the patient about the orthognathic surgical principles and to gain the patient's confidence. The importance of a comprehensive treatment plan developed by both the orthodontist and surgeon is explained. At this consultation, a systematic patient evaluation is conducted, and records are obtained if not previously sent from the orthodontist.

Definitive surgical consultation

The definitive surgical consultation is conducted once the orthodontist and surgeon have finalized a treatment plan. The need for orthodontic preparation before surgery is confirmed. The basic principles of the specific surgical treatment, general sequence of events of the surgical phase of treatment, hospitalization time, recovery period, and need for a soft food diet are discussed. The surgical objectives may be explained by treatment results of patients with similar dentofacial problems. A patient information brochure is provided, and the patient is reassured during the preoperative orthodontic phase that he or she is welcome to discuss with the surgeon any concerns regarding the planned surgery. The estimated costs, including costs of the planned surgery, hospitalization costs, and the anesthetization fee, should also be discussed at this time.

Consultation with Other Disciplines

Consultation with practitioners in other disciplines may be needed in the treatment of patients with a dentofacial deformity.

Periodontics

In general, most periodontal diseases should be treated prior to orthodontic banding. The teeth and periodontium should be sound before treatment. The importance of oral hygiene during the orthodontic treatment phase should be stressed, and the possibility of periodontal treatment after debanding should be mentioned to the patient.

Prosthodontics

Any work on fixed partial dentures is preferably performed after a period of orthodontic retention. However, it is often advantageous for the patient to consult with a prosthodontist before beginning treatment. The prosthodontist can contribute valuable insight into certain aspects of the surgical/orthodontic treatment and prosthodontic rehabilitation. For example, in a patient with congenitally missing lateral incisors, should the interdental spaces be closed, or should spaces be maintained and the missing teeth be replaced by implants or fixed partial dentures? For edentulous patients or those with a limited number of teeth that would not require orthodontic treatment, the preoperative prosthodontic consultation is mandatory.

Implant dentistry

It is often possible to place the necessary implants at the time of orthognathic surgery. It is important, however, to keep any postoperative orthodontic tooth movement in mind. Dental implants can often be placed more accurately after band removal and a short period of retention. However, it will be more expensive for the patient to undergo two separate surgeries. For patients requiring bone grafts before implants can be placed, the surgeon should consider placing the bone grafts during orthognathic surgery.

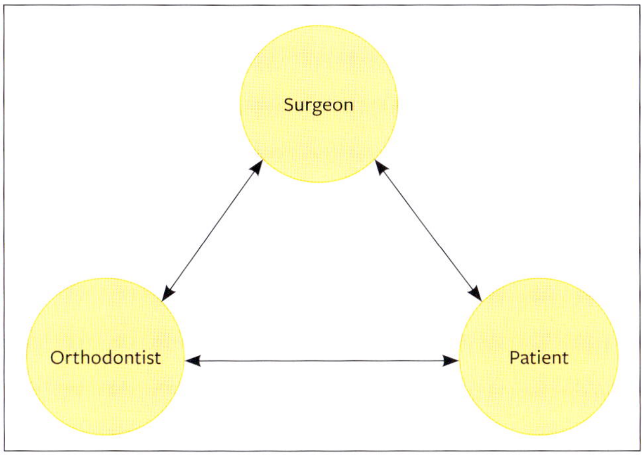

Fig 1-7 Kindness, communication, and free flow of information between the surgeon, orthodontist, and patient facilitate efficient and successful treatment and ensure patient confidence.

General dentistry

Problems such as dental caries, fractures, periodontitis, and poor-fitting crowns should be addressed before treatment begins. The condition of certain teeth may influence the decision of which teeth are extracted for orthodontic reasons. The initial referral to the orthodontist or surgeon is often made by the general practitioner, and it is important to keep him or her informed of the treatment plan and the progress of the patient's treatment. The general practitioner should be part of the treatment team.

Importance of communication

Accurate treatment planning and meticulous orthodontic and surgical practice are essential to the achievement of treatment objectives. Just as important, however, is communication between the clinician and the patient, as well as between clinicians. It is crucial to have adequate communication between the orthodontist, patient, and surgeon about the patient's main complaint and concerns, dentofacial diagnosis, treatment possibilities, and treatment objectives (Fig 1-7). The confident sharing of information with the patient will build trust between patient and clinician. Remember, people want to know how much you care before they care how much you know.

The communication between the surgeon and the orthodontist is equally important. Lack of communication here not only hampers the development of an efficient and sound treatment plan but also generally leads to poor treatment results. Patients are extremely concerned about poor or lacking communication between the orthodontist and the surgeon, and it can lead to confusion. Clinicians should refrain from sending messages to each other via the patient.

Treatment plan

The development of a treatment plan has three advantages:

1. It represents an agreement between the orthodontist and the surgeon on how the patient will be treated.
2. The treatment plan and objectives can confidently be presented to the patient without contradictions.
3. Although the treatment plan may be changed when indicated, it serves as a solid guideline.

The treatment plan may need to be revised or changed after the preoperative orthodontic treatment is under way. The reason for a change in treatment plan and the solution should be discussed by the orthognathic team so that there will be no surprises during the immediate preoperative surgical consultation. Superb orthodontic alignment of teeth and excellent surgical technique do not substitute for good clinical judgment, optimal decision making, proper communication, and empathy with patients.

Recommended Reading

Arnett GW, McLaughlin RP. Facial and Dental Planning for Orthodontists and Oral Surgeons. St Louis: Mosby, 2004.

Bell WH. Modern Practice in Orthognathic and Reconstructive Surgery, vol 1. Philadelphia: Saunders, 1992.

Enlow DH. Facial Growth, ed 3. Philadelphia: Saunders, 1990.

Epker BN, Stella JP, Fish LC. Dentofacial Deformities: Integrated Orthodontic and Surgical Correction, vol 1. St Louis: Mosby, 1994.

Gasparini G, Boniello MD, Moro A, Di Nardo F, Pelo S. Orthognathic surgery: A new preoperative informed consent model. J Craniofac Surg 2009;20:90–92.

Naini FB. Facial Aesthetics: Concepts & Clinical Diagnosis. Wiley-Blackwell, 2007.

Proffit WR, White RP. Surgical Orthodontic Treatment. St Louis: Mosby, 1990.

Sarver DM, Proffit WR, White RP. Contemporary Treatment of Dentofacial Deformities. St Louis: Mosby: 2002.

Spalding PM. Craniofacial growth and development. In: Miloro M, Ghali GE, Larsen P, Waite P (eds). Peterson's Principles of Oral and Maxillofacial Surgery, ed 3. Shelton, CT: People's Medical Publishing House-USA, 2012:1189–1238.

Wolford LM, Stevao ELL, Alexander CM, Goncalves JR, Rodrigues DB. Orthodontics for orthognathic surgery. In: Miloro M, Ghali GE, Larsen P, Waite P (eds). Peterson's Principles of Oral and Maxillofacial Surgery, ed 3. Shelton, CT: People's Medical Publishing House-USA, 2012:1263–1294.

2

Systematic Patient Evaluation

With contributions by Steven Sullivan, DDS

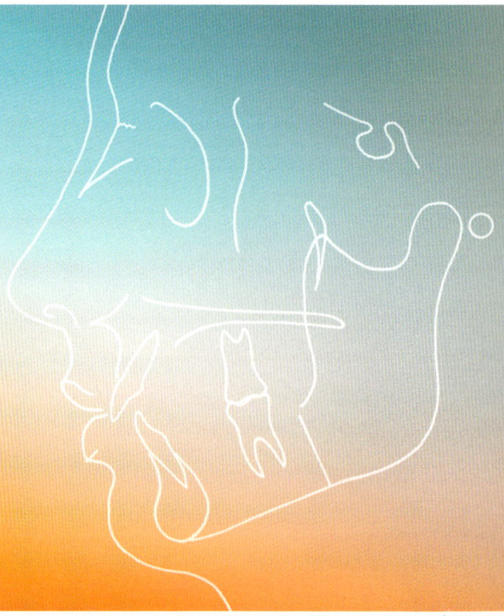

There must be clear and effective communication between the orthodontist and the maxillofacial surgeon from the outset of treatment to achieve the best results from surgical therapy. Through this close relationship, a full exchange of information and data can be made. Each practitioner involved in the patient's care should be familiar with the standard records required, and the data on the patient should be shared regardless of who actually performs the investigations. Treatment should commence only after both the orthodontist and the surgeon have consulted with the patient, a treatment plan has been jointly prepared, and both clinicians have a copy of the patient's records. Orthognathic surgeons should have a thorough understanding of orthodontic treatment principles to enable them to communicate sensibly, to plan realistically, and to know what can be expected from the orthodontic treatment. Conversely, orthodontists should understand the surgical possibilities, limitations, and requirements to make the partnership ultimately advantageous to the patient.

A systematic examination is necessary to adequately evaluate and plan treatment for patients with dentofacial deformities. In routine cases, this evaluation includes the following:

- General patient evaluation
- Sociopsychologic evaluation
- Esthetic facial evaluation
- Radiographic evaluation
  - Lateral cephalometric
  - Posteroanterior cephalometric
  - Full-mouth periapical
  - Panoramic
- Occlusion and study cast evaluation
- Temporomandibular joint evaluation

General Patient Evaluation

Hereditary tendencies in the development of dentofacial deformities

The term *dentofacial deformity* is generally used to describe a significant disproportion of the jaws in association with malocclusion. Jaw deformities are thought to be more common among individuals with genetic backgrounds that are crossed between different racial and ethnic groups as compared with those from isolated human populations. It is assumed that about one-third of children who present with a severe Class III malocclusion will have a parent with the same problem and that one-sixth of these children will have siblings with the same problem. A short face growth pattern with a deep bite malocclusion is more frequently found in Caucasians, while bimaxillary protrusion with anterior open bite and microgenia is more prevalent among individuals of African descent.

Knowledge and an understanding of normal facial growth and development as well as the effect of malformations on associated facial structures is useful in diagnosis and treatment planning as well as to limit complications during treatment. Factors that are known to alter facial growth and cause dental malocclusion and skeletal deformities may include the following: (1) syndromes, (2) hereditary factors, (3) environmental and neuromotor effects, (4) trauma, and (5) pathology (eg, tumors).

Medical history

The patient's medical history can be obtained by means of a questionnaire that the patient fills out at the first consultation. The questionnaire should be thorough so that no important areas are overlooked. The data are used to focus follow-up questions. Existing medical problems must be further evaluated and discussed with the appropriate physician or specialist. The potential for these medical problems to complicate general anesthesia or reconstructive surgery must be evaluated. Risk management and potential complications related to any medical problem should be discussed with the patient and carefully documented. Other medical specialists treating the patient should be consulted as necessary, and reports on existing conditions and drugs the patient may be taking should be obtained. It is also important to look for and recognize congenital syndromes because these patients may have unusual growth patterns and may respond unpredictably to orthodontic or surgical treatment.

Dental evaluation

History

Previous restorative, orthodontic, orthognathic surgery, periodontal, and facial pain treatment should be reviewed. The dental history is often an important barometer of the patient's probable commitment to future treatment.

General evaluation

Oral hygiene and previous dental treatment are good indications of the patient's "dental IQ" and motivation for future treatment. Caries, periodontal and periapical pathology, and the presence of unerupted and/or impacted teeth should be noted. The need for implants should be evaluated for possible inclusion in the final treatment plan. However, final prosthetic decisions are deferred until surgical orthodontic treatment has been completed.

Periodontal considerations

The prognosis for any periodontally affected teeth is established and the effect of orthodontic and surgical treatment considered. Periodontal disease and inadequately attached gingiva must be managed before commencement of orthodontic treatment. Long-term management, further periodontal treatment, and prognosis should be discussed with the periodontist and the patient.

Occlusal–oral function evaluation

Mastication, swallowing, mouth breathing, modified eating habits, and maximum mouth opening are documented. Snoring and breathing during sleep (eg, obstructive sleep apnea) should be noted and investigated. The effect of the dentofacial deformities on speech should be noted and the patient referred for pretreatment speech evaluation. Tongue thrust, thumbsucking, and lip-biting habits should be noted and their effect on the deformity evaluated.

Sociopsychologic Evaluation

Evaluation of the patient's sociopsychologic makeup is often neglected. It is important to consider the patient's motives for treatment and to determine the patient's expectations from treatment. There are two basic causes of patient dissatisfaction with the treatment outcome: (*1*) failure of the clinician to clearly inform the patient of realistic and probable treatment results (especially esthetic results), and (*2*) overoptimistic expectations of the patient regarding the results of treatment.

At the first consultation, the patient should be introduced to the concept of orthognathic surgery gently but confidently. It is imperative that from the start, the clinician provides the patient with a realistic and understandable overview of orthognathic treatment principles and general treatment possibilities in relation to the patient's specific dentofacial problem. Understanding the patient's concerns, motivations, and expectations will provide insight into the patient's psychologic health.

The clinician should refrain from overwhelming the patient with overt enthusiasm about the benefits of treatment, but rather should allow the patient to make his or her own decision. Some patients may need time to discuss future treatment with family or friends. Further counseling about realistic treatment expectations may be necessary, and it may even be best to delay treatment until the patient seeks psychologic guidance and is able to cope with treatment realities.

The perception of one's own appearance is often the "motor" behind direction in life. Surgical-orthodontic change of facial appearance inevitably has an effect on this motor. The following are some relevant questions for the patient to consider:

Sociopsychologic Evaluation

1	Who attends the first consultation?									
	Patient		Father		Mother		Spouse		Friend	
2	What does the patient think is wrong?									
	Function		Esthetics		Pain		Speech		None	
3	Patient's perception of esthetic severity:									
	1	2	3	4	5	6	7	8	9	10
	Mild				Moderate					Severe
4	Patient's perception of functional severity:									
	1	2	3	4	5	6	7	8	9	10
	Mild				Moderate					Severe
5	Patient's ability to define problem:									
	1	2	3	4	5	6	7	8	9	10
	Poor				With assistance					Good
6	Expectations of treatment:									
	1	2	3	4	5	6	7	8	9	10
	Unrealistic				Unclear					Realistic
7	Motivation									
	1	2	3	4	5	6	7	8	9	10
	Low				Moderate					High

Fig 2-1 Sociopsychologic evaluation form.

- *What does the patient (and/or the patient's parents) think is wrong?* Many individuals are able to identify, explain, and prioritize their concerns, which may vary from functional to esthetic problems. A patient is often referred by his or her dentist for treatment for conditions unfamiliar to the patient or family. The patient may be seen by the dentist not because of their own concerns but those of their parents. For these patients, it is paramount to explain their specific problems and the reasons for correction, including the risks of nontreatment, the treatment required, and the associated risks of treatment. It may come as a shock to the patient and family members that the patient may need surgery. It is therefore important to comprehensively discuss with the patient (and family when necessary) the concepts related to surgery combined with orthodontic treatment. The advantages and disadvantages of combining orthodontics with surgery, alternative treatments, and compromises should be discussed; if possible, results from previously treated patients should be reviewed. This information will help the patient and family to make an informed decision regarding treatment.
- *Why is treatment required?* The motivation for treatment is often a good predictor for the patient's cooperation during treatment.
- *Why is treatment required now?* The timing of seeking treatment is influenced by various factors including finances, onset of symptoms, and late diagnosis, among others.
- *What is expected from treatment?* The expectations and priorities of patients differ. For patients with severe facial deformities, the esthetic change is more important than functional occlusal correction. Patients who need correction of their malocclusion but prefer not to have any esthetic facial change can present a treatment challenge to the surgeon and the orthodontist.

Figure 2-1 shows a sociopsychologic evaluation form, which should give the clinician an overview of the patient's sociopsychologic status, indicating any existing problems and possible need for consultation with a psychologist.

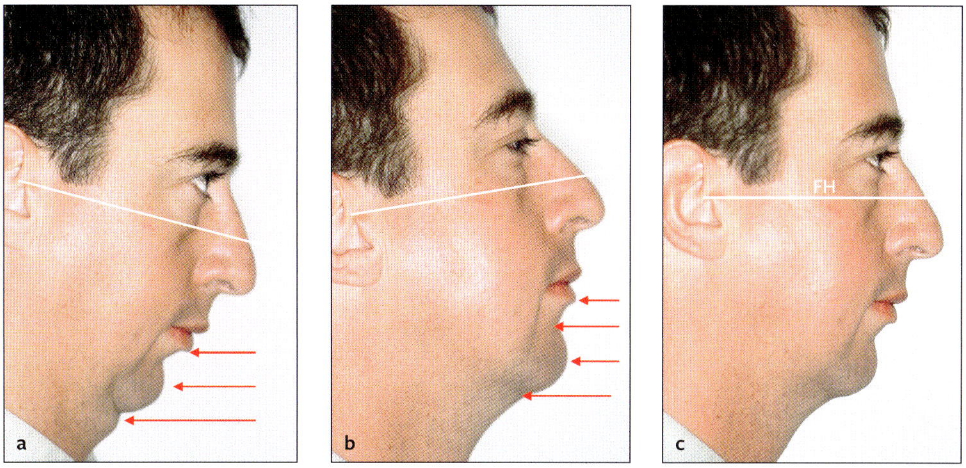

Fig 2-2 Clinical assessment of the chin and throat area is possible only when the head is in natural posture. Note the differences with the head tilted down (*a*), tilted up (*b*), and with the head in natural posture (*c*). The *white line* represents the Frankfort horizontal (FH) plane.

Esthetic Facial Evaluation

The clinical assessment of the face is probably the most valuable of all diagnostic procedures. The esthetic facial evaluation should be performed in a systematic fashion with the patient standing or seated comfortably. Primary emphasis should be placed on frontal esthetics because that is how people see themselves. Data should be recorded on a special form that can also serve as a checklist. Only abnormal and pertinent data should be recorded. Balance and proportion between the various facial structures in the individual are more important than numeric values. It is also important to compare the facial proportions with the patient's general build and posture (ie, corporofacial relationship).

The clinical examination of the face should always be done with two questions in mind:

1. Would orthodontic-surgical treatment be able to correct the dental, skeletal, and soft tissue structure diagnosed as abnormal?
2. How would the orthodontic-surgical correction of the abnormal structures influence the facial structures considered to be normal?

It is often possible to correct the malocclusion of patients with dentofacial deformities by means of *compromised orthodontic treatment*, meaning an orthodontic-dental compromise for a skeletal jaw discrepancy resulting in an acceptable long-term functional and stable occlusion and facial esthetics. The fear of surgery, financial issues, unsatisfactory surgical experience of the orthodontist, and feasibility of correction by compromised orthodontic treatment will influence the orthodontist to implement orthodontic treatment for a skeletal deformity.

The patient should be examined in natural head posture, with the teeth in centric occlusion and the lips relaxed. *Natural head posture* is the position in which the patient orients his or her head and that feels most natural. Figure 2-2 illustrates the profound effect a change in head posture may have, for example, on chin position, chin-throat angle, and chin-throat length. Skeletal and soft tissue changes can therefore only be planned with the head in natural posture and the lips relaxed to ensure appropriate soft tissue changes. Orthodontic and surgical treatment are planned to produce ideal function in centric occlusion. All examination data should therefore be recorded in centric occlusion. However, patients with vertical maxillary deficiency and severely closed bites are an exception to this rule. Because of the inadequate height of the maxilla, these patients' bites are overclosed, leading to distortion of their lips. To accurately evaluate these patients' lips and maxillary incisor–upper lip relationships, they should be evaluated in an open bite posture. A wax bite can be placed between the teeth to increase the vertical dimension until the lips just part. The lack of tooth exposure, lip shape and thickness, anteroposterior position of the chin, labiomental fold, upper lip length, nasolabial angle, and soft tissue thickness can now be assessed more meaningfully. Figure 2-3 illustrates the profound changes in soft tissue characteristics in a patient with vertical maxillary deficiency in centric relation and in the open bite position.

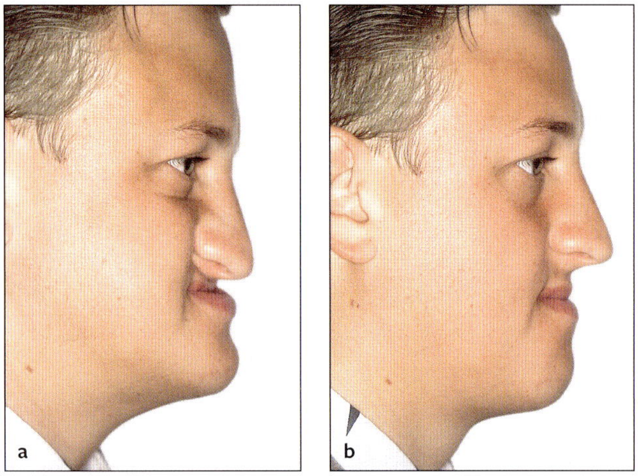

Fig 2-3 Individual with vertical maxillary deficiency. Note the change in the shape of the lips and lower facial height with the teeth in occlusion (*a*) and with the mandible rotated open until the lips just part (*b*).

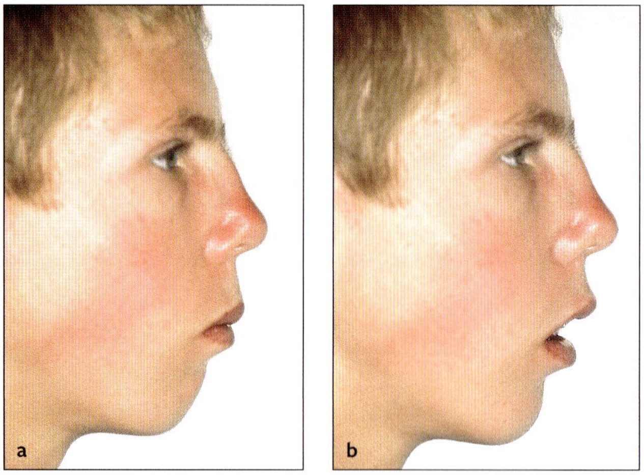

Fig 2-4 The profile of the lower third is profoundly different when the lips are forced together (*a*) versus in repose (*b*).

It is imperative that the patient be examined with the lips in a relaxed position, because it is impossible to assess the relationship between the soft tissue and the hard tissue when the lips are forced together. Figure 2-4 demonstrates the effect of muscular compensation on the lips and chin. Note the change in the interlabial gap, labiomental fold, chin and lip shape, and maxillary tooth exposure. The sella-nasion (S-N) plane and Frankfort horizontal (FH) plane have traditionally been used as horizontal planes of reference for various cephalometric and clinical assessments. However, patients do not carry their heads with the S-N or FH planes parallel to the floor. Cephalometric landmarks should not dictate head posture used for facial assessment and treatment planning. The clinical evaluation should therefore be carried out with the head in the natural posture.

Frontal analysis

From the frontal view, it is particularly important to assess facial form; transverse dimensions; facial symmetry; the vertical relationship in the upper, middle, and lower thirds of the face; the lips; and the nose.

Facial form

The relationship between the facial width and vertical height has a strong influence on facial harmony. Facial form and harmony should also be correlated with the patient's overall body build. When correcting facial form, the overall body build of the individual should be considered (ie, short and stocky versus long and thin). The height-to-width proportion of the face is 1.3:1 for females and 1.35:1 for males. The bigonial width should be approximately 30% less than the bizygomatic dimension (Fig 2-5). Short, square facial types are often associated with a Class II deep bite malocclusion, vertical maxillary deficiency, masseteric hyperplasia, and macrogenia, whereas long, narrow facial types are often associated with vertical maxillary excess, a narrow nose, mandibular anteroposterior deficiency, microgenia, a high palatal vault, and an anterior open bite malocclusion (Figs 2-6 and 2-7; Table 2-1).

Transverse dimensions

The rule of fifths is a convenient method for evaluating transverse facial proportions. The face is divided into five equal parts—each the approximate width of the eye—from helix to helix of the outer ears (Fig 2-8).

The outer fifths are measured from the center helix of the ears to the outer canthus of the eyes. Prominent ears may have a profound effect on facial proportions and can be corrected by otoplasty. In patients with masseter hypertrophy, the face appears square, and the gonial angles fall well outside the canthus line. A more harmonious facial form can be established in these patients by means of bilateral reduction of the masseter muscles and contouring the mandibular angles (Fig 2-9). Intergonial width can be increased by subperiosteal angle implants (Fig 2-10).

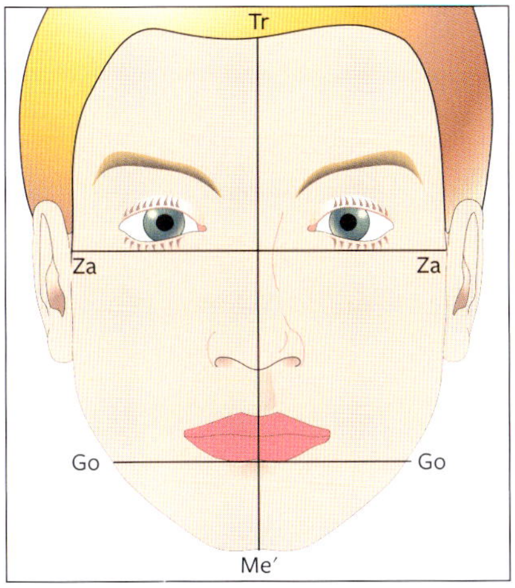

Fig 2-5 Facial form. The facial height (trichion [Tr]–soft tissue menton [Me′]):bizygomatic width (Za-Za) should be 1.3:1 (females) and 1.35:1 (males). The bigonial width (Go-Go) should be approximately 30% less than the bizygomatic width.

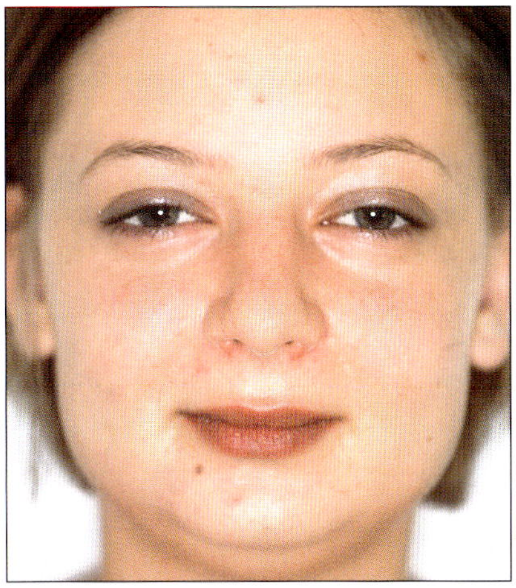

Fig 2-6 In this individual, the bigonial width is greater than the bizygomatic width because of bilateral masseter muscle hypertrophy.

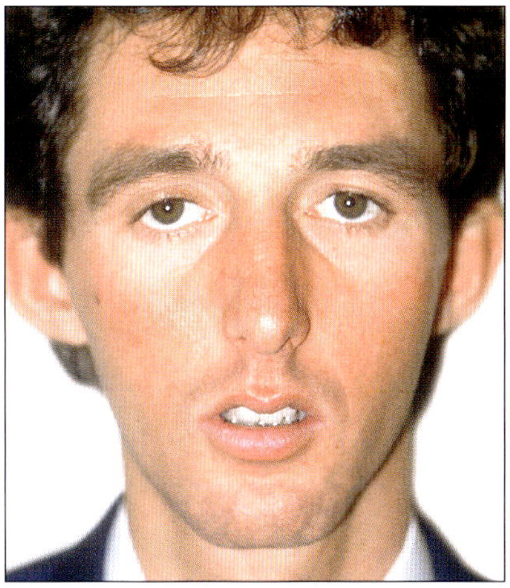

Fig 2-7 Individual with a long, narrow face. The bizygomatic width is more than 30% greater than the bigonial width.

Table 2-1 | Comparison of broad and narrow faces

	Broad face	Narrow face
Facial height	Square, short	Long
Bigonial width	Masseter hypertrophy	Decreased intergonial distance
Nose	Broad nose	Narrow nose
Chin	Macrogenia	Microgenia

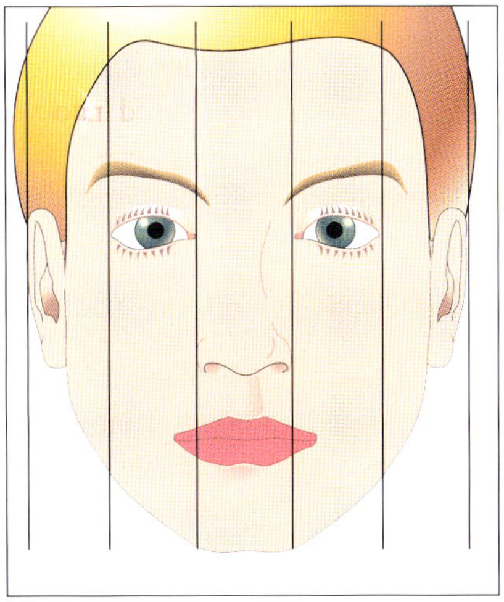

Fig 2-8 Transverse facial proportions.

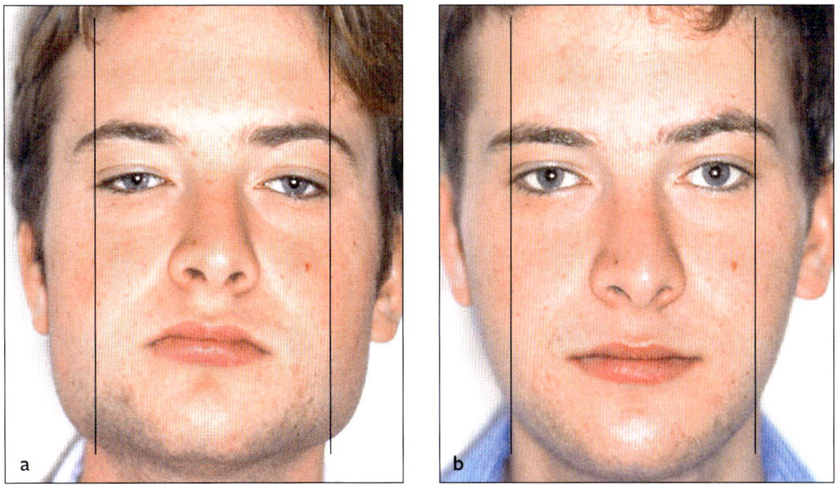

Fig 2-9 (*a*) The bigonial width is increased because of bilateral masseter muscle hypertrophy. The gonion falls lateral to a vertical line drawn through the outer canthus of the eye. (*b*) Transverse facial harmony has been restored by bilateral masseter muscle and mandibular angle reduction.

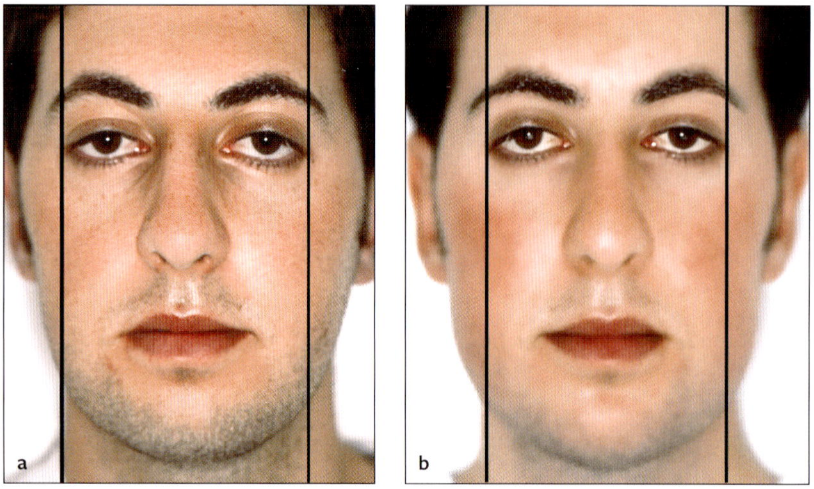

Fig 2-10 (*a*) This patient wanted to make his oval face more square. (*b*) The angles of the mandible were augmented by the placement of bilateral subperiosteal angle implants.

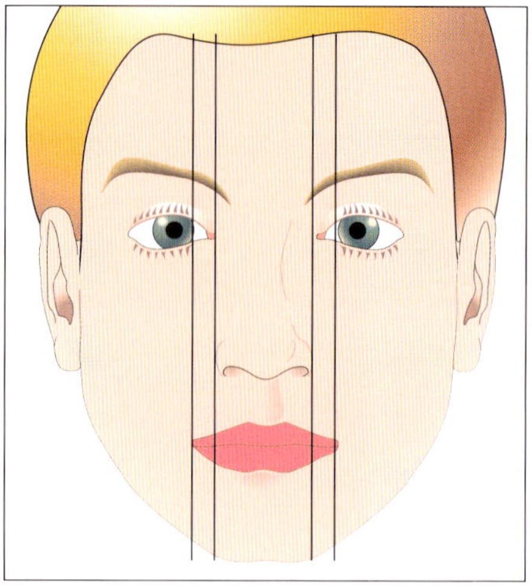

Fig 2-11 Vertical lines drawn through the medial canthi should coincide with the ala of the nose, whereas vertical lines drawn through the medial margins of the irises of the eyes should coincide with the corners of the mouth.

The medial three-fifths of the face are measured from the outer to the inner canthus of the eyes. The outer border should coincide with the gonial angles of the mandible. In patients with masseter muscle hypertrophy, the gonial angles will fall well lateral to this line (see Fig 2-9a). In patients with long faces, there will be a tendency for the gonial angles to be medial to these lines. It should be noted that the width of the mouth should approximate the distance between the inner margins of the irises of the eyes (Fig 2-11).

The middle fifth is delineated by the inner canthus of the eyes. In patients with hypertelorism, this fifth will be out of proportion with the other four-fifths. The ala of the nose should coincide with these lines (see Fig 2-11). For patients in whom maxillary advancement and/or superior repositioning is considered and the ala falls outside of the lines, control of alar width is indicated during surgery (see chapter 5).

Facial symmetry

To assess facial symmetry, an imaginary line is drawn through the soft tissue glabella (G′), pronasale (Pn), center of the philtrum of the upper lip and lower lip, and soft tissue pogonion (Pog′; Fig 2-12). For more accurate assessment, these points should be marked on the patient's face one at a time while other parts of the face are blocked out.

The maxillary and mandibular dental midlines should be assessed in relation to the facial midline, as well as in relation to each other. These observations will play an important role in the decision-making process regarding surgical or orthodontic correction of dental midlines. It is also important to evaluate the mandibular dental midline in relation to the midline of the chin. This information will assist in treatment planning for correction of mandibular asymmetry by means of mandibular surgery, genioplasty, or both. The presence of a transverse cant in the occlusal plane should be noted and correlated with the asymmetry. Surgical correction of an occlusal plane cant will often play a significant role in the total correction of facial asymmetry and should not be corrected orthodontically (see chapter 4).

No face is perfectly symmetric, but the absence of any obvious asymmetry is necessary for good facial esthetics. Posteroanterior cephalometric radiography or CBCT imaging for 3D virtual treatment planning are indicated in the presence of a clinically significant asymmetry. This will allow the clinician to distinguish between bone, soft tissue, or a combination of the two as etiologic factors.

Vertical relationship

In the vertical dimension, the face can be divided into three equal parts (Fig 2-13): (1) upper third (hairline [trichion] to the glabellar area), (2) middle third (glabellar area to subnasale [Sn]), and (3) lower third (Sn to soft tissue menton [Me′]).

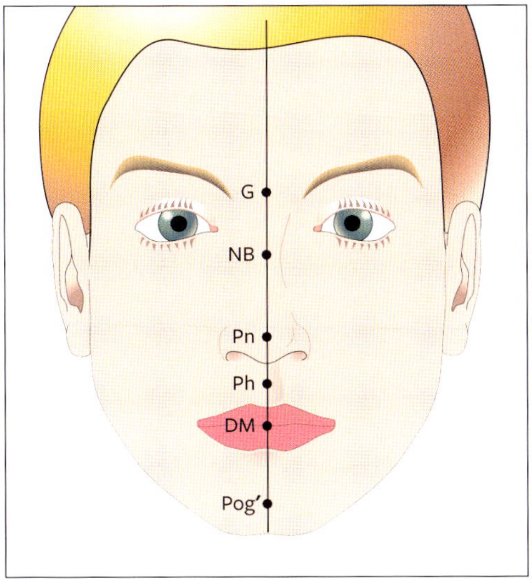

Fig 2-12 Facial symmetry. Important midline structures are the midpoint between the eyebrows (G), nasal bridge (NB), nasal tip (Pn), midpoint of the philtrum of the upper lip (Ph), dental midlines (DM), and midpoint of the chin (Pog′).

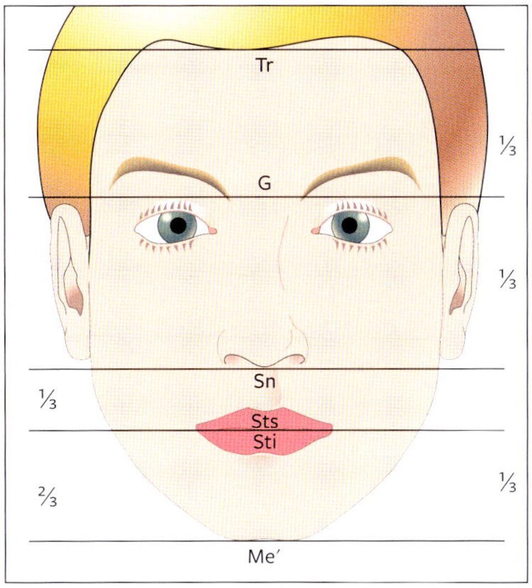

Fig 2-13 The face is divided into thirds by drawing horizontal lines through the trichion (Tr), G, subnasale (Sn), and soft tissue menton (Me′). The lower third can be divided into an upper third (from Sn to stomion superius [Sts]) and a lower two-thirds (from stomion inferius [Sti] to Me′).

Table 2-2 | Comparison of excessive and deficient midface dimensions

	Excessive middle third	Deficient middle third
Vertical maxillary dimension	Excessive	Deficient
Cheeks	Sallow	Full
Sclera showing	Visible below the iris	Normal
Cheekbones	Flat	Prominent, broad
Paranasal areas	Flat	Full
Nose	Narrow, long	Short, broad

Upper third of the face

Fortunately, deformities that exist in the upper third of the face can usually be masked by an appropriate hairstyle. However, it is important to record deformities in this area because they may indicate craniofacial deformities.

Middle third of the face

The nose, center of the lips, and middle of the chin (in the lower third of the face) should fall along a true vertical line (Table 2-2). Generally, no sclera is seen above or below the iris in a relaxed eyelid position with the patient looking straight ahead in natural head posture. Individuals with a midface deficiency tend to show sclera below the iris of the eye (Fig 2-14).

Sequential evaluation of the cheekbones, paranasal areas, alar eminences, and upper lip relation (in the lower third) should be performed. The cheekbone–nasal base–lip contour is a convenient contour line to evaluate the harmony of the structures of the midface (zygoma, maxilla, and nasal base) with the paranasal area and upper lip. This line starts just anterior to the ear, extends forward through the cheekbone, and then runs anteroinferiorly over the maxilla adjacent to the alar base of the nose, ending lateral to the commissure of the mouth. The line should form a smooth, continuing curve (Fig 2-15). An interruption of the curve may be an indication of an apparent skeletal deformity. Figure 2-16 illustrates a clear interruption of the line in the maxillary area, indicating maxillary antero-

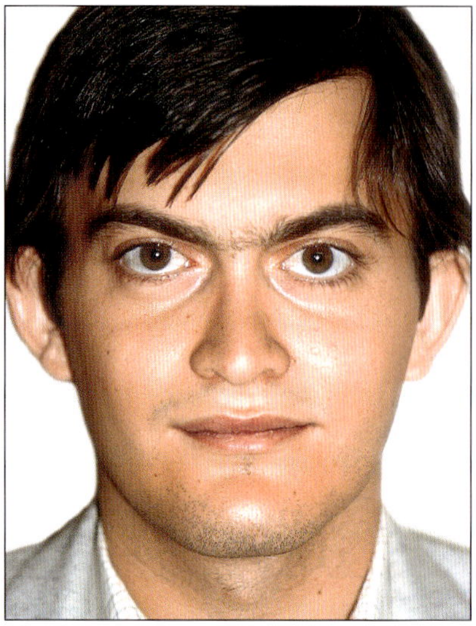

Fig 2-14 Sclera shows below the irises of the eyes in this individual with midface deficiency.

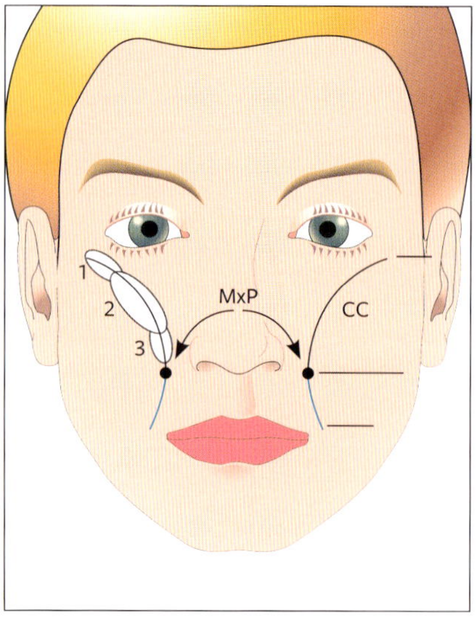

Fig 2-15 Cheekbone–nasal base–lip contour. The cheekbone area (CC) is divided into three parts: (1) zygomatic arch, (2) middle area, and (3) subpupillary area. The maxillary point (MxP) is the most medial point on the curve. The nasal base–upper lip contour (blue) extends inferiorly from MxP. The line should curve gently, without interruptions, ending lateral to the corner of the mouth.

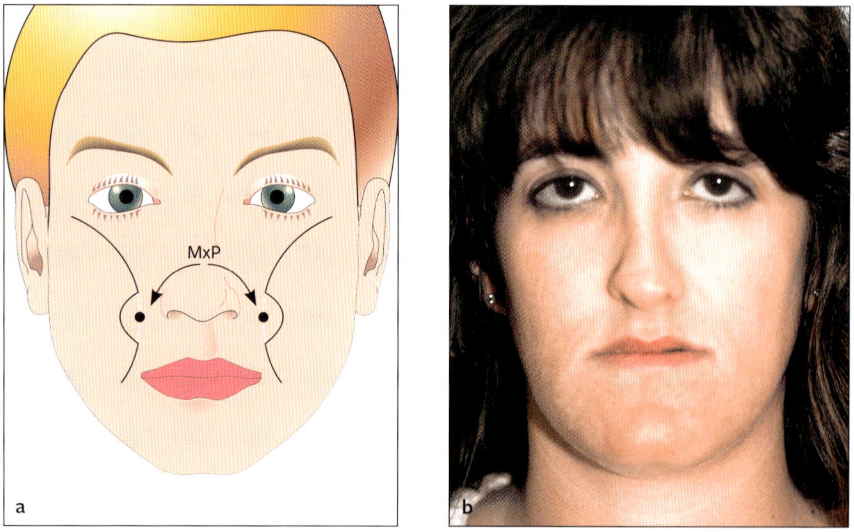

Fig 2-16 (*a*) Interruption of the curve at MxP. (*b*) Individual with maxillary anteroposterior deficiency. There is an interruption in the cheekbone–nasal base–lip contour at MxP.

posterior deficiency. In Fig 2-17, there is a double break with one indicating maxillary deficiency and the other an interruption in the lower part because of mandibular anteroposterior excess.

Lower third of the face

The middle third to lower third vertical height of the face should have a 5:6 ratio (Table 2-3). The length from Sn to stomion superius (Sts; called the *upper lip length*) should

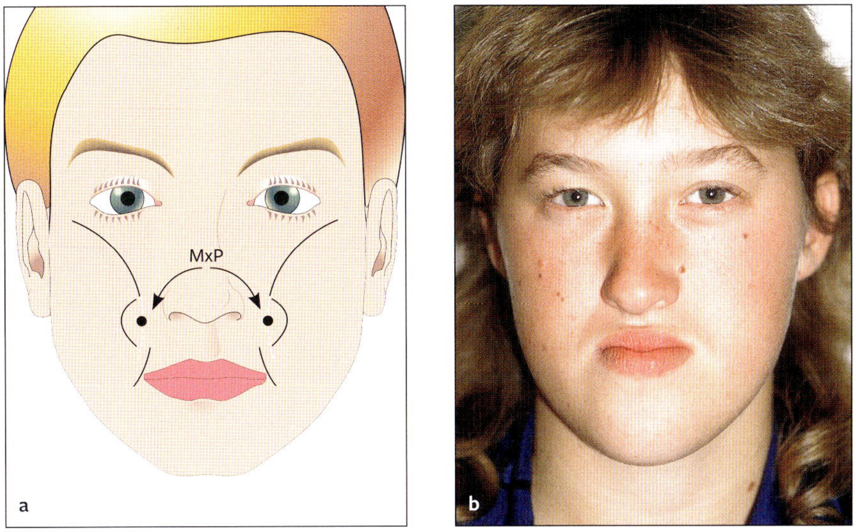

Fig 2-17 (*a*) Interruption of the curve at MxP and below MxP. (*b*) An individual with maxillary antero-posterior deficiency and mandibular prognathism. The cheekbone–nasal base–lip contour is interrupted with a double break, at MxP and also below MxP.

Table 2-3 | Comparison of excessive and deficient lower face height

	Excessive lower third	Deficient lower third
Vertical maxillary dimension	Excessive	Deficient
Lip appearance	Increased interlabial gap	Overclosed
Smile	Gummy	Toothless
Maxillary incisor exposure	Excessive	Little or none
Chin	Microgenia	Macrogenia
Malocclusion	Class II with or without anterior open bite	Class III closed bite or Class II deep bite

make up one-third of the lower third facial height. The distance from stomion inferius (Sti) to Me′, the *lower lip length*, should equal two-thirds of the lower third face height (see Fig 2-13).

Normal upper lip length is 20 ± 2 mm for females and 22 ± 2 mm for males, measured from Sn to upper lip inferior (Sts). If the upper lip is anatomically short, there is a tendency for the interlabial gap to be larger than normal and for increased maxillary tooth exposure with normal lower facial height. This condition should not be confused with skeletal vertical maxillary excess. The distance from lower lip superior (Sti) to Me′ is 40 ± 2 mm for females and 44 ± 2 mm for males. The lower lip may often appear short because of posture caused by maxillary incisor interference in patients with deep bite. The upper lip length should be related to lower anterior dental height.

With the patient's lips in repose, the amount of maxillary incisor exposure beneath the upper lip should be noted (Fig 2-18). For individuals in whom the maxillary incisors are not visible under the upper lip, the tooth-lip relation should be evaluated with the mandible rotated open until the lips just separate (Fig 2-19). The relation of the dental

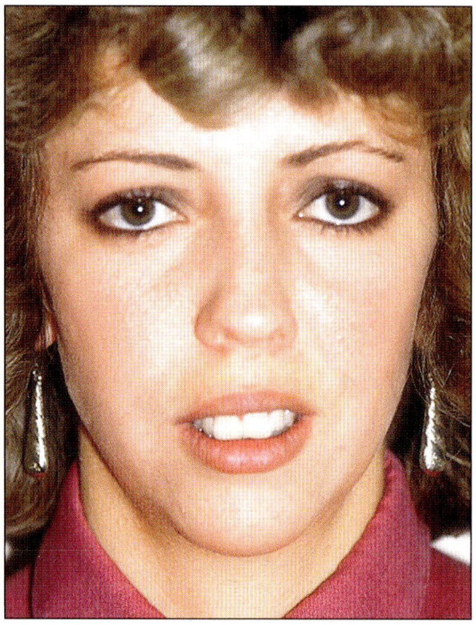

Fig 2-18 Excessive maxillary incisor exposure and increased interlabial gap. Normal maxillary incisor exposure under the upper lip is 1 to 4 mm. This measurement will be influenced by upper lip length, vertical maxillary length, lip thickness, and the angle and anteroposterior position of the maxillary incisors.

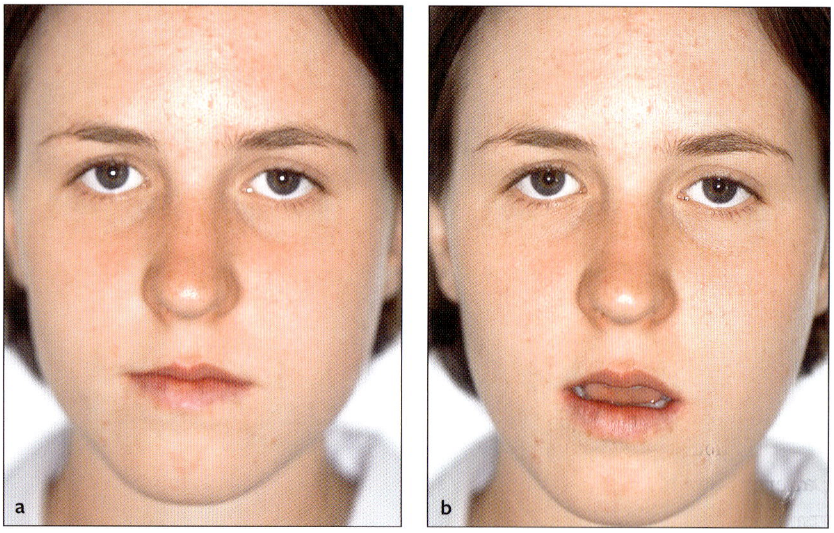

Fig 2-19 Individual with vertical maxillary deficiency. (*a*) It is not possible to assess maxillary incisor–lip relationship with the teeth in occlusion. (*b*) The lack of maxillary incisor exposure is evident with the mandible rotated open until the lips part and the upper lip is relaxed and not influenced by the lower lip.

midline to the facial midline is an important aspect to note because dental midlines can be coordinated and/or corrected either orthodontically or surgically. The etiology of dental midline shifts may be dental or skeletal. Dental factors that may cause midline shifts include spaces; missing teeth; tooth rotations; malpositioned teeth; crowding; crowns, fixed partial dentures, fillings, or implants (which can all change the size of teeth); and tooth size discrepancy.

In faces with asymmetry involving the mandible, it is critical to note the midline of the chin and its relation to the mandibular dental midline. The chin is evaluated for symmetry, vertical relation, and shape. The cant of the occlusal plane is evaluated, especially in individuals with facial asymmetry, by asking the patient to bite on a wooden spatula and then relating the occlusal plane to the interpupillary line (Fig 2-20). The maxillary dental arch level (between the maxillary canine tips) must be distinguished from the mandibular dental arch level (between the mandibular canine tips). However, with this assessment it is necessary to make sure that the orbits are on a horizontal plane because there may be an orbital deformity influencing this observation. Patients who present with facial asymmetry and a cant in the occlusal plane will require an anteroposterior cephalometric radiograph for further analysis.

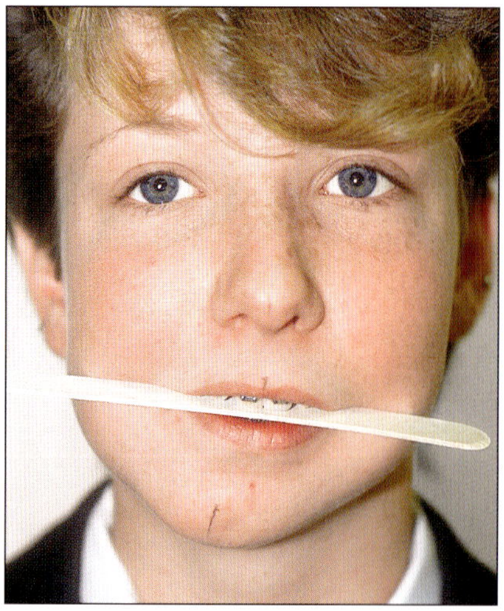

Fig 2-20 The cant in the occlusal plane can be evaluated in relation to the interpupillary line by asking the patient to bite on a wooden spatula. During this assessment, make sure that the interpupillary line is parallel to the floor.

The amount of gingiva exposed during smiling is also noted. The ideal tooth exposure during smiling is the full tooth crown to 2 mm of gingiva, which occurs in females more often than males. When examining the smile, it should be kept in mind that the amount of tooth exposure is influenced by (*1*) the vertical length of the maxilla, (*2*) lip length, (*3*) maxillary incisor crown length, (*4*) amount of lip action with smile, and (*5*) shape of Cupid's bow of the lip.

Surgical superior repositioning of the maxilla is indicated only when excessive gingival exposure is found in combination with an increased interlabial gap, increased maxillary incisor exposure, and increased vertical height of the lower third of the face. The amount of surgical superior repositioning will be dictated by the amount of tooth exposure, lip length, crown length, and age and sex of the patient. Keep in mind that superior repositioning of the maxilla will tend to shorten the upper lip. The upper lip will lengthen with age, especially in males. If necessary, surgical repositioning should err on the long side because overcorrection gives the patient a toothless and aged look.

One should never plan treatment based on the smile pattern. For example, an individual may exhibit a normal maxillary tooth–lip relationship (1 to 4 mm) that increases during smiling to expose up to 7 mm of gingiva ("gummy smile"). If superior repositioning is planned according to the amount of gingiva exposed during smiling, the maxilla will need to be superiorly repositioned by 6 mm to establish the ideal full tooth exposure. However, this will result in no tooth exposure and a toothless look in repose.

Lips

The lips are extremely critical to overall esthetics. Lip symmetry should be evaluated; if asymmetry exists, its etiology should be determined (eg, cleft lip, facial nerve dysfunction, underlying dentoskeletal asymmetry, scarring caused by previous trauma, or congenital unilateral microsomia or macrosomia).

The lower lip generally exhibits 25% more vermilion than the upper lip, and the lips should be 0 to 3 mm apart in repose. An increased overjet will result in an everted lower lip and excessive vermilion exposure due to the effect of the maxillary incisors on the lip. There are specific racial differences in lip thickness and shape that one must bear in mind for the purposes of treatment planning. To accurately evaluate the maxillary incisor–lip relationship in patients with closed bites, the lips should be relaxed and the jaws moved apart until the lips are slightly parted (closed bites may be the result of maxillary vertical deficiency or severe deep bites). Accentuation of Cupid's bow of the upper lip may lead to exposure of the maxillary central incisors only. This exposure of the maxillary central incisors will not be evident on a lateral cephalometric radiograph because only the central incisors can be seen. Therefore, the amount of superior repositioning of the maxilla in patients with vertical maxillary excess should be assessed clinically and not radiographically.

Nose

Although the nose has not always been considered part of orthognathic correction, it comprises an important aspect of the overall facial esthetics, and the form and function of the nose can be affected by orthognathic surgery. Many orthognathic surgeons also perform rhinoplasty as part of overall dentofacial correction. In many instances, nasal reconstruction may be part of the orthognathic treatment plan; sometimes, rhinoplasty and orthognathic surgery can be performed simultaneously. Control of the nasal form should also be considered, especially in patients requiring superior repositioning and/or advancement of the maxilla (see page 292.)

The functional and esthetic nasal evaluation should be included in the examination of the orthognathic patient. An intranasal examination should be performed to identify a possible existing deviated nasal septum, hypertrophied turbinates, or nasal polyps. Esthetic concerns should be noted, and the nose should be evaluated from a frontal and profile view.

A discussion of detailed esthetic parameters of the nose is beyond the scope of this text. However, important esthetic factors to consider are the width of the nasal base, the distance from the base of the nose to the anterior extent of the nares, and from the anterior aspect of the nares to the tip of the nose. The prominence of the dorsum, the shape of the nasal tip, and the acuteness of the supratip break must also be considered in relation to the intended orthognathic surgery and the physical and/or relative esthetic effects surgery may have on these structures. The length of the columella and the nasolabial angle as well as the projection and shape of the nares should be considered; these aspects may be negatively affected by maxillary surgery.

Because orthognathic surgery can have a relative and anatomical effect on nasal form and esthetics, simultaneous rhinoplasty and orthognathic surgery should be limited to small corrections to the nasal dorsum only. Formal rhinoplasty should be deferred to a second procedure. Figure 2-21 demonstrates the profound relative change of the nose following orthognathic surgical correction of a Class III malocclusion.

Although the face is divided into equal thirds to simplify clinical examinations and for schematic descriptive purposes, an orthognathic surgical procedure may affect the soft tissue in one or more of these thirds. Ferretti and Reyneke described the division of the face from the frontal view into five areas of surgical influence (Fig 2-22).

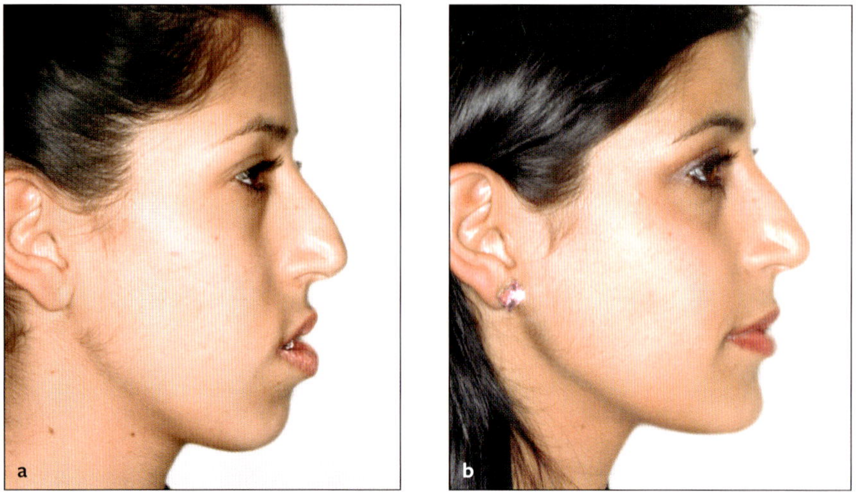

Fig 2-21 Corrective facial changes following orthognathic surgery may have a profound relative and/or anatomical effect on the nose. (*a*) Preoperative view showing a nose that appears large with a prominent dorsum. (*b*) The nose appears to have a normal shape and form following correction of a Class III occlusion by superior repositioning of the maxilla via a Le Fort I osteotomy, mandibular setback by means of a bilateral sagittal split osteotomy, and advancement genioplasty.

Profile analysis

Upper third of the face

The supraorbital rims normally project 5 to 10 mm beyond the most anterior projection of the globe of the eye. Frontal bossing, supraorbital hypoplasia, exophthalmos, or enophthalmos should be distinguished.

Middle third of the face

It is helpful to examine the middle and lower thirds of the face in isolation, and masking the lower third with a card eliminates any undue influence that this third may have on the perceptions of the face as a whole. The middle third of the face can also be blocked out to evaluate only the lower third in relation to the rest of the face (Fig 2-23). The nose, cheeks, and paranasal areas are sequentially evaluated.

Nose

The shape of the dorsum is noted as normal, convex, or concave. The projection of the nasal bridge should be anterior to the globes (5 to 8 mm). The appearance of the nasal tip is evaluated for the presence of a supratip break and for tip definition and projection (Fig 2-24). It is important to distinguish between a dorsal hump and a turned-down tip because each has different treatment implications. The possible effect of maxillary surgery on the nose should be kept in mind when evaluating the proportions of the base of the nose (Fig 2-25).

Cheeks

The globes generally project 0 to 2 mm ahead of the infraorbital rims, whereas the lateral orbital rims lie 8 to 12 mm behind the most anterior projection of the globes (Fig 2-26). The cheeks should exhibit a general convexity from the apex of the cheekbone to the commissure of the mouth. This line of convexity, called the *cheekbone–nasal base–lip curve contour*, requires simultaneous frontal and profile examination. This line starts just anterior to the ear, extending forward through the cheekbone, then anteroinferiorly over the maxilla adjacent to the alar base of the nose, and ending lateral to the commissure of the mouth (Fig 2-27). The line should form a smooth, continuing curve with no interruptions. An interruption of the curve may indicate an apparent skeletal deformity. Figure 2-28 illustrates a clear interruption of this line in the maxillary area, indicating maxillary anteroposterior deficiency. In Fig 2-29, the interruption in the line is in the maxillary area, indicating maxillary anteroposterior deficiency, and inferior to the upper lip section, indicating mandibular anteroposterior excess.

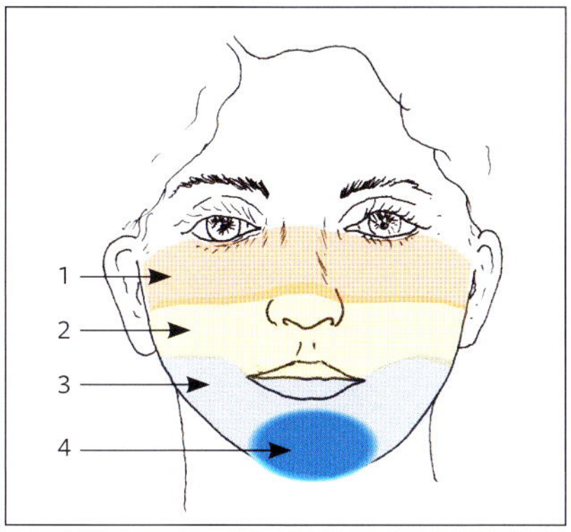

Fig 2-22 The face can be divided into oculonasal (1), maxillary (2), and mandibular (3) complexes. The mandibular complex includes the genial subcomplex (4).

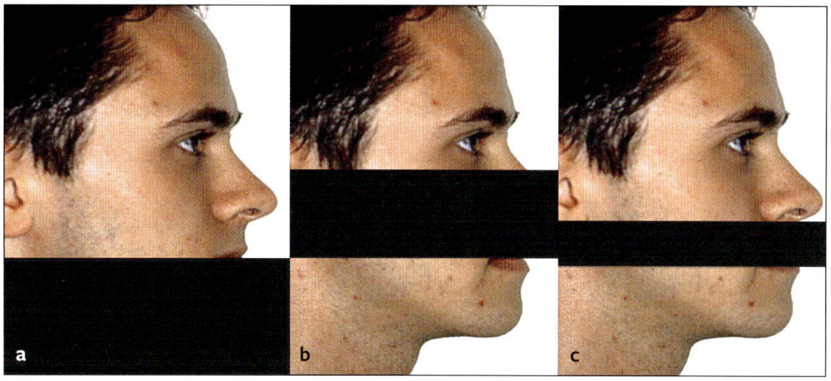

Fig 2-23 (*a*) The mandibular complex (including the chin) is blocked out, revealing the deficient paranasal flattening and poor upper lip support. (*b*) The middle third of the face is blocked out, showing the mandible and chin in good relation to the rest of the face. This observation is confirmed when only the upper lip and maxilla are blocked out (*c*).

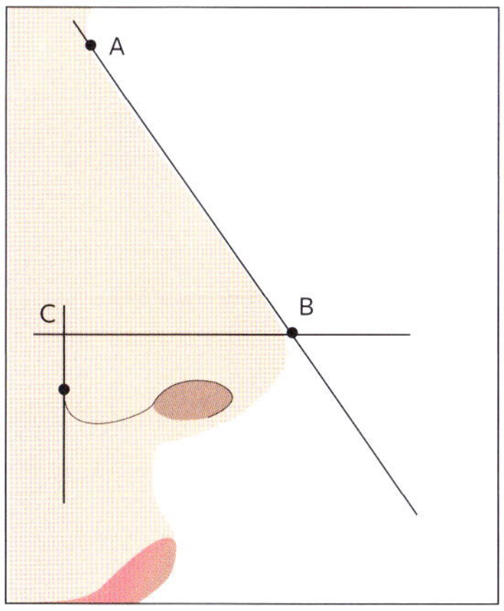

Fig 2-24 The nasal tip projection is evaluated by the Goode method. If BC is greater than 55% to 60% of AB, the nasal tip usually appears disproportionately overprojected.

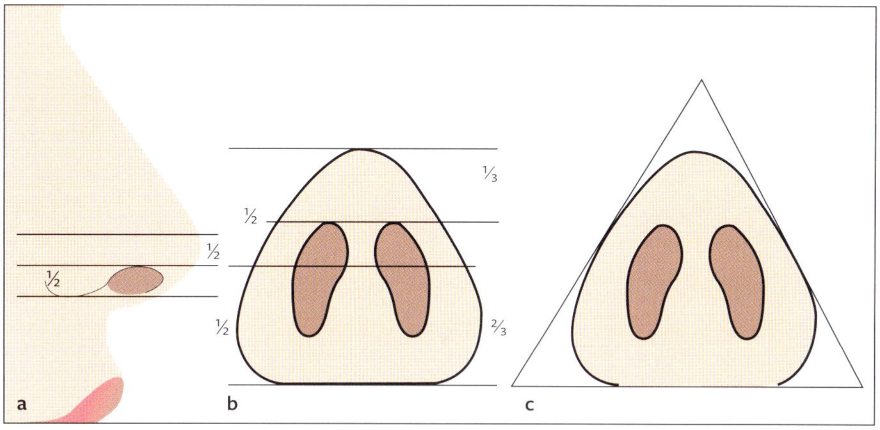

Fig 2-25 (*a*) Vertical ala-columella relationship. (*b*) Columella-lobule relationship with a ratio of approximately 2:1. (*c*) The general shape of the alar base should resemble an isosceles triangle, with the lobule neither too broad nor too narrow.

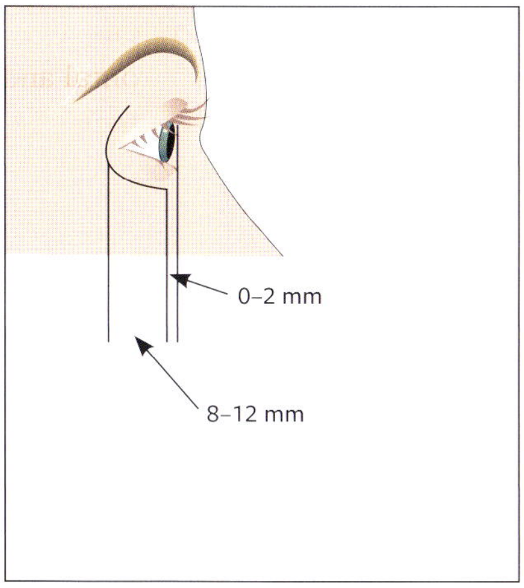

Fig 2-26 The lateral orbital rim lies 8 to 12 mm behind the globe, and the globe projects 0 to 2 mm ahead of the infraorbital rim.

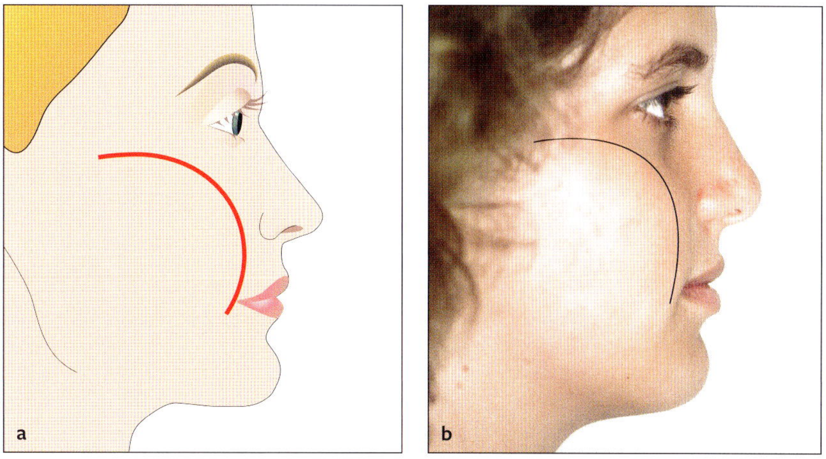

Fig 2-27 (*a*) Cheekbone–nasal base–lip curve contour. (*b*) Note the smooth, uninterrupted curve of the contour line in an individual with good facial proportions.

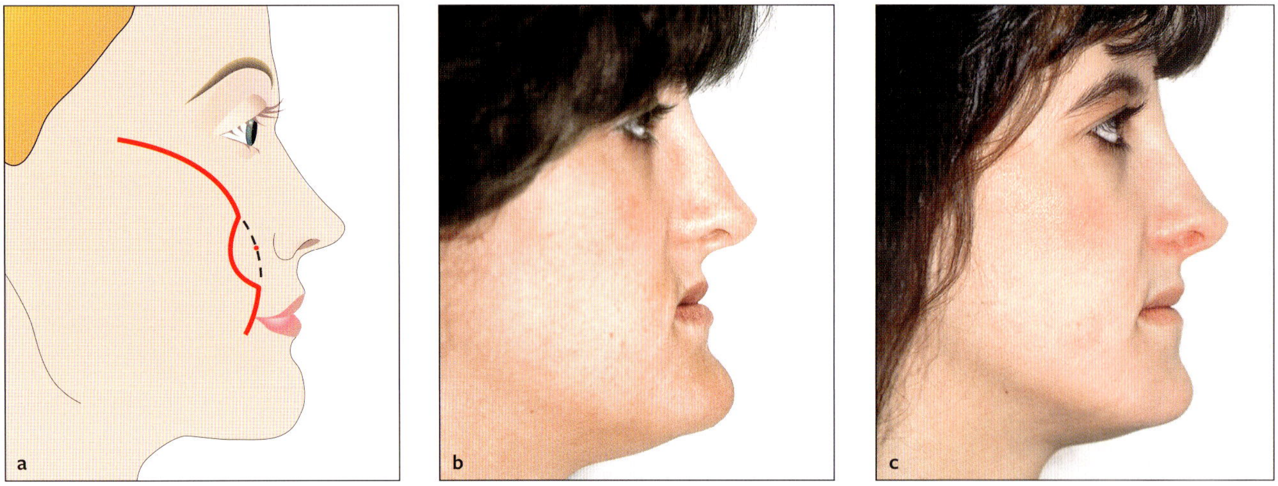

Fig 2-28 (*a and b*) An interruption in the curve of the contour line at MxP, indicating maxillary anteroposterior deficiency. (*c*) An improvement in the curve after advancement of the maxilla.

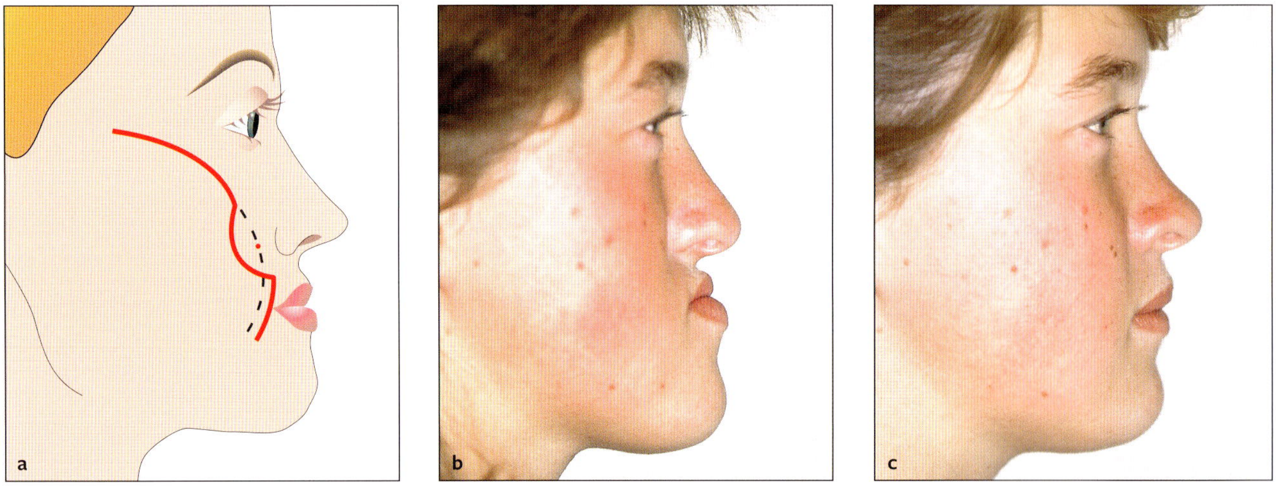

Fig 2-29 (*a and b*) A double break in the contour line in an individual with maxillary anteroposterior deficiency and mandibular anteroposterior excess. (*c*) The curve in the contour line is more harmonious after surgical advancement of the maxilla and mandibular setback.

Paranasal areas

The clinician should carefully assess the paranasal area because it plays an important role in distinguishing between middle third deficiency and mandibular anteroposterior excess. The ratio of the linear distance (horizontally) from nasal tip to Sn and from Sn to alar base crease is normally 2:1 (Fig 2-30). A ratio closer than 1:1 indicates maxillary anteroposterior deficiency. An increased ratio indicates decreased nasal projection. Patients with a Class III malocclusion, decreased nasal projection, and a short nose should be treated by mandibular setback rather than maxillary advancement. The possibility of rhinoplasty as a second procedure should be discussed with the patient.

Lower third of the face

A systematic examination of the lower third of the face includes evaluation of the lips, labiomental fold, nasolabial angle, chin, and chin-throat area.

Lips

The protrusion, retrusion, and soft tissue thickness of each lip is evaluated with the lips in repose. The upper lip usually

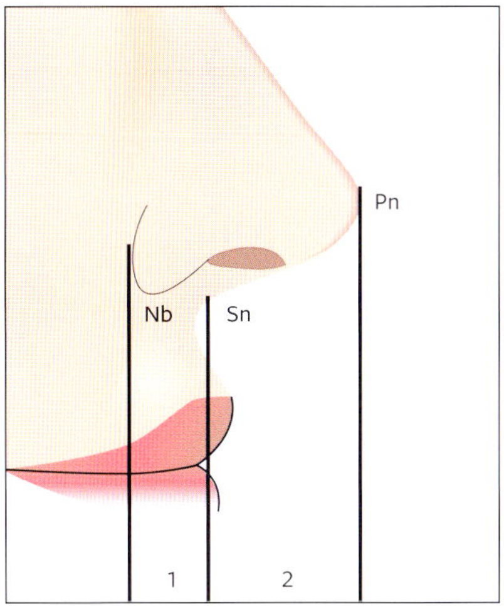

Fig 2-30 Nasal projection. The projection of the nose is measured horizontally from Pn to Sn and is normally 16 to 20 mm. From the nasal base (Nb), the ratio of Pn-Sn to Sn-Nb should be 2:1.

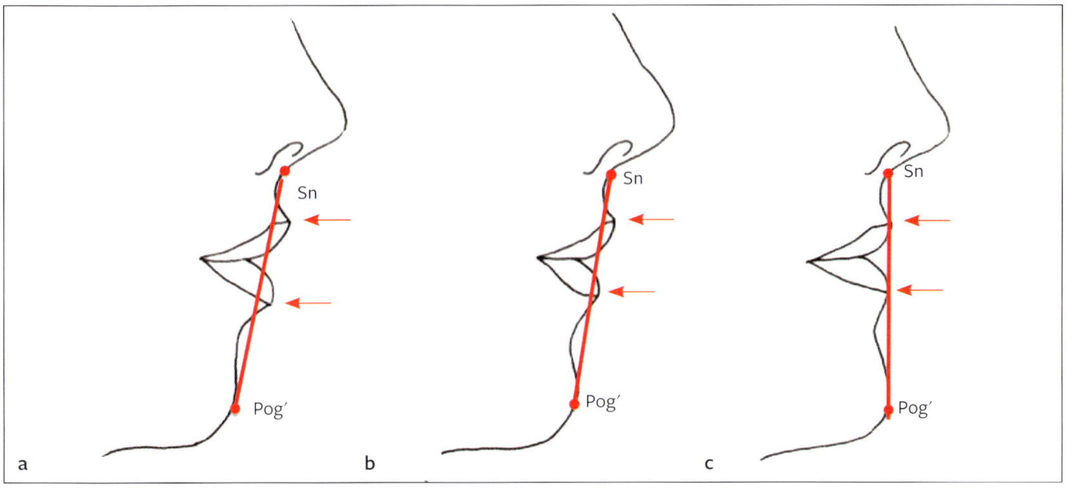

Fig 2-31 Effect of the chin position on the Sn-Pog′ line. (*a*) Effect in an individual with mandibular anteroposterior deficiency (lips ahead of the line). (*b*) With the chin in normal horizontal relationship to the maxilla, the upper lip should be 3.5 mm and the lower lip 2.5 mm ahead of Sn-Pog′. (*c*) Effect in an individual with mandibular prognathism (lips on the line). In all three cases, the upper lip position has not changed; however, a change in Pog′ position results in a change in the lip position relative to the Sn-Pog′ line.

projects slightly anterior to the lower lip. The position of the lips relates to the underlying dental position, such as maxillary dental protrusion or lack of upper lip support caused by, for example, Class II, division 2 malocclusion or excessive orthodontic retraction of maxillary incisors. An individual with an excessive increase in lower lip vermilion and a deep labiomental fold often also has a Class II, division 1 malocclusion.

The anteroposterior lip position may be assessed with the help of the esthetic line of Ricketts (E-line) or esthetic plane of Steiner (S-line) as guidelines (see the following sections on cephalometrics). The Sn-Pog′ line, also called the *lower facial plane*, is an important guide in assessing the lip position and planning orthodontic and surgical positioning of the incisors, as well as surgical positioning of the chin. The upper lip should be 3 ± 1 mm ahead of this line and the lower lip 2 ± 1 mm ahead of this line. Extractions followed by retraction of incisors behind the Sn-Pog′ line should be avoided. Keep in mind that this assessment is influenced by the anteroposterior position of the chin and the soft tissue thickness of the lips (Fig 2-31).

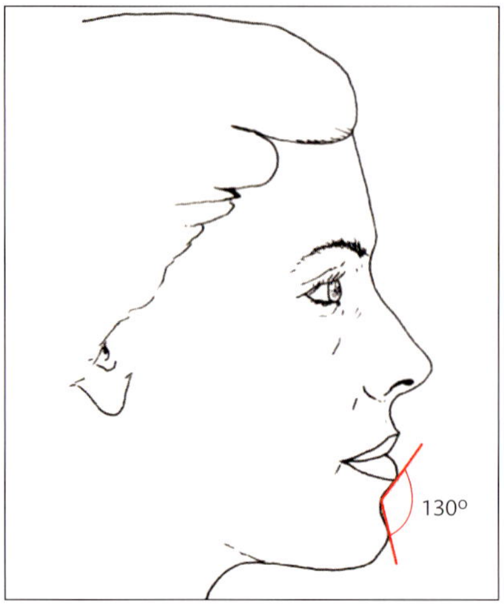

Fig 2-32 Labiomental fold. The lower lip–chin angle should be at least 130 degrees.

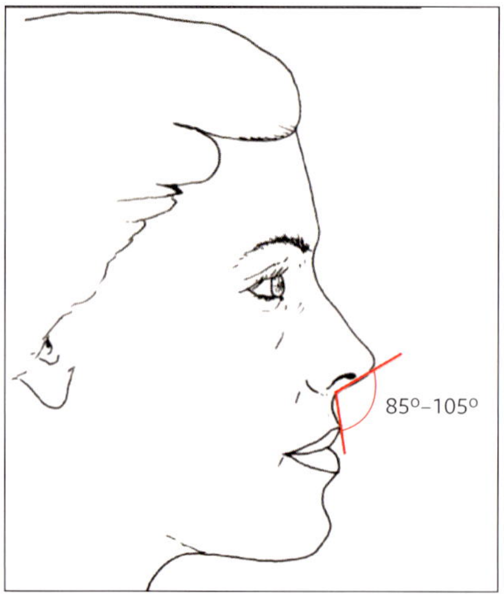

Fig 2-33 The nasolabial angle, measured between the inclination of the columella of the nose and the upper lip, should be 85 to 105 degrees.

Table 2-4 | Comparison of acute and obtuse nasolabial angles

	Acute angle	Obtuse angle
Maxillary incisor position	Protruding	Upright or retroinclined
Nasal projection	Drooping nasal tip	Prominent or hanging columella
Occlusion	Class III	Class II
Bite	Deep bite	Open bite
Maxillary vertical dimension	Deficient	Excessive

Labiomental fold

The lower lip–chin contour should have a gentle S-curve, with a lower lip–chin angle of at least 130 degrees (Fig 2-32). The angle is often acute in patients with Class II mandibular anteroposterior deficiency because of impingement of the maxillary incisor on the lower lip or macrogenia. The angle is flattened in individuals with microgenia or lower lip tension caused by Class III malocclusion. The surgeon considering genioplasty should assess not only the anteroposterior position of the Pog′ but also the chin shape and the labiomental fold.

Nasolabial angle

The nasolabial angle, which is measured between the inclination of the columella and the upper lip (Fig 2-33), should be in the range of 85 to 105 degrees (Table 2-4). In females, a slightly larger angle is acceptable; whereas in males, a smaller angle is considered esthetically pleasing. Patients with mandibular anteroposterior deficiency have increased nasolabial angles, and this angle is usually acute in individuals with Class III occlusion. Surgical or orthodontic retraction of maxillary incisors should be avoided in individuals with large nasolabial angles. Where crowding necessitates tooth extraction, the nasolabial angle should influence the decision to extract first versus second premolars. Surgical repositioning of the maxilla also affects the nasolabial angle. In general, the maxilla should never be moved posteriorly, especially in combination with superior repositioning. This surgical movement leads to loss of lip support, increase in nasolabial angle, increase in nasal projection, and flattening of the nasal base. These changes result in poor esthetics and a premature aging effect. The maxilla should be moved posteriorly only in individuals with true maxillary protrusion, which occurs very rarely.

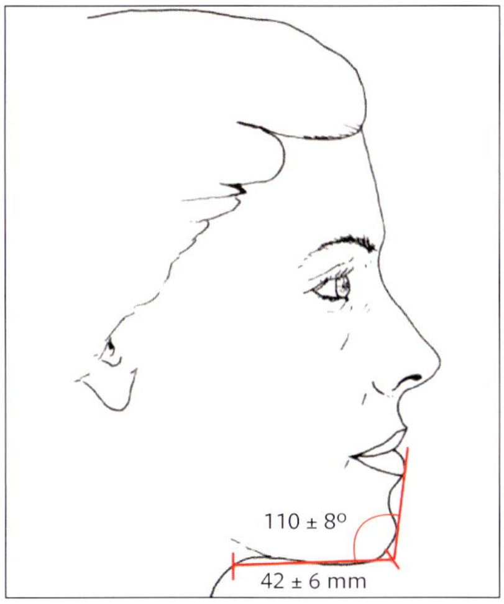

Fig 2-34 Lip-chin-throat angle and submandibular length.

Table 2-5 | **Comparison of acute and obtuse lip-chin-throat angles**

	Acute angle	Obtuse angle
Mandibular anterposterior dimension	Excessive	Deficient
Submandibular fat	None	Present
Occlusion	Class III	Class II

Chin

Although the chin forms a prominent esthetic feature of the face, it has no clearly defined function. Anatomically the chin is considered to be the soft tissue structure below the labiomental fold. Chin projection should be in good balance with the entire profile. The anteroposterior position of Pog′, however, is not the only determining factor for good chin esthetics. When examining the chin, the clinician should consider the entire complex of structures forming the lower third of the face from Sn to Me′. It is difficult to isolate individual parts constituting this complex because the examiner should evaluate the size, shape, and position of each structure in relation to the other structures as well as the chin complex in relation to the rest of the face. At this stage, the middle third of the face should be masked and the relationship of the chin to the rest of the facial structures evaluated. Various soft tissue cephalometric analyses are available to assist in clinical evaluation of the anteroposterior chin position. However, the chin should be evaluated in all three dimensions. The width of the chin should be assessed in relation to the overall facial shape. A narrow chin often has a knobby appearance, and if surgical advancement of the chin is planned, widening of the chin should be contemplated. The labiomental fold, chin shape, relationship to the dental midline, symmetry, and cant of the lower border should be considered.

Chin-throat area

The presence of a double chin and adipose tissue should be noted. The lower lip–chin-throat angle (normally 110 degrees) provides chin definition (Fig 2-34). The distance from the neck-throat angle to Pog′ (submandibular length) should be approximately 42 mm. These observations are pertinent when considering mandibular setback or advancement procedures, genioplasty (advancement or reduction), or submental liposuction (Table 2-5).

Radiographic Evaluations

Lateral Cephalometric Radiographic Evaluation

The information from lateral and (if indicated) posteroanterior cephalometric radiographs forms an important part of the database for orthognathic surgical treatment planning. Although clinical evaluation must be the primary diagnostic tool in determining surgical treatment of the orthognathic patient, cephalometric analysis is a helpful diagnostic guide. It enables the clinician to quantify, classify, and communicate dentofacial deformities; create a treatment plan via a visual treatment objective; help plan for tooth extractions; monitor progress during treatment; study specific changes during and after treatment to evaluate treatment results; and study facial growth.

The lateral cephalometric radiograph should be taken with the patient's head in a natural posture, the teeth in centric occlusion, and the lips in repose. There are three exceptions to this requirement:

1. Where there is a clinically significant difference between the centric occlusion and centric relation, a second radiograph should be taken with the teeth in centric relation.
2. In patients with maxillary vertical deficiency, a second radiograph should be taken with the mandible rotated open until the lips just part. The maxillary incisor–upper lip relationship, upper lip length and shape, and the amount of maxillary downgraft can be more accurately evaluated on this radiograph.
3. In patients with severe Class III malocclusion and overclosed bites, it is difficult to assess the lips, tooth-lip relationship, and the relationship between the maxilla and mandible. A second radiograph should be taken with the mandible rotated until the lips just part.

The primary objective of treatment is not to make the patient's cephalometric measurements normal, but rather to make the occlusal function normal and the facial appearance harmonious. For most patients, function and esthetics go hand in hand.

Cephalometric analysis involves measuring, comparing, and relating various linear and angular measurements of the hard and soft tissue structures of the face. The following analysis, a compilation of measurements useful in making a diagnosis and developing a treatment plan, is divided into lateral cephalometric analysis of soft tissue, hard tissue (skeletal analysis), and dental relationships.

Although soft tissue analysis is discussed as part of cephalometric analysis, it should be emphasized that the primary soft tissue examination of the facial esthetics guided by cephalometric analytic values should be done clinically. A patient's cephalometric analysis and photographs should be part of the permanent records, but controlled, reliable records of the clinical examination are necessary for accurate diagnosis and correct treatment. The diagnosis should not be based only on the examination of photographs and cephalometric analysis.

Soft tissue analysis

Soft tissue landmarks

Lateral soft tissue landmarks, shown in Fig 2-35, include the following:

- *Soft tissue glabella* (*G′*): The most anterior point of the forehead
- *Soft tissue nasion* (*N′*): The deepest point of concavity in the midline between the forehead and the nose
- *Pronasale* (*Pn*): The most anterior point of the nose
- *Subnasale* (*Sn*): The point at which the columella of the nose merges with the upper lip in the midsagittal plane
- *Labrale superior* (*Ls*): The mucocutaneous border of the upper lip vermilion
- *Stomion superius* (*Sts*): The lowest point of the vermilion of the upper lip
- *Stomion inferius* (*Sti*): The uppermost point of the lower lip vermilion
- *Labrale inferior* (*Li*): The mucocutaneous border of the lower lip
- *Soft tissue pogonion* (*Pog′*): The most anterior point of the chin in the midsagittal plane
- *Soft tissue menton* (*Me′*): The lowest point on the contour of the soft tissue chin, found by dropping a perpendicular line from a horizontal line through the skeletal menton

Soft tissue planes

Soft tissue planes are shown in Fig 2-36 and include the following:

- *Facial plane:* Extends from N′ to Pog′
- *Upper facial plane:* Extends from G′ to Sn
- *Lower facial plane:* Extends from Sn to Pog′

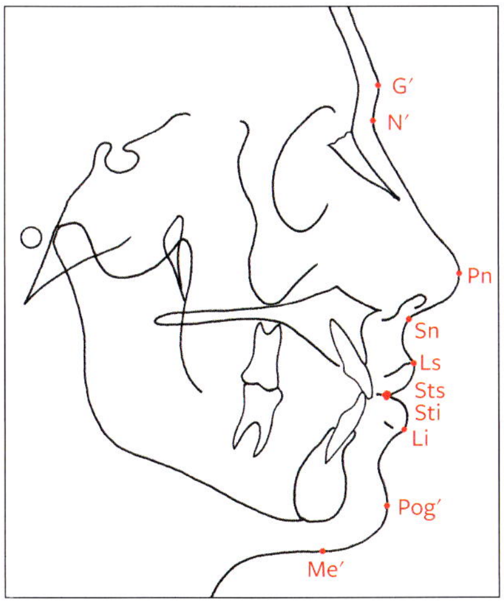

Fig 2-35 Soft tissue cephalometric landmarks.

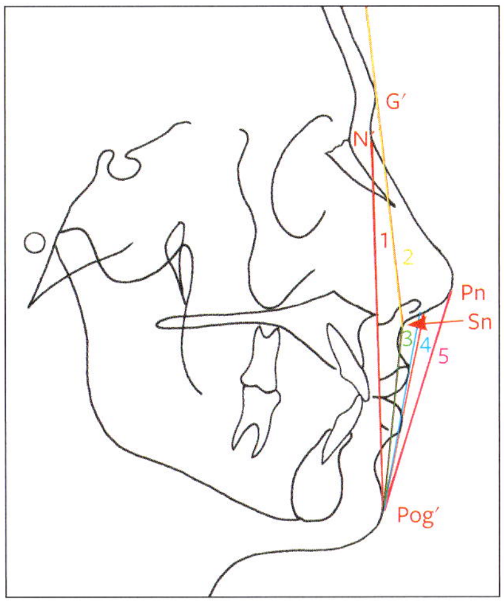

Fig 2-36 Soft tissue planes. (1) Facial plane. (2) Upper facial plane. (3) Lower facial plane. (4) S-line. (5) E-line (esthetic plane).

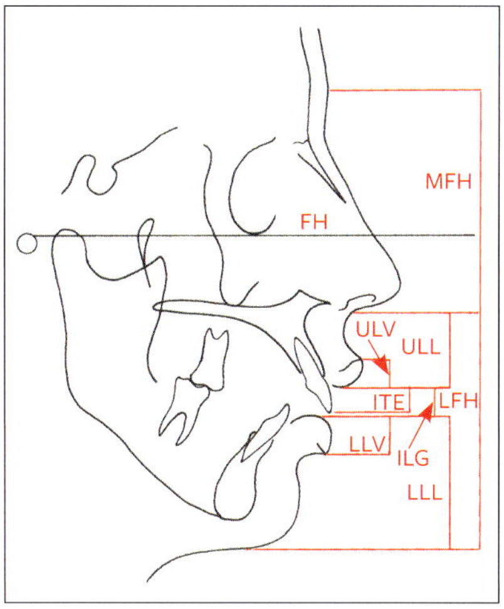

Fig 2-37 Soft tissue vertical evaluation. Vertical measurements are made perpendicular to the FH plane. MFH, middle facial third height; ULV, upper lip vermilion height; ULL, upper lip length; ITE, incisor tooth exposure; LFH, lower facial third height; LLV, lower lip vermilion height; ILG, interlabial gap; LLL, lower lip/chin length.

Table 2-6 | **Comparison of increased and decreased lip lengths**

	Increased lip length	Decreased lip length
Maxillary incisor exposure	Decreased	Increased
Differential diagnosis	Vertical maxillary deficiency	Vertical maxillary excess
Smile	Toothless	Gummy
Lip seal	Adquate	Increased interlabial gap

- *S-line:* Formed by connecting Pog′ to a point midway between Pn and Sn
- *E-line:* Extends from Pn to Pog′

Soft tissue vertical evaluation

Relationship of middle to lower facial third height

The distance from G′ to Sn (middle facial third height) and from Sn to Me′ (lower facial third height) is measured. The ratio should be approximately 1:1. In most orthognathic surgical patients, abnormalities are in the lower third of the face (Sn-Me′). In patients in whom the lower third of the face is increased in relation to the upper third, either vertical maxillary excess or an increase in the vertical anterior height of the mandible should be expected (Fig 2-37).

A decrease in lower vertical height could be caused by either vertical maxillary deficiency, vertical deficiency of the anterior mandible, or an overclosed bite.

Upper lip length

Upper lip length measured from Sn to Sts should be 22 ± 2 mm for males and 20 ± 2 mm for females (see Fig 2-37). Patients with relatively long upper lips tend to have less maxillary incisor exposure, whereas individuals with short upper lips tend to have an increased interlabial gap with increased maxillary incisor exposure (Table 2-6). When vertical repositioning of the maxilla is contemplated, upper lip length should be considered to plan the correct amount of superior repositioning of the maxilla for each individual.

Table 2-7 | Comparison of increased and decreased interlabial gaps

	Increased interlabial gap	Decreased interlabial gap
Maxillary incisor exposure	Increased (assess with teeth in occlusion and lips relaxed)	None or little
Smile exposure	Gummy	Less than the full incisor crown exposed
Lip competence	Mouth breathing	Overclosed appearance
Vertical maxillary dimesnion	Excessive	Deficient/deep bite
Upper lip	Short	Long
Vermilion exposure	Excessive	Less

Lower lip/chin length

The lower lip/chin length is measured from Sti to Me′ and should be 44 ± 2 mm for males and 40 ± 2 mm for females (see Fig 2-37). An increase in the vertical dimension may indicate an increased anterior vertical height of the mandible. In contrast, a decrease may indicate a short anterior mandibular height. This dimension may also be short in individuals with both deep bites and everted lower lips.

Ratio of upper lip length to lower lip/chin length

The upper lip length (Sn-Sts) should be approximately half the length of the lower lip and chin (Sti-Me′; see Fig 2-37). A decrease in the vertical relation indicates either a long upper lip or a vertical deficiency of the anterior mandibular height. An increase in the ratio may be caused by either a short upper lip or a vertical excess of the anterior mandible.

Interlabial gap

When the lips are relaxed, they should be touching slightly, although an interlabial gap of 1 to 3 mm is still considered normal (see Fig 2-37). An increased interlabial gap (ie, larger than 4 mm) is usually an indication of lip incompetence due to vertical maxillary excess. Patients with a short upper lip, however, also tend to have an increased interlabial gap (Table 2-7).

Maxillary incisor exposure

When the patient's lips are relaxed, 1 to 4 mm of the maxillary incisors should be visible under the upper lip. Lack of tooth exposure may be an indication of maxillary vertical deficiency; more than 4 mm of tooth exposure may indicate vertical maxillary excess (see Fig 2-37). The upper lip length should be kept in mind with this assessment.

Patients with relatively normal upper lips and excessive incisor exposure under the upper lip will have vertical maxillary excess. This assessment can be made only with the lips in repose. Lack of tooth exposure under an upper lip of normal length is an indication that the maxilla is vertically deficient. Vertical maxillary deficiency can be assessed only with the bite opened until the lips begin to part.

Upper and lower lip vermilion height

The upper lip vermilion height should be 25% less than the lower lip vermilion height. In short, the ratio of Ls-Sts to Sti-Li should be 3:4 (see Fig 2-37). Vermilion heights may vary depending on race, a fact that should be kept in mind during evaluation. Increased lower lip vermilion exposure may be due to lower lip eversion caused by lip incompetence in patients with vertical maxillary excess. The lower lip is also often everted in Class II deep bite cases or Class II, division 1 cases where the lower lip is rolled outward by the maxillary incisors.

Table 2-8 summarizes the vertical soft tissue relationships.

Soft tissue anteroposterior evaluation

Nasolabial angle

The *nasolabial angle* is formed by a line tangent to the columella and a line tangent to the upper lip. A value of 85 to 105 degrees is considered normal. In males, the angle is usually more acute, whereas in females, a more obtuse angle is considered to be attractive (Fig 2-38).

The nasolabial angle is influenced by the position of the upper lip supported by the maxillary incisors and the inclination of the columella of the nose. Excessive orthodontic retraction of the maxillary incisors will undermine upper lip support, leading to an unattractive increase of

Table 2-8 | **Summary of vertical soft tissue relationships**

Vertical relationship	Measurement	Normal value
Middle facial height: lower facial height (MFH:LFH)	G′-Sn:Sn-Me′	1:1
Upper lip length (ULL)	Sn–Sts	20 ± 2 mm (females) 22 ± 2 mm (males)
Lower lip/chin length (LLL)	Sti–Me′	40 ± 2 mm (females) 44 ± 2 mm (males)
Upper lip length: lower lip/chin length (ULL:LLL)	Sn–Sts:Sti–Me′ Sn–LLV:LLV–Me′	1:2 1:0.9
Interlabial gap (ILG)	NA	0 to 3 mm
Maxillary incisor tooth exposure (ITE)	Sts–Maxillary incisor tip	1 to 4 mm
Upper lip vermilion:lower lip vermilion (ULV:LLV)	Ls–Sts:Sti–Li	3:4

NA, not applicable.

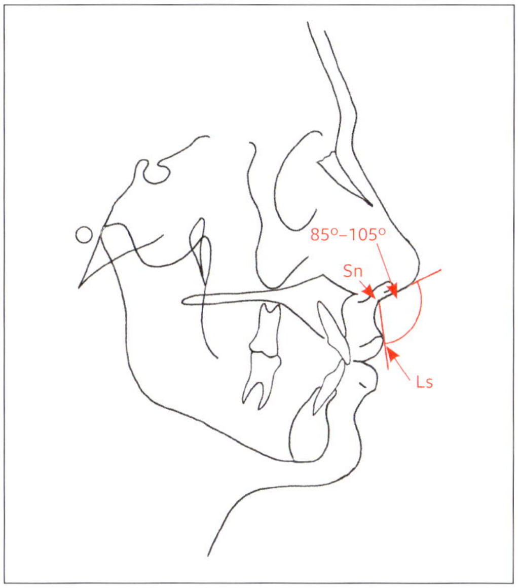

Fig 2-38 The nasolabial angle is formed by a line tangent to the columella and a line tangent to the upper lip (Sn-Ls).

the nasolabial angle. The angle is more acute in Class III cases and more obtuse in Class II cases. The following factors that may influence the nasolabial angle should be considered during treatment planning:

- *Lip support.* The existing maxillary incisor–upper lip relationship must be assessed.
- *Lip strain.* Strained lips tend to move posteriorly once tension has been released. Tense lips, however, move less anteriorly with tooth or bone movement.
- *Lip thickness.* Thin lips respond more readily than thick lips to tooth movement.
- *Magnitude of the overjet.* If orthodontic retraction of maxillary incisors is contemplated, the larger the overjet, the more retraction that will be necessary. This retraction may lead to an increase in the nasolabial angle and loss of lip support.

The final anteroposterior position of the maxillary incisors and anteroposterior lip position are affected by interdental crowding or spaces in the anterior maxillary dental arch, tooth size discrepancies (maxillary versus mandibular), extraction versus nonextraction, extraction pattern (first versus second premolars), and existing tooth angulation.

Lip prominence

A line is drawn from Sn to Pog′ (lower facial plane). The perpendicular distance of the Ls ahead of the Sn-Pog′ line should be 3 ± 1 mm, whereas the Li should be 2 ± 1 mm anterior to the Sn-Pog′ line (Fig 2-39a).

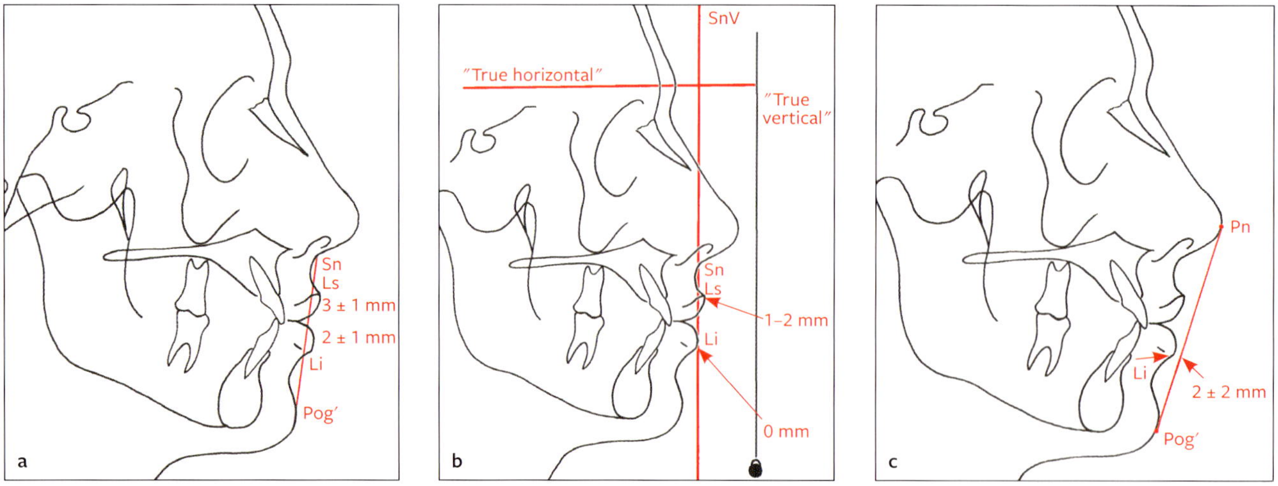

Fig 2-39 (*a*) Lip prominence in relation to the lower facial plane. The distance of Ls and Li to Sn-Pog′ is measured. Ls to Sn-Pog′: 3 ± 1 mm. Li to Sn-Pog′: 2 ± 1 mm. (*b*) Lip prominence in relation to SnV. The distances of Ls and Li are measured to the line drawn parallel to true vertical through the Sn. Ls to SnV: 1 to 2 mm. Li to SnV: 0 mm. (*c*) Lip prominence in relation to the E-line. Li should be 2 ± 2 mm behind Pn-Pog′.

The anteroposterior position of the upper lip is an indication of soft tissue support by the maxillary incisors and plays an important role in orthodontic or surgical positioning of the maxillary incisors. Thus, it should be kept in mind during treatment planning. The Li tends to be further ahead of Sn-Pog′ in Class II cases (with Pog′ posteriorly situated) and behind the line in Class III cases (with Pog′ anteriorly situated).

A vertical line drawn through the Sn perpendicular to "true horizontal" is called the *subnasale vertical* (SnV), and the upper lip should be 1 to 2 mm ahead of SnV. The lower lip should be on or just posterior to SnV (Fig 2-39b). In cases of mandibular anteroposterior deficiency, the lower lip tends to be more than 1 mm posterior to SnV. In patients with mandibular anteroposterior excess and/or maxillary anteroposterior deficiency, the lower lip will be anterior to the SnV. The distance of the most prominent part of the lower lip is measured to the E-line (Pn-Pog′). The lower lip should be 2 ± 2 mm behind the E-line (Fig 2-39c).

This evaluation is influenced by the nose and chin prominence and could also be used for planning the final chin position. The lower lip would tend to be ahead of this line in individuals with Class II mandibular anteroposterior deficiency, in whom Pog′ is situated posteriorly and the lower lip everted.

Maxillary and mandibular anteroposterior position

A vertical line perpendicular to the constructed horizontal plane is drawn through G′. Pog′ should be 1 to 4 mm behind the line. For maxillary anteroposterior assessment, Sn should be 6 ± 3 mm ahead of this line (Fig 2-40).

In patients with maxillary anteroposterior deficiency, Sn will be less than 3 mm ahead of the line, or in severe cases, even behind the line. Pog′ ahead of the line indicates possible mandibular anteroposterior excess. In mandibular anteroposterior deficiency, Pog′ will be more than 4 mm behind the line. It is important, however, to evaluate the anteroposterior position of the chin in conjunction with other features (particularly the shape of the chin) to distinguish among microgenia, macrogenia, and mandibular anteroposterior deficiency.

Chin prominence

Soft tissue chin prominence can be evaluated by measuring the distance to a line drawn through N′ perpendicular to the FH. This line is also known as *0-degree meridian*; Pog′ should be 0 ± 2 mm ahead of it (Fig 2-41). A more prominent chin would be more than 2 mm ahead of the 0-degree meridian, whereas a horizontally deficient chin would be more than 2 mm posterior to the line.

Another vertical line that is helpful in assessing the horizontal prominence of the chin is a line drawn perpendicular to FH through Sn. Pog′ should be 3 ± 3 mm behind this line (see Fig 2-41). A horizontally excessive chin would be on or ahead of the vertical line, whereas a deficient chin would be more than 6 mm posterior to this line.

It is extremely important, however, to use the above measurements only as a guide when assessing chin position. Chin prominence must be evaluated in conjunction

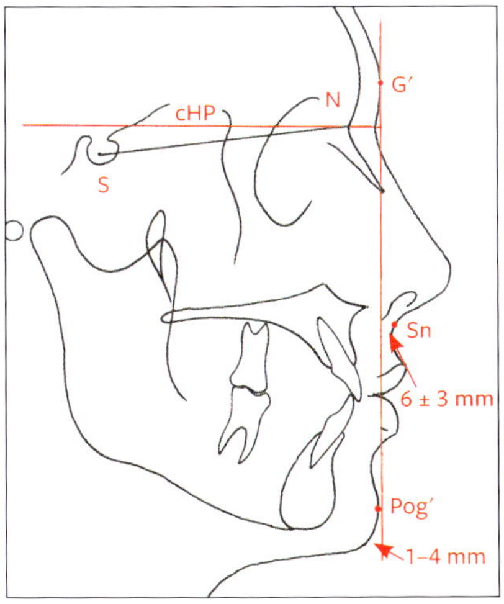

Fig 2-40 Maxillary and mandibular anteroposterior position. Sn should be 6 ± 3 mm ahead of the vertical line drawn through G′, and Pog′ should be 1 to 4 mm behind this line.

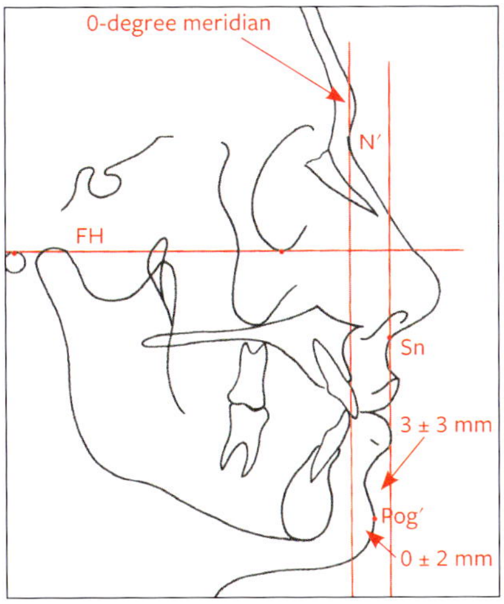

Fig 2-41 Chin prominence. Anteroposterior evaluation of the chin to the 0-degree meridian and to a line perpendicular to the FH through Sn. Pog′ should be 0 ± 2 mm ahead of the 0-degree meridian and 3 ± 3 mm behind the SnV.

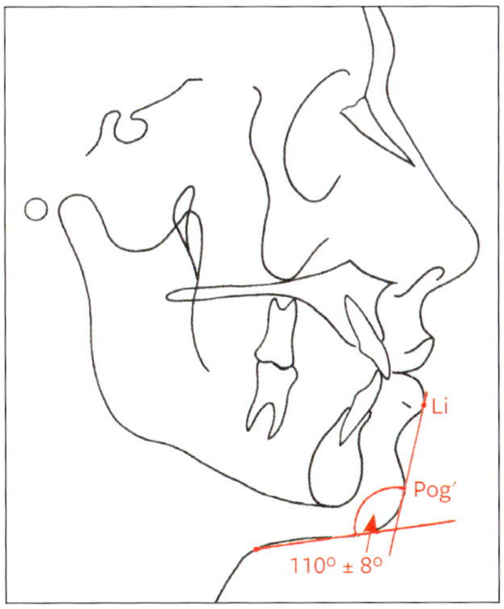

Fig 2-42 Lower lip–chin–throat angle.

Table 2-9 | **Comparison of increased and decreased chin-throat lengths**

	Increased chin-throat length	Decreased chin-throat length
Mandibular anteroposterior dimension	Excessive	Deficient
Occlusion	Class III	Class II
Chin	Macrogenia	Microgenia

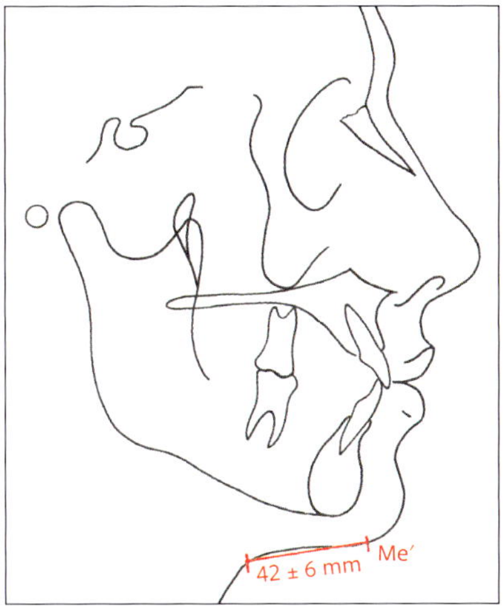

Fig 2-43 Chin-throat length.

with other factors, such as chin shape, depth of the labiomental fold, microgenia, macrogenia, lower lip position, and mandibular anteroposterior excess or deficiency.

Lower lip–chin–throat angle

The lower lip–chin–throat angle is contained between a line drawn from Li to Pog′ and a submental tangent line. An angulation of 110 ± 8 degrees is considered normal. For this assessment, the radiograph must be taken in natural head posture (Fig 2-42). This angle will be more acute in patients with mandibular anteroposterior excess and/or macrogenia. It will be more obtuse in cases of mandibular anteroposterior deficiency and/or microgenia.

Chin-throat length

The chin-throat length is measured from the angle of the throat to Me′ (Fig 2-43). A distance of 42 ± 6 mm is considered normal. This measurement is only meaningful with the patient's head in natural posture. The distance will be excessive in individuals with mandibular prognathism and short in those with a recessive mandible (Table 2-9). This measurement is significant in differentiating between mandibular anteroposterior excess and maxillary deficiency. Mandibular setback would obviously reduce this length.

Facial contour angle

The angle of facial convexity is formed by lines drawn from G′ to Sn and from Sn through Pog′. The line from

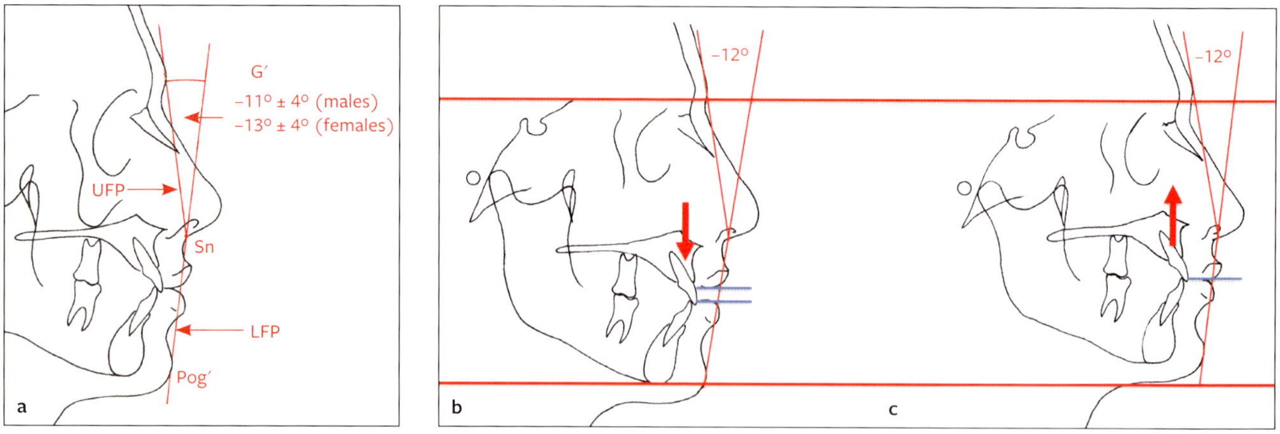

Fig 2-44 (*a*) Facial contour angle. (*b and c*) Both individuals have a facial contour angle of −12 degrees, but they have different vertical deformities. (*b*) Vertical maxillary excess. (*c*) Vertical maxillary deficiency.

G′ to Sn is also called the *upper facial plane*, whereas the *lower facial plane* is formed by the line from Sn to Pog′. The mean angulation is estimated to be −12 degrees. A clockwise angle is expressed as positive; a counterclockwise angle is negative. Males tend to have a straighter profile (−11 ± 4 degrees); a slightly more convex profile is considered esthetically pleasing for females (−13 ± 4 degrees; Fig 2-44a). It is important, however, to differentiate among the various facial deformities that may produce the same facial contour angle. The measurement of the angle does not reveal the localization of the deformity.

In Figs 2-42b and 2-44c, both individuals have normal anteroposterior relations according to the facial contour angle (ie, −12 degrees). However, the vertical height of one is long (see Fig 2-44b), and the mandible has rotated clockwise; the other has a short vertical height (see Fig 2-44c) due to maxillary anteroposterior deficiency with the mandible rotated counterclockwise.

In Figs 2-44d to 2-44f, all three patients have a Class II malocclusion and an increased facial contour angle (ie, −20 degrees). Their identical facial contour angles, however, are produced by entirely different skeletal patterns. Figure 2-44d shows mandibular anteroposterior deficiency. Figure 2-44e shows maxillary anteroposterior excess, and Fig 2-44f shows vertical maxillary excess, with clockwise (backward) rotation of the mandible.

Figures 2-44g to 2-44i show Class III malocclusion and a more concave profile with decreased facial contour angle (ie, −7 degrees) produced by three entirely different skeletal patterns. Figure 2-44g shows mandibular anteroposterior excess. Figure 2-44h shows maxillary anteroposterior deficiency, and Fig 2-44i shows a maxillary vertical deficiency with counterclockwise (forward) rotation of the mandible.

E-line (**Ricketts**)

In relation to the E-line (Pn to Pog′), the upper lip should lie approximately 4 mm behind it whereas the lower lip should lie about 2 mm behind it (Fig 2-45). The profile contained by this line should form a reasonably symmetric Cupid's bow. Dental support for the upper and lower lips will affect these values and distort the shape of the Cupid's bow. In the assessment, the clinician should keep in mind the effect of the anteroposterior chin position (Pog′).

S-line (**Steiner**)

The upper and lower lips should touch the S-line (drawn from Pog′ to the midpoint of the S-shaped curve between Sn and Pn; Fig 2-46). Lips behind this line may indicate lack of lip support or a prominent chin. Lips may fall ahead of this line because of dental protrusion or a deficient chin.

Z-angle (**Merrifield**)

The Merrifield Z-angle is formed by the intersection of FH and a line connecting Pog′ and the most protrusive lip point (upper or lower; Fig 2-47). The average Z-angle is 80 ± 9 degrees. An angle greater than 80 degrees is indicative of mandibular anteroposterior excess, whereas an angle of less than 80 degrees suggests an anteroposterior deficiency of the mandible. The Z-angle also indicates the relationship of the lips to the chin, as well as possible chin prominence or deficiency.

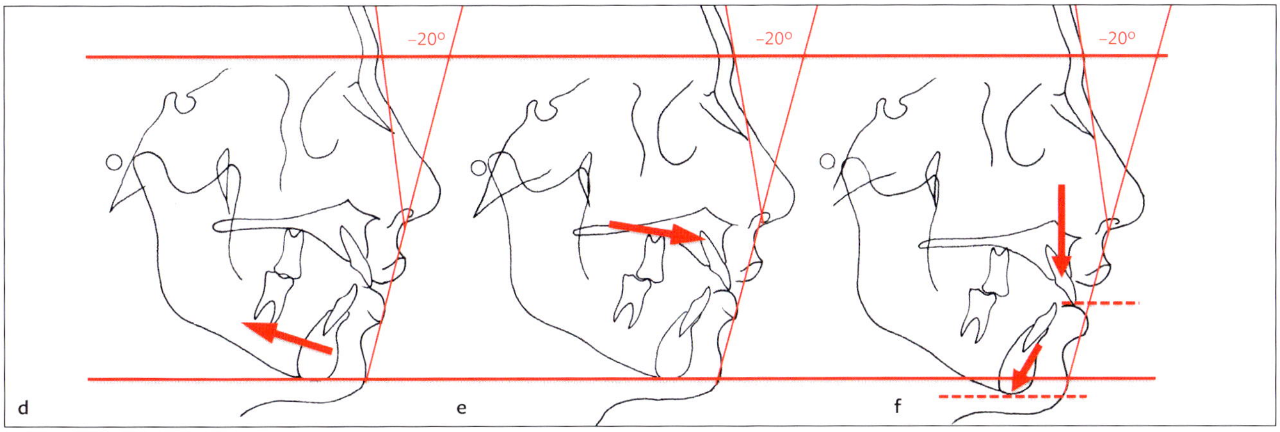

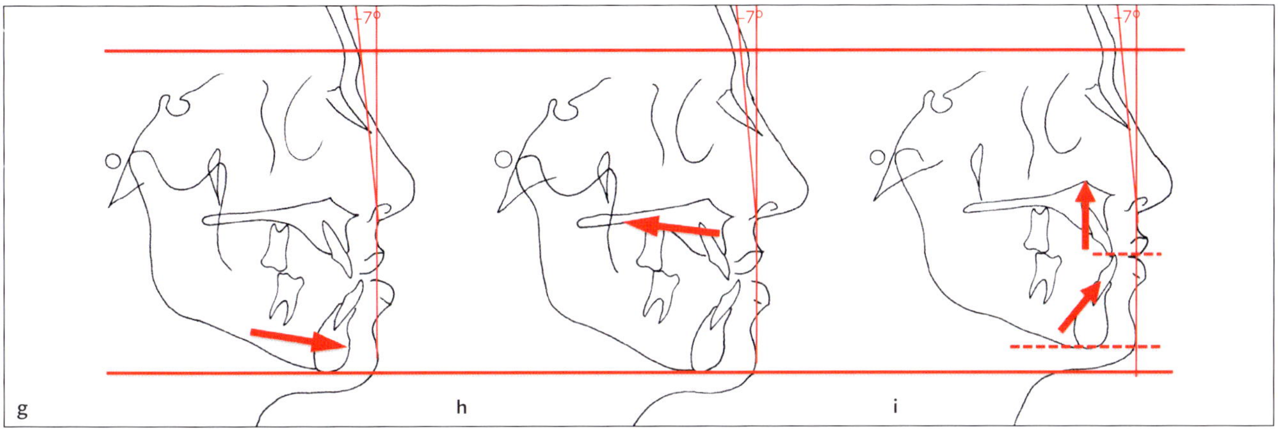

Fig 2-44 *(cont)* (*d to f*) The facial contour angle in all three individuals is –20 degrees, indicating a convex profile. The convexity, however, is caused by different deformities: (*d*) mandibular anteroposterior deficiency, (*e*) maxillary anteroposterior excess, and (*f*) vertical excess of the maxilla with clockwise mandibular rotation. (*g to i*) The facial contour angle in all three individuals is –7 degrees. This concavity is caused by different deformities: (*g*) mandibular anteroposterior excess, (*h*) maxillary anteroposterior deficiency, and (*i*) maxillary vertical deficiency with counterclockwise mandibular rotation.

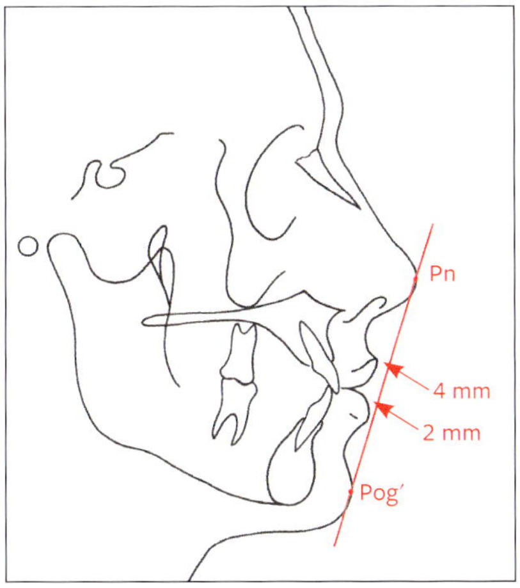

Fig 2-45 E-line (Pn-Pog′).

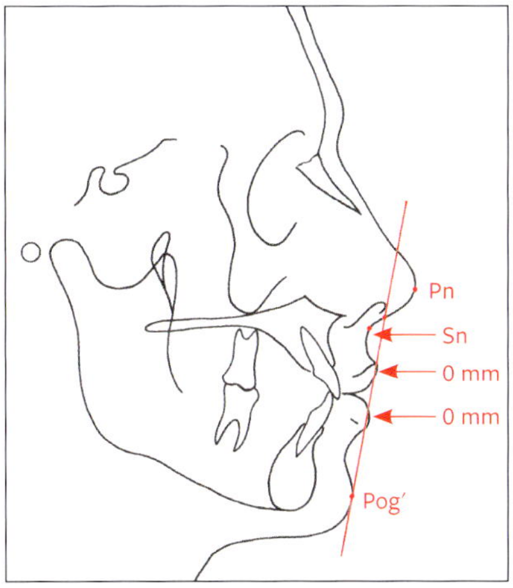

Fig 2-46 The S-line follows Pog′ to the midpoint of the S-shaped curve between Sn and Pn.

Lip thickness

Upper lip thickness is measured horizontally anterior to the bone from 2 mm below A-point to the anterior border of the upper lip (Fig 2-48). Upper lip strain is measured from the vermilion border to the labial surface of the maxillary central incisor and compared with lip thickness above this point.

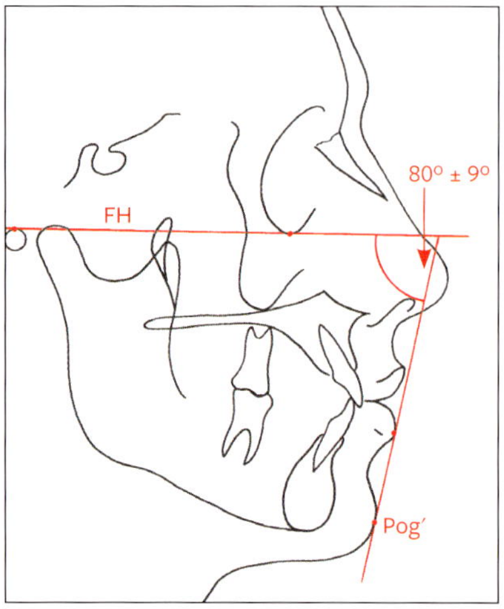

Fig 2-47 The Z-angle is formed by the intersection of FH and a line connecting Pog′ and the most protrusive lip point (upper or lower).

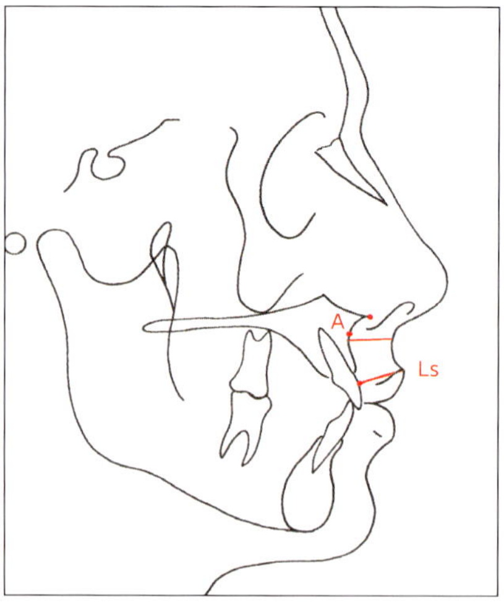

Fig 2-48 Soft tissue thickness of the upper lip.

Table 2-10 | Summary of anteroposterior soft tissue relationships

Anteroposterior relationship	Normal value
Nasolabial angle	85 to 105 degrees
Lip prominence:	
Ls to Sn-Pog′	3 ± 1 mm ahead
Li to Sn-Pog′	2 ± 1 mm ahead
Ls to SnV	1 to 2 mm ahead
Li to SnV	0 mm
Chin prominence:	
Pog′ to 0-degree meridian	0 ± 2 mm ahead
Pog′ to Sn (perpendicular to FH)	3 ± 3 mm ahead
Lower lip-chin-throat angle	110 ± 8 degrees
Chin-throat length	42 ± 6 mm
Facial contour angle	−11 ± 4 degrees (males) −13 ± 4 degrees (females)
E-line to Ls	−4 mm
E-line to Li	−2 mm
S-line to Ls	0 mm
S-line to Li	0 mm
Z-angle	80 ± 9 degrees

The two measurements above should be within 1 mm of each other. A distance between the vermilion border and tooth surface that is more than 1 mm less than the upper lip thickness is indicative of upper lip strain, which may be caused by maxillary dental protrusion. The difference reflects the strain factor and gives the clinician an indication of how far the incisors would have to be retracted before the lip would assume normal form and thickness and start responding to incisor retraction by moving posteriorly. Thin lips would respond more readily than thick lips to orthodontic tooth movements. Racial differences in facial soft tissue thickness should be taken into account.

Anteroposterior soft tissue relationships are summarized in Table 2-10.

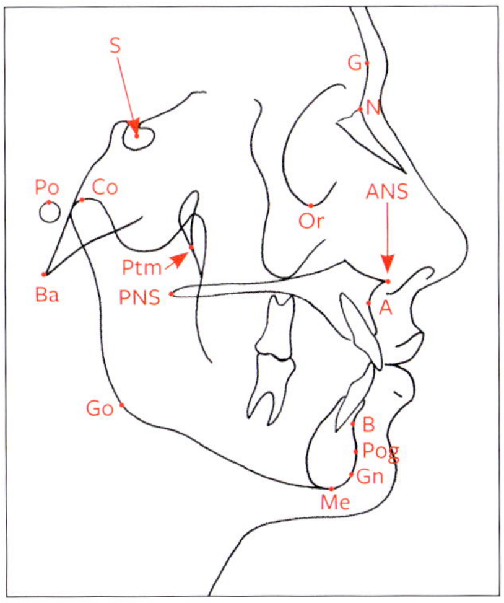

Fig 2-49 Hard tissue cephalometric landmarks.

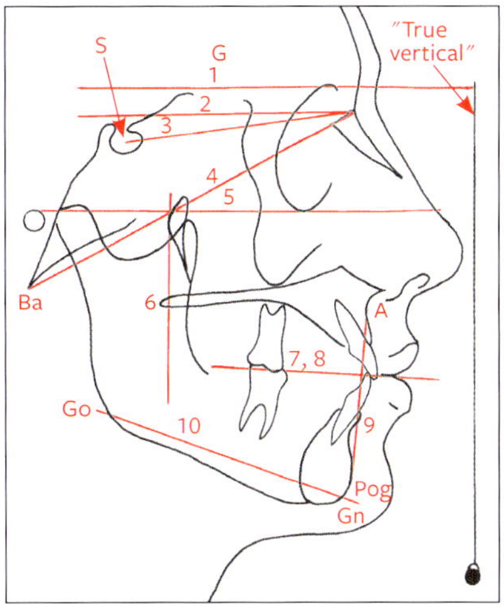

Fig 2-50 Hard tissue planes. (1) True horizontal plane (HP). (2) Constructed horizontal plane (cHP). (3) Anterior cranial base (S-N). (4) Basion-nasion (Ba-N) plane. (5) Frankfort horizontal (FH) plane. (6) Pterygoid vertical (Ptv). (7) Functional occlusal plane. (8) Occlusal plane. (9) Dental plane (A-Pog). (10) Mandibular plane (Go-Gn).

Skeletal analysis

Hard tissue landmarks

Hard tissue landmarks, shown in Fig 2-49, include the following:

- *Glabella* (*G*)*:* The most anterior point of the frontal bone
- *Nasion* (*N*)*:* The most anterior point on the frontal nasal suture in the midsagittal plane
- *Orbitale* (*Or*)*:* The lowest point on the inferior orbital rim
- *Sella* (*S*)*:* The center of the sella turcica, as on the lateral cephalogram, which is located by inspection
- *Pterygomaxillare* (*Ptm*)*:* The apex of the teardrop-shaped pterygomaxillary fissure (lowest point of the opening)
- *Basion* (*Ba*)*:* The point where the median sagittal plane of the skull intersects the lowest point in the anterior margin of the foramen magnum
- *Anterior nasal spine* (*ANS*)*:* Anterior tip of the nasal spine
- *Posterior nasal spine* (*PNS*)*:* The most posterior aspect of the palatal bone
- *A-point, or subspinale:* The most posterior midline point in the concavity where the lower anterior edge of the anterior nasal spine meets the alveolar bone overlying the maxillary incisors
- *B-point, or supramentale:* The most posterior midline point in the concavity of the mandible between the alveolar bone overlying the mandibular incisors (infradentale) and the pogonion
- *Pogonion* (*Pog*)*:* The most anterior point of the chin
- *Gonion* (*Go*)*:* The point defined by using two lines, one tangent to the inferior border of the mandible and the other tangent to the posterior border of the ramus; found by bisecting the angle formed by the two lines and extending the bisector through the curvature of the mandible
- *Gnathion* (*Gn*)*:* The lowest, most anterior midline point on the symphysis of the mandible (midway between the Me and the Pog)
- *Menton* (*Me*)*:* The most inferior point on the symphysis of the mandible in the midline
- *Porion* (*Po*)*:* The most superior point of the external auditory meatus (anatomical point); the machine porion is the uppermost point on the outline of the rods of the cephalometer
- *Condylion* (*Co*)*:* The most posterosuperior point on the head of the condyle

Hard tissue planes

Hard tissue planes, shown in Fig 2-50, include the following:

- *True horizontal plane* (*HP*)*:* A line perpendicular to a plumb line on the radiograph will be the HP for a specific patient.
- *Constructed horizontal plane* (*cHP*)*:* A horizontal plane constructed by drawing a line through N at an angle of 7 degrees to S-N (see point 2 in Fig 2-48). This plane tends to be close to true horizontal.

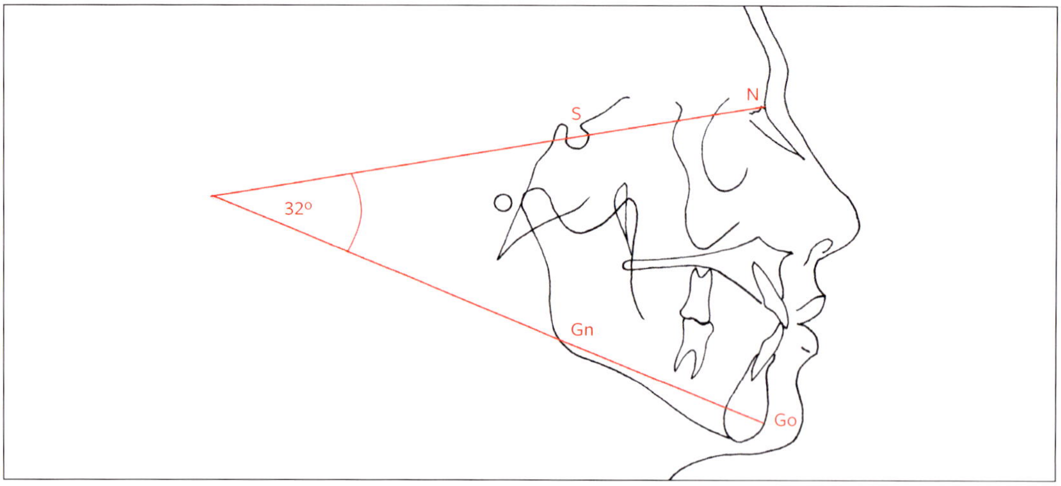

Fig 2-51 Mandibular plane angle is formed by the intersection of the mandibular plane and the anterior cranial base (S-N).

- *Anterior cranial base* (*S-N*): Formed by a line drawn from S to N.
- *Basion-nasion* (*Ba-N*) *plane*: Extends between Ba and N and divides the face and the cranium.
- *Frankfort horizontal* (*FH*) *plane*: Extends from Po to Or.
- *Pterygoid vertical* (*Ptv*): A vertical line perpendicular to the FH and drawn through the distal outline of Ptm fissure.
- *Functional occlusal plane*: A line through the cusp contacts of the molars and premolars.
- *Occlusal plane*: Formed by a line drawn through the mesial cusp contact of the molars and dividing the incisor overbite.
- *Dental plane*: Extends between A-point and Pog.
- *Mandibular plane*: Extends from Go to G.

Skeletal anteroposterior relationships

Mandibular plane angle (Steiner)

The mandibular plane is drawn between Go and Gn. The mandibular plane angle is formed between the mandibular plane and the anterior cranial base (S-N). Its mean is 32 degrees (Fig 2-51). This angle interprets the difference between anterior and posterior facial heights. Individuals with high mandibular plane angles tend to have Class II malocclusions, vertical maxillary excess, and anterior open bites. Patients with low mandibular plane angles tend to be vertically deficient and have deep bites.

SNA angle (Steiner)

The SNA angle is formed between the anterior cranial base (S-N) and a line drawn through N and A-point. Its mean is 82 degrees (Fig 2-52). The SNA angle gives an indication of the anteroposterior position of the maxilla relative to the anterior cranial base. An angle less than 82 degrees is indicative of maxillary anteroposterior deficiency, whereas an increased angle may indicate maxillary protrusion.

SNB angle (Steiner)

The SNB angle is formed between the anterior cranial base (S-N) and a line drawn through N and B-point. Its mean is 80 degrees (see Fig 2-52). The angle gives an indication of the anteroposterior position of the mandible relative to the anterior cranial base. Patients with mandibular anteroposterior excess will have an angle greater than 80 degrees. Those with mandibular deficiency will have a decreased angle.

ANB angle (Steiner)

The ANB angle is formed between A-N and N-B. Its mean is 2 degrees (see Fig 2-52). The angle provides an idea of the anteroposterior discrepancy between the maxilla and the mandible. In Class III cases, the angle is less than 2 degrees or even negative; in Class II cases, the angle is increased.

In spite of its shortcomings, Steiner analysis continues to be a popular method of evaluating the anteroposterior relationship of the maxilla and mandible. However, this analysis should not be used to make an absolute diagnosis of sagittal skeletal disharmony because vertical and rotational jaw dimensions relative to the anterior cranial base often have a significant effect on the measurements (see the next section).

Wits appraisal

Most cephalometric analyses, like Steiner analysis, relate the maxillary and mandibular anteroposterior position to the cranium. Measurements from the cranial base, however,

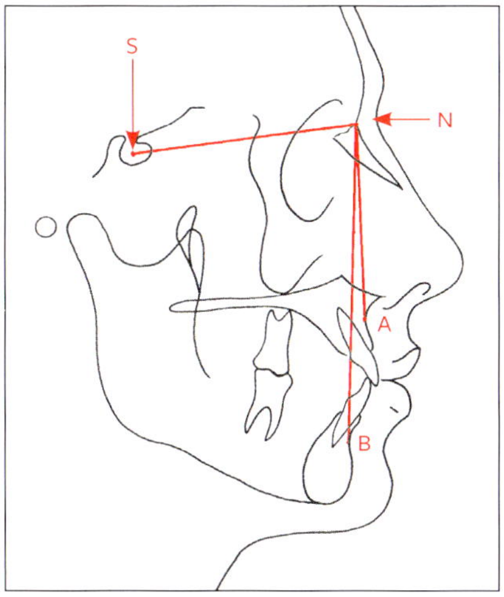

Fig 2-52 Steiner analysis for maxillary and mandibular anteroposterior positions relative to the anterior cranial base (S-N). SNA is 82 degrees. SNB is 80 degrees. The maxillomandibular relationship is indicated by the ANB angle (mean, 2 degrees).

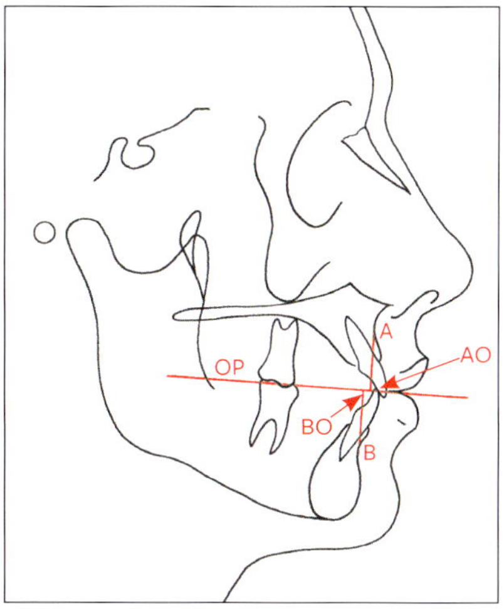

Fig 2-53 Wits appraisal. Vertical lines are drawn perpendicular to the occlusal plane (OP) from A-point and B-point. The points of contact on the OP are labeled AO and BO, respectively.

do not always provide a reliable expression of the anteroposterior relationship between the maxilla and mandible. The Wits appraisal is a linear measurement between the maxilla and mandible and is not influenced by the cranium.

Points BO and AO are established by dropping perpendicular lines from the A-point and B-point, respectively, onto the occlusal plane (Fig 2-53). The mean in males is BO 1 mm ahead of AO. In females, BO and AO coincide. The measurement between BO and AO indicates the anteroposterior discrepancy between the maxilla and the mandible. A small discrepancy may indicate that a patient can be treated orthodontically, whereas a large discrepancy may indicate that surgical correction will be required.

Clockwise or counterclockwise rotations of the maxillomandibular complex relative to the anterior cranial base do not affect the Wits appraisal measurements. However, these rotations significantly affect Steiner analysis. This is a good example of how two cephalometric analyses may render quite contradictory measurements; however, the observations assist in treatment planning. Figures 2-54a to 2-54c illustrate three cases with the same Wits measurements (0 mm) but ANB angles of +2, +8, and –2 degrees and very different facial profiles. Surgical rotation of the maxillomandibular complex may be indicated for correction in the cases depicted in Figs 2-54b and 2-54c. The case in Fig 2-54d has an ANB angle of –1 degree, indicating a mild Class III discrepancy between the jaws. The Wits appraisal for this case, however, is 8 mm, indicating a substantial jaw discrepancy; the patient could not be treated by orthodontic means alone.

Facial angle (Downs)
The facial angle is the inferior inside angle in which the facial line (N-Pog′) intersects the FH. Its mean is 82 to 95 degrees (Fig 2-55). The facial angle indicates the relative anteroposterior position of the mandible to the cranium.

Maxillary depth (McNamara)
The maxillary depth is the horizontal distance between N and A-point. It is calculated by drawing a line through N perpendicular to FH until A-point is reached (Fig 2-56). Its mean is 0 mm. A-point is expressed as a positive value anterior to the line and as a negative value posterior to the line. The maxillary depth is an indication of the anteroposterior position of the maxilla in relation to the cranium.

Anteroposterior and vertical relationships (McNamara)
The lower anterior facial height is measured from ANS to Me, and the midfacial length is measured from Co to A-point. The distance from Co to Gn constitutes the mandibular length (Fig 2-57). There should be a correlation between the lower anterior facial height (ANS-Me), the length of the midface (Co-A), and the mandibular length (Co-Gn). The correlations are listed in Table 2-11.

Maxillary-mandibular anteroposterior relationship (McNamara)
The clinician should be aware that in McNamara analysis, the effective lengths of the midface and the mandibular length are related and are expressed as *small*, *medium*, and *large*. The maxillomandibular differential is determined by

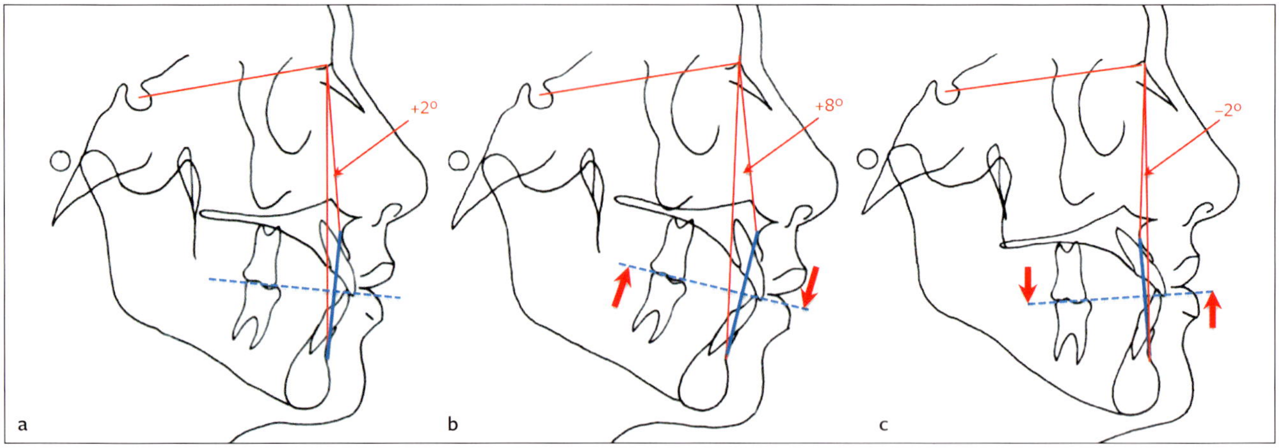

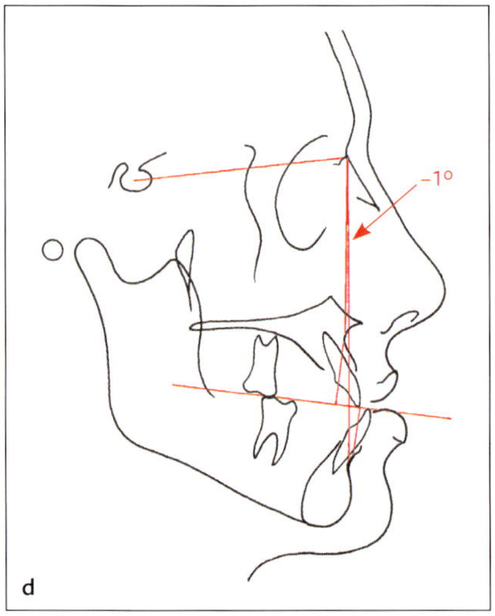

Fig 2-54 The effect of rotation of the maxillomandibular complex relative to the anterior cranial base and the ANB angle. (*a*) Normal relation: ANB angle is +2 degrees. (*b*) Counterclockwise rotation resulting in an ANB angle of +8 degrees. (*c*) Clockwise rotation with an ANB angle of −2 degrees. In all three cases, the Wits appraisal (*blue line*) indicates a normal relationship (0 mm) between the maxilla and mandible. (*d*) An ANB angle of −1 degree indicates a mild Class III jaw relationship (Steiner). According to the Wits appraisal, the discrepancy between the maxilla and mandible is severe (8 mm).

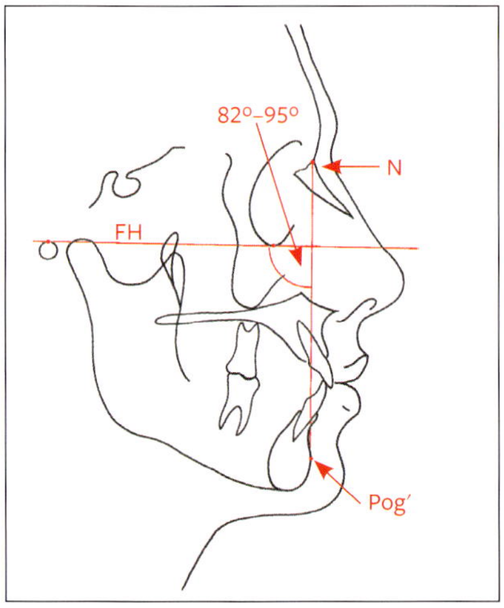

Fig 2-55 Facial angle. The mean is 82 to 95 degrees.

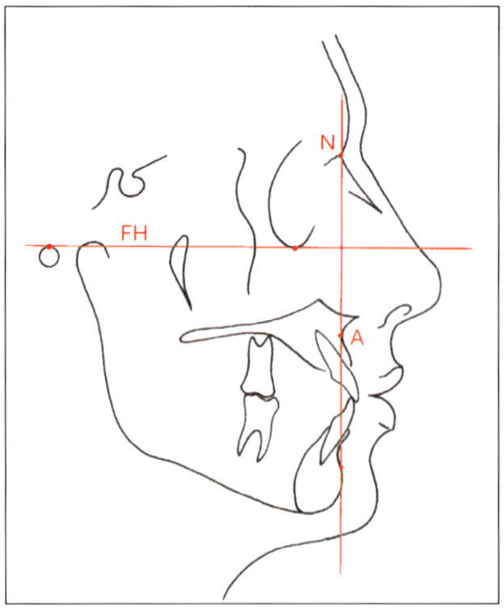

Fig 2-56 Maxillary depth. A line is drawn through N perpendicular to FH. A-point (maxillary position) is expressed as positive anterior to the line and as negative posterior to the line.

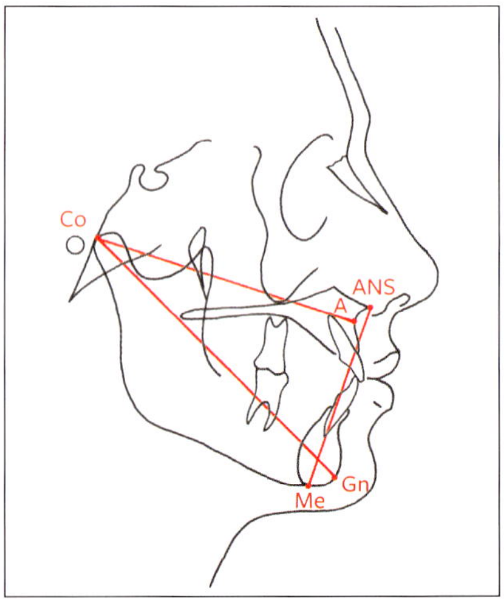

Fig 2-57 Lower anterior facial height: ANS-Me. Midfacial length: Co-A. Mandibular length: Co-Gn.

Table 2-11 | Normative standards (mm) in McNamara analysis

Midfacial length (Co-A)	Mandibular length (Co–Gn)	Lower anterior facial height (ANS–Me)
80	97–100	57–58
81	99–102	57–58
82	101–104	58–59
83	103–106	58–59
84	104–107	59–60
85	105–108	60–62
86	107–110	60–62
87	109–112	61–63
88	111–114	61–63
89	112–115	62–64
90	113–116	63–64
91	115–118	63–64
92	117–120	64–65
93	119–122	65–66
94	121–124	66–67
95	122–125	67–69
96	124–127	67–69
97	126–129	68–70
98	128–131	68–70
99	129–132	69–71
100	130–133	70–74
101	132–135	71–75
102	134–137	72–76
103	136–139	73–77
104	137–140	74–78
105	138–141	75–79

subtracting the midfacial length from the mandibular length. In small individuals (mixed dentition stage), the difference should be 20 to 23 mm. In medium-sized individuals, there should be a difference of 27 to 30 mm, and in large individuals, the difference should be 30 to 33 mm (Fig 2-58).

The graph in Fig 2-59 illustrates the relationship between midfacial length, mandibular length, and lower anterior facial height. A discrepancy greater or smaller than the normative values would indicate a disharmonious relationship between the maxilla and mandible. Alternative analysis should be used to identify which jaw is at fault. The midfacial length is measured from Co to A-point, whereas the mandibular length is measured from Co to the anatomical Gn. The linear relationship between the midfacial length and the length of the mandible is called the *ratio of effective maxillary to mandibular length*. Any specific maxillary (midfacial) length will correspond to a specific mandibular length within a given range (see Table 2-11).

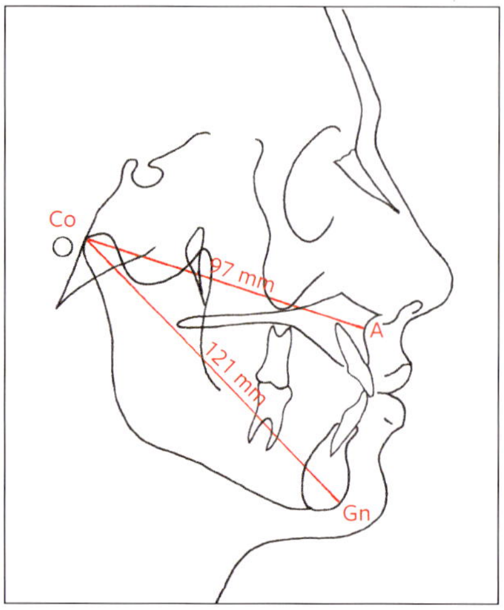

Fig 2-58 Maxillomandibular anteroposterior relationship. The maxillomandibular differential of 24 mm shown here would be ideal for a small to medium individual. The maxillomandibular ratio of 1:1.24, however, indicates a discrepancy in the relationship between the jaws. According to McNamara's normative standards (see Table 2-11), a midfacial length of 97 mm would be better related to a mandibular length of 126 to 129 mm. This may indicate a slight anteroposterior deficiency of the mandible.

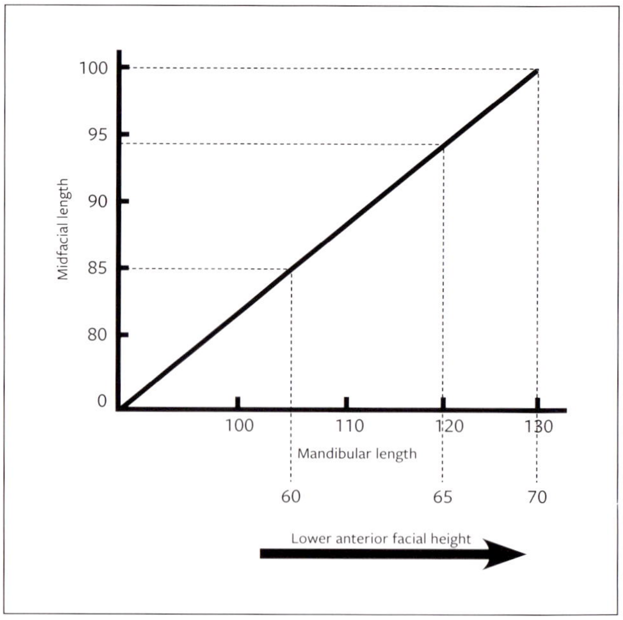

Fig 2-59 The relationship between midfacial (maxillary) length and mandibular length is generally linear and dependent on size rather than on age or sex. An individual with a maxillary length of 100 mm should have an effective mandibular length of 130 mm. The difference between the maxillary and mandibular lengths in this instance would be 30 mm. (Adapted from McNamara and Brudon, 1993, with permission).

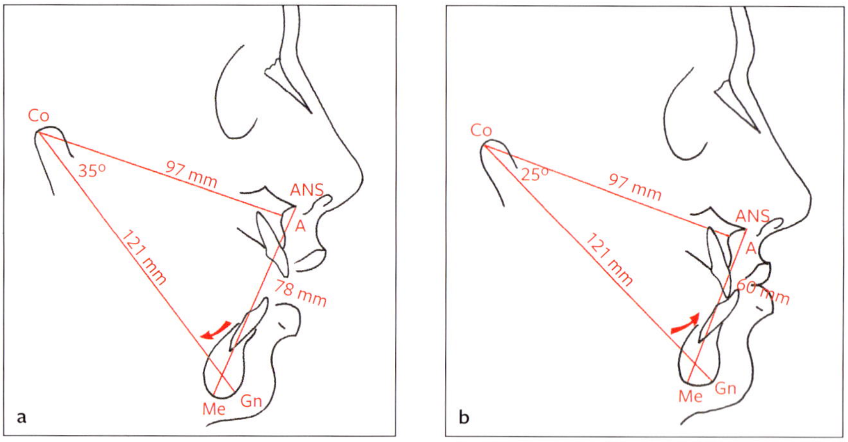

Fig 2-60 The esthetic effect of the change in lower anterior facial height and backward (*a*) and forward (*b*) rotation of the chin. In both *a* and *b*, the midfacial lengths (97 mm) and mandibular lengths (121 mm) are the same. In *a*, the lower anterior facial height (ANS-Me) is 78 mm, whereas in *b*, it is 60 mm. The angle between Co-A and Co-Gn is 35 degrees in *a* but 25 degrees in *b*.

The normal adult ratio should be maxilla (Co-A) to mandible (Co-Gn) = 1:1.3.

During normal growth, the ratio decreases from 1:1.25 for an 8-year-old child to the adult value. The effective mandibular length increases faster than the length of the maxilla, at the rate of 0.005 mm per year (ratios of 1:1.26 at 10 years of age, 1:1.27 at 12 years, 1:1.28 at 14 years, and 1:1.29 at 16 years). The clinician should be aware that a change in this value may indicate disproportionate growth, but it does not indicate which jaw is at fault.

The esthetic effect of the effective maxillary and mandibular lengths is closely related to the anterior facial height and, therefore, the angle formed between A-point, Co, and Gn. This angle normally decreases as an individual ages (Fig 2-60).

Skeletal anteroposterior relationships are summarized in Table 2-12.

Table 2-12 | **Summary of skeletal anteroposterior relationships**

	Anteroposterior relationship	Normal value
Maxilla		
	To anterior cranial base (SNA)	82 degrees
	To mandible (ANB)	2 degrees
	To mandible (Wits appraisal)	AH 1 mm behind BO (males) AO and BO coincide (females)
	Maxillary depth: A-point to N perpendicular to FH	0 mm
	To mandibular length: Co-A:Co-Gn	1:1.3
Mandible		
	Mandibular plane angle S-N to Go-Gn	32 degrees
	To anterior cranial base (SNB)	80 degrees
	To maxilla (ANB)	2 degrees
	To maxilla (Wits appraisal)	BO 1 mm ahead of AO (males) BO and AO coincide (females)
	To maxillary length: Co-Gn:Co-A	1.3:1

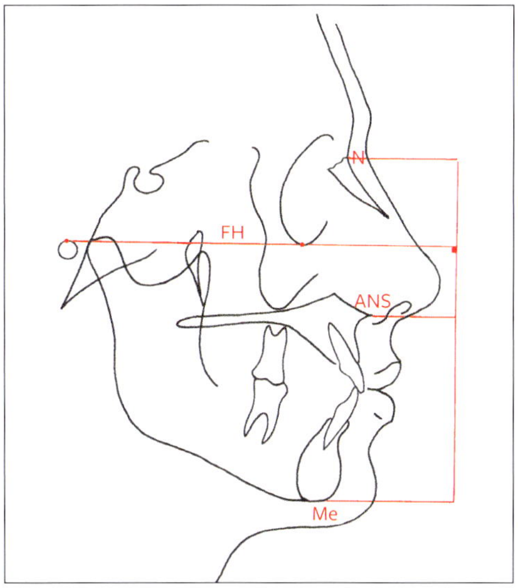

Fig 2-61 Midface and lower face skeletal heights. N-ANS:ANS-Me = 5:6.

Skeletal vertical relationships

Midface to lower face skeletal height

Skeletal vertical relationships are measured from N to ANS and from ANS to Me. A vertical line is drawn perpendicular to the FH anterior to the face. In turn, perpendicular lines are drawn to the vertical line from N, ANS, and Me, and the distance is measured from N to ANS and from ANS to Me (Fig 2-61). The normal values are 53 mm from N to ANS and 65 mm from ANS to Me. However, the relationship between the vertical heights is more important than the measurement. A ratio of 5:6 is normal. In most individuals with vertical dentofacial deformities, the lower measurement (ANS-Me) will be affected, which in turn will affect the relationship with the upper measurement (N-ANS). The ANS-Me distance will be increased in individuals with vertical maxillary excess, vertical mandibular excess, and open bites. The lower measurement (ANS-Me) will be decreased in individuals with vertical maxillary deficiency, closed bites, deep bites, and vertical mandibular deficiency.

Analysis of dental relationships

Maxillary incisor evaluation

Maxillary incisor position

Steiner analysis. According to the Steiner analysis, the relative location of the maxillary incisor is determined by relating the angulation of the incisor to the N-A line. The most anterior point of the maxillary incisors should be 4 mm ahead of N-A, with an axial inclination of 22 degrees to this line (Fig 2-62a).

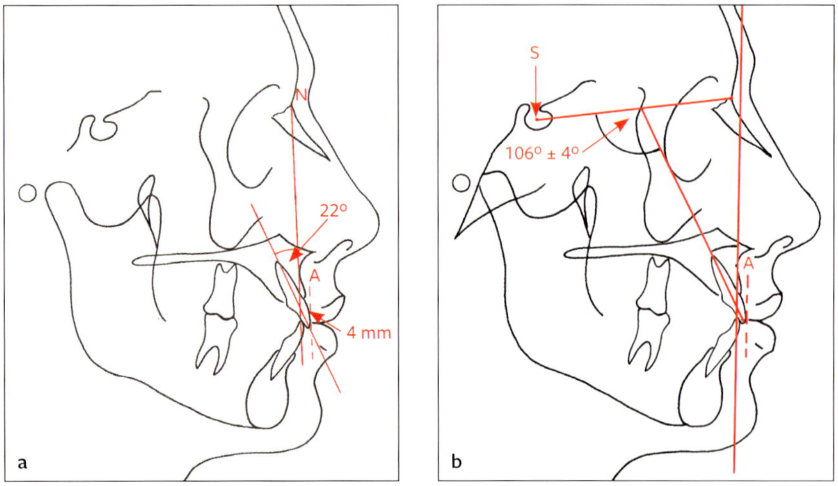

Fig 2-62 (*a*) Maxillary incisor position (Steiner): 22 degrees to N-A, 4 mm ahead of N-A. (*b*) An alternative measurement of maxillary incisor angulation. The angle between the cranial base (S-N) and maxillary incisor (apex to incisor tip) should be 106 ± 4 degrees.

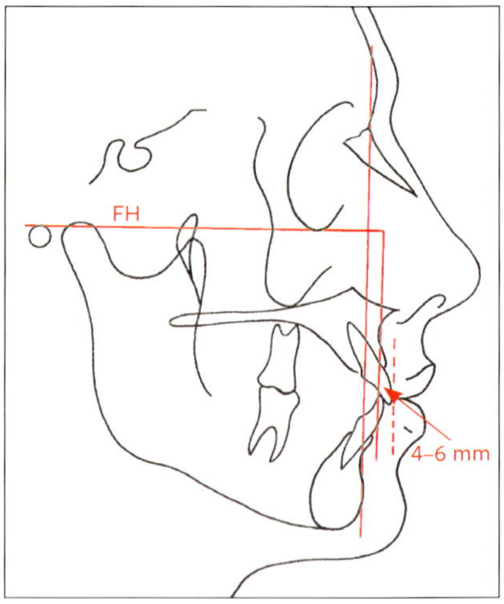

Fig 2-63 Maxillary incisor position (McNamara). The labial surface of the incisor should be 4 to 6 mm ahead of the vertical line through A-point.

The linear relationship of the incisor tip to N-A provides information on the anteroposterior position of the incisor to the maxilla, but not to the entire facial complex. In orthognathic cases, this measurement can be helpful in determining the preoperative positioning of the tooth if the relation of the maxilla to the cranial base is also considered. In individuals with dentofacial deformities, the N-A line is often not a reliable basis to assess the incisor position because of the skeletal disharmony between cranial base and maxilla. In these cases, a vertical line through A-point should be substituted for N-A (Fig 2-62b). A helpful additional measurement is the angulation between a line through the maxillary incisor (apex to incisor tip) and a line through the anterior cranial base (S-N), which should be 106 ± 4 degrees (see Fig 2-62b).

McNamara analysis. An important relationship, especially in orthognathic patients, is that of the incisors to the underlying basal bone of each jaw. In the McNamara analysis, the position of the maxillary incisors to their respective bone bases is determined by drawing a vertical line through A-point parallel to N and perpendicular to FH. The facial surface of the maxillary incisor should be 4 to 6 mm ahead of the line (Fig 2-63).

In maxillary dental protrusion cases, the incisor will be more than 6 mm ahead of the vertical line through A-point and will be an indication for orthodontic retraction. Where the maxillary incisors are upright (eg, in Class II, division 2 malocclusions), the incisor tip will be less than 4 mm ahead of this line or may be even behind it.

Mandibular incisor evaluation

Mandibular incisor position

Steiner analysis. The relative location of the mandibular incisors is determined by its relation to the N-B line (Fig 2-64). According to the Steiner analysis, the mandibular incisor angulation to the N-B line should be 25 degrees, and the most labial portion of the tooth crown should be 4 mm anterior to the line. However, the N-B line often is not reliable to assess the mandibular incisor position in patients with dentofacial deformities because of a lack of harmony between the mandible and the cranial base.

The angular and linear measurements give an indication of the relationship of the mandibular incisors to the mandible. In individuals with Class III malocclusions and compensated incisors, the angle will be smaller and the incisor tip closer to the N-B line or even behind it. Protrusive incisors would produce a larger angle, and the labial surface would be more than 4 mm ahead of N-B. These measurements can also serve as a guide in planning for extractions and preoperative orthodontic positioning of the mandibular incisors.

McNamara analysis. As in the maxilla, in the mandible, it is important to determine the relationship of the mandibular incisors to the mandibular bony base. According to the McNamara analysis, the labial surface of the mandibular incisors should be 4 mm ahead of a true vertical line drawn through the B-point and at an angle of 25 degrees to the line (Fig 2-65a).

An increase in this measurement indicates mandibular dental protrusion. In some racial groups, this measure-

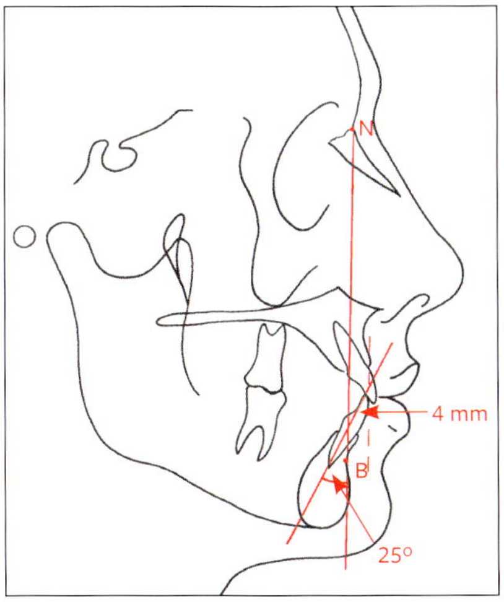

Fig 2-64 Mandibular incisor position (Steiner): 25 degrees to N-B line, and 4 mm ahead of N-B.

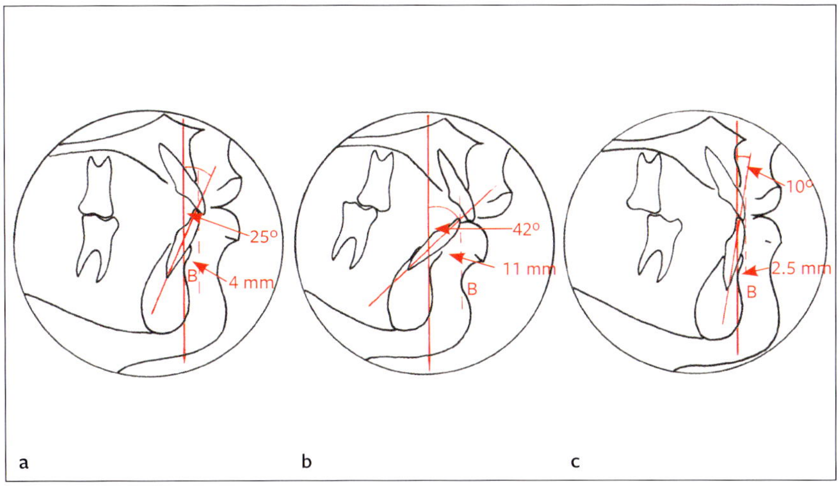

Fig 2-65 (*a*) Class I occlusion; incisor to vertical line through B-point: 4 mm and 25 degrees. (*b*) Class II malocclusion with mandibular incisor protrusion; incisor to vertical line through B-point: 11 mm and 42 degrees. (*c*) Class III malocclusion with compensated mandibular incisors; incisor to vertical line through B-point: 2.5 mm and 10 degrees.

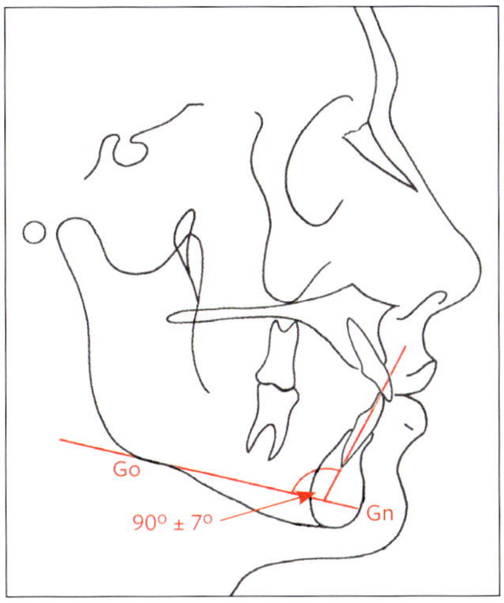

Fig 2-66 Mandibular incisor position (Downs). The axial inclination of the mandibular incisor to the mandibular plane (Go-Gn) is 90 ± 7 degrees.

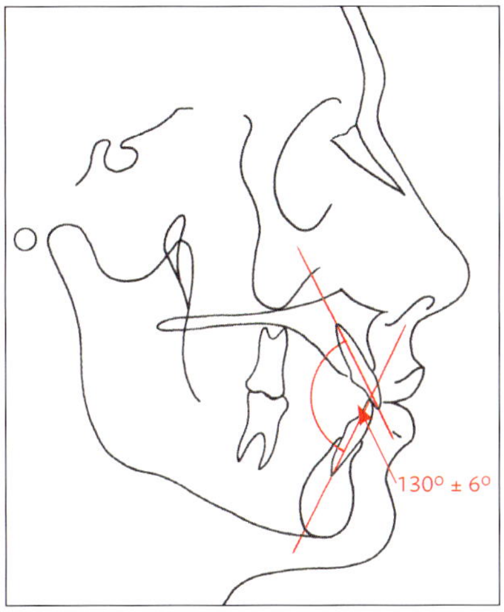

Fig 2-67 Interincisal angle.

ment may be normal, but in Caucasians, it is often seen in Class II malocclusion with mandibular skeletal deficiency (Fig 2-65b). In Class III dental and skeletal relationships, the mandibular incisors are often compensated and are closer to this line or even behind it (Fig 2-65c).

Downs analysis. According to the Downs analysis, the ideal inclination of the long axis of the mandibular incisors to the mandibular plane is 90 ± 7 degrees (Fig 2-66). In individuals with Class III malocclusion and compensated mandibular incisors, this angle tends to be small. It tends to be larger when the lower incisors are protrusive (eg, in bimaxillary protrusion or Class II, division 1 malocclusion).

Interincisal angle (Downs)

The interincisal angle is formed by a line through the incisal edge and the apex of the root of the maxillary and mandibular central incisors (130 ± 6 degrees; Fig 2-67). The more protrusive the incisors, the smaller the angle. Low angles indicate protrusion of the incisors and are often associated with Class II, division 1 malocclusions. High angles are frequently associated with Class II, division 2 deep bites.

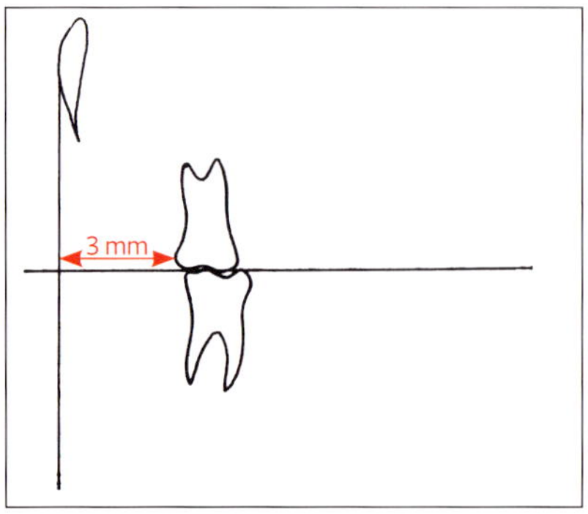

Fig 2-68 Maxillary molar position. The distance from Ptv to the first molar should be the patient's age + 3 mm.

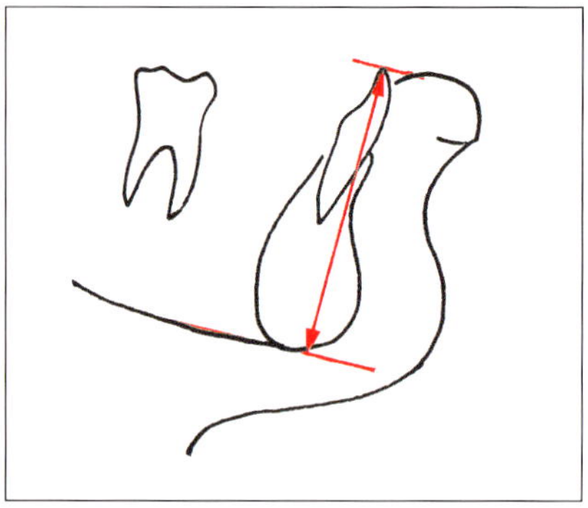

Fig 2-69 Mandibular anterior dental height: 44 ± 2 mm for male patients and 40 ± 2 mm for female patients.

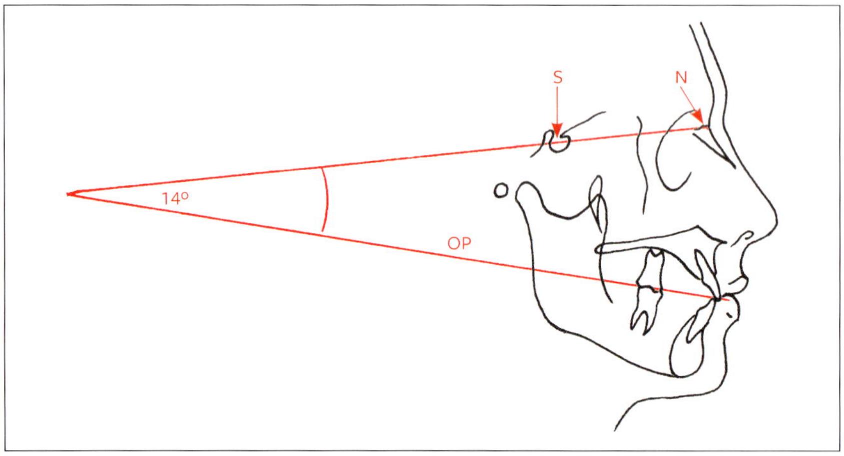

Fig 2-70 Occlusal plane angle. Angle between OP and anterior cranial base (S-N).

Maxillary molar to pterygoid vertical (Ricketts)

The distance from the pterygoid vertical (back of the maxilla) to the distal surface of the maxillary first molar (Fig 2-68) should be equal to the patient's age + 3 mm. The distance will increase as the maxilla grows forward. For example, a 12-year-old child has a normal distance of 15 mm; an 18 year-old adult, 21 mm. It stabilizes at 24 mm in the adult, around age 21. This measurement helps determine whether a malocclusion is due to the maxillary or mandibular molar position. It is also useful in deciding whether extractions or headgear may be indicated and is indicative of the anteroposterior position of the maxilla. A small value indicates that the molar is too far distal, and thus headgear and distalization should be avoided; large values indicate the opposite. This measurement is influenced by previous maxillary tooth extractions allowing mesial drifting of the molar.

Mandibular anterior dental height

The mandibular anterior dental height is measured from the mandibular incisor tip to the inferior border of the mandible. The average mandibular dental height is 44 ± 2 mm for males and 40 ± 2 mm for females (Fig 2-69). An increase in the mandibular vertical height of the face of a patient with normal upper lip length and normal maxillary incisor exposure may be caused by the anterior vertical height of the mandible. In this patient, vertical reduction genioplasty may be indicated.

Occlusal plane angle

According to the Steiner analysis, the occlusal plane angle is formed between a line drawn through the region of the overlapping cusps of the first premolar and first molar bisecting the incisal overbite (the occlusal plane [OP]) and the anterior cranial base (S-N). The mean angle is 14 degrees (Fig 2-70). According to the Downs analysis, the angle is measured between the occlusal plane and the FH plane and should be 9 degrees.

Table 2-13 | Summary of dental relationships

	Dental relstionship	Normal value
Maxillary incisor	Angle to N-A Distance to N-A Distance to A-point vertical	22 degrees 4 mm ahead 4 to 6 mm ahead
Mandibular incisor	Angle to N-B Distance to N-B Distance to B-point vertical Angle to mandibular plane	25 degrees 4 mm ahead 4 mm ahead 90 ± 7 degrees
Interincisal angle	Maxillary to mandibular incisor	130 ± 6 degrees
Maxillary first molar	Molar to Ptv	Patient's age + 3 mm in growing individuals
Mandibular anterior dental height	Incisor tip to mandibular border	44 + 2 mm (males) 40 + 2 mm (females)
Occlusal plane angle	Occlusal plane to S-N Occlusal plane to FH	14 degrees 9 degrees

The occlusal, palatal, and mandibular plane angles are often used in describing an individual as "high angle" or "low angle." High-angle individuals tend to have relatively long anterior facial heights, whereas low-angle individuals tend to have vertically short anterior facial heights.

The numeric values of tooth positions given in Table 2-13 should be considered a guide to diagnosing abnormal tooth positions and to determining final dental, skeletal, and soft tissue positions. The clinician must subjectively evaluate the positioning of the teeth to determine whether they are positioned in the central trough of bone.

Posteroanterior Cephalometric Radiographic Evaluation

In addition to lateral cephalometric radiography, individuals with facial asymmetry require posteroanterior radiographic evaluation of the facial bones. It would certainly be advantageous to obtain a CBCT image or multislice CT to facilitate virtual treatment planning (Fig 2-71). CBCT allows images to be obtained with the patient in a standing or seated position with the teeth in the preferred occlusion and the soft tissue in repose. As always, accurate image acquisition also applies here. Multislice CT scanning is performed with the patient in supine position, which will inherently falsify the 3D facial soft tissue mask of the patient, and gravity may distort the facial soft tissue in this position and interfere with the accuracy of the image. Also, careful attention should be paid to the wax-bite or registration device so the lip position or morphology will not be disturbed when taking a CT scan. (See "Virtual Surgical Planning" in chapter 3.)

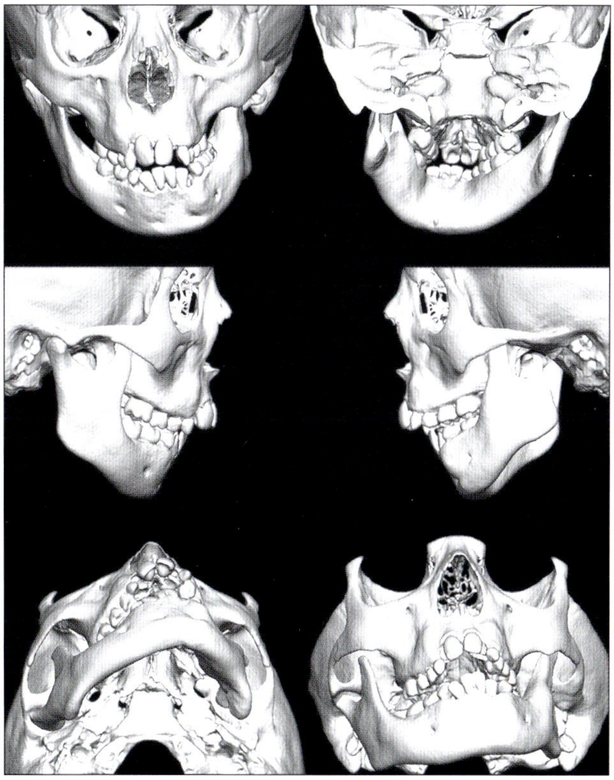

Fig 2-71 The 3D CT scanned image of a patient with hemifacial microsomia. The skeletal asymmetry and agenesis of the left mandibular ramus and condyle is clearly demonstrated and allows for accurate virtual treatment planning.

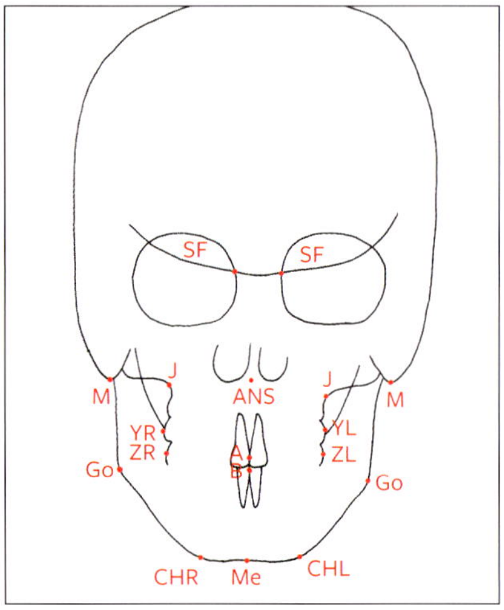

Fig 2-72 Posteroanterior hard tissue cephalometric landmarks.

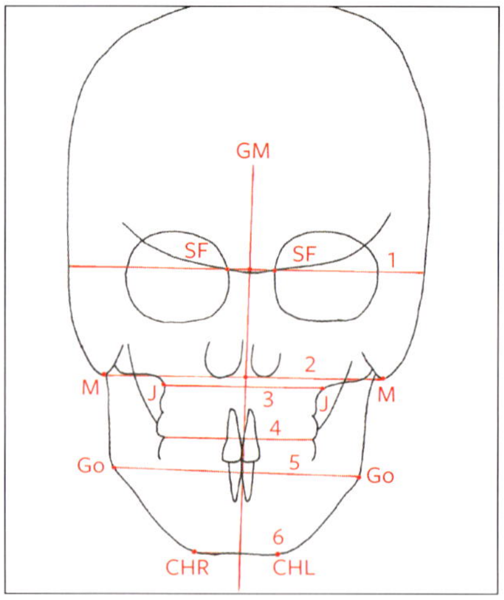

Fig 2-73 Transverse posteroanterior and vertical planes. (1) Cranial base plane. (2) Mastoid plane. (3) J-plane. (4) Occlusal plane. (5) S-plane. (6) Chin plane.

Hard tissue cephalometric landmarks

Posteroanterior hard tissue landmarks, shown in Fig 2-72, include the following:

- *Spheno-frontal (SF) point:* Where the smaller wing of the sphenoid bone crosses the medial orbital ridge
- *ANS:* The center point at the base of the nose
- *Jugulare (J):* The most superior and medial point on the zygomatic buttress
- *Mastoid (M):* The most inferior point on the mastoid bone
- *A:* The contact area between the maxillary incisors. Note: This is distinct from A-point.
- *B:* The contact area between the mandibular incisors. Note: This is distinct from B-point.
- *Y:* The most lateral point on the buccal surface area of the first maxillary molar (YL on the left and YR on the right)
- *Z:* The most lateral point on the buccal surface area of the first mandibular molar (ZL on the left and ZR on the right)
- *Go:* The most inferior posterior point at the angle of the mandible
- *Me:* The most inferior point at the anterior mandibular area
- *CH:* The most inferior lateral point on the anterior inferior border of the mandible (CHL on the left and CHR on the right)

Transverse posteroanterior cephalometric planes

Transverse posteroanterior cephalometric planes, shown in Fig 2-73, include the following:

- *Cranial base plane (C-plane):* A horizontal line connecting the left and right SF points and extending laterally to the cranium
- *Mastoid plane (D-plane):* A line connecting the left and right mastoid points
- *S-plane:* The connecting line between the left and right Go of the mandible
- *J-plane:* A line drawn from the left J-point to the right J-point, which is divided into two halves (IR and IL) by the geometrically constructed vertical axis (GM)
- *Occlusal plane:* A plane formed by a line connecting the occluding points of the maxillary and mandibular buccal cusps left and right
- *Chin plane (CHP):* A line drawn on the inferior border of the chin at maximum bone contact, through Me

Vertical posteroanterior cephalometric line

The vertical cephalometric line is called the *geometrically constructed vertical axis* (GM; see Fig 2-73). It is constructed by dividing the C-plane and the D-plane, connecting these two midpoints, and extending this line to the chin.

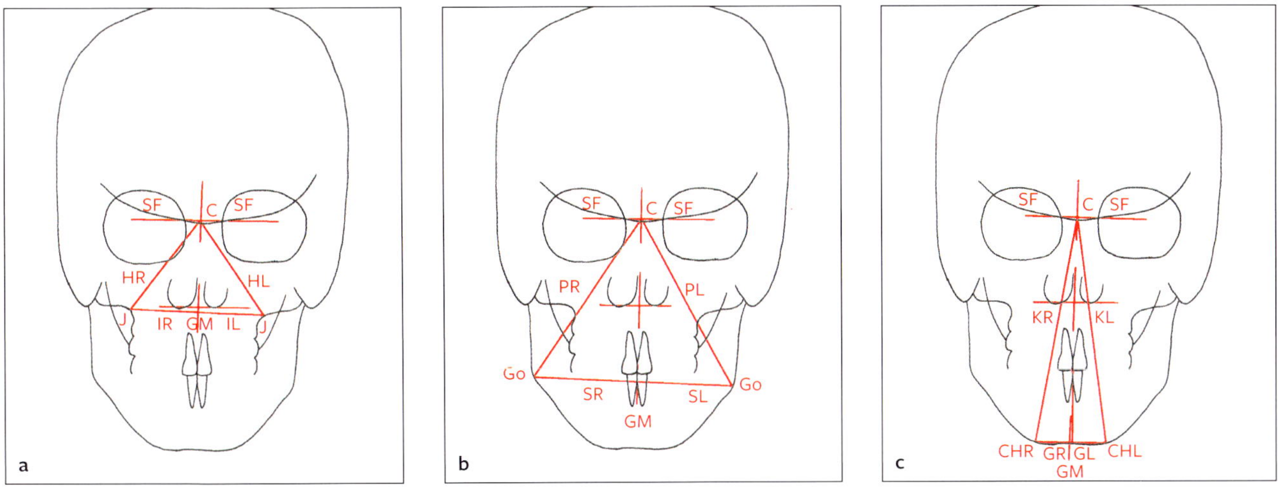

Fig 2-74 (*a*) Maxillary triangle. (*b*) Mandibular triangle. (*c*) Chin triangle and vertical line through B-point perpendicular to CHP.

Triangular analysis

Triangles are constructed for evaluation of the symmetry of the maxilla, mandible, and chin. The maxillary triangle is constructed by connecting the midpoint of the C-plane (C-point) with points J on either side of the GM. These connecting lines are called the *HR line* and the *HL line*. The base of the triangle is divided in two halves, IR and IL, by GM (Fig 2-74a).

The mandibular triangle is constructed by connecting C-point with Go bilaterally using lines PR and PL. The base of the mandibular triangle is halved into SR and SL by GM (Fig 2-74b).

The chin triangle is constructed by connecting the C-point with CHR and CHL; the long legs of the triangle are called *KR* and *KL*. A line is drawn from B-point perpendicular to CHP to evaluate the mandibular incisor midline in relation to the midline of the chin. The base of this triangle is divided into two halves, GR and GL, by GM (Fig 2-74c).

By measuring the long legs of the triangles, cants in the maxilla, mandible, and chin can be evaluated in relation to the cranial base, as well as to each other. By comparing the left and right sides of the bases of the triangles, transverse discrepancies on rotations can be assessed. Midline asymmetries of the nasal spine, Me, and dental midlines can be evaluated. Any discrepancy between the mandibular dental midline and the midpoint of the chin can be evaluated by the vertical line perpendicular to CHP (see Fig 2-74c).

Vertical and transverse dentoalveolar assessment

The vertical relationship between the basal bones and the dental and alveolar structures is evaluated by dropping perpendicular lines from the J-plane at YR and YL to the occlusal plane and from the S-plane to the occlusal plane at ZR and ZL. Transverse discrepancies are assessed by measuring the distances both from YR and YL and from ZR and ZL to the GM line. Vertical discrepancies are assessed by measuring the vertical heights from the J-plane to the occlusal plane, comparing left and right side heights. Mandibular dentoalveolar vertical discrepancies can be examined by measuring the vertical heights from the occlusal plane to the S-plane at ZR and ZL (Fig 2-75).

The posteroanterior cephalometric analysis is helpful in assessing facial asymmetry. Also, in combination with the lateral cephalometric analysis, it gives the clinician a better dimensional understanding of dentofacial deformities. The lateral and posteroanterior cephalometric analyses of an individual with severe facial asymmetry involving the maxilla, mandible, and chin are demonstrated in Fig 2-76.

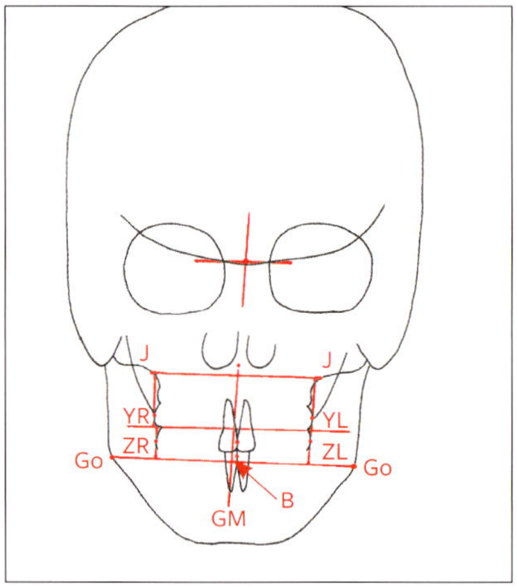

Fig 2-75 Vertical dentoalveolar assessment.

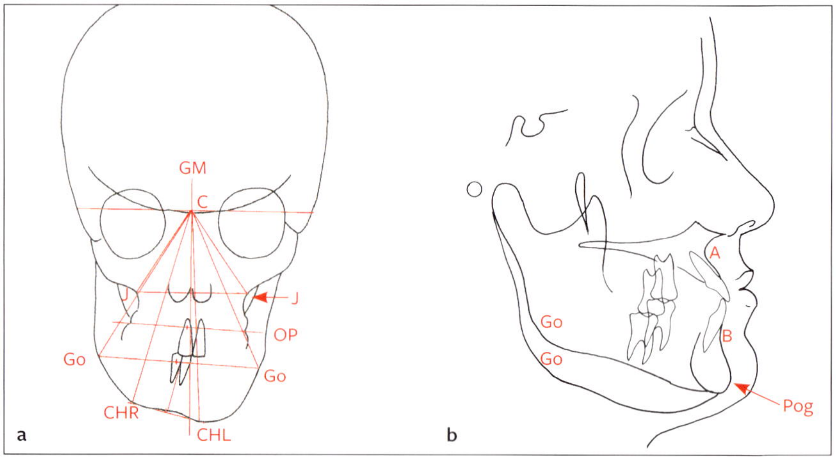

Fig 2-76 (*a*) Severe facial asymmetry. Note the severe rotation of the triangles. (*b*) The severe asymmetry is also evident on the lateral cephalometric tracing. The 3D nature of the facial asymmetry, a common finding in such cases, is well demonstrated.

Limitations of Cephalometric Analysis

Although cephalometric analysis is important in both diagnosis and development of a treatment plan, it has the following limitations:

- Most individuals with dentofacial deformities have anatomical variations in the location of the cephalometric landmarks used as a baseline in many analyses, such as S, N, and Or. These anatomical variations often lead to incorrect conclusions from the analysis.
- The clinician must not base interpretations on single cephalometric measurements.
- The clinician must recognize the limitations as well as the advantages of cephalometry and be sure to integrate measurements with clinical findings.
- The art of cephalometric interpretation lies in understanding abnormal findings and identifying the etiologic factors behind these cephalometric abnormalities in patients with dentoskeletal deformities.
- Although cephalometric analysis forms an important part of the database for diagnosis and treatment planning, it should not take precedence over the clinical evaluation of the patient.

Full-Mouth Periapical Radiographic Evaluation

If a patient has any indication of periapical or periodontal pathology and/or dental caries, periapical radiographs should be taken to obtain a more detailed understanding of the pathologic condition. Periapical radiography can also more accurately assess the deviation of roots in areas of intended interdental osteotomies.

Panoramic Radiographic Evaluation

Panoramic radiography is an excellent means to establish an overview of the paranasal sinuses, bony temporomandibular joint (TMJ), periapical and periodontal pathology, dental caries, position of the inferior alveolar canal, position of the lingula, position of the mental foramen, tooth root lengths in relation to the maxillary sinus, and mandibular symphysis. Any suggestion of temporomandibular pathology should be further investigated by more specific radiographic examination. In addition, the panoramic radiograph can detect root deviations in areas of intended interdental osteotomies (although not as accurately as can a periapical radiograph), unerupted and/or impacted teeth, and previously undetected pathologic conditions. The information obtained is valuable not only in the pretreatment assessment but also in the determination of the relative position of anatomical structures, which is important

Panoramic Radiographic Evaluation		
Absent teeth		
Unerupted teeth		
Impacted teeth		
Dental caries		
Periodontal pathology		
Maxillary sinus pathology	Left:	Right:
Tempormandibular joint pathology	Left:	Right:
Bone pathology	Maxilla:	Mandble:

Fig 2-77 Panoramic radiographic evaluation form. This evaluation should be used during the pretreatment assessment, at the presurgical examination, and at the time of surgery.

during the actual surgical procedure. Figure 2-77 shows a panoramic radiographic evaluation form. It is essential that an immediate preoperative panoramic radiograph is available at the time of surgery because it gives the surgeon a valuable overview of anatomical structures relevant in most orthognathic surgical procedures (eg, position of the inferior alveolar canal, mental foramen, tooth roots, impacted third molars [if present], and maxillary sinuses).

Occlusion and Study Cast Evaluation

Occlusal functional evaluation

The basic aims of occlusal functional evaluation are to determine the compatibility of centric occlusion (CO) and centric relation (CR); to note the difference between CO and CR, if present; to note any bite of convenience or occlusal slide; and to note interocclusal rest space. Figure 2-78 is a sample functional evaluation form.

Study cast analysis

Intra-arch relationship

In the study cast analysis, arch form and symmetry, missing teeth, tooth rotations, and overerupted teeth are noted. Maxillary and mandibular occlusal curves are studied. Crowding and the need for extractions are determined. Bolton discrepancies of tooth sizes are studied. Any tooth size discrepancies should be noted and compensated for during the preoperative orthodontic treatment stage. Tooth size discrepancy influences arch compatibility and leads to poor occlusal fit at surgery.

Interarch relationship

The study cast analysis also includes examination for incisor overjet and overbite, as well as Angle classification for molars and canines. The clinician evaluates coordination of dental midlines and crossbites while moving the dental casts into a Class I malocclusion to get an idea of general arch compatibility.

If the possibility of establishing an acceptable occlusion, accommodating the teeth, or providing for tooth size discrepancies is at all questionable, a Kesling diagnostic setup should be used. This setup also can be used to test for various extraction patterns.

If a crossbite exists with the teeth in CO and it is corrected when the dental casts are moved into a Class I occlusion, the crossbite is considered relative. If the crossbite still exists after the dental casts have been positioned in a Class I relationship, the crossbite is considered absolute (see chapter 5, Fig 5-38).

A sample form for study cast analysis is presented in Fig 2-79.

Functional Evaluation	
Difference between centric occlusion and centric relation	
Premature contact	
Occlusal slide	
Freeway space	
Tooth attrition	
Bite of convenience	

Fig 2-78 Functional evaluation form.

Study Cast Analysis Evaluation			
Intra-arch evaluation:			
Arch form: Maxilla			
Mandible			
Missing teeth			
Impacted/unerupted teeth			
Occlusal plane cant			
Occlusal curve			
Crowding: Maxillary arch	mm:		
Mandiblular arch	mm:		
Tooth rotations			
Overeruption of teeth			
Interarch relations:			
Molar	Left:	Right:	
Canine	Left:	Right:	
Overjet	mm:		
Open bite	mm:		
Maxillary-to-mandibular dental midline	mm:		
Crossbite	Absolute:	Left:	
	Relative:	Right:	
Location of crossbite			
Tooth size discrepancy			

Fig 2-79 Study cast analysis form.

Temporomandibular Joint Evaluation		
Maximal mouth opening	mm:	
Deviation on mouth opening	Left:	Right:
Maximal protrusion	mm:	
Deviation on protrusion	Left:	Right:
Temporomandibular joint signs:		
Clicking/popping	Left:	Early(< 10 mm) Late (> 10 mm)
	Right:	Early (< 10 mm) Late (> 10 mm)
Pain	Left:	Joint: Muscles(s):
	Right:	Joint: Muscle(s):
Crepitations	Left:	Right:
Previous treatment		

Fig 2-80 TMJ evaluation form.

TMJ Evaluation

The TMJ is an important component of the orthognathic mechanism and should be examined with care. Pathologic conditions may be present in the joint at the outset, may develop during treatment, or may even develop long after treatment. Therefore, the clinician should diagnostically and prognostically evaluate the joint before orthodontic-surgical treatment begins. A basic TMJ examination evaluates three areas: (1) mandibular movements, (2) TMJ signs and symptoms, and (3) mouth opening and deviations.

Careful documentation of TMJ pretreatment status is very important (Fig 2-80). The correct positioning of the condyle in the fossa is a critical aspect of the orthognathic surgical procedure, and information gathered at the pretreatment evaluation may be useful during surgery. The patient should also understand that correction of the dentofacial deformity and malocclusion will not necessarily correct a TMJ problem. Some clinicians believe it to be advantageous to perform TMJ surgery and orthognathic surgery simultaneously.

According to an evidence-based systematic review of temporomandibular dysfunction, Rinchuse and McMinn came to the following conclusions:

- There is evidence-based support for the use of occlusal splints and biofeedback to treat temporomandibular joint disorders (TMDs).
- There is no evidence supporting the treatment of TMDs by occlusal adjustments in orthodontic patients.
- Occlusion, which was once considered to be the primary and sole cause of TMDs, now is only recognized as having a secondary role in causing it (if any role at all).
- Orthodontic treatment to improve the occlusion does not cause TMDs.

Several clinicians studied the effect of orthognathic surgery on patients with signs and symptoms of TMDs.

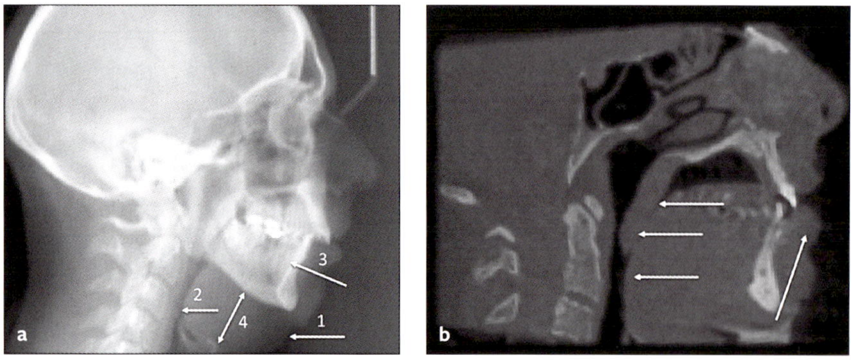

Fig 2-81 (*a*) Note short chin-throat length (1), narrow oropharyngeal airway (2), and mandibular retrusion (3) and large distance from hyoid cartilage to mandible (4) in a patient with an obstructed airway. (*b*) CBCT scan shows significant narrowing at the base of the tongue in the naso and oropharynx region (*arrows*). The patient's head is up here, but a head-down position results in near complete obstruction.

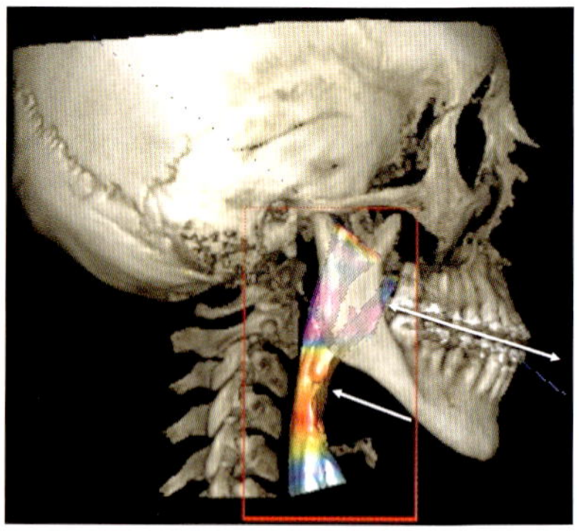

Fig 2-82 Patients with a high mandibular plane and Class III malocclusion often have good chin projection but narrowed airways (*arrow*). Linear movements can exacerbate airway problems, especially with the mandible moving backward along a steep occlusal plane.

When comparing and contrasting their findings, some observations can be made (Onizawa et al 1995, Panula et al 2000, Dervis et al):

- Patients scheduled for orthognathic surgery did not have significantly different TMD signs and symptoms than patients in the control group.
- TMD signs and symptoms frequently improved in patients following orthognathic surgery.
- Not all TMD patients improved following orthognathic surgery. For some patients, the signs and symptoms got worse.
- Masticatory muscle and joint tenderness frequently improved following orthognathic surgery.
- In most patients, the maximum mouth opening decreased following orthognathic surgery; however, this was clinically insignificant.

Airway Considerations in Orthognathic Surgery

It has been estimated that anywhere between 9% to 24% of men and 4% to 9% of women between the ages of 30 to 60 years are affected by obstructive sleep apnea (OSA). It is further estimated that 80% to 90% of those affected remain undiagnosed. Though, historically, cephalometric evaluations and clinical evaluations have been relied on in treatment planning for corrective jaw surgery with an end result of dental stability, skeletal stability, and a pleasing esthetic outcome, the impact on the airway must now be factored in for all treatment plans. Orthognathic surgery can either dramatically improve the airway or potentially compromise it.

Features of patients with compromised airways include those with maxillary and/or bimaxillary retrusion, lower facial height, large tongue, elongated soft palate, inferior hyoid position, and those who tend to have a head-up posture in an effort to dilate the airway in addition to one of these other symptoms (Fig 2-81).

Individuals with high mandibular plane angles in addition to steep occlusal planes are often accompanied by a skeletal Class II pattern. However, it is possible to have a skeletal Class III high-angle skeletal structure with a short chin-throat dimension that may also present with a narrow oropharyngeal airway dimension (Fig 2-82). Lateral cephalometric analysis has been the most widely reported in the literature for evaluating the posterior airway space (PAS); however, an intraoperative fiber-optic pharyngoscopy can be used as well. With the prevalence of CBCT scanning, volumetric area measurements are possible, and these can also be correlated with compromised airways.

Landmarks and measurements

Cephalometric airway analysis reveals that the soft palate anteroposterior (AP) dimension in a normal individual is approximately 10.0 mm. A retrognathic patient will have 7.4 mm of PAS, and a prognathic patient will typically have 12.5 mm or more. The dimensions of the tongue base are

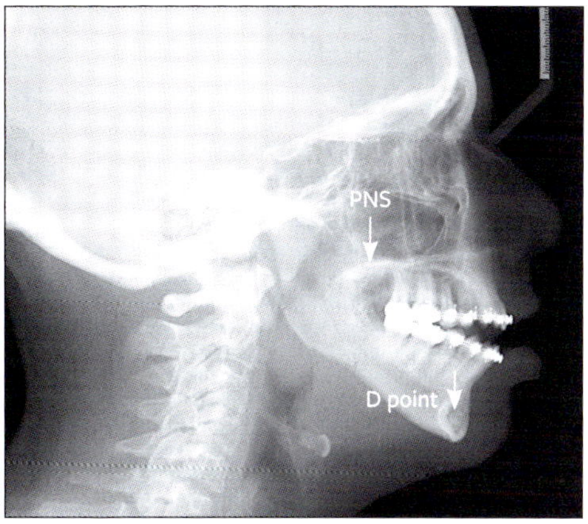

Fig 2-83 Important anatomical landmarks when treatment planning include the PNS and D-point, which corresponds to the approximate position the genioglossal tubercles though centered in the symphysis (*arrows*). Movement of PNS downward and D-point upward and forward have positive effects on airway volume.

11.0 mm, 8.3 mm, and 12.8 mm, respectively, for normal, retrognathic, and prognathic patients. Early studies indicate that a PAS less than 11.0 mm and a mandibular plane to hyoid distance of greater than 15.4 mm was associated with OSA. Those with a posterior airway space of less than 5.0 mm and a hyoid distance of greater than 24.0 mm tended to demonstrate the worst respiratory deficiencies. Recent studies disputed this and indicated that no one skeletal or soft tissue parameter can be directly linked to OSA; however, it is important that one pay close attention to airway dimensions so that treatment planning can be used to achieve positive effects on the airway, if warranted, or to at least minimize the effects of surgical movements.

Important cephalometric landmarks to be mindful of are the potential changes in the vertical and AP positions of the PNS and D-point (Fig 2-83). Recent studies have demonstrated that significant airway volume changes occurred when PNS moved vertically and D-point (which essentially corresponds to the genial tubercles) moved in a horizontal or an upward vertical direction. The data further indicated that there was an increase or decrease of 2% of the total airway volume for every millimeter of directional change in these points. Furthermore, certain vertical and horizontal movements tend to impact various areas of the airway differently. When PNS was moved inferiorly, the oropharynx tended to have a smaller total volume; however, the nasopharynx enlarged. If PNS moved superiorly, then airway volume increased, but it was at the expense of the nasopharyngeal airway; when the airway lengthened, the nasopharyngeal airway narrowed as a result. With this in mind, one needs to be cautious with maxillary movements that result in the PNS moving upward. These should be offset with advancement of both jaws to promote airway increases as well as increases in the minimal cross-sectional area. Simple autorotation of the mandible after a posterior impaction of the maxilla is not nearly as predictable relative to its impact on improving the airway as is a mandibular advancement in the correction of the skeletal Class II malocclusion. Therefore, it may be strongly considered that both jaws be surgically corrected in patients with airway issues.

Vertical movements of the genial tubercles, or D-point, significantly affect the oropharyngeal airway in total airway volume, largely due to the positional changes of the suprahyoid musculature. It appears, however, that more sagittal movements of D-point have the greatest impact on Class II patients, and vertical movements have the greatest impact on Class III patients. With these changes in mind, it is important that the surgeon's treatment plan take into consideration the skeletal geometry of their movements and how they will affect the airway. According to Steiner, a mandibular plane angle of 32 degrees (SN-mandibular plane; see Fig 2-51) is considered normal. As an example, a high angle (> 40 degrees) Class II malocclusion is best treated from an airway standpoint, with a counterclockwise rotation of the maxillomandibular complex, because this results in all of the favorable skeletal movements that have been shown to increase airway volume and minimal cross-sectional area, namely movement of PNS downward and D-point forward and upward (Fig 2-84).

Class II patients

Some amount of maxillary advancement is often incorporated. Two-jaw surgery in Class II patients has a predictable improvement in the airway when the mandible is advanced. This improvement is even more pronounced when both jaws come forward or are rotated in a counterclockwise direction. (Chapter 3 discusses these treatment planning concepts in more detail.) In patients with Class II skeletal deformities, orthognathic surgery is used both to give the patient a better esthetic appearance and to alleviate airway concerns from a retrognathic mandible. Hernández-Alfaro et al (2011) performed a study on this topic. A retrospective evaluation of 30 patients who underwent maxillomandibular advancement, maxillary advancement, or mandibular advancement was performed. Three groups of 10 subjects each were established: group 1, bimaxillary surgery (Le Fort I maxillary osteotomy and mandibular bilateral sagittal split osteotomy with maxillomandibular advancement); group 2, maxillary advancement (Le Fort I maxillary osteotomy); and group 3, mandibular advancement (bilateral sagittal split osteotomy). Pre- and postoperative CBCT scans were taken in each case, and the changes in pharyngeal airway volume were compared.

A statistically significant increase in the pharyngeal airway volume occurred systematically. The average percentage of increase was 69.8% in group 1 and 78.3% in group 3. Group 2 exhibited a lower magnitude of increase (37.7%).

Class III patients

Class III patients are far more complicated because the skeletal deformity may have a mixed nature. In addition, the situation might include isolated maxillary hypoplasia, isolated mandibular hypoplasia, or a combination of maxillary hypoplasia and mandibular hyperplasia. The goal of a recent study by Rosário et al (2016) was to investigate whether advancement of the maxilla alone would affect the volume of the upper airway. CBCT scans were taken before and after surgery in 14 patients with a Class III skeletal deformity undergoing maxillary advancement exclusively. The effects of the procedure led to a mean increase in volume of 3.22 cm^3. Patient age and sex were not factors in the results.

As one might expect, mandibular setback surgery demonstrates a decrease in airway volume. In a study by Tselnik and Pogrel (2000), 14 patients had their pharyngeal airway space evaluated after mandibular setback surgery. Lateral cephalograms were obtained before surgery, immediately after surgery, and at long-term follow-up between 6 months and 2 years. The mean setback distance was 9.7 mm, which resulted in a long-term mean decrease in tongue base to posterior pharyngeal wall length of 4.77 mm. The area of the pharyngeal airway space decreased long-term an average of 1.52 cm^2. It was observed that outcome measurements increased at the immediate postoperative radiograph before decreasing at the long-term follow-up radiograph. This was thought to be from forward movement of the hyoid bone after surgery to preserve airway opening in the immediate postoperative period to prevent airway collapse. It is clear that individuals with short necks, obese individuals, or those with large tongues who have mandibular setbacks may be predisposed to the development of OSA, and patient selection should be carefully managed when planning isolated mandibular surgeries in those populations.

Given that there is improvement in the airway with isolated maxillary advancement and worsening of the airway dimensions with isolated mandibular setback, the better approach is strong consideration for two-jaw procedures. A small amount maxillary advancement can be effectively used to mitigate the negative impact of the mandibular setback. With that in mind, the authors rarely perform isolated mandibular procedures but instead opt for isolated maxillary advancement in those that can esthetically tolerate the surgical movement or a two-jaw procedure in those Class III patients who cannot.

Class III patients with normal mandibular plane angles can often be treated with linear movements. Class III patients with a high or low mandibular plane angle malocclusion can be more complicated and often require rotational movements. Low-angle (SN-mandibular plane < 22 degrees; see Fig 2-51) Class III patients often have overprojected chins due to vertical deficiency and/or overclosure. High-angle Class III patients, on the other hand, often have a short chin-throat dimension but a well-shaped chin. This scenario of course can lead to inadequate skeletal support for the airway. Low-angle Class III patients esthetically benefit from clockwise movements to deemphasize the chin and magnify the movement of the midface, but high-angle Class III patients often benefit esthetically from counterclockwise movements. Though this sounds counterintuitive, a counterclockwise rotation point around the incisors or B-point results in minimal chin movement and proportionately more posterior incisor movement. The D-point is often superior movement, which has a very positive effect on airway dimensions (Fig 2-85).

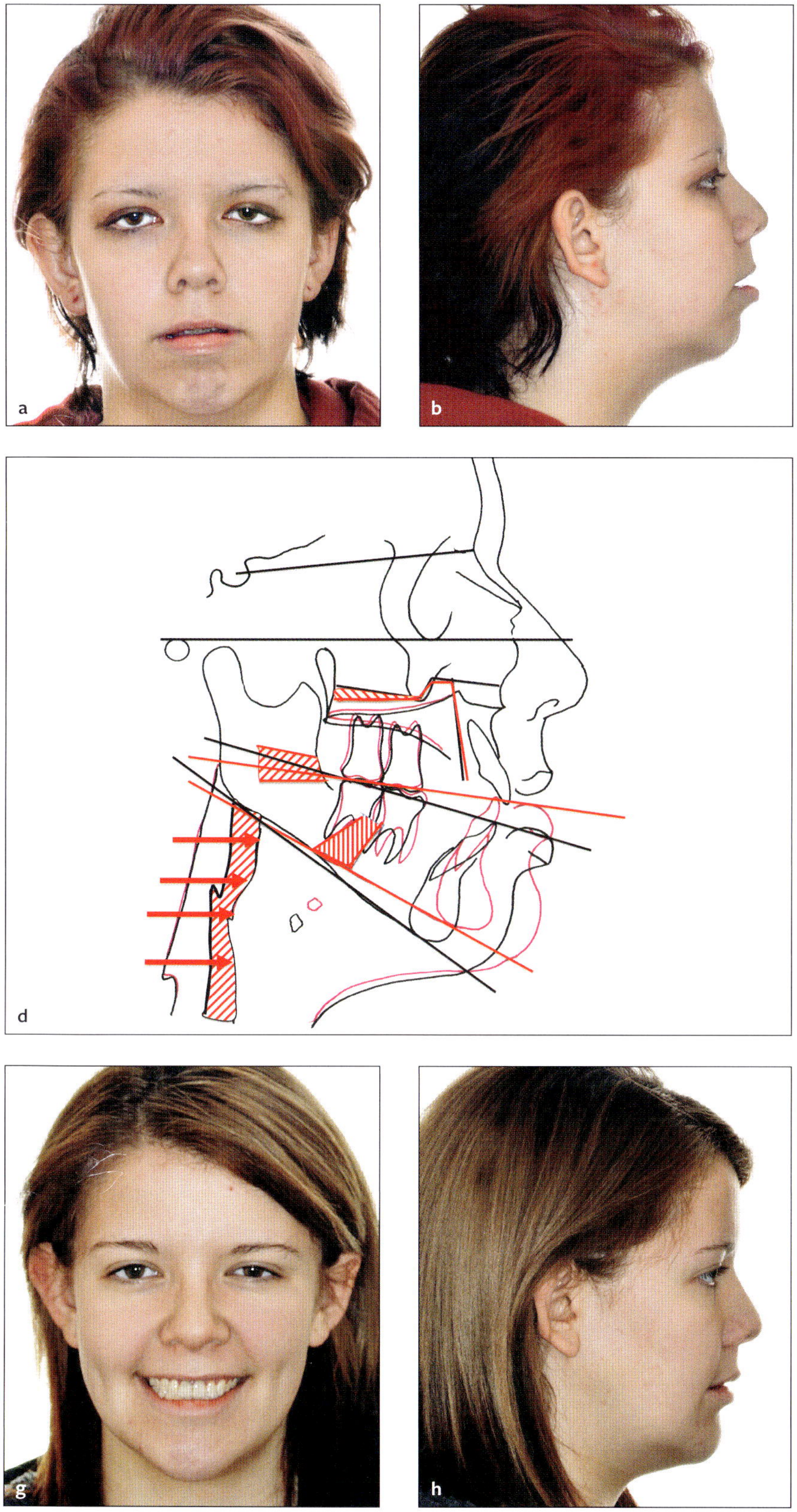

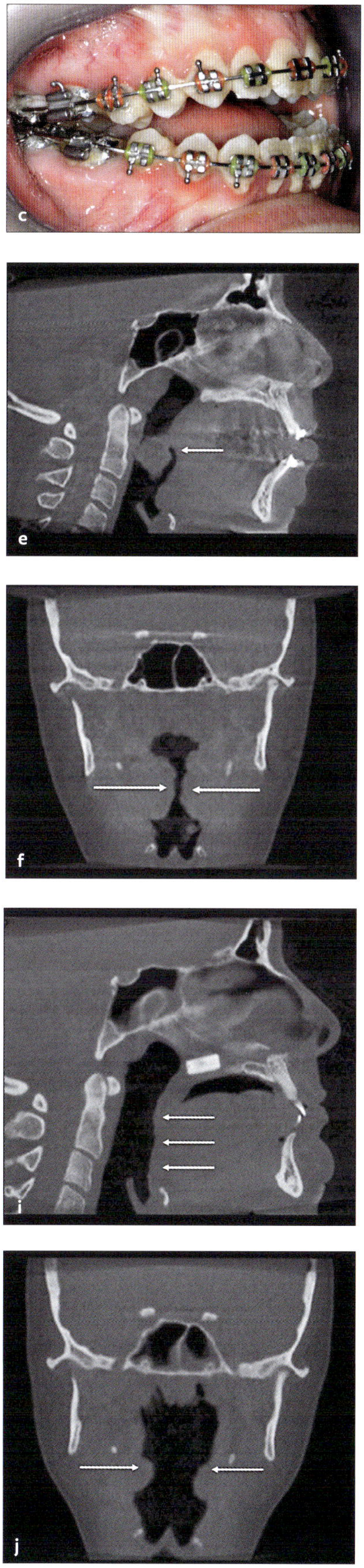

Fig 2-84 This patient had severe OSA. (*a*) Presurgical frontal view. (*b*) Presurgical profile view. (*c*) Presurgical occlusion. (*d*) The surgical plan consists of a large counterclockwise rotational advancement, closing the open bite in the mandible. (*e and f*) CBCT images confirm marked airway compromise. (*arrows*). (*g and h*) The upward and forward movement of the mandible restulted in significant postsurgical facial and skeletal changes. (*i and j*) The postoperative CBCT scans confirm a significant improvement in the airway anatomy (*arrows*).

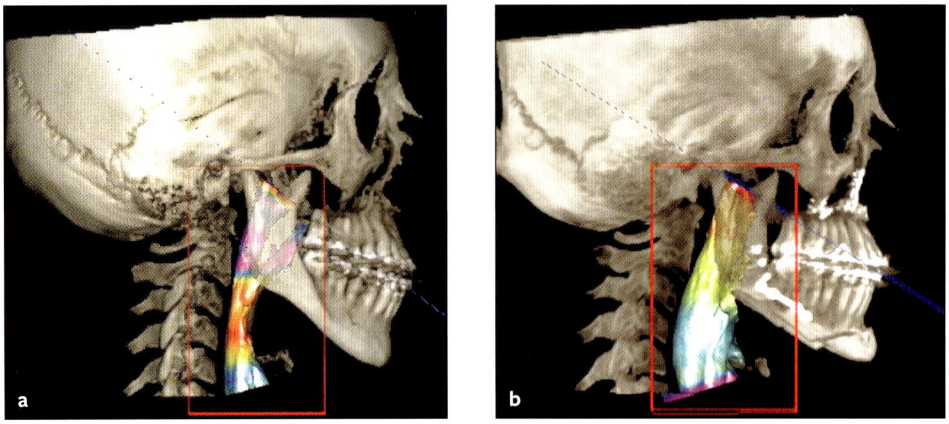

Fig 2-85 Patients with high mandibular plane angle Class III occlusion treated with counterclockwise rotation of the maxillomandibular and advancements benefit because the D-point moves upward and forward, the incisors move backward, and the airway is enhanced. Presurgical (*a*) and postsurgical (*b*) CBCT scans demonstrate the advantage of this approach (*red rectangles*).

Orthognathic surgery can impact the airway whether or not a patient has OSA, so the changes in the airway must be carefully considered during treatment planning.

Conclusion

Generations of surgeons have focused mainly on the original three pillars of orthognathic surgery treatment planning: dental decompensation and stability, skeletal correction and stability, and a pleasing esthetic outcome. Now there is a fourth pillar of treatment planning: providing skeletal support of the airway and surgical movements that enhance the airway or at least mitigate any deleterious effects.

Recommended Reading

Abramson Z, Susarla SM, Lawler M, Bouchard C, Troulis M, Kaban LB. Three-dimensional computed tomographic airway analysis of patients with obstructive sleep apnea treated by maxillomandibular advancement. J Oral Maxillofac Surg 2011;69:677–686.

Ackerman JL, Proffit WR. The characteristics of malocclusion: A modern approach to classification and diagnosis. Am J Orthod 1969;56:443–454.

Aquilino SA, Matteson SR, Holland GA, Phillips C. Evaluation of condylar position from temporomandibular joint radiographs. J Prosthet Dent 1985;53:88–97.

Arnett GW, Bergman RT. Facial keys to orthodontic diagnosis and treatment planning, Part I. Am J Orthod Dentofacial Orthop 1993;103:299–312.

Arnett GW, Bergman RT. Facial keys to orthodontic diagnosis and treatment planning, Part II. Am J Orthod Dentofacial Orthop 1993;103:395–411.

Barbosa AL, Marcantonio E, Barbosa CE, Gabrielli MF, Gabrielli MA. Psychological evaluation of patients scheduled for orthognathic surgery. J Nihon Univ Sch Dent 1993;35:1–9.

Becker OE, Avelar RL, Göelzer JG, Dolzan Ado N, Haas OL Jr, De Oliveira RB. Pharyngeal airway changes in Class III patients treated with double jaw orthognathic surgery—Maxillary advancement and mandibular setback. J Oral Maxillofac Surg 2012;70:e639–e647.

Burstone CJ, James RB, Legan H, Murphy GA, Norton LA. Cephalometrics for orthognathic surgery. J Oral Surg 1978;36:269–277.

Burstone CJ. Lip posture and its significance in treatment planning. Am J Orthod 1967;53:262–284.

Burton PR, Tobin MD, Hopper JL. Key concepts in genetic epidemiology. Lancet 2005;366:941–951.

Bütow KW, van der Walt PJ. The "Stellenbosch"—Triangle analysis of posteroanterior and basilar cephalograms. J Dent Assoc S Afr 1981;36:461–467.

Bütow KW, van der Walt PJ. The use of the triangle analysis for cephalometric analysis in three dimensions. J Maxillofac Surg 1984;12:62–70.

Butterfield KJ, Marks PL, McLean L, Newton J. Linear and volumetric airway changes after maxillomandibular advancement for obstructive sleep apnea. J Oral Maxillofac Surg 2015;73:1133–1142.

Czarnecki ST, Nanda RS, Currier GF. Perceptions of a balanced facial profile. Am J Orthod Dentofacial Orthop 1993;104:180–187.

Downs WB. Analysis of the dentofacial profile. Angle Orthod 1956;26(4):191–211.

Dervis E, Tuncer E. Long-term evaluation of temporomandibular disorders in patients undergoing orthognathic surgery compared wit a control group. Oral Surg Oral Med Oral Pathol Oral Radiol Endod 2002;94:554-560.

Ellis E 3rd, McNamara JA Jr. Cephalometric reference planes—Sella nasion vs Frankfort horizontal. Int J Adult Orthodon Orthognath Surg 1988;3:81–87.

Epker BN, Fish LC. Dentofacial Deformities: Integrated Orthodontic and Surgical Correction, vol 1. St Louis: Mosby, 1986.

Epker BN, Stella JP. Systematic aesthetic evaluation of the neck for cosmetic surgery. Atlas Oral Maxillofac Surg Clin North Am 1990;2(3):217.

Epker BN. Evaluation of the face. In: Fonesca RJ, Marciani RD, Turvey TA (eds). Oral and Maxillofacial Surgery, vol 3, ed 2. Philadelphia: Saunders, 2009:1–57.

Fishman LS. Radiographic evaluation of skeletal maturation. A clinically oriented method based on hand-wrist films. Angle Orthod 1982;52:82–112.

Frost DE. Database collection for orthognathic surgery. In: Peterson LJ (ed). Principles of Oral and Maxillofacial Surgery, vol 3. Philadelphia: Lippincott, 1992:1279–1305.

Garvill J, Garvill H, Kahnberg KE, Lundgren S. Psychological factors in orthognathic surgery. J Craniomaxillofac Surg 1992;20:28–33.

Grave KC, Brown T. Skeletal ossification of the adolescent growth spurt. Am J Orthod 1976;69:611–619.

Greulich WW, Pylers I. Radiographic Atlas of Skeletal Development of the Hand and Wrist, ed 2. Stanford, CA: Stanford UP, 1959.

Hart PS, McIntyre BP, Kadioglu O, et al. Postsurgical volumetric airway changes in 2-jaw orthognathic surgery patients. Am J Orthod Dentofacial Orthop 2015;147:536–546.

Henzi A. Effects of different orthognathic surgery procedures on pharyngeal airway space: A single center study [thesis]. Zurich: University of Zurich, 2012.

Hernández-Alfaro F, Guijarro-Martínez R, Mareque-Bueno J. Effect of mono- and bimaxillary advancement on pharyngeal airway volume: Cone-beam computed tomography evaluation. J Oral Maxillofac Surg 2011;69:e395–e400.

Holdaway RA. A soft tissue cephalometric analysis and its use in orthodontic treatment planning. Part I. Am J Orthod 1983;84:1–28.

Holdaway RA. A soft tissue cephalometric analysis and its use in orthodontic treatment planning. Part II. Am J Orthod 1984;85:279–293.

Hulsey CM. An esthetic evaluation of lip-teeth relationships present in the smile. Am J Orthod 1970;57:132–144.

Jacobson A. The "Wits" appraisal of jaw disharmony. Am J Orthod 1975;67:125–138.

Kennedy B. Systematic aesthetic evaluation of the eyes and periorbital area for cosmetic surgery. Atlas Oral Maxillofac Surg Clin North Am 1990;2(2):393.

Kiyak HA, Hohl T, Sherrick P, West RA, McNeill RW, Bucher F. Sex differences in motives for and outcomes of orthognathic surgery. J Oral Surg 1981;39:757–764.

Kiyak HA, Vitaliano PP, Crinean J. Patient's expectations as predictors of orthognathic surgery outcomes. Health Psychol 1988;7:251–268.

Laskin JL. Clinical history and physical examination. In: Laskin DM (ed). Oral and Maxillofacial Surgery, vol 1. St Louis: Mosby, 1980:399.

Legan HL, Burstone CJ. Soft tissue cephalometric analysis for orthognathic surgery. J Oral Surg 1980;38:744–751.

Li KK, Riley RW, Powell NB, Guilleminault C. Patient's perception of the facial appearance after maxillomandibular advancement for obstructive sleep apnea syndrome. J Oral Maxillofac Surg 2001;59:377–380.

Lindhe J. Textbook of Clinical Periodontology. Copenhagen: Munksgaard, 1983.

McNamara JA Jr. A method of cephalometric evaluation. Am J Orthod 1984;86:449–469.

McNamara JB, Brudon WL. Orthodontic and Orthopedic Treatment in the Mixed Dentition. Ann Arbor, MI: Needham, 1993.

Merrifield LL. The profile line as an aid in critically evaluating facial esthetics. Am J Orthod 1966;52:804–822.

O'Ryan F, Schendel SA, Carlotti AE Jr. Nasolabial esthetics and maxillary surgery. In: Bell WH (ed). Modern Practice in Orthognathic and Reconstructive Surgery, vol 1. Philadelphia: Saunders, 1992: 284–317.

Okeson JP. Fundamentals of Occlusion and Temporomandibular Disorders. St Louis: Mosby, 1985.

Onizawa K, Schmelzen R, Vogt S. Alteration of temporomandibular joint symptoms after orthognathic surgery comparison with healthy volunteers. J Oral Maxillofac Surg 1995;53:117–121.

Panula K, Somppi M, Finne K, Oikarinen K. Effects of orthognathic surgery on temporomandibular joint dysfunction: A controlled prospective 4-year follow-up study. Int J Oral Maxillofac Surg 2000;29:183–187.

Park JW, Kim NK, Kim JW, Kim MJ, Chang YI. Volumetric, planar, and linear analyses of pharyngeal airway change on computed tomography and cephalometry after mandibular setback surgery. Am J Orthod Dentofacial Orthop 2010;138:292–299.

Parsi GK, Alsulaiman AA, Kotak B, Merhra P, Will LA, Motro M. Volumetric changes of the upper airway following maxillary and mandibular advancement using cone beam computed tomography. Int J Oral Maxillofac Surg 2019;48:203–210.

Posnick JC. Orthognathic Surgery: Principles & Practice. St Louis: Elsevier, 2014.

Powell N, Humphreys B. Proportions of the Aesthetic Face. New York: Thieme-Stratton, 1984.

Proffit WR, White RP. Surgical Orthodontic Treatment. St Louis: Mosby, 1990.

Resnick CM, Kim S, Yorlets RR, Calabrese CE, Peacock ZS, Kaban LB. Evaluation of Andrews' analysis as predictor of ideal maxillary positioning in orthognathic surgery. J Oral Maxillofac Surg 2018;76:2169–2176.

Reyneke JP, Evans WG, McCollum AGH. Introduction to Orthognathic Surgery: A Color Atlas. St Louis: Ishiyaku Euro America, 1990.

Reyneke JP, Ferretti C. Correction of dentofacial deformities. In: Pogrel MA, Khanberg K-E, Anderson L (eds). Essentials of Oral and Maxillofacial Surgery. London: Wiley-Blackwell, 2014:315–330.

Reyneke JP, Ferretti C. Diagnosis and treatment planning for orthognathic surgery. In: Anderson L, Khanberg K-E, Pogrel MA (eds). Oral and Maxillofacial Surgery. London: Wiley-Blackwell, 2010:973–1012.

Reyneke JP, Tsakiris P, Kienle F. A simple classification for surgical treatment planning of maxillomandibular asymmetry. Br J Oral Maxillofac Surg 1997;35:349–351.

Reyneke JP. The surgical correction of dentofacial deformities. Contin Med Educ J 1995;13:661–668.

Ricketts RM. Cephalometric analysis and synthesis. Angle Orthod 1961;31:141–156.

Rinchuse DJ, McMinn JT. Summary of evidence-based systematic reviews of temporomandibular disorders. Am J Orthod Dentofacial Orthop 2006;130:715–720.

Rosário HD, de Oliveira BG, Pompeo DD, de Freitas PH, Paranhos LR. Surgical maxillary advancement increases upper airway volume in skeletal Class III patients: A cone beam computed tomography-based study. J Clin Sleep Med 2016:12:1527–1532.

Rothberg S, Fried N, Kane J, Shapiro E. Predicting the "Wits" appraisal from the ANB angle. Am J Orthod 1980;77:636–642.

Scheideman GB, Bell WH, Legan HL, Finn RA, Reisch JS. Cephalometric analysis of dentofacial normals. Am J Orthod 1980;78:404–420.

Schudy FF. Cant of the occlusal plane and axial inclinations of teeth. In: The Occlusal Plane: Its Origin, Development and Correction. Houston: Armstrong, 1992.

Shin JH, Kim MA, Park IY, Park YH. A 2-year follow-up of changes after bimaxillary surgery in patients with mandibular prognathism: 3-dimensional analysis of pharyngeal airway volume and hyoid bone position. J Oral Maxillofac Surg 2015;73;340.e1–340.e9.

Showfety KJ, Vig PS, Matteson S. A simplified method for taking natural-head-position cephalograms. Am J Orthod 1983;83:495–500.

Solberg WK, Clark GT. Abnormal Jaw Mechanics: Diagnosis and Treatment. Chicago: Quintessence, 1984.

Sperry TP, Speidel TM, Isaacson RJ, Worms FW. Differential treatment planning for mandibular prognathism. Am J Orthod 1977;71:531–541.

Steiner CC. Cephalometrics for me and you. Am J Orthod 1953;39:729–755.

Steiner CC. The use of cephalometrics as an aid to planning and assessing orthodontic treatment. Am J Orthod 1960;46:721.

Swennen GRJ (ed). 3D Virtual Treatment Planning of Orthognathic Surgery: A Step-by-Step Approach for Orthodontists and Surgeons. Berlin: Springer, 2017.

Tanner JM, Whitehouse RH. Standards for Skeletal Maturity Based on the Study of 3000 British Children: The Scoring System for All 28 Bones of the Hand and Wrist. London: University of London Institute of Child Health, 1959.

Todres JI. Static and Continuing Measurement of Head Posture: A Comparative Investigation [thesis]. Johannesburg: University of the Witwatersrand, 1993.

Tselnik M, Pogrel MA. Assessment of the pharyngeal airway space after mandibular setback surgery. J Oral Maxillofac Surg 2000;58:282–285.

Wolford LM, Karras SC, Mehra P. Concomitant temporomandibular joint and orthognathic surgery: A preliminary report. J Oral Maxillofac Surg 2002;60:356–363.

Wolford LM. Concomitant temporomandibular and orthognathic surgery. J Oral Maxillofac Surg 2003;61:1198–1204.

Worms FW, Isaacson RJ, Spiedel TM. Surgical orthodontic treatment planning: Profile analysis and mandibular surgery. Angle Orthod 1976;46:1–25.

Wylie GA, Fish LC, Epker BN. Cephalometrics: A comparison of five analyses currently used in the diagnosis of dentofacial deformities. Int J Adult Orthodon Orthognath Surg 1987;2:15–36.

Yen P. Identification of landmarks in cephalometric radiographs. Angle Orthod 1960;30:35–41.

Zylinski CG, Nanda RS, Kapila S. Analysis of soft tissue profile in white males. Am J Orthod Dentofacial Orthop 1992;101:514–518.

3

Diagnosis and Treatment Planning

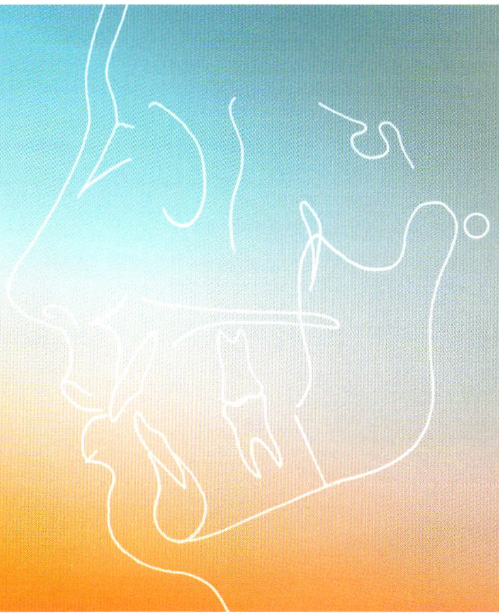

The information from the systematic patient evaluation forms a database that the practitioner can use to compile a short problem list, which in turn leads to an initial diagnosis of the patient's dentofacial deformity. Careful assessment and consideration of soft tissue along with skeletal and dental positions are necessary to differentiate between various dentofacial deformities that can have similar patterns. For example, a patient with a Class III malocclusion may have the skeletal characteristics of anteroposterior deficiency of the maxilla, anteroposterior excess of the mandible, maxillary vertical deficiency with overclosure of the mandible, or any combination of these. Figure 3-1 provides a schematic guide to the differential diagnosis of various dentofacial deformities and their interrelationships. Figure 3-2 illustrates the treatment pathway—starting at the gathering of information, followed by the recording of a database, which leads to a problem list and diagnosis, and ending with the development of a treatment plan.

The following section uses a specific case to demonstrate systematic evaluation, the formation of a database, the diagnostic process, and the treatment-planning pathway. Although the specific treatment of patients has not yet been discussed in the text, the visual treatment objectives along with treatment and posttreatment results of this patient are included here to give the reader an idea of where the cumbersome initial stages of examination and treatment planning are leading.

Case Overview

General patient evaluation

Age: 16 years.
Medical history: Not pertinent.
Dental history: Orthodontic treatment by her general dental practitioner for 18 months; currently wearing a fixed lingual retention appliance in the mandibular incisor area. Four impacted third molars are present.
Main complaints: She finds it increasingly difficult to bite through food with her incisors. Her left mandibular lateral incisor is malpositioned. She thinks she has a "toothy" look. She has to strain to move her lips together. She is unhappy following the treatment received from her general dentist.
Motivation: Internal (self).
Psychologic assessment: Good parental support; low self-confidence.

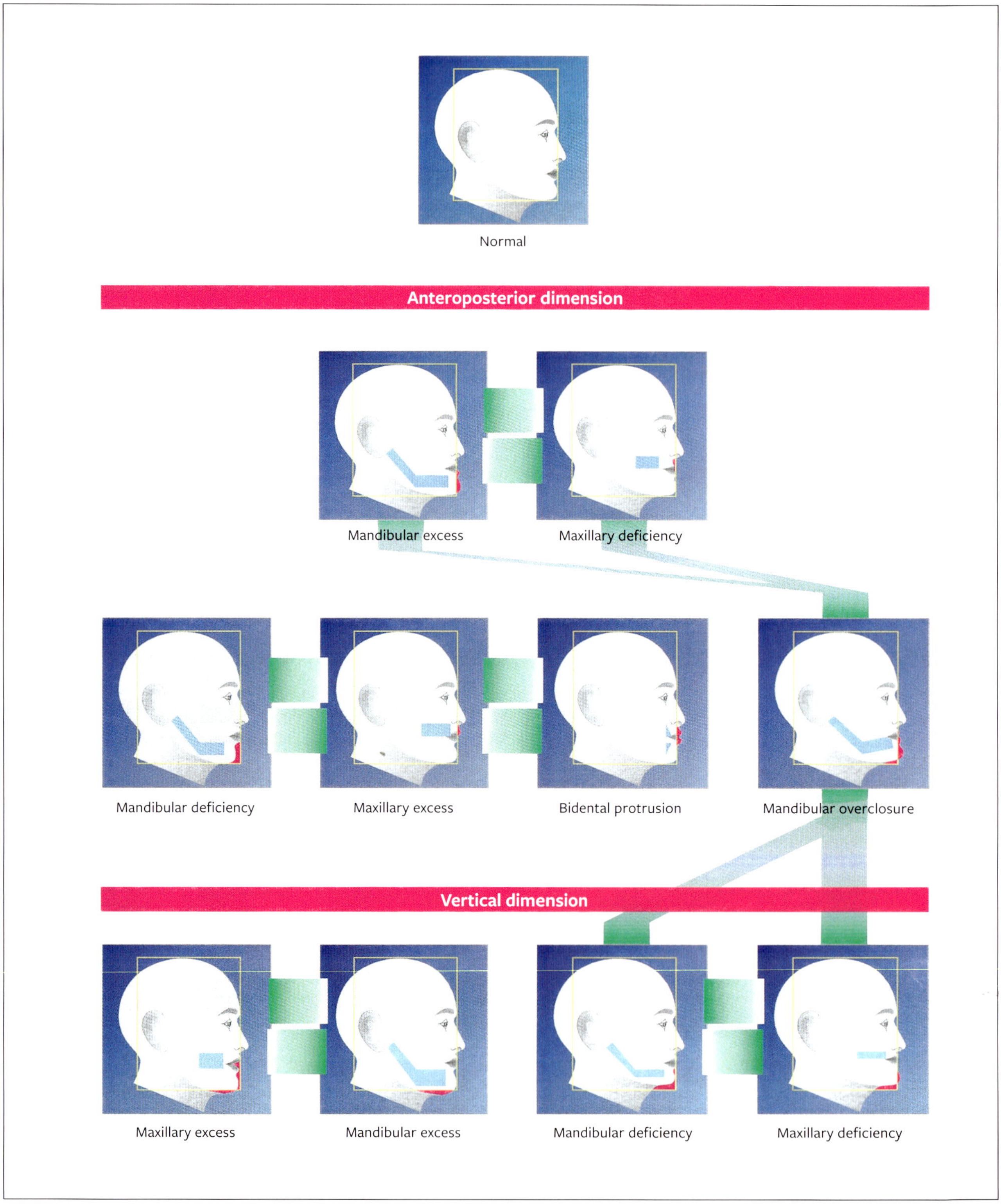

Fig 3-1 Schematic guide to the differential diagnosis of dentofacial deformities and their interrelationships.

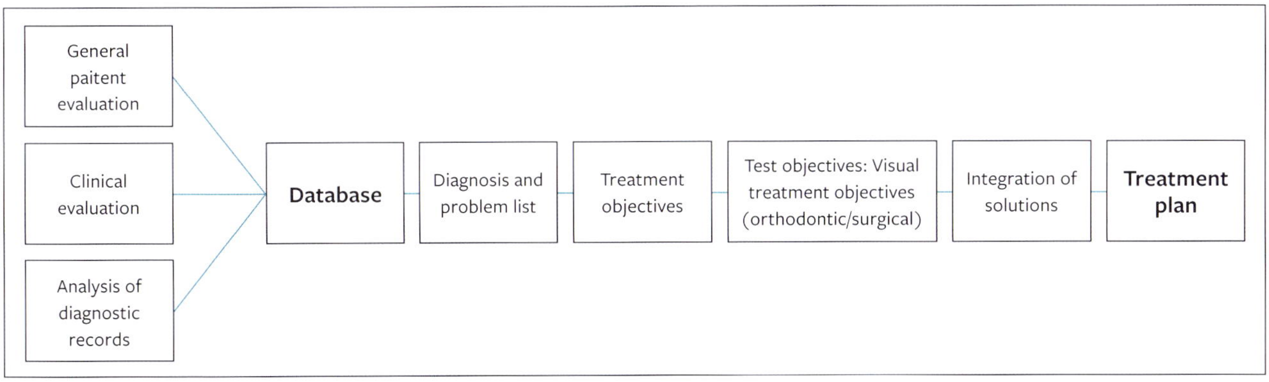

Fig 3-2 Flowchart illustrating the systematic gathering of data leading to a diagnosis and eventually the development of a treatment plan.

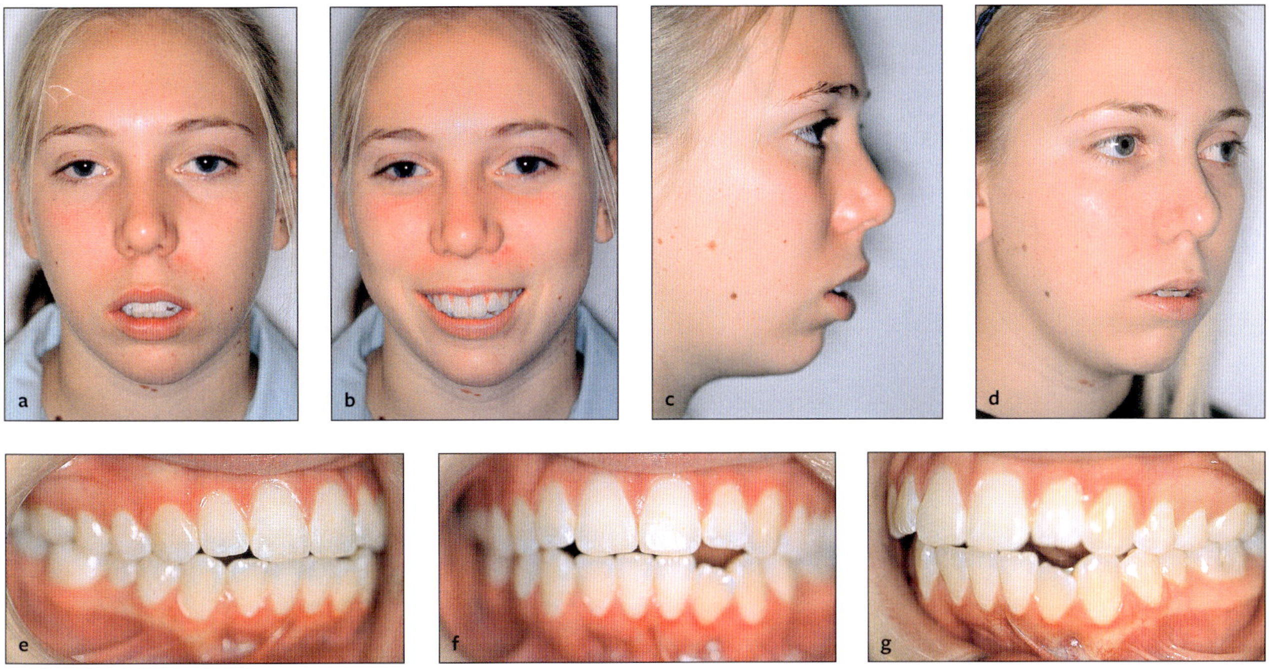

Fig 3-3 Preoperative evaluation. (*a*) Frontal view. (*b*) Frontal view, smile. (*c*) Profile view. (*d*) Three-quarter view. (*e*) Occlusion, right. (*f*) Occlusion, center. (*g*) Occlusion, left.

Clinical evaluation

1. Extraoral examination
   - Frontal view (Figs 3-3a and 3-3b)
     - Increased lower facial height
     - Increased interlabial gap
     - Excessive maxillary incisor exposure
     - "Gummy smile"
     - Slightly flattened paranasal areas
     - Narrow alar base
     - Excessive lower lip vermilion exposure
     - Mandible asymmetric to the left
   - Profile view (Fig 3-3c)
     - Convex profile
     - Anteroposterior chin deficiency
     - Anteroposterior mandibular deficiency
     - Everted lower lip
     - Increased interlabial gap
     - Increased lower facial height
   - Three-quarter view (Fig 3-3d)
     - Paranasal flattening
     - Ill-defined chin
     - Narrow alar base
     - Poor nasal tip definition
2. Intraoral examination (Figs 3-3e to 3-3g)
   - Mandibular arch
     - Crowding in the incisor area
     - Incisor protrusion

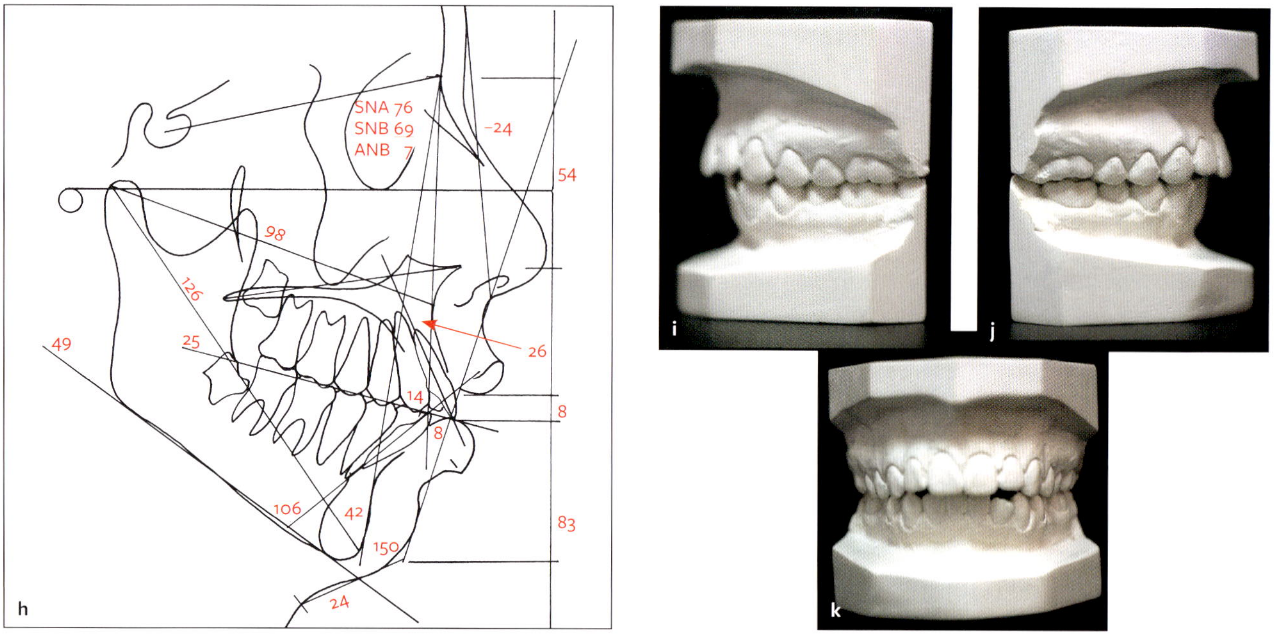

Fig 3-3 (cont) (*h*) Pretreatment cephalometric analysis. (*i to k*) Study cast: left, right, and center.

  - Serrated incisor edges
  - Narrow area of attached gingiva in the incisor area
- Maxillary arch
  - Incisor protrusion
  - Slight crowding
- Interarch area
  - Class I malocclusion
  - Anterior open bite
  - Bidental protrusion
  - Mandibular dental midline 1.5 mm to the left

3. Other
   - Slight marginal gingivitis in the incisor areas
   - Mouth breathing

Special investigations

Radiographic evaluation

1. Cephalometric analysis
   - Soft tissue analysis (Fig 3-3h)
   - Increased facial contour angle (−24 degrees)
   - Increased interlabial gap (8 mm)
   - Increased maxillary incisor exposure (8 mm)
   - Increased lip-chin-throat angle (150 degrees)
   - Decreased chin-throat length (24 mm)
   - Skeletal analysis (see Fig 3-3h)
     - Increased ANB angle (7 degrees)
     - Increased mandibular plane angle (49 degrees)
     - Increased vertical height (83 mm [midface, 54 mm])
     - Decreased mandibular length (126 mm [maxilla, 98 mm])
     - Mandible rotated clockwise
   - Dental analysis
     - Maxillary incisor protrusion (26 degrees)
     - Mandibular incisor protrusion (42 degrees, 14 mm)
     - Anterior open bite
2. Panoramic evaluation: Impacted third molars
3. Posteroanterior cephalographic analysis
   - Mandibular asymmetry to the left
   - Mandibular dental midline to the left
4. Dental radiographic analysis: No relevant finding
5. Occlusal plane radiographic analysis: No relevant findings
6. Other: No relevant findings

Dental cast analysis

The cast analysis (Figs 3-3i to 3-3k) confirms the clinical assessment.

Diagnosis and problem list

1. Skeletal diagnosis and problems
   - Vertical maxillary excess
   - Mandibular anteroposterior deficiency
   - Microgenia
   - Mandibular asymmetry to the left
2. Soft tissue diagnosis and problems
   - Convex profile
   - Mandibular anteroposterior deficiency

Table 3-1 | Orthodontic treatment objectives and solutions

Treatment objective	Solutions
Reduce lip prominence	Retract maxillary and mandibular incisors
Correct bimaxillary protrusion	Retract incisors
Reduce crowding	Extract premolars
Facilitate surgical advancement of the mandible	Extract maxillary second premolars and slightly retract maxillary incisors Extract mandibular first premolars, retract incisors, and increase overjet
Ensure orthodontic stability	Make no attempt to close open bite orthodontically

Table 3-2 | Surgical treatment objectives and solutions

Treatment objective	Solutions
Correct facial convexity	Advance the mandible
Improve chin prominence	Advance the chin
Reduce vertical maxillary excess	Reposition the maxilla superiorly
Correct open bite	Reposition the posterior maxilla superiorly
Create a lip seal	Reposition the maxilla superiorly
Correct mandibular asymmetry	Reposition the mandible to the right

- Deficient chin
- Increased interlabial gap
- Everted lower lip

3. Dental diagnosis and problems
   - Crowding in both arches
   - Bidental protrusion
   - Impacted third molars
   - Mandibular dental midline to the left
4. Other diagnoses and problems
   - Mouth breathing

Treatment objectives

1. Soft tissue treatment objectives
   - Correct facial convexity
   - Improve chin prominence
   - Create lip seal
   - Reduce lip prominence slightly
2. Skeletal treatment objectives
   - Reduce vertical maxillary excess
   - Advance mandible
   - Advance chin
3. Dental treatment objectives
   - Correct bimaxillary protrusion
   - Correct anterior open bite
   - Reduce crowding

Testing objectives

The clinician should now move on to set specific treatment objectives for the case. When considering the final treatment plan, three basic questions should be kept in mind:

1. What are the esthetic objectives, and which surgical procedures are indicated?
2. What specific orthodontic treatment is required to facilitate the proposed surgery?
3. What is the best sequence of treatment—taking into account dental, periodontal, prosthodontic, and orthodontic treatment; surgical needs; and other requirements—to obtain the desired result in the shortest length of time?

Orthodontic treatment objectives and possible solutions are shown in Table 3-1. Surgical treatment objectives and possible solutions are shown in Table 3-2.

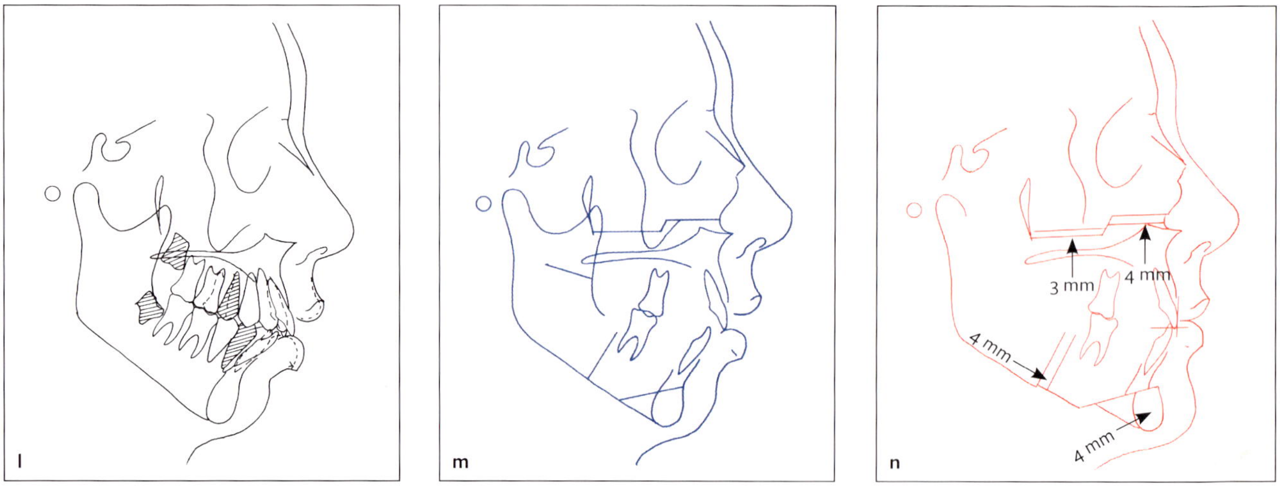

Figs 3-3 *(cont)* (*l*) Orthodontic visual treatment objective: surgical removal of all four third molars and extraction of both maxillary second premolars and both mandibular first premolars. Retraction of incisors and creation of a Class II malocclusion. (*m*) Visual treatment objective of completed preoperative orthodontics. (*n*) Surgical visual treatment objective: superior repositioning of the maxilla (4 mm anterior and 3 mm posterior), advancement of the mandible (4 mm), and advancement of the chin (4 mm).

Treatment plan

Preoperative orthodontics

The expected dental and soft tissue changes to be effected by the preoperative orthodontic treatment are predicted and illustrated by the cephalometric tracing and orthodontic visual treatment objective (Figs 3-3l and 3-3m).

In the maxillary arch:

- Surgically remove both third molars and extract both second premolars.
- Retract the incisors slightly and maintain upper lip support.
- Align the arch in one piece and close the extraction spaces.
- Establish a good arch form to be compatible with the mandibular arch.

In the mandibular arch:

- Surgically remove both third molars and extract both first premolars.
- Retract the incisors to increase the overjet and create a Class II malocclusion.
- Level and align the arch, and establish a good arch form to be compatible with the maxillary arch.
- Make no attempt to close the open bite by extrusion of incisors or intrusion of molars.

Surgery

The surgical visual treatment objectives, outlined here, are shown in Fig 3-3n:

- Le Fort I maxillary osteotomy (one piece) to superiorly reposition the maxilla in order to establish ideal tooth-lip relationship and allow the mandible to autorotate and close the open bite
- Bilateral sagittal split osteotomy to advance the mandible
- Genioplasty to advance the chin

Postoperative orthodontics

- Light 3.5-oz quarter-inch elastics with slight Class II vector to guide the occlusion
- After 3 to 4 weeks, heavier up-down elastics (6-oz, 0.25-inch elastics)
- Finalization of the occlusion

Retention

- Mandibular fixed intercanine retainer
- Removable maxillary appliance

Results

The achievement of the preoperative orthodontic goals is illustrated in Figs 3-3o to 3-3s. The end result of treatment is demonstrated in Figs 3-3t to 3-3aa.

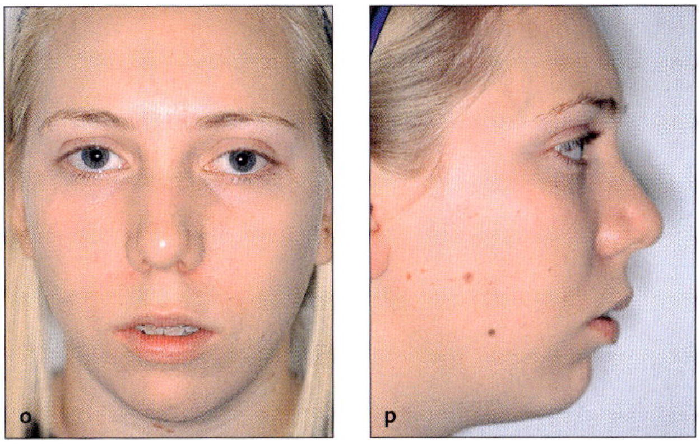

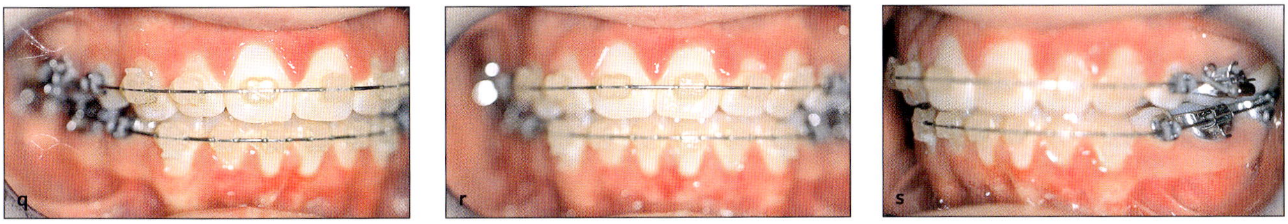

Fig 3-3 *(cont)* Immediate preoperative views. (*o*) Frontal view. (*p*) Profile view. (q) Occlusion, right. (*r*) Occlusion, center. (*s*) Occlusion, left.

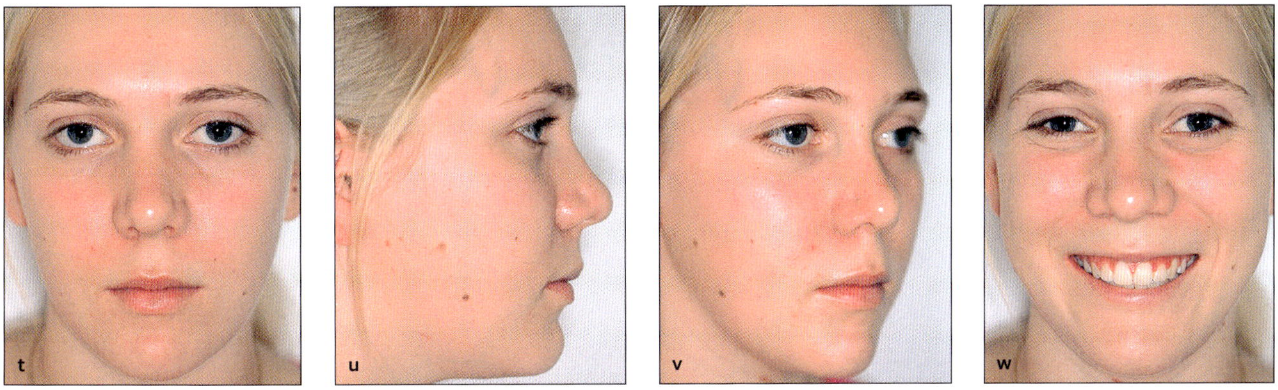

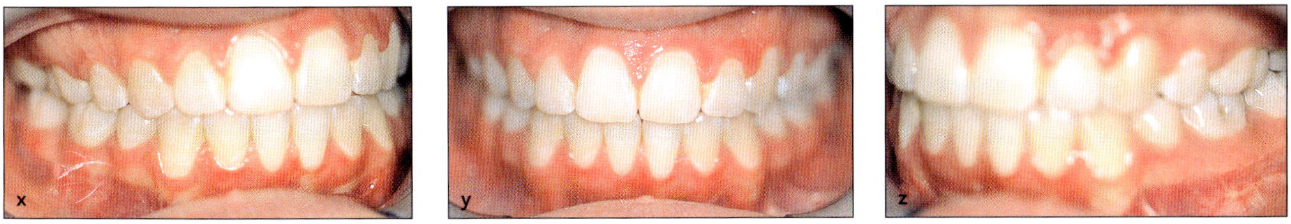

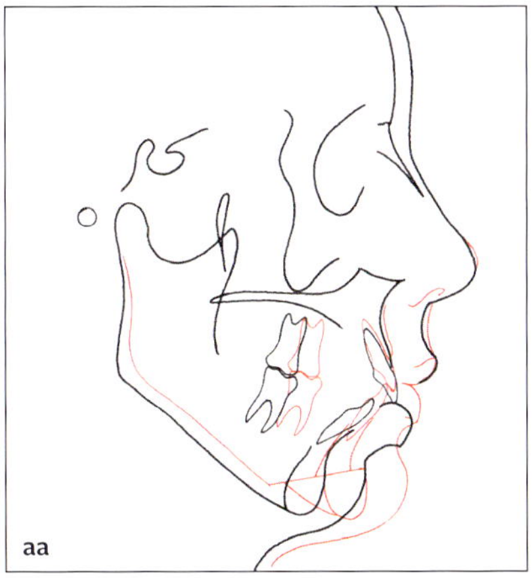

Fig 3-3 *(cont)* End result of treatment. (*t*) Frontal view. (*u*) Profile view. (*v*) Three-quarter view. (*w*) Frontal view, smile. (*x*) Occlusion, right. (*y*) Occlusion, center. (*z*) Occlusion, left. (*aa*) Pretreatment and posttreatment composite cephalometric tracing illustrating the soft tissue, skeletal, and dental changes.

This case demonstrates a systematic approach that is achieved by listing the problems under the following categories: soft tissue, skeletal, dental, and other. For treatment planning to be successful, the interaction of the specific solutions, the sequence of the various steps, and the impact the steps are likely to have on one another must all be considered.

Facial Changes Associated with Skeletal Repositioning

The correction of a dentofacial deformity with orthognathic surgery will result in altered facial esthetics. To decide on the correct surgical procedure and be able to predict the soft tissue changes, the clinician must have an in-depth knowledge of the soft tissue reactions subsequent to the different surgical movements of the jaws. The basic reactions are summarized in the following outline.

1. Mandibular advancement
   - Frontal changes
     - Induces a vertical increase in lower-third facial height (more in cases with a high mandibular plane angle than in low-angle cases)
     - Reduces lower lip eversion (effect of maxillary incisor on lower lip reduction)
     - Reduces labiomental fold (lower lip rolls back)
     - Improves neck-chin definition
   - Profile changes
     - Increases chin prominence
     - Decreases lower vermilion exposure (lower lip rolls back)
     - Increases lower lip fullness
     - Decreases chin-throat angle
     - Decreases labiomental fold
2. Mandibular setback
   - Frontal changes
     - Decreases mandibular prominence
     - Makes upper lip vermilion more prominent
     - Decreases lower-third facial height (more in cases of high mandibular plane angle than in low-angle cases)
   - Profile changes
     - Decreases mandibular anteroposterior prominence
     - Reduces lower lip vermilion exposure
     - Reduces chin-throat length
     - Increases chin-throat angle
3. Maxillary advancement
   - Frontal changes
     - Increases alar base width (controllable)
     - Increases upper lip fullness
     - Increases upper lip vermilion exposure
     - Increases paranasal fullness
   - Profile changes
     - Increases paranasal area fullness
     - Elevates nasal tip (controllable)
     - Increases upper lip fullness
     - Decreases prominence of chin and nose (relative)
4. Maxillary superior repositioning
   - Frontal changes
     - Reduces maxillary incisor exposure
     - Reduces upper lip vermilion exposure
     - Reduces interlabial distance
     - Reduces upper lip length (controllable)
     - Reduces lower-third facial height
     - Reduces gingival exposure when smiling
     - Increases alar base width (controllable)
   - Profile changes
     - Elevates nasal tip (controllable)
     - Reduces lower-third facial height
     - Reduces interlabial distance
     - Increases mandibular anteroposterior prominence (autorotation)
     - Increases paranasal fullness
5. Maxillary inferior repositioning
   - Frontal changes
     - Increases lower-third facial height
     - Increases upper lip length
     - Increases upper lip vermilion exposure
     - Increases maxillary tooth exposure
   - Profile changes
     - Increases upper lip prominence
     - Makes nasolabial angle more obtuse
     - Makes mandible less prominent anteroposteriorly (autorotation)

Esthetic Objectives and Surgical Indications

The choice of surgical procedure is dictated by the esthetic goals, which are determined by the patient's main complaint and the facial examination (of both hard and soft tissues). The esthetic goals can be attained by developing the orthodontic and surgical visual treatment objectives. Close collaboration between the orthodontist and the surgeon is necessary for effective planning and successful execution of the treatment plan.

Consider a patient with the esthetic requirement of increasing the mandibular prominence. The shape of the chin plays an important role in the decision-making process. Chin surgery is indicated only when the chin is too flat (microgenia) and there is an obtuse labiomental fold. The possible surgical solutions for increasing chin prominence are (1) surgical advancement of the chin, (2) surgical advancement of the mandible, and (3) surgical advancement of the chin and mandible. The choice of surgery is influenced by the dental occlusion, mandibu-

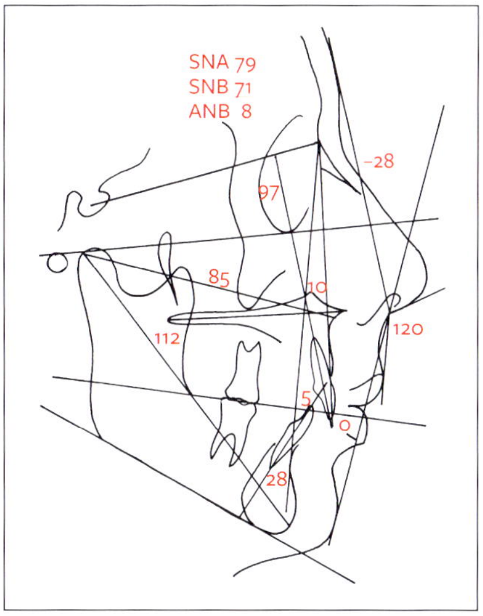

Fig 3-4 Cephalometric analysis of a patient with a Class II malocclusion and mandibular anteroposterior deficiency. The maxillary first premolars and mandibular second premolars have been removed and the maxillary incisors retracted excessively, decreasing upper lip support and overjet. This will limit the surgical advancement of the mandible and result in a compromised esthetic result. The favorable shape of the chin and normal labiomental fold do not allow the surgeon to perform a genioplasty without making the chin too prominent and accentuating the poor lip support.

lar skeletal base position, and chin shape. The following discussion illustrates how these variables influence treatment possibilities in various scenarios.

Class II malocclusion

Scenario 1

The patient has a Class II malocclusion, mandibular anteroposterior deficiency, and good chin shape. The solution is orthodontic alignment of the teeth and making the malocclusion more Class II, if necessary. Surgical advancement of the mandible is then performed. The orthodontic challenge and art lie in establishing an incisor overjet that will facilitate the required amount of surgical advancement of the mandible (determined by esthetics; see Fig 3-5).

Scenario 2

In this scenario, the patient has a Class II malocclusion, mandibular anteroposterior deficiency, and microgenia. The solution is orthodontic alignment of the teeth along with surgical advancement of the mandible and chin. Alternatively, the clinician could decide to accept the Class II malocclusion and recommend surgical advancement of the chin. However, genioplasty is not a substitute for mandibular surgery. Keep in mind that chin shape is more important than chin projection (see Fig 3-5).

Class I malocclusion

Scenario 1

This patient has a Class I malocclusion, mandibular anteroposterior deficiency, and good chin shape. The solution is to use orthodontics to create a Class II malocclusion, followed by surgical advancement of the mandible.

Scenario 2

In this scenario, the patient has a Class I malocclusion, mandibular anteroposterior deficiency, and microgenia. One solution would be to advance the chin, but again, genioplasty does not achieve the same result as mandibular surgery. A second solution, which would be useful in cases of more severe deformity, would be to use orthodontics to create a Class II malocclusion and then surgically advance the mandible and chin.

Specific Orthodontic Treatment Required to Facilitate Surgery

It is as important for the surgeon to understand the orthodontic decision-making process as it is for the orthodontist to have a good understanding of the presurgical orthodontic requirements. Knowledgeable practitioners not only maintain good interprofessional communication but also achieve improved treatment results.

The preoperative positioning of the teeth dictates the nature and extent of the surgical procedure and influences the final esthetic result. Poor orthodontic preparation, dental compensation for a skeletal discrepancy, or failure to follow the treatment plan will lead to surgical compromise (Fig 3-4). It may also force the surgeon to perform adjunctive procedures that were not initially part of the surgical treatment plan in an attempt to achieve a more acceptable functional and esthetic result (eg, segmental surgery, genioplasty, or even rotation of the maxillomandibular complex). The treatment result is usually a compromise rather than an ideal solution.

The orthodontic treatment objectives, extraction patterns, and mechanics used in surgical-orthodontic cases

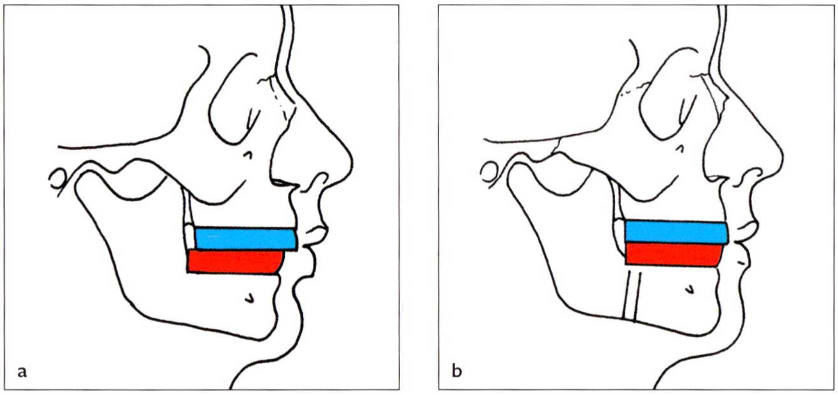

Fig 3-5 (*a*) Class II malocclusion and mandibular anteroposterior deficiency. (*b*) The orthodontically prepared maxillary arch and favorable position of the mandibular incisors allow the surgeon to advance the mandible into a Class I occlusion and an ideal esthetic position.

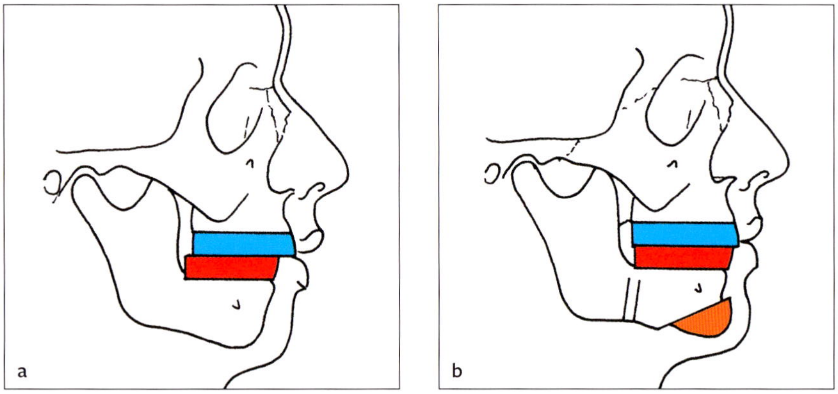

Fig 3-6 (*a*) Class II malocclusion, mandibular anteroposterior deficiency, and microgenia. (*b*) The esthetic requirements demand a surgical advancement of the mandible and chin.

often differ or may be opposite to those used in nonsurgical orthodontic cases. When developing an orthodontic treatment plan for the surgical-orthodontic correction of a dentofacial deformity, a few basic surgical treatment scenarios should be considered. Guidelines to assist in the orthodontic and surgical decision-making process are presented in this section in various treatment scenarios involving one or both jaws. When surgical correction requires repositioning of only one jaw, the dentition of the unoperated jaw will determine the final position of the jaw to be repositioned.

Mandibular repositioning

The maxillary dentition, especially the incisors, will determine the new vertical, anteroposterior, and transverse positions of the mandible (Fig 3-5). The anteroposterior and vertical positions of the chin may be altered by means of a genioplasty. These positions will be influenced by the prominence and shape of the chin as well as the labiomental fold.

For example, when a patient has a Class II malocclusion and mandibular anteroposterior deficiency combined with microgenia, the chin should be advanced by means of a genioplasty (Fig 3-6).

A second example is a patient with a Class II malocclusion who has either a mandibular dentoalveolar process that is anteroposteriorly deficient (Fig 3-7a) or macrogenia. The surgeon should consider two alternatives:

1. Advancement of the mandible by means of a bilateral sagittal split osteotomy combined with a reduction genioplasty (Fig 3-7b).
2. A total subapical mandibular osteotomy with advancement of the dentoalveolar process (Fig 3-7c). However, the author finds this surgical procedure cumbersome with a greater risk of inferior alveolar nerve damage.

Orthodontic considerations

Patients with mandibular anteroposterior deficiency and a Class II malocclusion should not undergo excessive retraction of the maxillary incisors because that approach would reduce

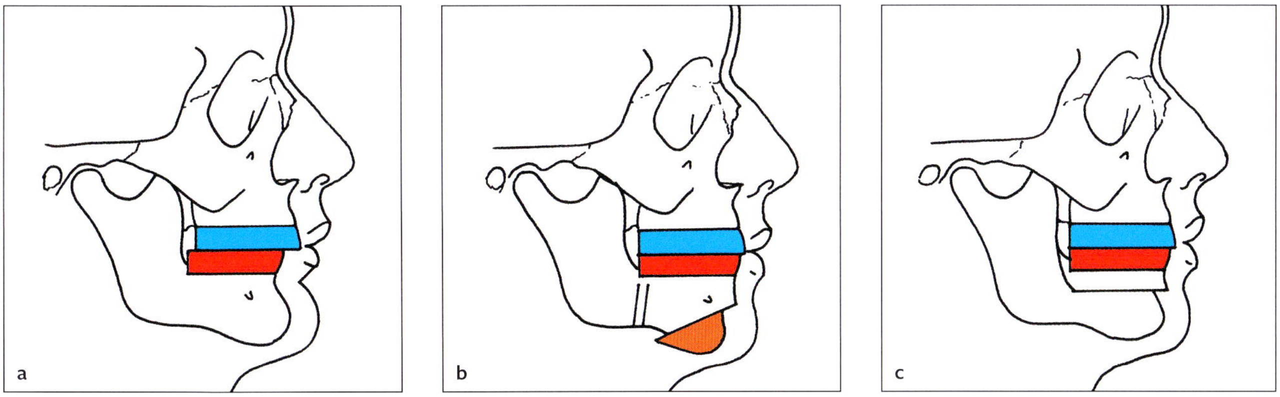

Fig 3-7 (*a*) Dentoalveolar anteroposterior deficiency. (*b*) Surgical advancement of the mandible combined with reduction genioplasty. (*c*) Advancement of the dentoalveolar part of the mandible by means of total subapical osteotomy. In both surgical options, the maxillary incisors determine the amount of surgical advancement and final esthetic shape of the chin area (either by the amount of chin reduction necessary or the amount of lower lip advancement resulting from the advanced dentoalveolar segment).

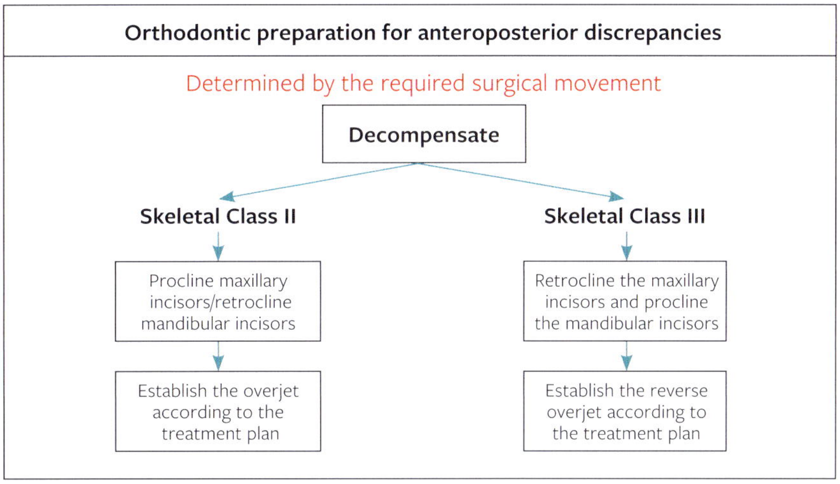

Fig 3-8 A flowchart illustrating the difference in orthodontic dental decompensation in preparation for surgical anteroposterior correction.

the upper lip support, increase the nasolabial angle, and limit mandibular advancement. The desired soft tissue position of the lips and chin, as determined by the visual treatment objective, should show the orthodontist where to place the maxillary and mandibular incisors. From this placement, the orthodontist can deduce the linear extent of the mandibular advancement. The desired incisor position will also help determine the correct extraction pattern, if extractions are indicated.

Patients with a Class III malocclusion and mandibular anteroposterior excess may require the mandibular incisors and molars to be decompensated. Once again, the desired soft tissue position, as determined by the visual treatment objective, will indicate the linear extent of the setback. This information will help the orthodontist determine the ideal incisor position (Fig 3-8).

In patients with mandibular anteroposterior deficiency, there is often dental crowding and an accentuated curve of Spee in the mandibular arch, and these conditions require tooth extractions. Three extraction patterns may be implemented, depending on the conditions:

1. *Crowding in the anterior mandible and no crowding in the maxilla.* The mandibular first premolars should be extracted. After mandibular advancement, a Class III molar and Class I canine relationship will result. Extraction of the first premolars will also allow for more retraction of the mandibular incisors, where required.
2. *Crowding in the posterior mandible and no crowding in the maxilla.* The mandibular second premolars should be extracted. This will allow less retraction of the mandibular incisors. This extraction pattern will result in a Class III molar and Class I canine relationship after surgical advancement.

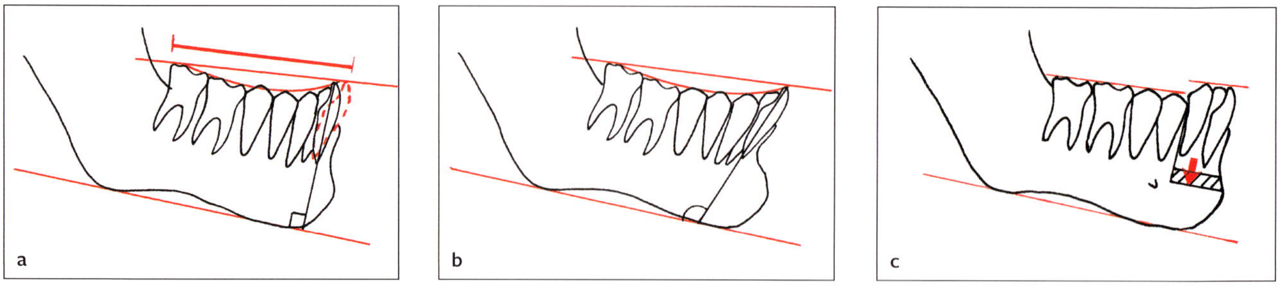

Fig 3-9 (*a*) An accentuated curve of Spee is present, and the incisors are upright. Labial movement of the incisors would create the extra space needed to level the arch. (*b*) The unfavorable position of the incisors does not allow arch leveling. Extractions are indicated. (*c*) Segmental alignments of the mandibular dental arch allow surgical leveling as an alternative. This does not require any additional arch length.

3. *Crowding in both dental arches, requiring extraction.* In patients requiring a large overjet, the maxillary second premolars and mandibular first premolars should be extracted. Keeping in mind the principles discussed in the two previous extraction patterns, the first or second premolars in both arches should be extracted.

Arch leveling requires arch length. Additional arch length will be necessary with crowding. For each 1 mm of leveling of the curve of Spee, the mandibular arch length will increase by 1 mm. Additional arch length will also be required when crowding is present. Further considerations include the angle of the mandibular incisors and the quality and amount of attached gingiva in the incisor region. If the mandibular incisors are angled lingually, improving the angulation by labial movement will create the space needed for arch leveling (Fig 3-9a). If the mandibular incisors are protrusive and crowding is present, extractions will be necessary (Fig 3-9b). The mandibular arch may be leveled surgically. This will not require additional arch length (Fig 3-9c). In Class II deep bite cases requiring mandibular advancement, the curve of Spee is not routinely leveled before surgery (see chapter 4).

Ensuring that the maxillary dental midline of the unoperated jaw coincides with the facial midline is another orthodontic consideration. Finally, the maxillary arch should be leveled, any arch rotations should be managed, and the dental arches should be compatible.

Maxillary repositioning

When the maxilla is advanced, the mandible (ie, the unoperated jaw)—especially the mandibular incisors—determines the new anteroposterior position of the maxilla (Fig 3-10). However, the surgeon may also alter the anterior facial height by inferior or superior repositioning of the maxilla. When the maxilla is superiorly repositioned (vertical maxillary excess) or downgrafted (vertical maxillary deficiency), the mandible will autorotate around a point at the condyle. Following any vertical changes, the anteroposterior position of the maxillary incisors will be determined by the anteroposterior position of the mandibular incisors after autorotation.

Correction of vertical maxillary excess by superior repositioning of the maxilla will result in superior and anterior rotation of the mandibular incisors caused by the autorotation of the mandible. It will make the occlusion more Class III and may require maxillary advancement in addition to superior repositioning (Fig 3-11). If necessary, the orthodontist should compensate the incisors for this added advancement of the maxilla. This may entail a slight retraction of the mandibular incisors or may necessitate two-jaw surgery if the anteroposterior discrepancy becomes too large to be treated by maxillary surgery only. Secondary anteroposterior changes following superior repositioning of the maxilla are summarized in Table 3-3.

Increasing the height of the maxilla by downgrafting will lead to clockwise rotation of the mandible (downward and backward). This secondary anteroposterior change will make the occlusion more Class II and may require orthodontic proclination of the mandibular incisors or even necessitate two-jaw surgery. Maxillary setback in these circumstances is not a good option and will worsen the esthetic outcome. Secondary anteroposterior changes following inferior repositioning (downgrafting) of the maxilla are summarized in Table 3-4.

Transverse discrepancies between the two dental arches can be surgically corrected. Narrowing or widening of the maxillary arch, vertical occlusal plane discrepancies (open bites), and interdental spaces in the maxillary arch may be corrected by segmental surgery (see chapter 4).

Orthodontic considerations

The orthodontic and surgical visual treatment objectives determine the ideal maxillary and mandibular incisor posi-

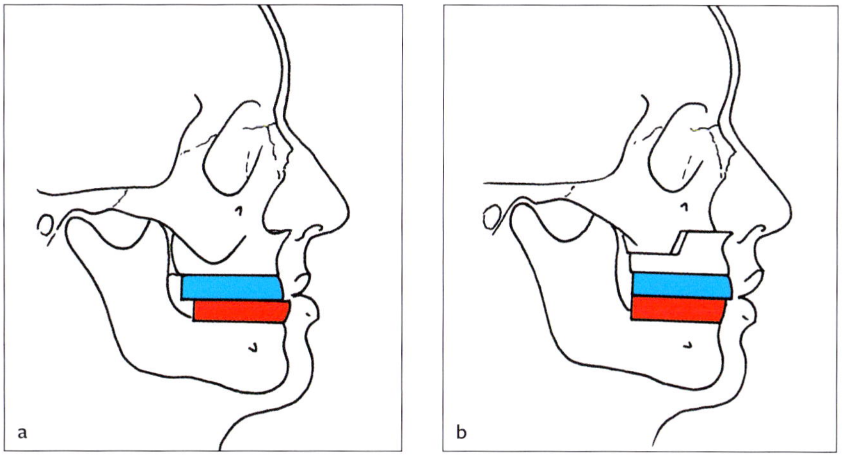

Fig 3-10 (*a*) Anteroposteriorly deficient maxilla with a Class III dental relationship. (*b*) The maxilla will be advanced to a Class I malocclusal relationship determined by the anteroposterior position of the mandibular incisors.

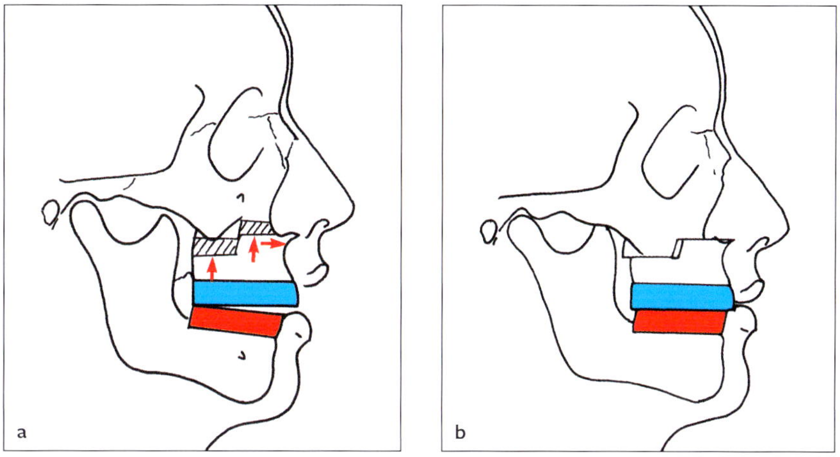

Fig 3-11 (*a*) Vertical maxillary excess and an anterior open bite malocclusion. (*b*) The bite is closed by surgical superior repositioning of the maxilla with autorotation of the mandible. Because of the anterior component of the autorotation, the maxilla needs to be advanced as well.

Table 3-3 | **Secondary anteroposterior changes following superior repositioning of the maxilla**

Following superior repositioning of the maxilla	Surgical correction of secondary skeletal anteroposterior problems	Orthodontic correction of secondary dental anteroposterior problems
Class I will rotate to Class III	Mandibular setback/maxillary advancement/genioplasty	Procline maxillary incisors/retract mandibular incisors
Class II will rotate to Class I	Genioplasty	Coordinate incisor positions
Super Class II will rotate to Class II	Mandibular advancement/genioplasty	Procline mandibular incisors/retract maxillary incisors
Class III will rotate to Super Class III	Maxillary advancement/mandibular setback/ genioplasty	Retract mandibular incisors/procline maxillary incisors

Table 3-4 | **Secondary anteroposterior changes following inferior repositioning (downgraft) of the maxilla**

Following maxillary inferior repositioning (downgraft)	Surgical correction of secondary skeletal anteroposterior problems	Orthodontic correction of secondary dental anteroposterior problems
Class I will rotate to Class II	Advance mandible/genioplasty (maxillary setback not recommended)	Procline mandibular incisors/retract maxillary incisors
Class II will rotate to Super Class II	Advance mandible/genioplasty	Procline mandibular incisors/retract maxillary incisors
Class III will rotate to Class I	Genioplasty	Coordinate incisor positions

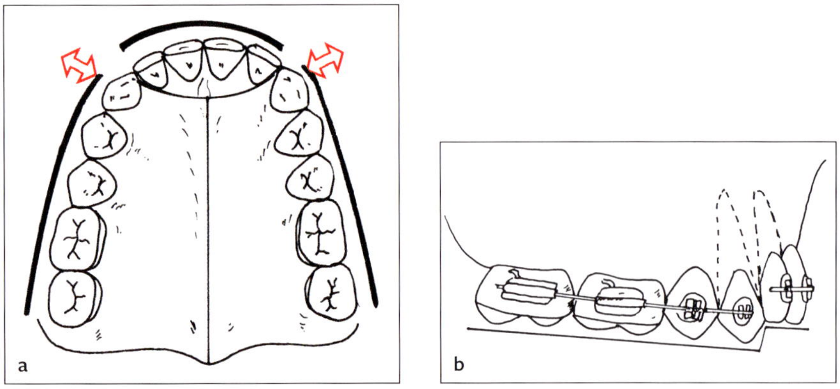

Fig 3-12 (*a*) Three-piece Le Fort I maxillary osteotomy, with the interdental osteotomy between the maxillary lateral incisors and canines. (*b*) Step in the occlusion between the anterior segment (the incisors) and posterior segments (canines through second molars bilaterally). The roots of the canine and lateral incisor are deviated. A shorter period of postsurgical orthodontics is required to correct the canine root positions.

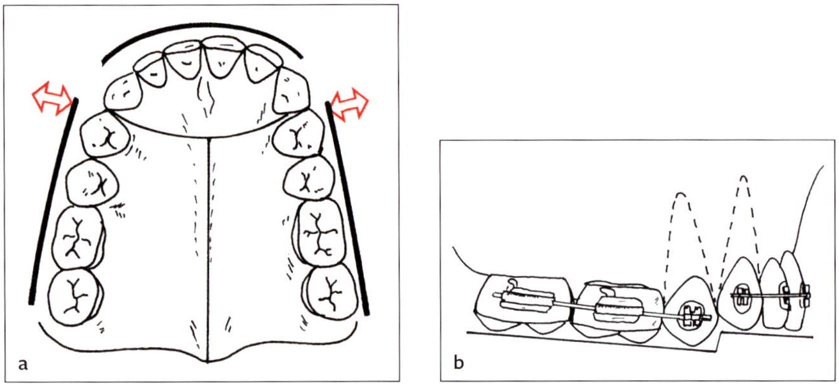

Fig 3-13 (*a*) Three-piece Le Fort I maxillary osteotomy, with the interdental osteotomy between the canines and premolars. (*b*) Step in the occlusion between the anterior segment (canines and incisors) and posterior segments (second premolars through second molars). The roots of the canine and second premolar are deviated. A longer period of postsurgical orthodontics is required to move the large canine root into a more correct distal inclination.

tions. Bear in mind that autorotation of the mandible will alter the anteroposterior position of the incisors.

Maxillary anteroposterior deficiency often results in crowding in the maxillary arch, and extractions may be necessary to accommodate all the teeth. Three extraction patterns may be implemented depending on the conditions:

1. Crowding in the anterior maxilla and no crowding in the mandible. Extraction of the maxillary first premolars will result in a Class II molar and Class I canine relationship after surgery. Extraction of the first premolars will also allow more retraction of the maxillary incisors.
2. Crowding in the posterior maxilla and no crowding in the mandible. Extraction of the maxillary second premolars will also result in a Class II molar and Class I canine relationship after surgery.
3. Crowding in both arches. The principles described in the two previous extraction patterns also apply here. Additionally, where a large overjet is required, the maxillary first premolars and mandibular second premolars should be extracted.

In patients for whom segmental surgery of the maxilla is planned (eg, for the surgical correction of open bites), extraction of the first premolars is preferred because it makes the orthodontic segmental alignment easier. The interdental osteotomy may be placed in one of two positions: between the deviated roots of the lateral incisors and canines or between the deviated roots of the canines and first premolars.

Placing the osteotomy between the deviated roots of the lateral incisors and canines has significant advantages (Fig 3-12). The surgeon has control over the intercanine width, which ensures a good Class I canine relationship. Furthermore, before surgery, the canine root is deviated distally, away from the interdental osteotomy site, to achieve the distalized canine root angulation that most clinicians aim for in their completed cases. This is important in the postsurgical orthodontic phase because a large canine root that requires distal movement can add many months to the finishing phase of orthodontics. Finally, with this method, the surgical site is more accessible and the interdental osteotomy is easier because the alveolar bone is thinner in this region.

Placing the osteotomy between the deviated roots of the canines and first premolars also has its advantages (Fig 3-13). This site is sometimes preferred when a natural step exists here in the pretreatment maxillary arch. Even though this site may be a more appropriate place for the segmental osteotomy, it necessitates significant postsurgical orthodontic work because the canine root must be tipped forward, away

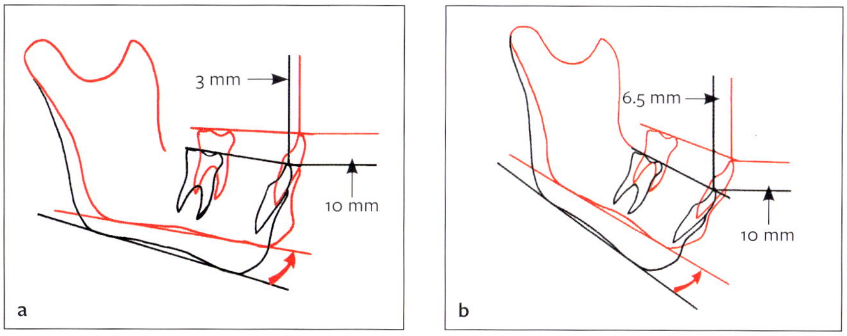

Fig 3-14 (*a*) Low-angle case with 10-mm superior repositioning of the maxilla. The mandible will rotate 10 mm superiorly and 3 mm anteriorly. (*b*) High-angle case. A 10-mm superior repositioning will result in a 6.5-mm anterior rotation of the mandibular incisors.

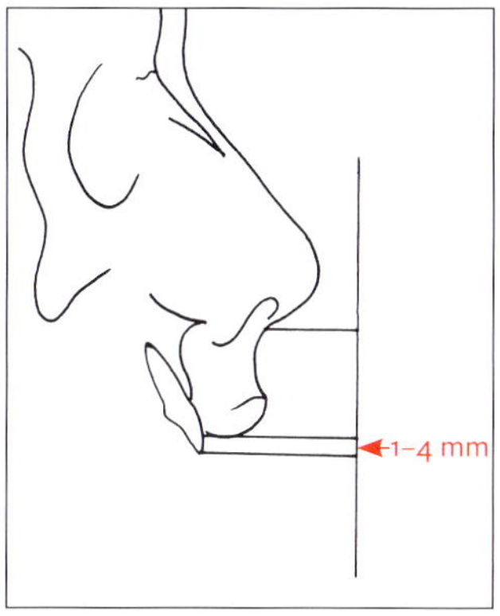

Fig 3-15 The ideal amount of maxillary tooth exposure under the relaxed upper lip should be 1 to 4 mm (less exposure in patients with long upper lips and more exposure in patients with short upper lips). Normal upper lip length is 20 ± 2 mm in females and 22 ± 2 mm in males.

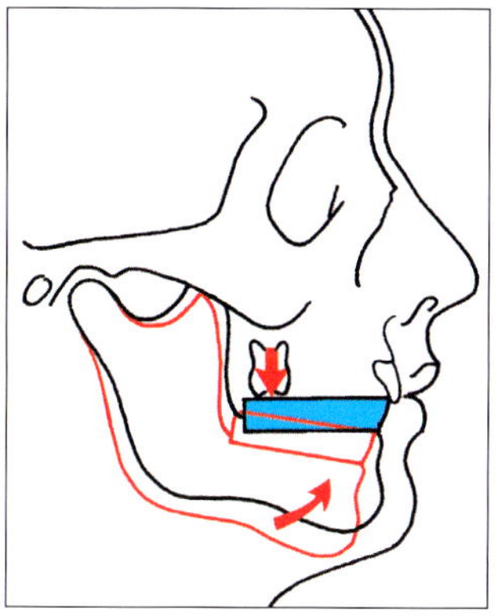

Fig 3-16 The final occlusal plane is determined by the mandibular occlusal plane once the vertical position of the anterior maxilla/mandible has been established. The vertical position of the posterior maxillary teeth will therefore be dictated by the posterior mandibular teeth (after autorotation).

from the osteotomy site, and this root angulation then must be corrected. This site is also preferred when first premolar extraction spaces are to be closed surgically. The orthodontist must ensure that the intercanine dimensions are coordinated because the surgeon has control over the width of the posterior segments only (unless further segmentalization of the maxilla is done). Bear in mind that residual extraction spaces in the maxilla may be closed by segmental surgery.

Counterclockwise rotation of the mandible will rotate the mandibular incisors anteriorly (more so in high-angle cases than in low-angle cases; Fig 3-14), whereas clockwise rotation will rotate the incisors posteriorly. This will have a significant effect on the final anteroposterior position of the maxilla.

The clinician must ensure that the dental midline of the mandible (ie, unoperated jaw) coincides with the facial midline. The maxillary dental midline can be corrected by the surgery. Finally, when segmental surgery is indicated (for narrowing, widening, vertical change, or closure of interdental spaces), the roots of the teeth adjacent to the interdental osteotomy should be deviated.

Two-jaw surgery: Maxillary and mandibular repositioning

With this scenario, the surgeon's "responsibility" increases. When two-jaw surgery is performed, surgery on the maxilla is usually performed first; however, it is the surgeon's choice as to which jaw will be repositioned first. The final position of the second jaw to be operated on will be determined by the jaw repositioned first, and the principles of single-jaw surgery then apply. The demand for surgical accuracy is obvious because any small inaccuracies during positioning of the first jaw will be accentuated when the second jaw is repositioned.

Surgical decisions

When maxillary surgery will be performed first in two-jaw surgery, several important decisions regarding the position of the maxilla need to be made:

- *Vertical positioning of the anterior maxilla.* This position is determined by the relationship between the maxillary incisors and the upper lip (Fig 3-15).
- *Vertical positioning of the posterior maxilla.* This position is determined by the mandibular molars after the mandible has autorotated, unless rotation of the maxillomandibular complex is indicated (Fig 3-16).
- *Vertical changes of the right and left sides of the maxilla.* These changes are relevant where a transverse maxillary occlusal plane cant exists (usually associated with facial asymmetry). The cant should be corrected, usually according to the interpupillary line. However, the interpupillary line may not always be in the horizontal plane and should be

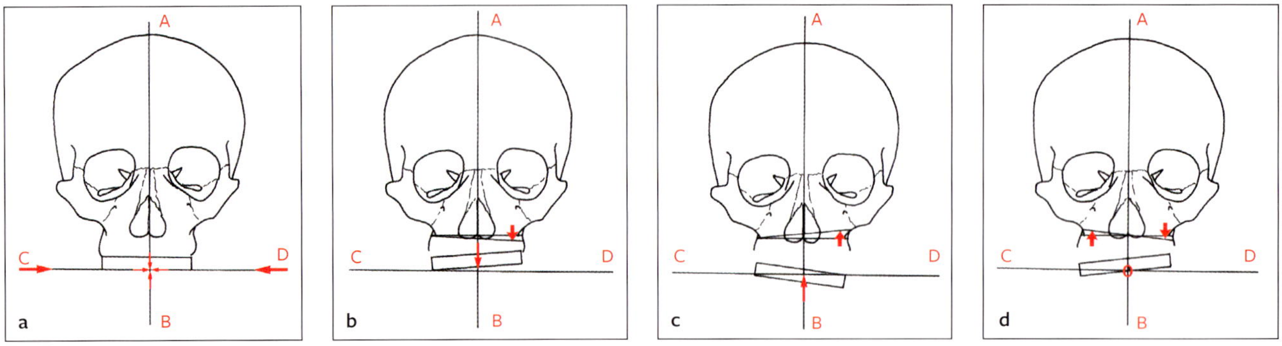

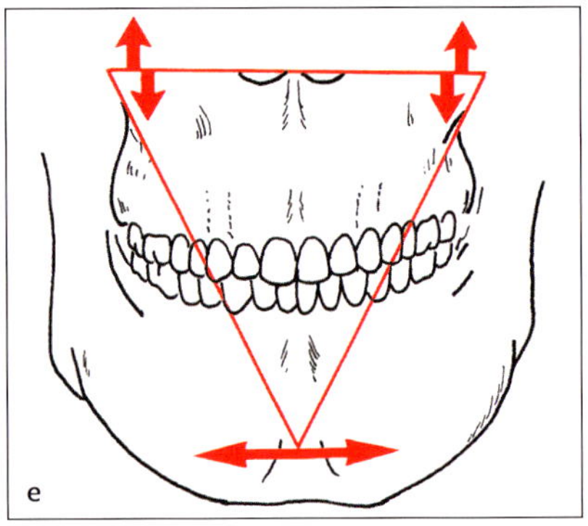

Fig 3-17 (*a*) Surgically correcting the transverse cant of the occlusal plane and, at the same time, ensuring ideal vertical and transverse position of the maxillary incisors. A-B represents the facial midline. C-D indicates the ideal vertical height of the maxillary incisors. (*b*) The left side of the maxilla is downgrafted. (*c*) The left side of the maxilla is superiorly repositioned. (*d*) The left side of the maxilla is downgrafted, and the right side is superiorly repositioned. (*e*) The constructed triangle illustrates the effect that change in the transverse occlusal cant may have on mandibular symmetry.

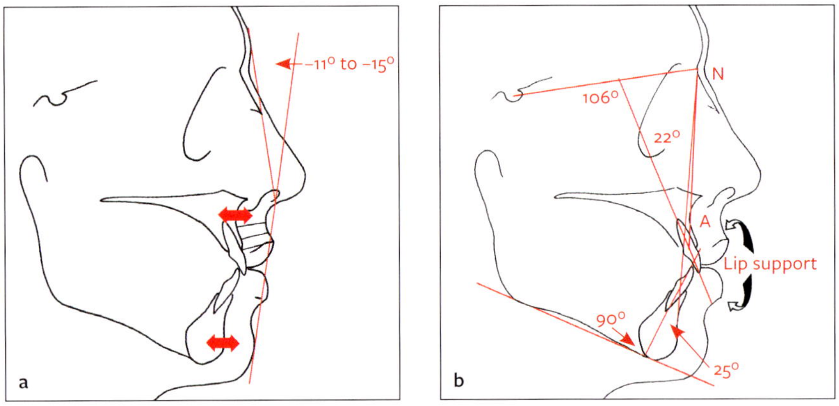

Fig 3-18 (*a*) The ideal facial contour angle (or angle of facial convexity) is –11 to –15 degrees. A maxilla positioned too far forward or a mandible positioned too far posteriorly would increase this angle, and vice versa. Class II cases will be more convex and Class III cases more concave. (*b*) The support rendered by the maxilla and maxillary incisors to the upper lip is mandatory for good esthetics. The position and angle of the maxillary incisors are also determining factors for the nasolabial angle. Normal angulation of the maxillary incisor to the N-A line is 22 degrees, with the incisal tip 4 mm ahead of N-A. A nasolabial angle of 90 to 110 degrees is considered ideal.

noted. Keep the vertical maxillary incisor–lip relationship in mind with the correction (Figs 3-17a to 3-17d). An alteration in the transverse cant of the occlusal plane in two-jaw surgery may have a profound effect on mandibular symmetry, and it is often integral in the correction of facial asymmetry involving both jaws (Fig 3-17e). 3D virtual treatment planning is certainly indicated when planning correction of facial asymmetry involving two-jaw surgery and simultaneous correction of an occlusal cant.

- *Anteroposterior position of the maxilla.* This position is determined by the maxillary incisor–lip relationship (lip support), paranasal form, and facial contour (Fig 3-18). It is preferable that arch symmetry and rotations be managed by the orthodontist during the presurgical orthodontic phase. However, this dimension should be noted by the surgeon before surgery and can be corrected during surgery if needed. However, the surgeon should take care not to build asymmetry into the result by neglecting this dimension.
- *Anteroposterior position of the left and right sides of the maxilla.* Any arch rotations will determine the changes in this dimension (Fig 3-19).
- *Transverse position of the maxilla.* This position is determined by the midline of the face. In two-jaw surgery, it is the surgeon's responsibility to position the dental midlines of both jaws and to ensure that the dental midlines and facial midlines coincide. Therefore, the orthodontist should not waste treatment time by correct-

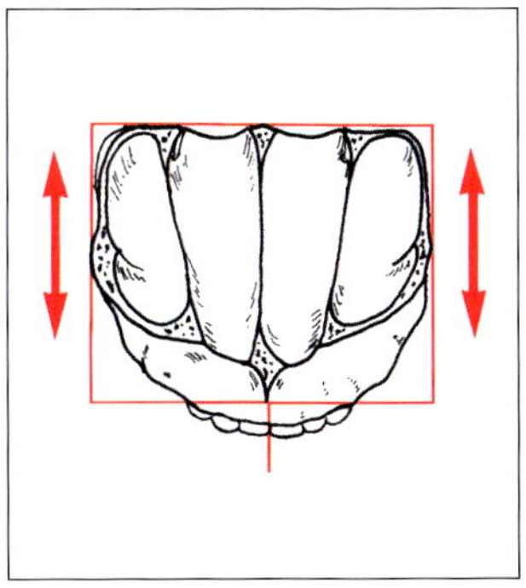

Fig 3-19 Arch relationships (compatibility) should not be confused with arch form, and both should be corrected orthodontically. However, the maxillary arch form may be altered surgically. In two-jaw surgery, the surgeon should ensure symmetrical positioning of the left and right sides of the maxilla.

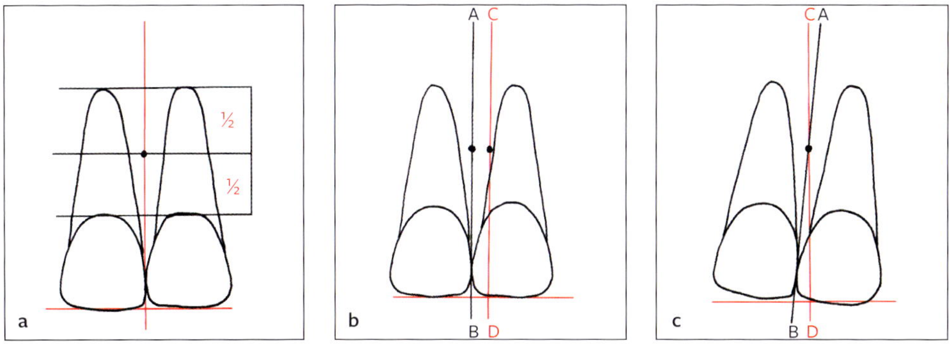

Fig 3-20 (*a*) The apical base midline is the central point vertically halfway between the central incisor roots. (*b*) The maxillary incisors are correctly angulated; however, the apical base midline (A-B) is asymmetric in relation to the facial midline (C-D). The maxillary midline should be surgically corrected. (*c*) Although the apical base midline (A-B) is central to the facial midline (C-D), the incisors are angled, and the maxillary dental midline is not centered. The midline should be corrected orthodontically in the preoperative orthodontic phase.

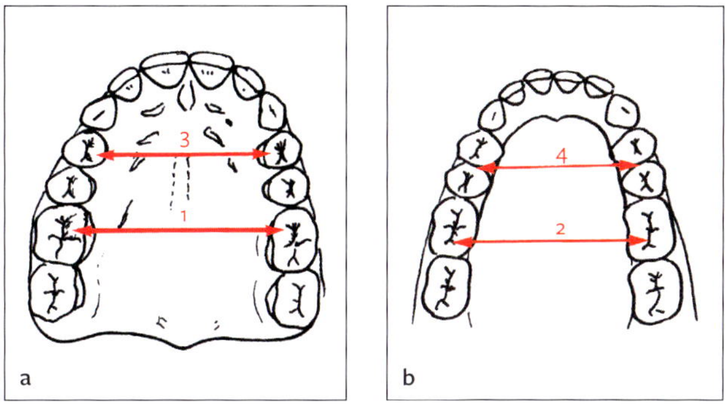

Fig 3-21 (*a and b*) Dental arch width may be assessed preoperatively by diagnostic casts or by measuring and comparing the distance between the mesiolingual cusps of the maxillary first molars (1) versus the central fossae of the mandibular first molars (2) and the distance between the lingual cusps of the maxillary first premolars (3) versus the centers of the distal marginal ridges of the mandibular first premolars (4).

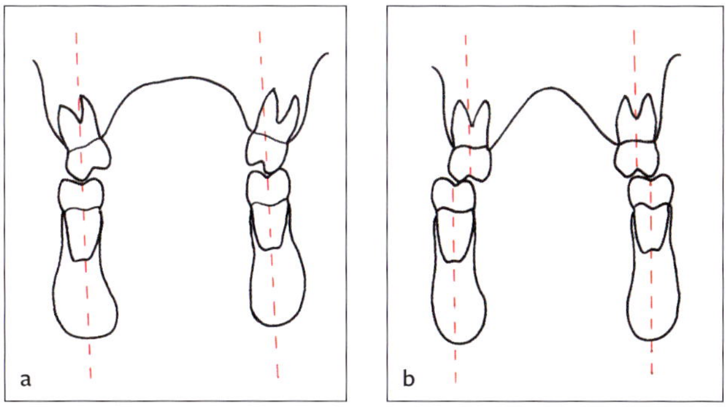

Fig 3-22 (*a*) The maxillary molars are tipped lingually although the skeletal maxillary width is adequate. The crossbite should be corrected orthodontically. (*b*) The crossbite is caused by a skeletal transverse deficiency of the maxilla and should be corrected surgically.

ing dental midlines. Keep in mind that in the mandible, the dental midline and the midline of the chin may not coincide, and genioplasty may have to be considered to correct the symmetry of the chin. In patients with chin asymmetry, the clinician should distinguish between dental midline and apical base midline (Fig 3-20).

- *Transverse dimension of the maxilla.* This dimension is determined by the width of the mandibular dental arch unless surgical change in the mandibular arch dimension is contemplated (Fig 3-21). A narrow maxillary dental arch caused by dental tipping should be corrected orthodontically. Skeletal transverse deficiency must be corrected by rapid palatal expansion in children or by surgically assisted orthodontics or segmental surgical expansion in adults (Fig 3-22; see chapter 4).

Repositioning of the maxilla entails accurate planning and meticulously performed surgery to establish the basis for mandibular repositioning.

Orthodontic considerations

The orthodontist should ensure that the maxillary dental arch is leveled. It is very difficult for the surgeon to place the anterior and posterior maxilla in the correct vertical position when there is an existing curve in the occlusal plane. In cases with an existing step in the occlusal plane, the dental arch should be orthodontically leveled in segments. The occlusal plane will then be leveled by means of segmental surgery.

Tooth extraction patterns in two-jaw surgery are influenced by the following: crowding (anterior or posterior), the amount of incisor discrepancy (overjet or crossbite) required to obtain optimal esthetics, the need to place teeth in a stable position in the central trough of bone, the curve of Spee, and the possibility of surgically closing residual extraction spaces. Here are some basic rules regarding orthodontic procedures for two-jaw surgery:

- The leveling of a transverse occlusal plane cant should not be attempted orthodontically in patients with facial asymmetry. The cant should be leveled surgically as part of the surgical correction of the facial asymmetry.
- Correct angulation and position of the maxillary incisors should be ensured. The position of the maxillary incisors (and their relationship to the upper lip) will determine the final anteroposterior position of the maxilla.
- A good arch form should be established. The orthodontist should not waste treatment time correcting anteroposterior and vertical discrepancies of the left or right side of the maxilla. These discrepancies can be corrected surgically.
- The maxillary dental midline should be corrected surgically as long as a good arch form exists.
- Transverse discrepancies involving dental tipping should be corrected orthodontically, whereas transverse skeletal discrepancies should be corrected surgically. Any orthodontic expansion in the maxilla beyond the skeletal base will have a strong tendency to relapse. Because the maxillary arch width is determined by the mandibular arch width, it is necessary to establish the mandibular arch form before surgery (eg, by decompensation of anterior and posterior teeth). When surgery on the maxilla is performed first, the anteroposterior, vertical, and transverse positions of the mandible will be determined by the maxilla after surgical repositioning. In contrast, the occlusal plane of the maxilla will be dictated by the occlusal plane of the mandible after autorotation.

Two-jaw surgery: Rotation of the maxillomandibular complex

Rotation of the maxillomandibular complex with consequent alteration of the angulation of the occlusal plane is a surgical treatment designed to achieve esthetic and functional results that cannot be achieved by conventional treatment. In this treatment scenario, the occlusal plane of the mandible (after autorotation) will not be the final occlusal plane (see chapter 4). Therefore, the surgeon has two additional decisions that must be made before positioning the maxilla:

1. Determine the new occlusal plane angle and the direction of rotation of the maxillomandibular complex. This decision will be influenced by the anteroposterior position of the chin, paranasal anatomy, and facial contour.
2. Determine the point around which the maxillomandibular complex will be rotated. By constructing a triangle involving the anterior nasal spine, posterior nasal spine, and pogonion (Pog) and varying the point of rotation or the direction of rotation, functional and esthetic possibilities can be investigated (Fig 3-23a). The position of the rotation point will be determined by the surgical cephalometric prediction tracing and will be influenced by the following:
   - The anteroposterior position of the chin (Pog). The higher and more anterior the point of rotation (ie, the closer to the anterior nasal spine), the more pronounced the anteroposterior movement of the chin (Fig 3-23b).
   - Paranasal flattening. The lower the rotation point (ie, the closer to Pog), the more pronounced the anteroposterior movement of the anterior nasal spine (Fig 3-23c).

The principles of the rotation of the maxillomandibular complex (alteration of the occlusal plane) are comprehensively discussed in chapter 4.

Orthodontic considerations

The orthodontic principles outlined in the previous section on two-jaw surgery with maxillary and mandibular repositioning also apply here. The practitioner should pay close attention to the angulation of the incisors and remember that it will change as a consequence of changing the angle of the occlusal plane. If necessary, the orthodontist should compensate for this expected change in angulation.

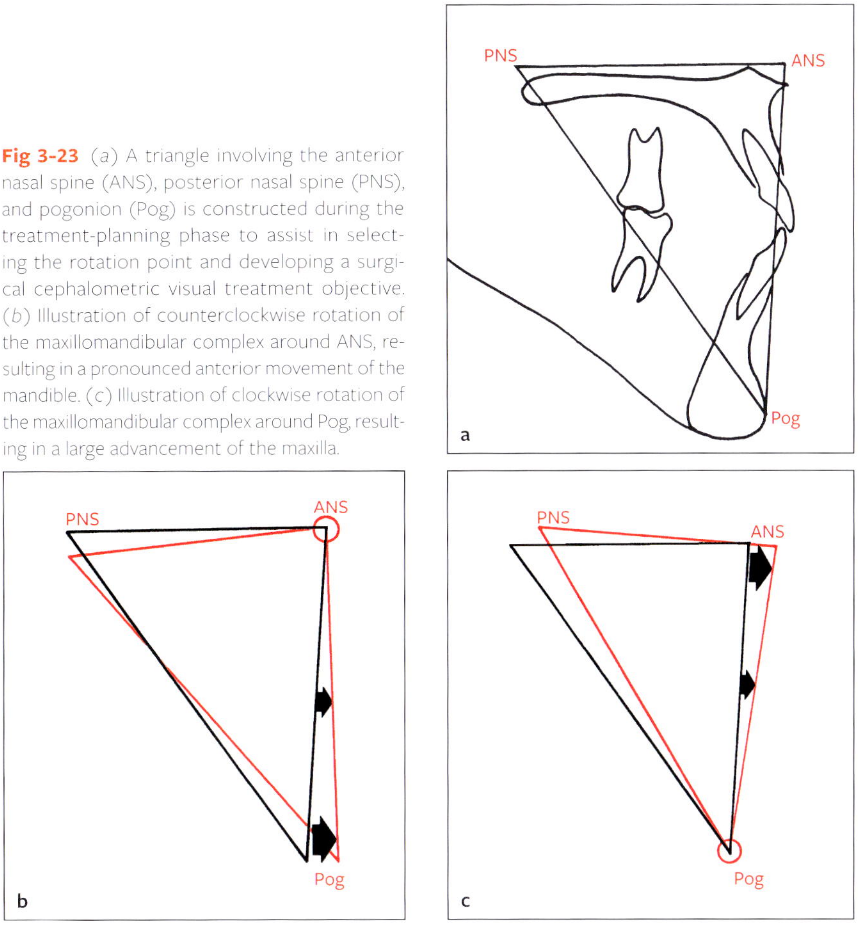

Fig 3-23 (*a*) A triangle involving the anterior nasal spine (ANS), posterior nasal spine (PNS), and pogonion (Pog) is constructed during the treatment-planning phase to assist in selecting the rotation point and developing a surgical cephalometric visual treatment objective. (*b*) Illustration of counterclockwise rotation of the maxillomandibular complex around ANS, resulting in a pronounced anterior movement of the mandible. (*c*) Illustration of clockwise rotation of the maxillomandibular complex around Pog, resulting in a large advancement of the maxilla.

Best Treatment Sequence to Obtain the Desired Result

The timing and sequencing of when orthognathic surgery should be performed may be influenced by several factors; such as development and growth of the patient; psychosocial conditions; temporomandibular joint (TMJ) ankylosis; the type of malocclusion (severe Class II deep bites, scissors bite); condylar pathology (resorption, hyperplasia, craniofacial syndromes); and sleep apnea. A growth modification approach to treatment is frequently considered by an evaluating orthodontist for a preadolescent child presenting with skeletal mandibular deficiency. In 2006, Cossa et al published a report following a systematic literature review on the efficacy of functional appliance use for enhancing mandibular growth in subjects with Class II malocclusion. They used a MEDLINE database and reviewed 704 articles published from January 1966 to January 2006. Only 22 articles qualified for final analysis, and only 4 were found to be scientifically worthy of inclusion in the study. It is interesting to note that none of the 4 trials found clinically significant changes in mandibular length induced by the functional appliance. Cossa et al (2006) are of the opinion that there are limited indications for a growth modification approach for patients with Class II malocclusion and in the early mixed dentition.

The goals of growth modification are frequently stated to be restraining maxillary forward growth while encouraging mandibular forward growth. However, this rationale often incorporates dental compensation for skeletal deformity, resulting in esthetic compromise (Fig 3-24). Most orthognathic surgical procedures should be delayed until completion of growth; however, the best time to perform the surgery during the surgical/orthodontic treatment is influenced by several factors (Fig 3-25).

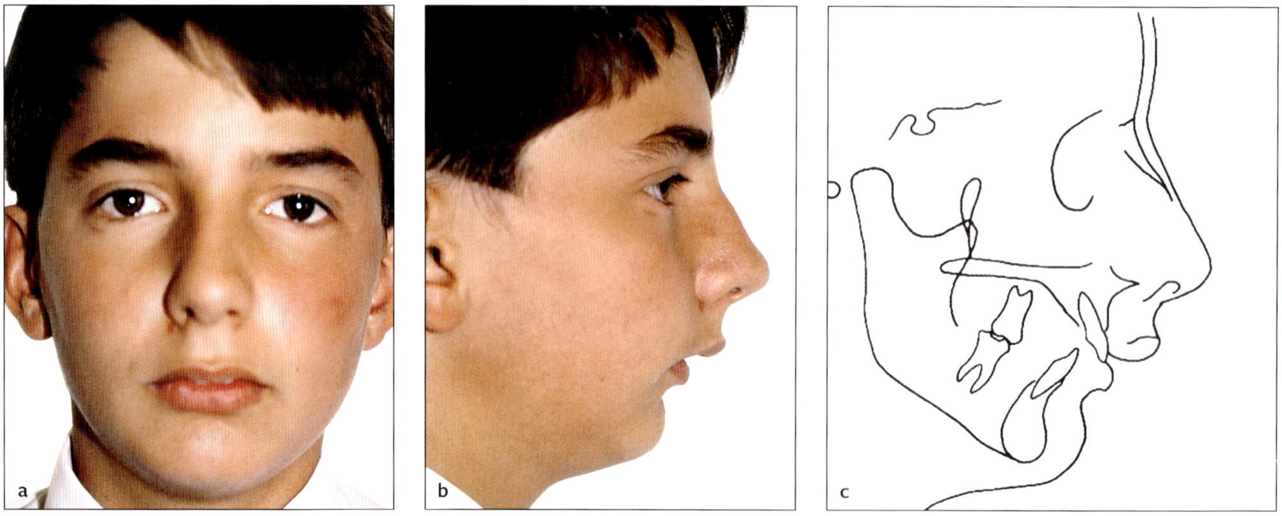

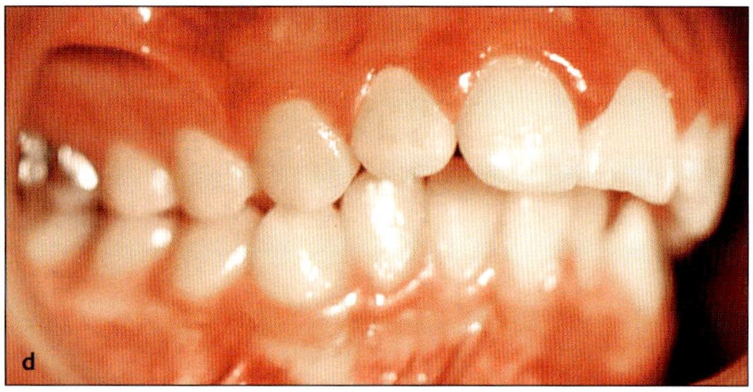

Fig 3-24 The frontal view (*a*), profile view (*b*), cephalometric tracing (*c*), and occlusion (*d*) of a 12-year-old boy following 2 years of growth modification. The treatment was further compromised by extraction of all four first premolars followed by orthodontic compromise for the severely deficient mandible. The poor result is demonstrated in frontal view (e), profile view (*f*), cephalometric tracing (*g*), and occlusion (*h*).

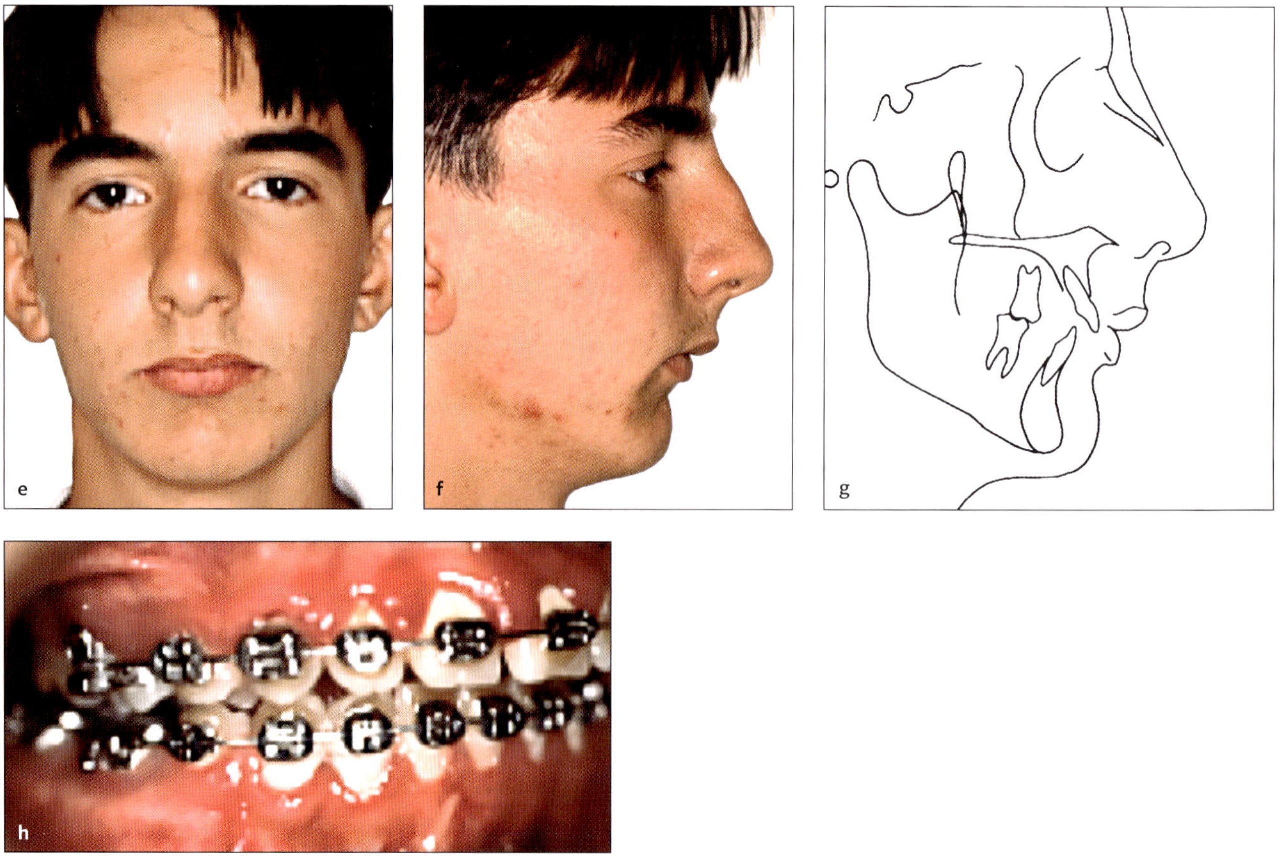

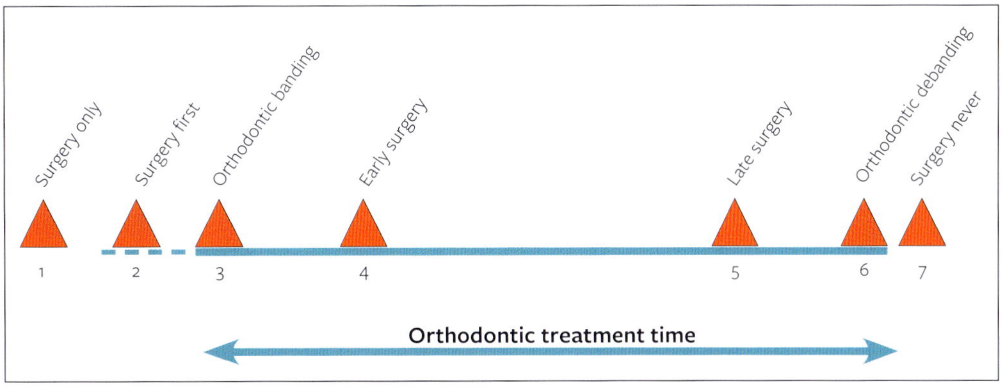

Fig 3-25 A schematic presentation of the timing of orthognathic surgery for patients with dentofacial deformities. The blue line represents the orthodontic treatment time. (1) Surgery is performed for patients not requiring any orthodontic alignment of their dentition. (2) Surgery first is performed before any orthodontic tooth alignment, and all the orthodontic tooth movements will take place after surgical correction of the jaw relationship. (3) Orthodontic banding occurs in the beginning of treatment. (4) Surgery is performed early in the orthodontic phase. (5) Surgery is performed once the dentition has been orthodontically prepared to enhance surgical accuracy and the occlusion. (6) The orthodontic appliances are removed and the retention phase starts. (7) In some cases, surgery is postponed indefinitely for various reasons (eg, medical, financial, psychologic).

Surgery without orthodontics

The indications to perform orthognathic surgery without orthodontic treatment are limited. The following groups of patients may be candidates for surgical intervention without presurgical orthodontic preparation:

1. Patient with severe obstructive sleep apnea and a Class I occlusion who require maxillomandibular advancement
2. Adolescent patients with TMJ ankylosis
3. Patients with certain syndromes (eg, hemifacial microsomia)

Surgery first

This approach involves performing the orthognathic surgery first with the specific intention to complete the treatment by orthodontically aligning the dentition in a second phase. Indications for surgery first are limited, and preliminary treatment planning is very demanding, requiring experienced clinicians.

Hernández-Alfaro and Guijarro-Martínez (2014) suggest that performing orthognathic surgery first should be considered (1) in cases with a skeletal malocclusion if no tooth extractions are required or (2) if the patient's motivation for treatment is esthetic improvement or to resolve a sleep disorder. They also state that the treatment should be managed by an experienced orthodontist. Exclusion factors for surgery first include active periodontal disease, active TMJ disorders (TMDs), severe 3D facial asymmetry, Class II deep bite malocclusions, and transverse maxillary deficiency requiring surgically assisted rapid palatal expansion (SARPE).

Surgery early in the orthodontic phase

In some instances, it would be advantageous to perform surgery early in the orthodontic phase of treatment and to facilitate and enhance the orthodontic treatment. Some examples include the following:

1. Patients with a scissors crossbite
2. Patients with a Class II deep bite
3. Alveolar cleft patients
4. Patients with severe crowding
5. Patients with certain syndromes (eg, hemifacial microsomia)
6. Patients requiring minimal orthodontic preparation and exhibiting an occlusion that would be acceptable following surgery soon after banding

Surgery later in the orthodontic phase

Some patients require tooth movements to allow for surgical jaw repositioning to be accurate and the planned occlusion to be achieved. In cases like this, surgery is performed later in the orthodontic treatment phase. It is usually preferable to perform basic restorative dental and periodontal treatment before beginning the preoperative orthodontic phase. This sequence will ensure that the dentition and supporting dental tissues are sound. It is also preferable to remove any impacted teeth at this stage. It is advantageous to achieve stable interdigitation of the teeth at the time of surgery for two reasons: (1) A good occlusion enhances postoperative stability and (2) it allows the orthodontist to finalize the occlusion in a relatively short time. The patient's enthusiasm for continued orthodontic treatment is likely to dwindle after surgery.

In general, the surgery should not be performed too early in the orthodontic phase for the following reasons:

- Delaying surgery allows the surgeon to position the jaws more accurately.
- Stability will improve because better interdigitation of the teeth can be achieved if the dental arches are better prepared.
- After surgery, the patient's appearance improves; as a consequence, motivation for correction of small orthodontic discrepancies diminishes and cooperation falters.

Surgery performed before presurgical orthodontic goals have been achieved will often lead to compromised surgical treatment, increased postoperative orthodontic treatment time, questionable stability, and unfavorable esthetics. Most orthodontic "mistakes" can be solved with orthodontic means, but surgical "mistakes" can and should be corrected by surgery (ie, reoperation).

In most cases, orthognathic surgery is performed once the planned presurgical orthodontic dental alignment has been completed. This will allow the surgeon to achieve the planned occlusion and usually only requires a relatively short period of postoperative orthodontic refinement. It is advantageous not to extend the postoperative orthodontic treatment beyond 3 to 6 months. If the postoperative orthodontic phase takes longer than anticipated, the orthodontist should reassess the case, possibly with new records, to determine the reason for the prolonged postoperative orthodontic treatment. Possible reasons may include poor patient cooperation, inaccurate surgery requiring longer orthodontic correction, skeletal relapse, and/or orthodontic relapse. The orthodontist should not attempt to correct significant skeletal relapse with orthodontics, but rather refer the patient back to the surgeon for reassessment.

In determining placement of dental implants, overall functional and esthetic results should be carefully considered. Implants can be placed during orthognathic surgery, saving the patient a second surgical procedure. Keep in mind that placement of dental implants during orthognathic surgery will limit any orthodontic tooth movement after surgery. However, the ideal time for placement of implants is after an orthodontic retention period of approximately 3 months. If bone grafting is required for the implants, the grafts can be placed during the orthognathic surgery. Prosthodontic restoration of dental implants should begin as soon as is practical. Early restoration will improve orthodontic stability and reduce the possibility of prepared spaces closing, should patients not cooperate in wearing retainers.

Development of Visual Treatment Objectives

During the last two decades, technological advances have had a major impact on the planning and efficiency of orthognathic surgery. Virtual surgical planning has become an increasingly important tool, especially for two-jaw surgery, correction of facial asymmetry, TMJ replacement, treatment of syndromic cases, and more. However, it is still necessary to be able to (1) develop an orthodontic prediction of tooth movement and (2) use cephalometric tracing to surgically reposition the jaws. Understanding these basic concepts is an important step in visualizing the orthognathic treatment.

Accurate and realistic visual treatment objectives are developed from the lateral cephalometric radiograph tracing in combination with all the data obtained from the systematic patient evaluation. There are two types of visual treatment objectives: the pretreatment visual treatment objective and the immediate presurgical prediction tracing.

The pretreatment visual treatment objective is developed once the primary surgical procedure has been selected. The following questions are used in its development:

- Will the selected surgical procedure produce the required facial esthetic changes?
- Will it be physically possible to create the skeletal change within the biologic boundaries?
- Will it be possible to orthodontically produce the tooth movements called for by the proposed surgery?

The pretreatment visual treatment objective is used for overall treatment planning. It consists of (1) an orthodontic prediction tracing illustrating the desired presurgical orthodontic tooth movement and the resulting soft tissue changes and (2) a surgical prediction tracing predicting the surgical repositioning of the jaws and subsequent soft tissue changes. The magnitude of the surgical movements of the jaws is not important at this stage as long as the procedure falls within the boundaries of good surgical technique. If more than one surgical or orthodontic option is under consideration, a series of prediction tracings should be made and all advantages and disadvantages of each treatment possibility analyzed. Where possible, simple treatment is best.

The immediate presurgical prediction tracing, which is created a few days before surgery, plans the definitive surgical movements and predicts the soft tissue changes. The presurgical orthodontic treatment is complete, and accurate tracing and measurement of surgical movements is now paramount.

The visual treatment objective has several advantages:

- It can accurately predict the soft tissue profile that will result after the proposed orthodontic tooth movements and surgical skeletal repositioning. The predicted soft tissue profile can be assessed and the treatment plan adjusted, if necessary.
- It enables the orthodontist and surgeon to investigate treatment options and evaluate the advantages and disadvantages of each option before treatment starts.
- It helps analyze the need for tooth extractions and indicates which teeth to extract.
- It helps assess the need for adjunctive surgical procedures (eg, genioplasty).
- It monitors the progress of orthodontic treatment using the orthodontic prediction.
- It helps assess the postsurgical skeletal movements.
- It acts as a communication medium between the orthodontist and the surgeon, as well as between the clinician and the patient.

Orthodontic Prediction Tracing

The presurgical position of the teeth dictates the surgical movement of the jaws and, ultimately, the soft tissue facial balance. Correct planning of orthodontic tooth positioning before surgery and accurate execution of the presurgical orthodontic plan will enhance the surgical potential and therefore the esthetic result. Because of the myriad treatment possibilities, it is impossible to discuss method and development for every conceivable treatment objective. Thus, the following sections demonstrate the development of a few prediction tracings that will be helpful in most treatment planning.

Mandibular advancement

Figure 3-26 shows the pretreatment cephalometric analysis of a patient who will benefit from a mandibular advancement. Cephalometric parameters, discussed in chapter 2, may be used as indicators of the dental, soft tissue, and hard tissue objectives. As has been noted, the cephalometric values should be used as a guide, and compromise (dental, skeletal, or soft tissue) may be necessary in formulating the best possible treatment for each patient.

When mandibular advancement is contemplated, the shape of the chin should be assessed as part of the orthodontic treatment planning. Esthetic planning of the soft tissue of the chin should assess the horizontal position of the soft tissue pogonion (Pog′), but the actual shape of the chin is more important in the overall esthetics. The following factors should be considered in the assessment of chin esthetics (Fig 3-27): vertical height of the chin, lower lip length, amount of lower lip vermilion exposed, depth of the labiomental fold, lower lip–chin–throat angle, chin-throat length, curvature of the chin, and horizontal relation of the labrale inferior (Li) and Pog′.

Figure 3-28 illustrates chin shape in three patients with ideal incisal relationships and Pog′ in the same horizontal position. Because of the variation in the shapes of their chins, however, the three patients have different esthetic appearances.

Therefore, when there is a clear indication for genioplasty to improve the shape of the chin, it should be incorporated in the orthodontic prediction tracing so the presurgical orthodontic tooth positioning will allow for the correct amount of mandibular advancement and incorporate the planned amount of chin advancement for the best esthetic result.

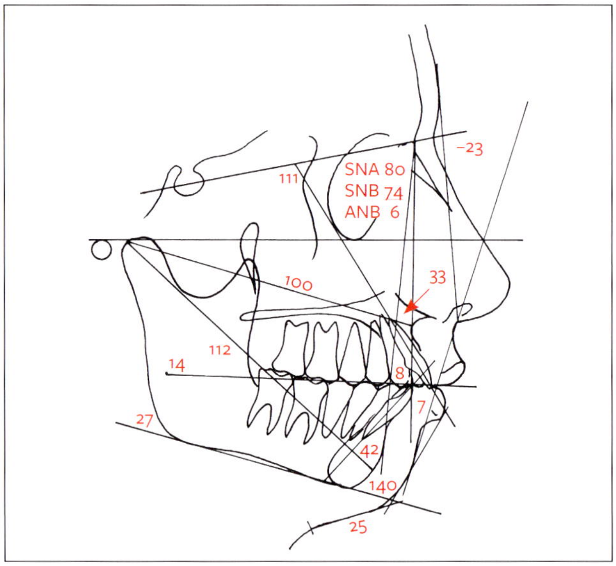

Fig 3-26 The pretreatment cephalometric analysis of a patient with the following diagnostic summary: 17-year-old girl whose main complaint is that her chin appears deficient. Skeletal: mandibular anteroposterior deficiency and microgenia. Dental: Class II, division 1 malocclusion; slightly narrow maxillary arch; slight maxillary incisor protrusion; mandibular incisor protrusion; and crowding in the mandibular incisor area. Soft tissue: convex profile, deficient chin, and short chin-throat length.

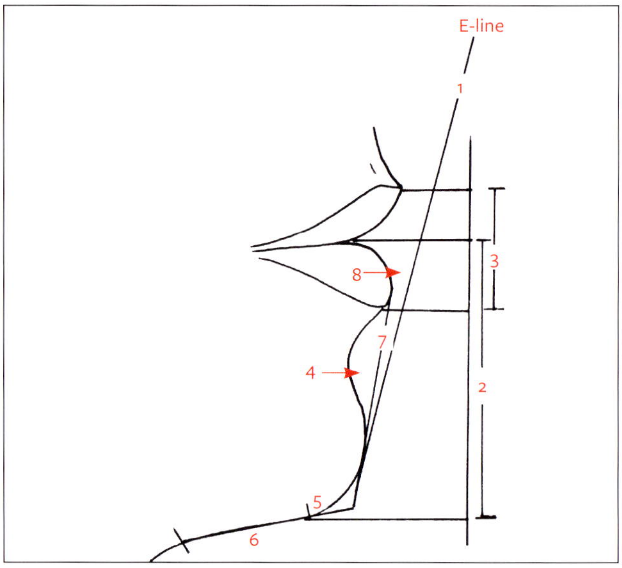

Fig 3-27 Parameters used in the evaluation of the overall esthetics of the chin. The esthetic line (E-line) (1) is drawn from nasal tip (Pn) to Pog′. The height of the chin (2) should be equivalent to two-thirds of the lower third of the face (subnasale-stomion:stomion–soft tissue menton = 1:2). Also known as *lower lip length*, chin height should be 40 ± 2 mm (females) and 44 ± 2 mm (males). Vermilion exposure (3): The lower lip exhibits approximately 25% more vermilion than the upper lip. Depth of the labiomental fold (4): The labiomental fold should have a smooth, concave curve connecting the lower lip with the chin. Mandibular-prognathic cases often exhibit flat labiomental folds, whereas mandibular-deficient cases often have deep folds. Lower lip–chin–throat angle (5): 110 ± 8 degrees. This angle tends to be smaller than normal in mandibular prognathism and larger than normal in mandibular deficiency cases. Chin-throat length (6): normal, 42 ± 6 mm. An advancement genioplasty will clearly increase this distance. The distance will decrease when the chin is set back. Curvature of the chin (7): The shape of the chin is enhanced if the profile forms a smooth S shape from stomion inferius to soft tissue menton. The lower lip should be 2 ± 2 mm behind the E-line (8).

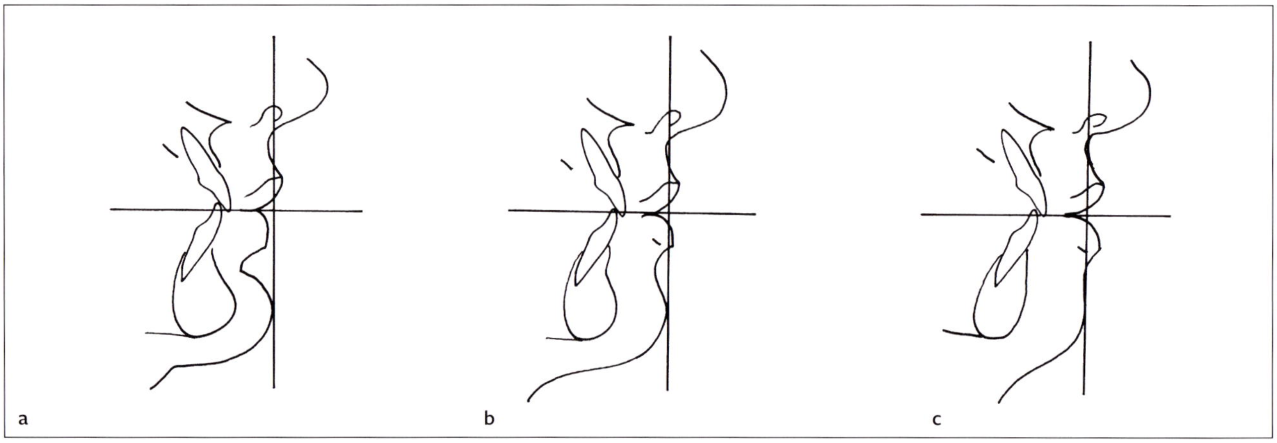

Fig 3-28 The fact that chin shape is more important than the horizontal position of Pog′ in overall esthetics is demonstrated in individuals with the following characteristics: (*a*) a deep labiomental fold and a knobby chin, (*b*) an esthetically well-shaped chin, and (*c*) an obtuse labiomental fold that gives the chin a flat appearance. All three individuals have Pog′ in exactly the same horizontal position.

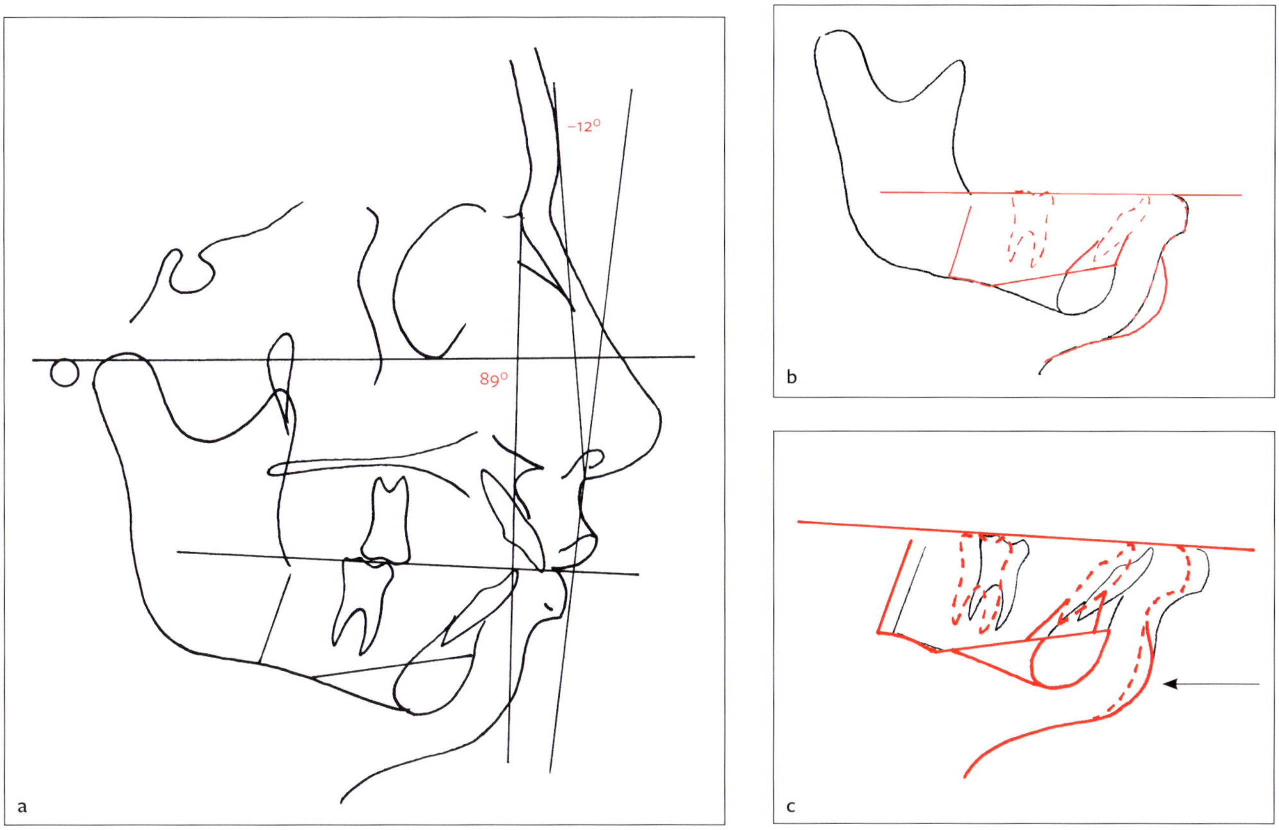

Fig 3-29 (*a*) Step 1: The original tracing. (*b*) Step 2: The prediction tracing. (*c*) Prediction of bony advancement of the chin (ratio of soft tissue to hard tissue advancement = 0.9:1.0) is done after the prediction tracing is moved to the left until predicted soft tissue at Pog′ coincides with that of the original tracing (*arrow*).

Step 1

Create the original tracing by tracing the hard and soft tissue, without analysis lines, on a separate sheet of acetate. In this case, the facial depth angle and facial contour angle are used as indicators of the "ideal" hard and soft tissue positions, respectively. The facial depth angle is formed by passing a line from nasion (N) through A-point and the Frankfort horizontal (FH) plane (with the maxilla in good position: males, 90 degrees; females, 89 degrees). An extension of the N-A line should go through Pog′. The facial contour angle is formed between the upper facial plane (UFP) and lower facial plane (LFP) and should be –11 to –15 degrees for males and –13 to –17 degrees for females. Also, draw a vertical line on the mandible posterior to the second molar, representing the vertical osteotomy line of the sagittal split osteotomy; draw a horizontal line on the chin, representing the genioplasty osteotomy line (Fig 3-29a).

Step 2

In this case, clinical and cephalometric assessment of the chin shape indicates an advancement genioplasty. Begin the prediction tracing by tracing the mandible anterior to the vertical osteotomy line and above the horizontal osteotomy line in red on a clean piece of acetate. The teeth, lower lip, and chin are traced in dotted lines. Draw the ideal soft tissue chin shape on this tracing (Fig 3-29b). Bearing in mind that soft tissue change in relation to hard tissue repositioning of the chin is 0.9:1.0, draw in the actual required bony advancement by sliding the prediction tracing to the left until the predicted soft tissue coincides with the soft tissue on the original tracing. The Pog′ should now be at, or very close to, the desired horizontal position, and the shape of the chin should be esthetically pleasing. Trace the occlusal plane (Fig 3-29c).

In this case, the mandibular occlusal plane is level. However, patients with Class II malocclusion often have deep bites with an accentuated curve of Spee. Preoperative versus postoperative leveling of the curve of Spee should be considered carefully because the choice affects facial esthetics, the amount of surgical advancement, and the need for genioplasty. An excessive curve of Spee should be leveled before surgery in the following cases:

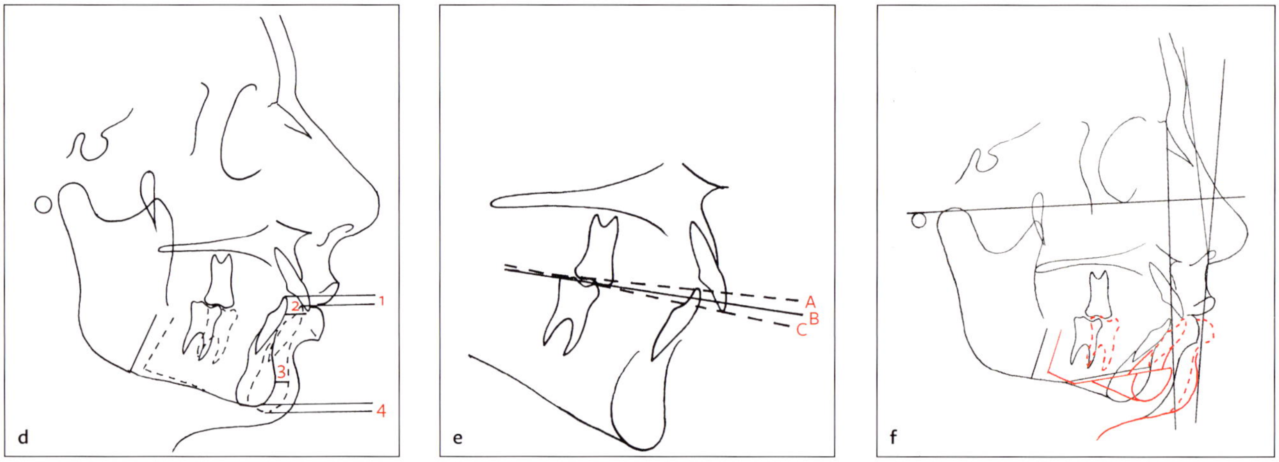

Fig 3-29 *(cont)* (*d*) The curve of Spee is not leveled, and as the mandible is advanced, the mandible will rotate clockwise. The incisors will advance (2) more than the Pog′ (3), whereas correction of the deep bite (1) will increase the vertical height of the chin (4) by the same amount. (*e*) Three occlusal planes: the molar-incisor plane of the mandible (A), the functional occlusal plane (B), and the molar-incisor plane of the maxilla (C). (*f*) Step 3.

- When the chin needs to be advanced the same distance as the mandibular incisors
- When little vertical increase in the lower facial height is indicated; in high-angle cases, the vertical increase is slightly more than in low-angle cases because of the steepness of the occlusal plane
- When less decompensation of the incisors will be necessary to achieve the desired chin projection

The curve of Spee should not be leveled prior to surgery when a clockwise rotation of the distal portion of the mandible will be advantageous (Fig 3-29d); for example:

- When the incisors need to be advanced more than the chin
- When the anterior vertical height of the lower third needs to be increased by the amount of excess of the overbite
- When a deep labiomental fold (usually present with deep bites) will improve because of the advancement of the mandibular incisors and downward rotation of the chin

Taking these factors into account, the clinician should choose the plane of advancement. The mandible can be advanced along one of three occlusal planes (Fig 3-29e): (1) the functional occlusal plane, (2) the molar-incisor plane of the maxilla, or (3) the molar-incisor plane of the mandible (in this case, all three planes are the same).

Step 3

Slide the prediction tracing to the right along the chosen occlusal plane (in this case, the functional occlusal plane) until the Pog coincides with the facial depth line and the Pog′ coincides with the LFP line (or best fit; Fig 3-29f). The soft tissue should take precedence because it will determine the esthetic result.

Step 4

Trace the rest of the facial structures. The maxillary teeth are drawn in dotted lines (Fig 3-29g). It is now clear that the mandibular advancement has resulted in an anterior crossbite. Can the teeth be orthodontically positioned in their ideal relationship to bone and to each other in the new jaw relationship? The clinician has various options:

- Retraction of the mandibular incisors with or without extractions
- Advancement of the maxillary incisors
- Less advancement of the mandible and more advancement of the chin

Step 5

Various cephalometric parameters may now be used on the prediction tracing to place the teeth in their ideal position in each arch and in relation to each other. Draw the incisors in their best possible position on the prediction tracing (Fig 3-29h).

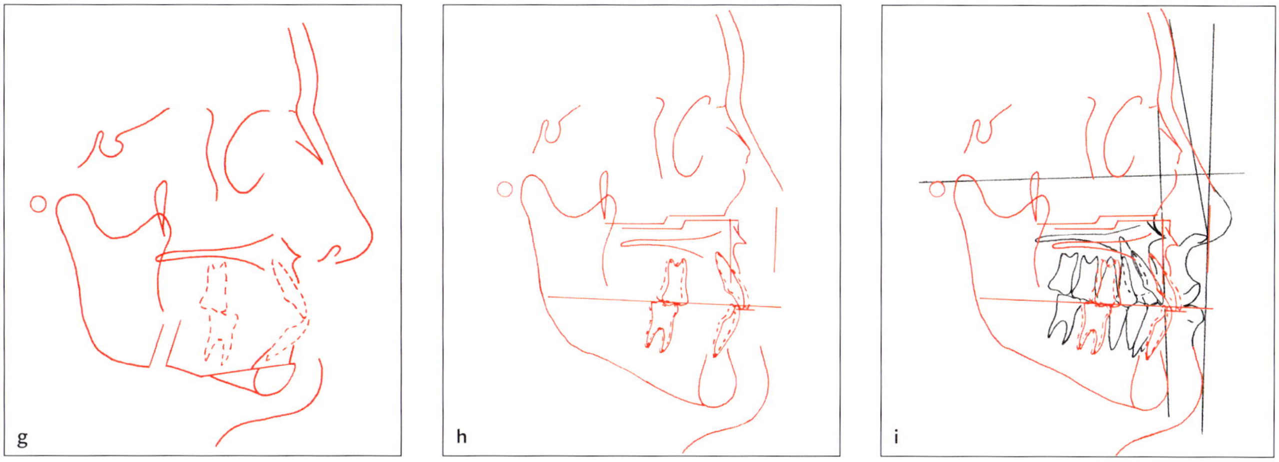

Fig 3-29 *(cont)* (*g*) Step 4. (*h*) Step 5. (*i*) Step 7.

Step 6

The predicted incisor positions are now carefully studied. In this case, the mandibular incisors will have to be retracted. However, the clinician should keep in mind not to excessively retract the maxillary incisors, because this would undermine lip support and limit mandibular advancement. The maxillary arch in Class II cases often needs some expansion to accommodate the mandibular arch after advancement. This expansion, in turn, often offers sufficient space for ideal positioning of the maxillary incisors. Extraction of premolars (first or second) may be indicated where crowding and an occlusal curve are present. Every 1 mm of arch leveling will increase the anteroposterior arch length by 1 mm. However, there will be an approximate 1-mm increase in arch length for every 1 mm of expansion of the arch at the canine area and a 4-mm increase for a 1-mm arch expansion in the molar area. The clinician can make a decision regarding tooth extraction by taking the following factors into account:

- Current incisor position
- Required incisor position to facilitate the correct amount of mandibular advancement
- Amount and area of crowding
- Extent of the occlusal curve
- Need for arch expansion
- Possibility of interdental stripping

Step 7

The required arch length can now be established. If tooth extractions are indicated, the width of the teeth to be extracted should be subtracted from the existing arch length. The remainder of space (if any) can be closed by advancing the molars. The feasibility of the predicted position of the incisors will now be evident. In some cases, it may be necessary to make small dental compromises because of lack of arch length (even with tooth extractions), thin mandibular symphysis limiting tooth movement, or increase in treatment time. In this case, two premolars should be extracted to achieve the amount of mandibular incisor retraction indicated on the prediction tracing. The remaining space will be made up by advancing the molars.

The molar relationship can also be established. In this case, where extractions are not indicated in the maxillary arch, the maxillary molar does not move and is placed in a Class III relationship to the mandibular molar. The mandibular molar is advanced slightly to close the remaining extraction space once the incisor has been retracted sufficiently (Fig 3-29i).

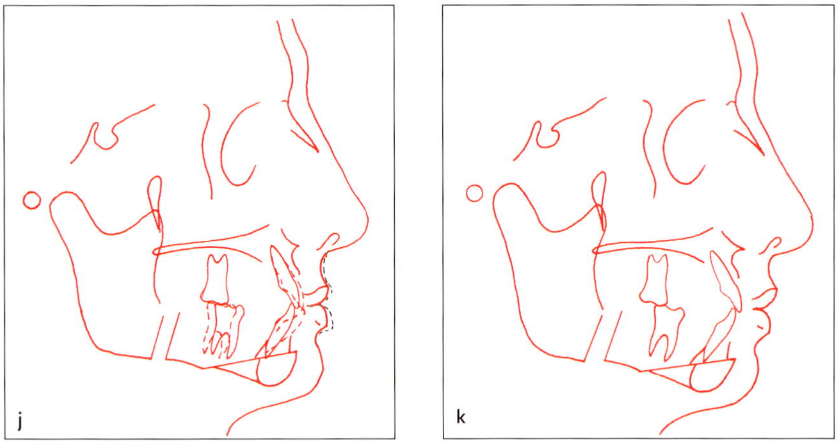

Fig 3-29 *(cont)* (*j*) Step 8. (*k*) Completed prediction tracing.

Step 8

The soft tissue profile prediction can now be completed. The upper lip will change very little because of the small amount of maxillary incisor retraction. In contrast, the lower lip will roll back subsequent to retraction (decompensation) of the mandibular incisors, as well as because of the elimination of the effect of the maxillary incisors on the lower lip. The rotation of the lower lip affects the soft tissue superior to the labiomental fold. Generally, the lower lip has the same thickness as the upper lip (Fig 3-29j).

Figure 3-29k illustrates the completed prediction tracing (visual treatment objective stage). The tracing indicates the intended orthodontic tooth movement, the surgical repositioning of the mandible and chin, and the expected soft tissue result.

Maxillary advancement

Figure 3-30a illustrates a cephalometric tracing and analysis of a patient who will benefit from a maxillary advancement procedure. Begin the original tracing by tracing all the relevant hard and soft tissues on a clean piece of acetate. Also trace all the teeth because this will assist in the prediction of the orthodontic tooth movement. Draw the Le Fort I osteotomy line on the maxilla as well as the mandibular occlusal plane. The following lines are drawn and angles constructed to assist in the ideal positioning of the teeth and in the surgical repositioning of the maxilla (Fig 3-30b):

- The facial depth line is drawn by dropping a line perpendicular to FH from N. The line should be tangent to A-point, as well as to Pog. In this case, however, the line is 5 mm ahead of the A-point, confirming the diagnosis of maxillary anteroposterior deficiency.
- The ideal position of subnasale (Sn) is predicted by constructing the ideal facial contour angle for the patient. In this case, a facial contour angle of −13 degrees is chosen. The UFP and the LFP are drawn at an angle of 13 degrees with the help of a protractor. The glabella (G) and Pog′ are static; Sn is advanced.

Step 1

Trace all the facial structures that will not be affected by the surgery on a clean piece of acetate. Trace the cranial base, soft tissue chin below the labiomental fold, hard tissue above the Le Fort I osteotomy line, mandible, mandibular occlusal plane, forehead, and soft tissue of the nose above the supratip break. The mandibular teeth (molar and incisor) are drawn in a dotted line. Trace the facial depth line and LFP in the midface region. The facial depth line is an indicator of the required A-point position on the maxilla, and the LFP indicates the required position of Sn. This tracing will develop into the prediction tracing (Fig 3-30c).

Step 2

Slide the prediction tracing to the left. The original tracing will move to the right, advancing the maxilla. Advance the maxilla on the original tracing until A-point is tangent to the facial depth line and Sn is tangent to LFP or best fit. In this case, A-point is moved just past the facial depth line whereas Sn falls short of LFP. Place the maxillary incisor tip on the horizontal incisor line (Fig 3-30d). Now draw the maxillary molars and incisors with dotted lines on the prediction tracing (Fig 3-30e).

The prediction tracing can now be carefully studied and the following observations made:

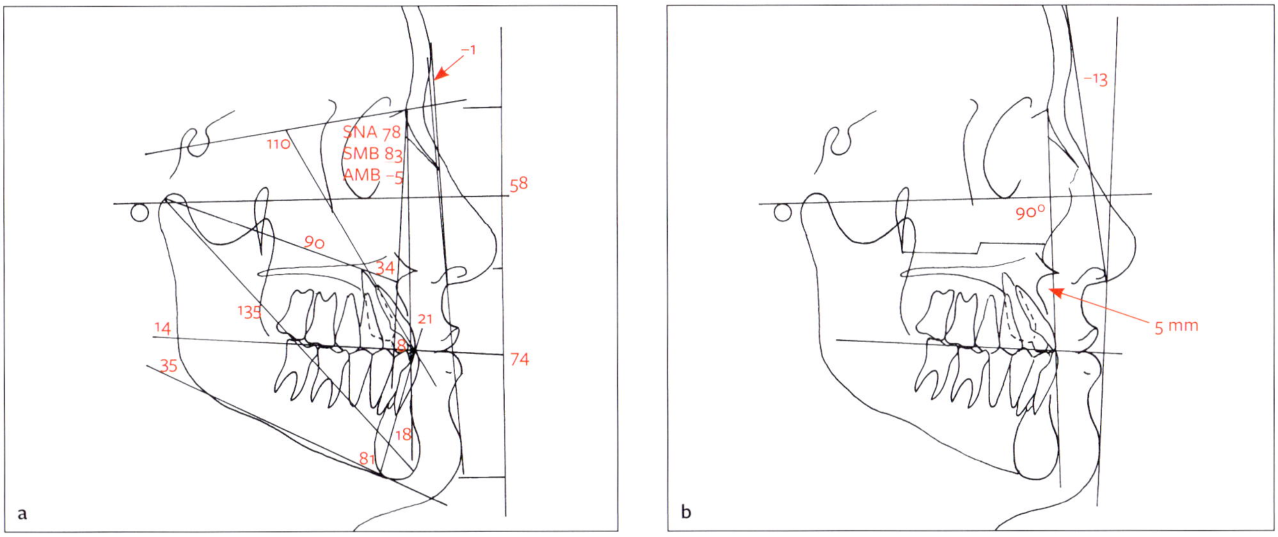

Fig 3-30 (*a*) The cephalometric analysis of a patient with the following diagnostic summary: 19-year-old man referred for the correction of a Class III malocclusion. Skeletal: maxillary anteroposterior deficiency and a tendency to vertical maxillary deficiency (clinically there is a 1-mm maxillary exposure under the upper lip with the lips slightly apart). Dental: Class II malocclusion, crowding in the maxillary arch (the maxillary canines are partially blocked out labially), and mandibular incisors slightly compensated. Soft tissue: lack of upper lip support, concave profile, and flat paranasal area. (*b*) The facial depth line, facial contour angle, occlusal plane, and Le Fort I maxillary osteotomy line on the original tracing.

- An increased incisor overjet is present.
- The maxilla is advanced by 6.5 mm.
- The maxilla is inferiorly repositioned by 2 mm.
- The molars are now in a Class II relationship.

The clinician has the following options:

- Advance the maxilla less to get a better occlusal relationship, and retract the maxillary incisors. However, there is still crowding in the maxillary arch. A small advancement would compromise the esthetic result.
- Extract the maxillary first premolars and retract the maxillary incisors, improving their angulation. The remaining space will be taken up by advancement of the molars. Decompensate the mandibular incisors. Keep the maxillary advancement at 6.5 mm.

It is clear that the second treatment option will achieve the better result. Trace the maxillary hard tissue and the Le Fort I osteotomy line (Fig 3-30f). Figure 3-30g illustrates what the prediction tracing should look like at this stage.

Step 3

Draw the maxillary incisor on the prediction tracing with the aid of cephalometric guidelines, keeping the tooth in the central trough of bone. Draw in the maxillary molar by advancing it slightly (the first premolars have been extracted), closing the remaining space. Decompensate the mandibular incisor by moving it slightly labially; then draw the tooth on the prediction tracing. The mandibular molar position will change very little (Fig 3-30h).

Step 4

The prediction tracing is now superimposed on its position on the original tracing. The surgical change in the position of the maxilla is clear (Fig 3-30i). The soft tissue changes subsequent to the repositioning of the maxilla can now be drawn in:

- Vermilion (stomion superius): 50% to 75% of horizontal movement
- Nasolabial angle: decreases 1 to 4 degrees per 1-mm advancement
- Nasal tip: advances 30% (variable) and can be controlled

First, draw the predicted soft tissue change with a dotted line (Fig 3-30j). When you are satisfied with the prediction, complete the line. Draw the soft tissue of the lower lip above the labiomental fold. Because of the effect of the upper lip on the lower lip, slight curling of the lower lip is expected (see Fig 3-30j).

Step 5

Complete the visual treatment objective by measuring the horizontal and vertical change between the two Le Fort I maxillary osteotomy lines, and note the orthodontic tooth movements (Fig 3-30k).

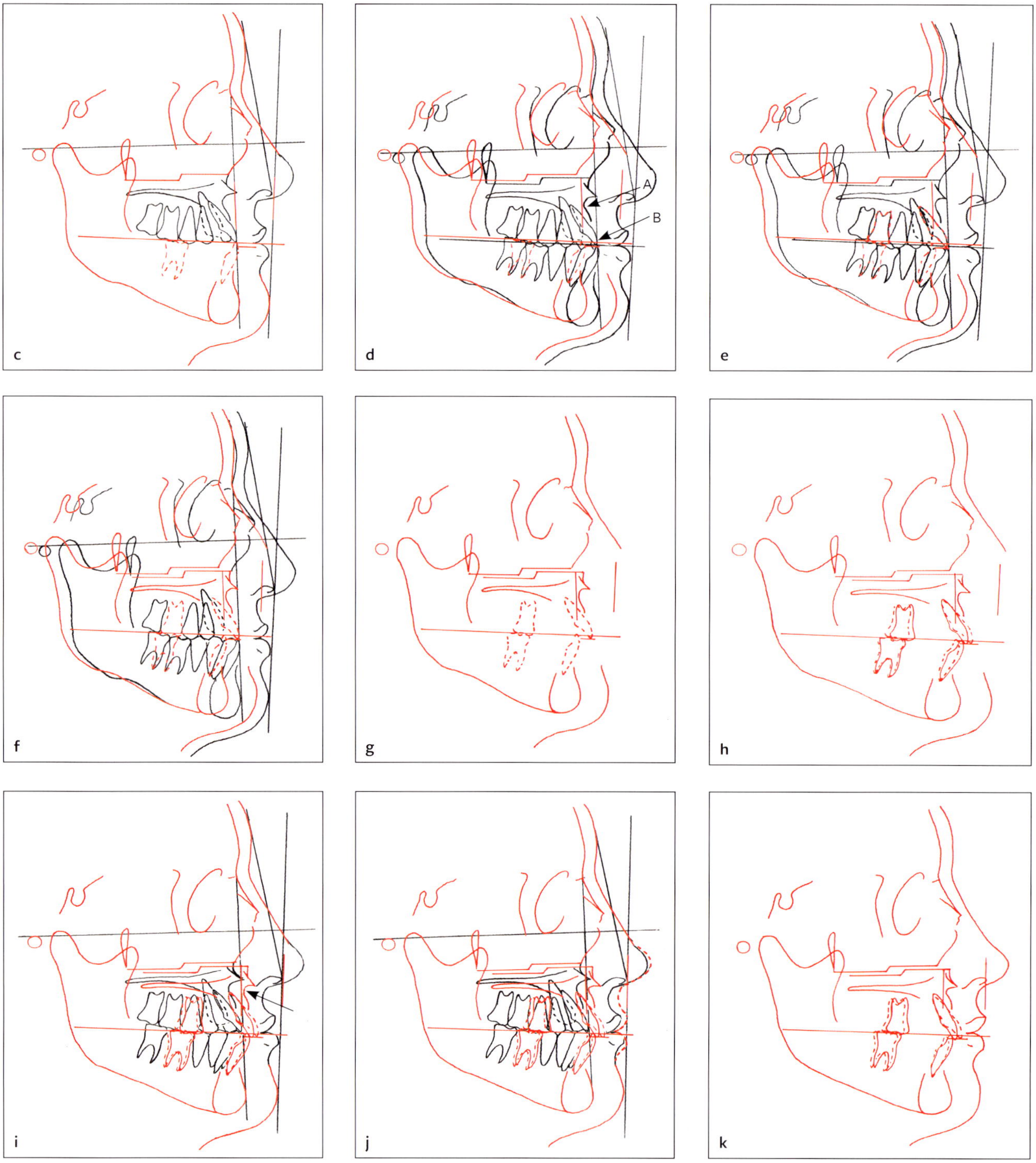

Fig 3-30 *(cont)* (*c*) Step 1: The prediction tracing. All facial structures that will not be affected by the surgery are traced in red. (*d*) Step 2: The prediction tracing is moved to the left and slightly upward until A-point is just anterior to the facial depth line (A) and the maxillary incisor is at the chosen vertical height (B). (*e*) The treatment possibilities can be studied at this stage. Note the increased incisor overjet, amount of maxillary advancement (6.5 mm), amount of inferior repositioning of the maxilla (2 mm), and Class II molar relationship. (*f*) The intended surgical repositioning is apparent by comparing the Le Fort I osteotomy lines. (*g*) The maxilla has been advanced and slightly inferiorly repositioned. The dental and soft tissue prediction should be done now. (*h*) Step 3: Prediction of incisor and molar positions. Note the Class II molar relationship. (*i*) By comparing the position of A-point on the prediction tracing and the original tracing (*arrow*), the amount of bone advancement can be seen (6.5 mm in this case). (*j*) Soft tissue prediction. (*k*) Completed pretreatment prediction tracing.

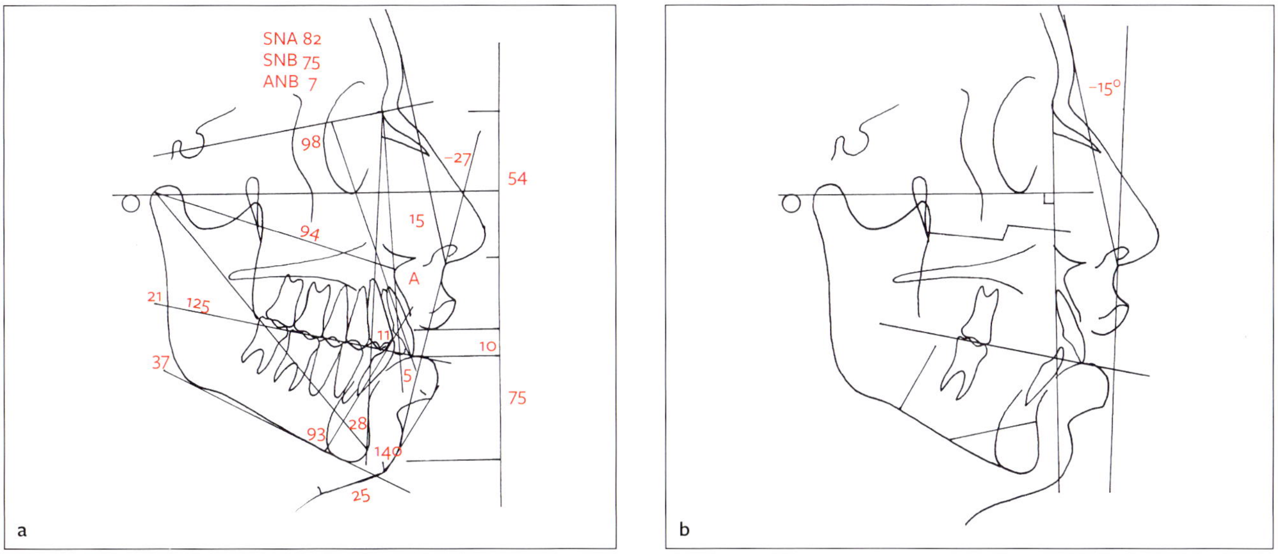

Fig 3-31 (*a*) Pretreatment cephalometric tracing of a 16-year-old boy with the following diagnostic summary. Skeletal: vertical maxillary excess and mandibular anteroposterior deficiency. Dental: Class II malocclusion and accentuated curve of Spee. Soft tissue: increased interlabial gap, excessive maxillary incisor tooth exposure, and increased lower third of the face. (*b*) The facial depth line and the facial contour angle on the original tracing will act as cephalometric guidelines to evaluate the horizontal position of the maxilla and the Pog′ and to plan the required position of A-point and the soft tissue of the chin, respectively.

Superior repositioning of the maxilla, advancement of the mandible, and advancement genioplasty

Figure 3-31a shows the pretreatment cephalometric tracing of a patient with a Class II malocclusion, vertical maxillary excess, mandibular anteroposterior deficiency, and microgenia. The clinician must ensure that the teeth are in centric relation and the lips are in repose during radiography.

Start the prediction by tracing the hard and soft tissues on clean acetate, deleting the analysis lines (the original tracing). To assist in developing the prediction, construct the following lines and angles on the original tracing (Fig 3-31b):

- The facial depth line is drawn through N and A-point and should be perpendicular to the FH plane. In this case, the line is constructed through N perpendicular to FH, and it is clear that A-point is slightly ahead of the line. This line is an indicator of the final position of the bony chin (Pog). Therefore, plan for Pog also to be slightly ahead of this line.
- The facial contour angle is formed by UFP and LFP and should be –11 to –15 degrees in males and –13 to –17 degrees in females. In this case, a –15-degree facial contour angle is chosen and constructed to show the clinician where the soft tissue chin (Pog′) should be.
- This patient will benefit from a Le Fort I maxillary osteotomy (superior repositioning), a bilateral sagittal split mandibular osteotomy (advancement), and genioplasty (advancement). For accuracy of measurement later, draw the osteotomy lines as close as possible to the areas where the osteotomies will be performed.

Step 1

On a clean piece of acetate, trace all the facial structures that will not be affected by the treatment: the cranial base, soft tissue of the forehead, and soft tissue of the nose above the supratip break. This tracing will develop into the prediction tracing. The ideal vertical position of the maxillary incisors is indicated by a horizontal line approximately 3 mm inferior to the upper lip. This decision is based on the required amount of incisor exposure under the upper lip after maxillary superior repositioning, as discussed in chapter 2. Bear in mind that there will be some lip shortening. A vertical line indicating the ideal anteroposterior position of the labial surface of the maxillary incisor is drawn crossing the horizontal line. (The decision of where to draw these lines is based on the soft tissue requirements of each case.) Trace the inferior part of the constructed LFP (Fig 3-31c).

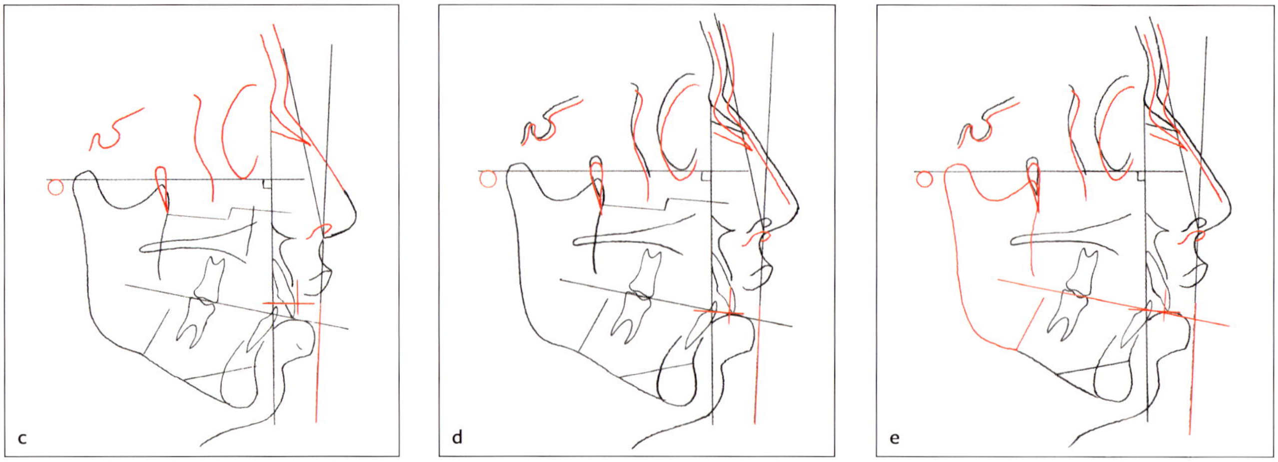

Fig 3-31 *(cont)* (*c*) Step 1. All the structures that will not be affected by the surgery are now traced in red. The desired horizontal and vertical positions of the maxillary incisor are drawn, and the inferior part of the LFP is traced. (*d*) The maxillary incisor is now in the ideal vertical position; however, it is still slightly ahead of the chosen horizontal position. (*e*) The mandibular ramus has autorotated and is traced in.

Step 2

Apply finger pressure just posterior to the condylion on the prediction tracing, and rotate the tracing counterclockwise around the condylion. In this case, the patient has a deep bite and an accentuated curve of Spee that will need to be leveled before surgery. Therefore, the maxillary occlusal plane will be the occlusal plane of choice.

Rotate the tracing until the maxillary incisor is tangent to the horizontal line (Fig 3-31d). Draw the mandibular ramus proximal to the vertical osteotomy line as well as the maxillary occlusal plane (Fig 3-31e).

Step 3

Slide the prediction tracing to the left along the occlusal plane until the soft tissue of the chin (Pog′) is tangent to the predicted LFP. After careful study of the distal section of the mandible on the original tracing in relation to the prediction tracing, three observations can be made (Fig 3-31f):

1. The mandibular incisor is ahead of the vertical line, indicating the desired labial surface of the maxillary incisor.
2. The mandibular incisor edge is 3 mm above the horizontal line, indicating the vertical position of the maxillary incisor edge.
3. The vertical osteotomy line is 8 mm ahead of the osteotomy line on the original tracing, indicating that an 8-mm surgical advancement is required to achieve the predicted chin position.

The clinician has the following options:

- Retraction of the mandibular incisors. In this case, the angle of the mandibular incisors is acceptable. Any retraction will make the teeth very upright and require teeth to be extracted.
- Leveling the curve of Spee. This option will increase the mandibular arch length and thus necessitate slight advancement of the mandibular incisors. Extraction of teeth may be indicated.
- Less advancement of the mandible. This option will compromise the esthetics.
- Less advancement of the mandible combined with an advancement genioplasty. The patient has a small chin and a large, everted lower lip. An advancement of the chin will benefit the patient.

From these considerations, it is clear that the best option is to level the mandibular arch without tooth extractions. The mandibular incisors will move slightly forward. Advance the mandible less, and combine the mandibular surgery with an advancement genioplasty. Steps 4 through 9 are taken to test this decision.

Step 4

Place a clean piece of acetate over the original tracing. Trace the distal part of the mandible anterior to the vertical osteotomy. Do not trace the mandible inferior to the genio-

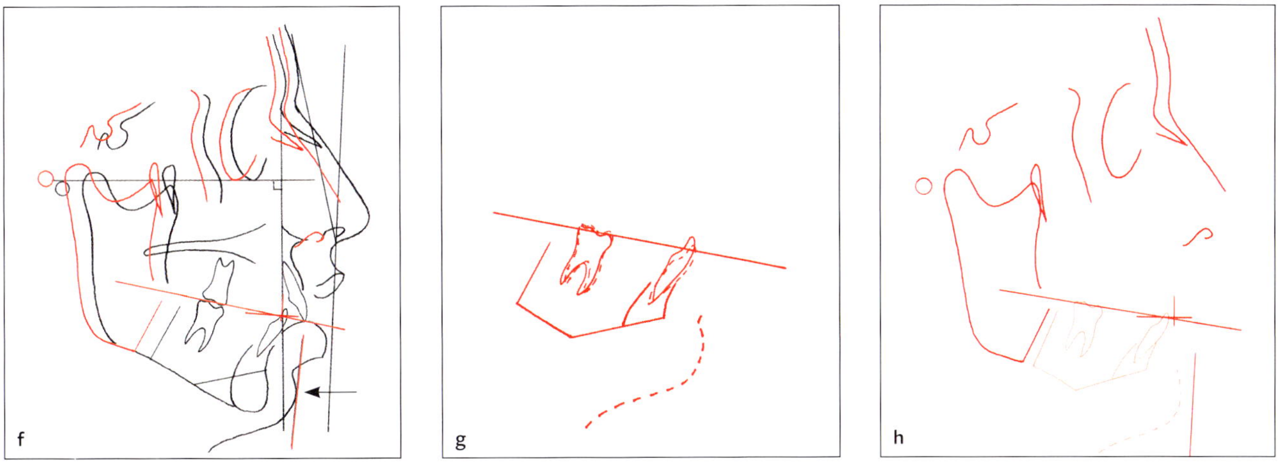

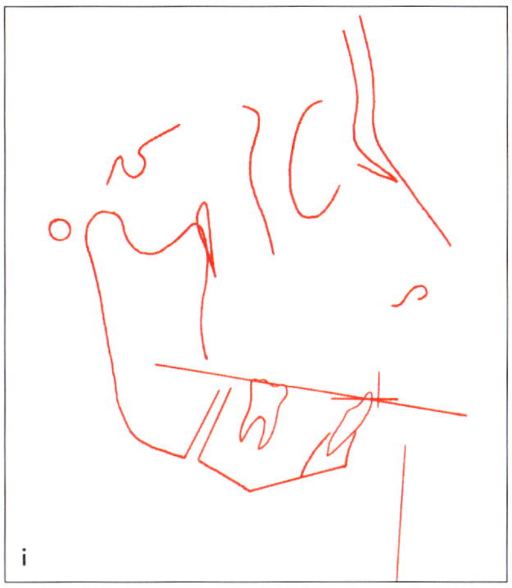

Fig 3-31 *(cont)* (*f*) Step 3. The prediction tracing is moved to the left along the occlusal plane. Pog′ is now tangent to the predicted LFP (*arrow*). Note that the mandibular incisor is ahead of the vertical line, indicating the desired anteroposterior position of the maxillary incisor; the mandibular incisor is 3 mm above the horizontal line, indicating the desired vertical position of the maxillary incisor edge; and an 8-mm mandibular advancement is necessary to achieve the predicted chin position. (*g*) Step 4. (*h*) Step 5. (*i*) Step 6.

plasty line. Trace the soft tissue of the chin below the depth of the labiomental fold using a dotted line. The curve of Spee will be leveled before surgery (for reasons discussed previously). Trace the maxillary occlusal plane. The first molar is extruded and the incisor intruded and moved slightly labially to facilitate leveling of the mandibular arch. This tracing is called the *mandibular tracing* (Fig 3-31g).

Step 5

Superimpose the prediction tracing on the mandibular tracing, and slide the prediction tracing to the left along the occlusal plane until the mandibular incisors are positioned 1 mm to the left of the vertical line. This will allow the maxillary incisors to fit between the mandibular incisor and the vertical line, indicating the labial surface of the maxillary incisor. The dotted line indicating the soft tissue of the chin is behind the predicted LFP, indicating the need for an advancement genioplasty (Fig 3-31h).

Step 6

Trace the distal part of the mandible (the mandibular tracing) on the prediction tracing. The amount of surgical advancement is indicated by the distance between the two vertical osteotomy lines (Fig 3-31i).

Step 7

Superimpose the prediction tracing on the original tracing with the occlusal planes coinciding and the first molars in a Class I relationship. The increased overjet of the incisors is clear (Fig 3-31j). The clinician must now determine whether it is possible to retract the maxillary incisors to achieve an ideal incisal relationship. In this case, it was found to be a feasible option. Now trace the maxillary incisor in its ideal relationship to the mandibular incisor, then trace the Le Fort I osteotomy line (Fig 3-31k). These two lines indicate the maxillary superior repositioning (it is typical that the superior movement is more in the anterior

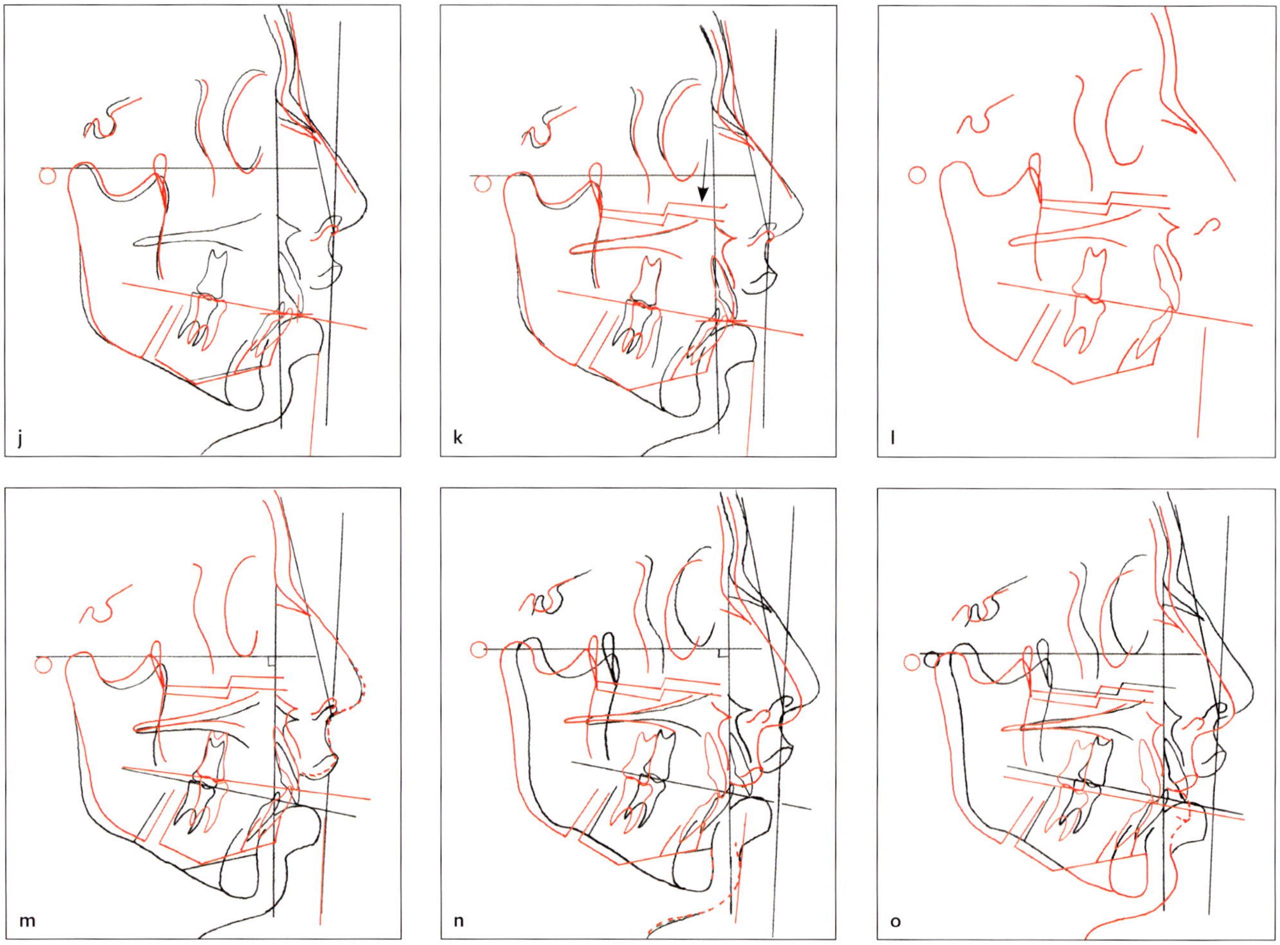

Fig 3-31 *(cont)* (*j*) The maxillary incisor is 2 mm ahead of the vertical line. (*k*) The amount of superior repositioning of the maxilla is indicated by the distance between the two Le Fort I osteotomy lines (*arrow*). (*l*) The soft tissue of the nasal tip, the upper lip, the sliding genioplasty, and the soft tissue of the chin must still be predicted. (*m*) Prediction of the nasal tip and upper lip. (*n*) Prediction of the chin. (*o*) Lower lip prediction.

region than the posterior region). Figure 3-31l illustrates the prediction tracing at this stage, with no soft tissue prediction below the Sn and the unfinished genioplasty. The LFP indicates the required anteroposterior position of the soft tissue chin.

Step 8

The next step is prediction of the upper lip and nasal tip. Superimpose the prediction tracing and the original tracing with unaffected tissues coinciding. Draw the upper lip using the original lip position as a guide, bearing in mind that there will be lip shortening (10% to 20% of total maxillary superior repositioning). The Sn will move slightly forward, and the lip curve will fill out. The tip of the nose below the supratip break will advance slightly (Fig 3-31m).

Step 9

To predict the hard and soft tissue of the chin and the lower lip, place the prediction tracing over the original tracing with the mandibular skeletal tissues. Slide the prediction tracing to the left along the genioplasty osteotomy line until the soft tissue of the chin (dotted line) is tangent to the LFP line (Fig 3-31n). Trace the soft tissue of the chin below the depth of the labiomental fold as well as the hard tissue below the genioplasty osteotomy line. Draw the lower lip, bearing in mind that the effect of the maxillary incisors on the lower lip is eliminated. The lip will rotate backward, reducing the vermilion exposure (Fig 3-31o).

Figure 3-31p illustrates the final visual treatment prediction of hard and soft tissue.

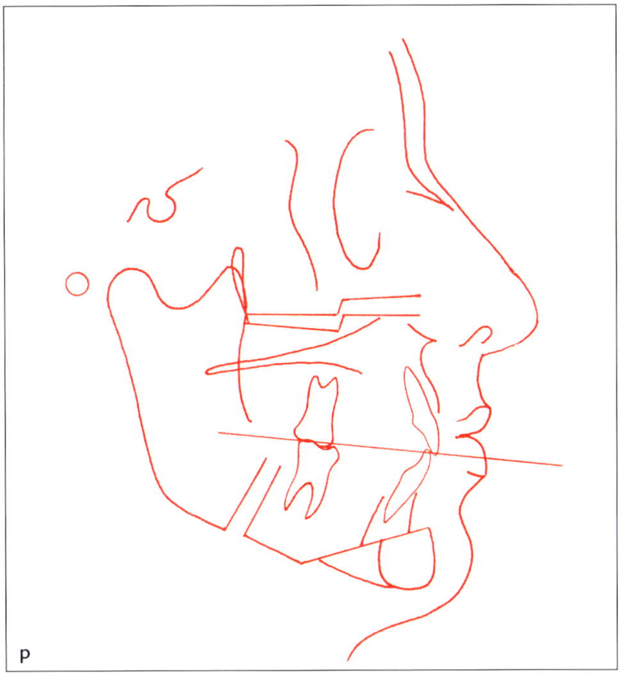

Fig 3-31 (*cont*) (*p*) Completed visual treatment objective.

Final Surgical Visual Treatment Prediction

The surgical visual treatment objective is based on the immediate preoperative cephalometric radiograph. The preoperative orthodontic preparation is now completed, and the immediate preoperative radiograph will accurately determine the skeletal surgical movements necessary to achieve the functional and esthetic treatment goals. The visual treatment objective can also be used after surgery to check whether the predicted surgical results have been achieved.

Because of the extreme diversity of surgical procedures and the combination of procedures used in the surgical correction of dentofacial deformities, it is impossible to illustrate the method of developing the cephalometric prediction tracing for every conceivable deformity. By creating the visual treatment predictions through trial and error and comparing the actual soft and hard tissue treatment results with the predicted results, surgeons will develop their own data for soft tissue predictions to perfect their prediction tracing techniques.

A few days before surgery, a cephalometric radiograph is obtained with the patient's teeth in centric relation and the lips in repose. To create the original tracing, the radiograph is accurately traced to demonstrate all the relevant hard and soft tissue structures. All the dental structures are also traced to accurately demonstrate the crowns and roots of the teeth. The analysis lines are not drawn on this tracing. The tracing is removed from the radiograph for better visualization when constructing the prediction tracing.

Advancement genioplasty

Step 1

The patient shown in the original tracing in Fig 3-32a will benefit from an advancement genioplasty. Draw a line on the original tracing representing the osteotomy cut on the chin. Bear in mind anatomical structures, such as the mental foramen and roots of the teeth. Also remember that the angle at which the osteotomy is performed will influence the vertical dimension of the chin as it is advanced (see chapter 5). Draw the facial contour angle formed by the upper and lower facial planes. Construct a predicted lower facial plane (in this case, an angle of −15 degrees to the upper facial plane is chosen) using dotted lines (Fig 3-32b).

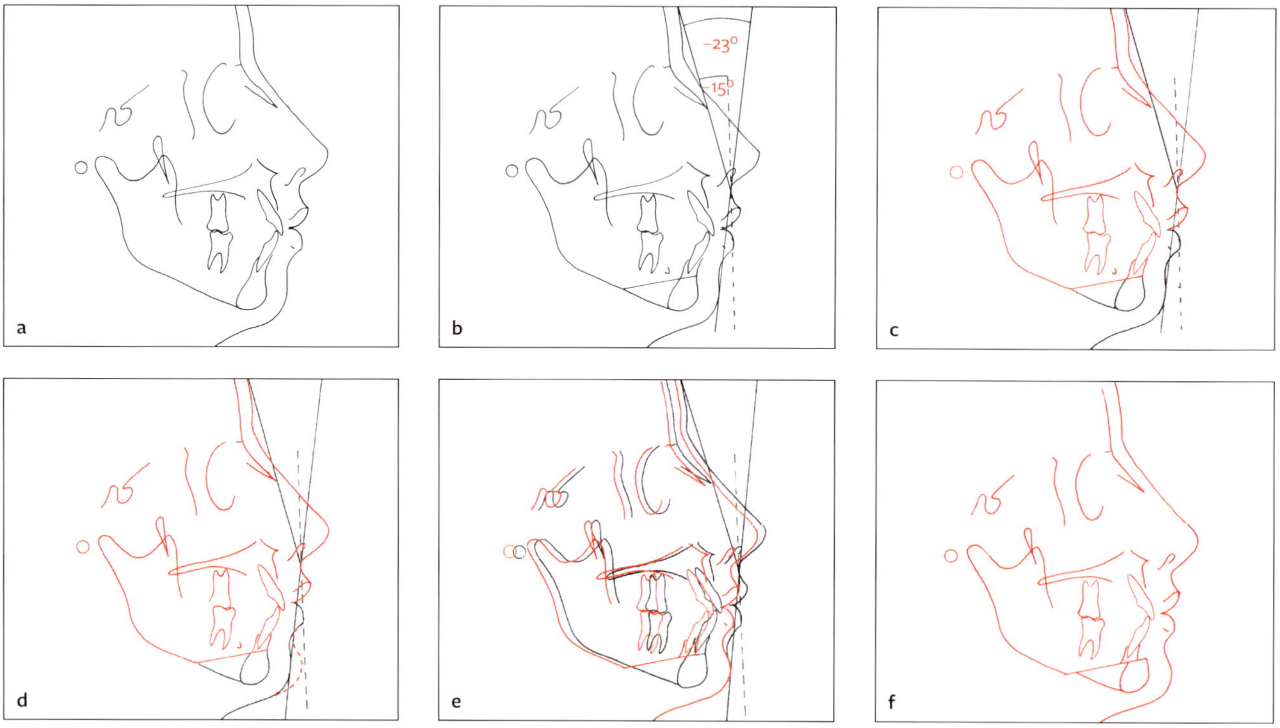

Fig 3-32 (*a*) Original tracing. (*b*) No vertical change of the anterior mandibular vertical height is required. The osteotomy for genioplasty is therefore made horizontal. (*c*) Step 2. All structures that will not be affected by the surgery are traced in red. (*d*) Step 3. Soft tissue prediction. (*e*) Step 4. Hard tissue prediction. (*f*) Completed prediction tracing.

Step 2

Place a clean sheet of acetate over the original tracing. Trace the osteotomy line and all skeletal and soft tissue structures that will remain unchanged by the surgical procedure—in this case, everything above the genioplasty line. This tracing is called the *prediction tracing* (Fig 3-32c).

Step 3

The clinician, guided by all the available references for the ideal soft tissue position of the chin (in this case, the facial contour angle is used) and an artistic sensibility, draws the soft tissue of the chin on the prediction tracing (Fig 3-32d).

Step 4

The prediction tracing is now moved toward the left until soft tissue chin line of the original tracing is tangent to, or just ahead of, soft tissue chin line of the prediction tracing (soft tissue change to hard tissue movement is 90% to 100%). Trace the skeletal change as superimposed on the original tracing (Fig 3-32e). Vertical changes can now be made where indicated (eg, ostectomy to vertically shorten the chin, downgrafting for vertical increase, or changing the angulation of the osteotomy so that the chin will slide superiorly when advanced or slide more horizontally when reduced). The skeletal advancement can be measured and recorded on the completed prediction tracing (Fig 3-32f).

Mandibular advancement

Step 1

Trace all the hard and soft tissue structures on a clean piece of acetate without the analysis lines. Draw a line just posterior to the second molar on the body of the mandible representing the vertical cut of the bilateral sagittal split osteotomy. This tracing is called the *original tracing* (Fig 3-33a).

Step 2

Place a clean sheet of acetate over the original tracing, and trace all skeletal and soft tissues that will not be affected by

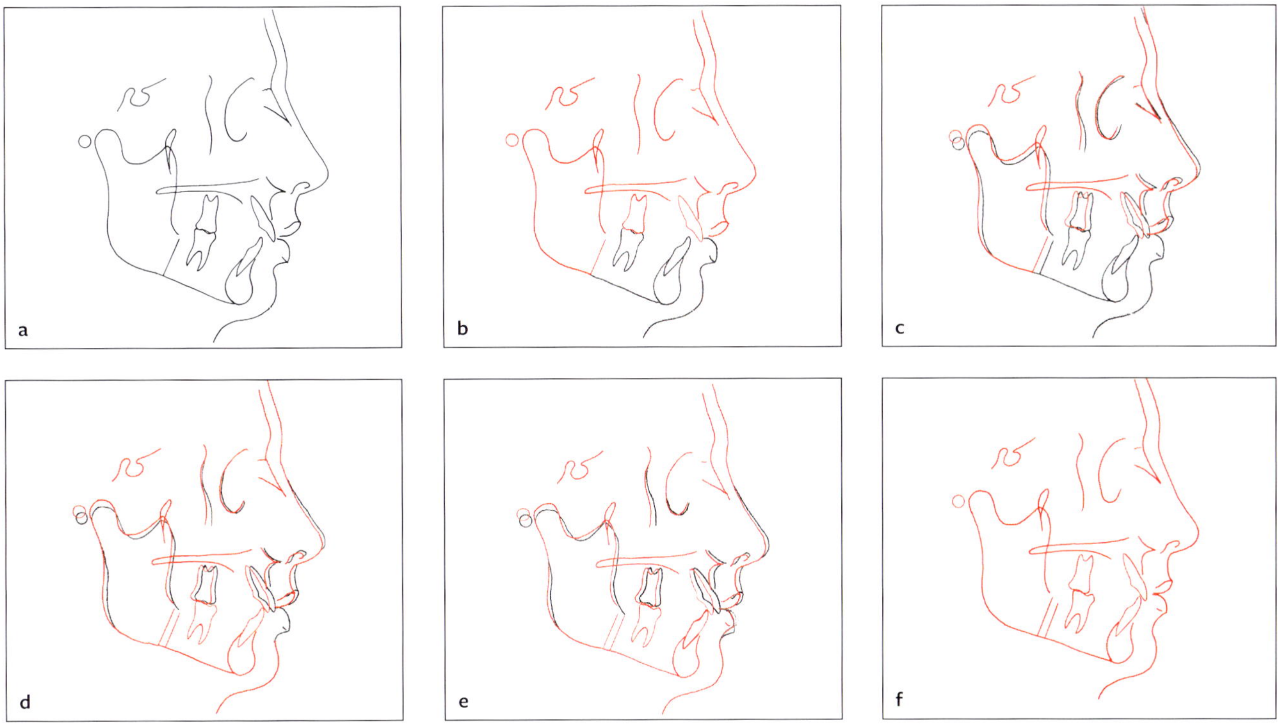

Fig 3-33 (*a*) Original tracing of a patient requiring advancement of the mandible. (*b*) Step 2. All structures that will not be affected by the surgery are traced in red. (*c*) The mandibular teeth on the original tracing are now in a Class I molar relationship and in the ideal incisor overbite and overjet with the maxillary teeth on the prediction tracing. (*d*) Step 3. The mandibular skeletal structures and teeth and the soft tissue of the chin below the labiomental fold are traced. (*e*) Step 4. The everted lower lip will rotate back as the effect of the maxillary incisor is eliminated. (*f*) Completed prediction tracing.

the surgery. Do not trace the hard and soft tissue structures of the mandible distal to the vertical osteotomy line. This tracing will develop into the prediction tracing (Fig 3-33b).

Step 3

Slide the prediction tracing to the left (the original tracing structures will move to the right). Position the mandibular teeth of the original tracing in the best interincisal and molar relationship with the maxillary teeth on the prediction tracing (Fig 3-33c). Trace the mandibular skeletal structures and the teeth. Also trace the soft tissue of the chin below the labiomental fold (the pogonion response to hard tissue advancement is 0.9:1.0 to 1:1; Fig 3-33d).

Step 4

Now trace the lower lip, keeping in mind how soft tissue will respond to hard tissue changes (Fig 3-33e). The labiomental fold flattens, and the lower vermilion advances 75% (66% to 100%) of horizontal skeletal movement. The effect of the maxillary incisor on the lower lip is now removed, and the lower lip will curl back, reducing the vermilion exposure. Figure 3-33f shows the completed prediction. The amount of mandibular advancement can be determined by measuring the distance between the two vertical osteotomy lines.

Mandibular setback

Step 1

Draw a line on the original tracing to represent the vertical cut of the bilateral sagittal split osteotomy on the body of the mandible. This line should be drawn as close as possible to where the actual osteotomy will be performed (Fig 3-34a).

Step 2

Place a clean sheet of acetate over the original tracing, and trace all skeletal and soft tissues that will not be affected by the surgery. Do not trace the upper lip or the hard and soft tissues distal to the mandibular osteotomy line (Fig 3-34b).

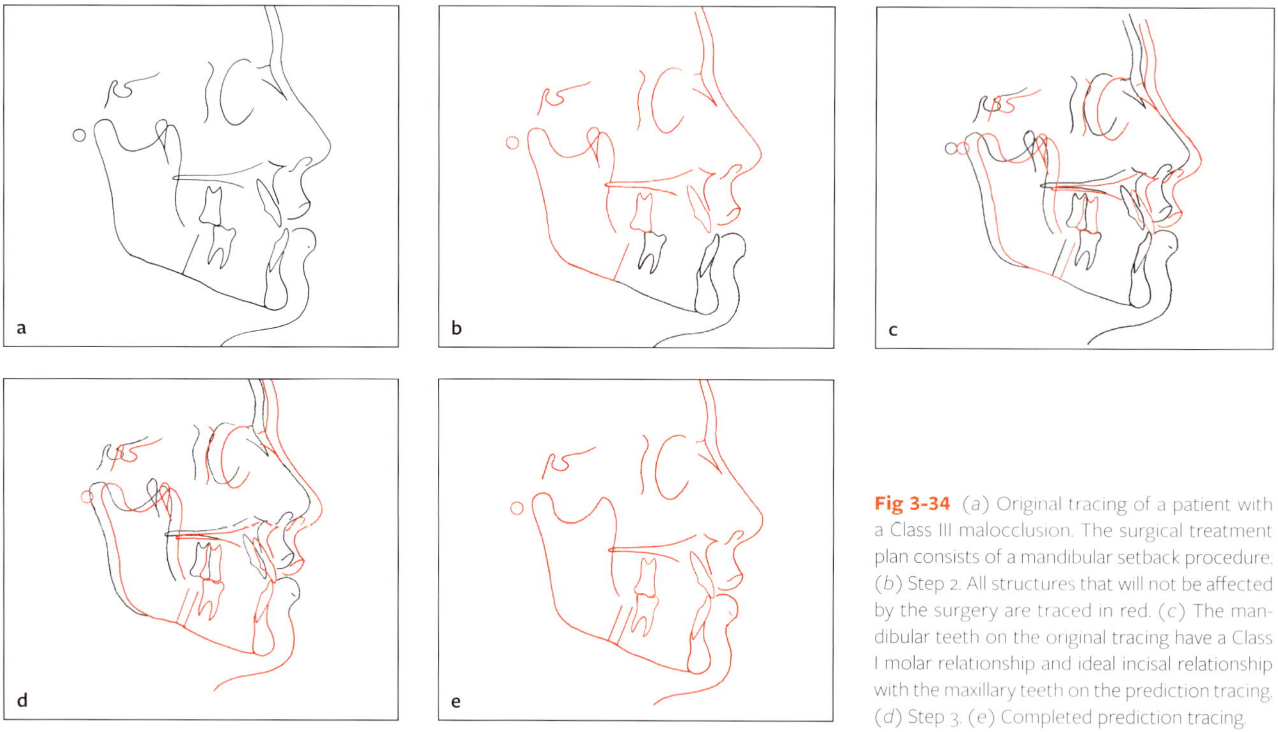

Fig 3-34 (*a*) Original tracing of a patient with a Class III malocclusion. The surgical treatment plan consists of a mandibular setback procedure. (*b*) Step 2. All structures that will not be affected by the surgery are traced in red. (*c*) The mandibular teeth on the original tracing have a Class I molar relationship and ideal incisal relationship with the maxillary teeth on the prediction tracing. (*d*) Step 3. (*e*) Completed prediction tracing.

Step 3

Slide the prediction tracing to the right (the distal mandible will move to the left) until the best interincisal and molar relationship is achieved (Fig 3-34c). Trace the skeletal tissue as well as the osteotomy line of the distal segment. Trace the soft tissue of the chin below the labiomental fold (soft tissue change to hard tissue movement is 90% to 100% at the pogonion; Fig 3-34d).

Step 4

The effect of the mandibular incisor on the upper lip (Class III deep bite cases) is now removed, and the lip will move back slightly. Draw the new position of the upper lip. In some Class III cases (eg, open bite cases), the mandibular incisors will have no effect on the upper lip. When this is true, as in this case, the lower lip can be traced in from the start. Thus, with the prediction tracing still in the same position, draw the lower lip. In Class III deep bite cases (overclosure), the lower lip will change in response to the influence of the upper lip and maxillary incisor. The amount of mandibular setback can now be determined on the completed prediction tracing by measuring the distance between the two vertical osteotomy lines (Fig 3-34e).

Maxillary advancement

Step 1

The original tracing of a patient with a Class III malocclusion is illustrated in Fig 3-35a. Draw a line on the original tracing to represent the Le Fort I maxillary osteotomy. This line should be drawn as close as possible to where the actual osteotomy will be performed on the maxilla; it makes the measurement of maxillary repositioning more accurate.

The line should be parallel to the occlusal plane of the maxilla so that the maxilla will be advanced along this plane. If the line is angled upward, the height of the maxilla will be reduced; if bone contact is maintained, the bite will open anteriorly. If the line is angled inferiorly, the maxilla will slide downward. In a Le Fort I advancement procedure, the final anteroposterior position of the maxilla is dictated by the mandibular dentition. However, the vertical position of the maxilla is controlled by the surgeon. The mandible will autorotate (clockwise subsequent to an increase in the maxillary height and counterclockwise subsequent to superior repositioning of the maxilla). The clinician can therefore decide on the final vertical position

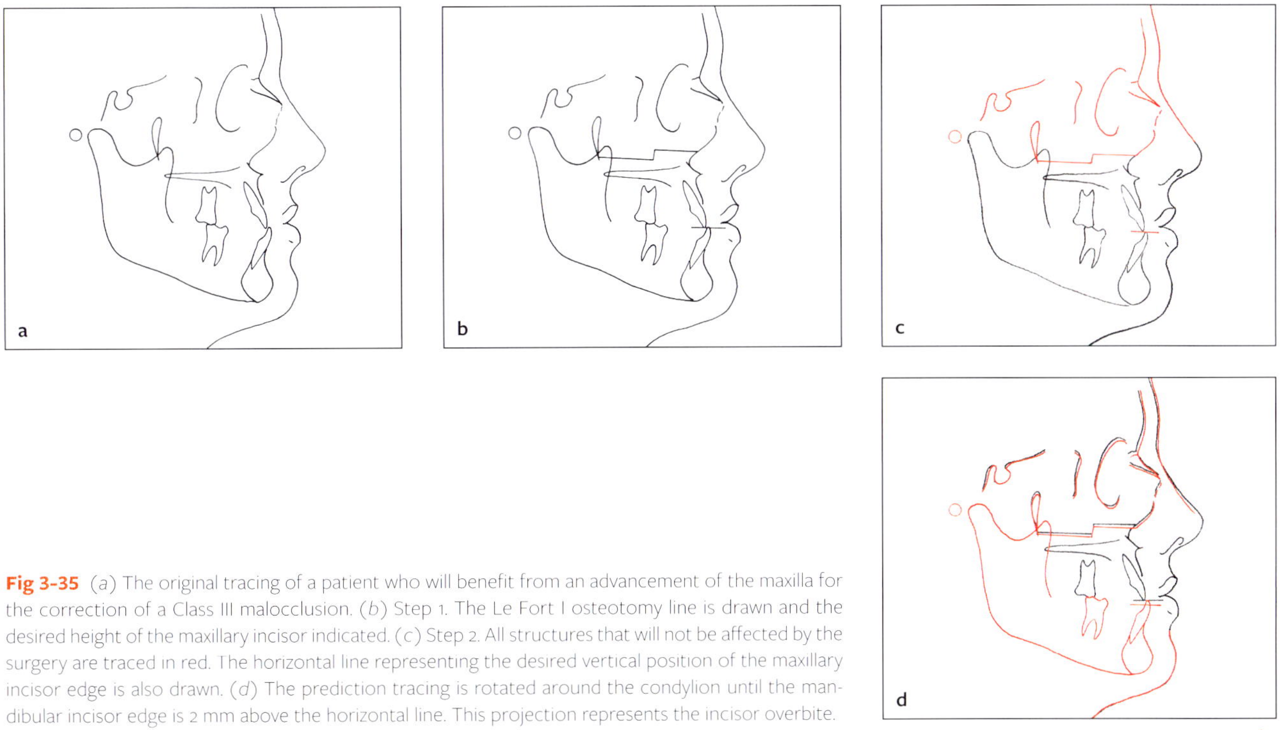

Fig 3-35 (*a*) The original tracing of a patient who will benefit from an advancement of the maxilla for the correction of a Class III malocclusion. (*b*) Step 1. The Le Fort I osteotomy line is drawn and the desired height of the maxillary incisor indicated. (*c*) Step 2. All structures that will not be affected by the surgery are traced in red. The horizontal line representing the desired vertical position of the maxillary incisor edge is also drawn. (*d*) The prediction tracing is rotated around the condylion until the mandibular incisor edge is 2 mm above the horizontal line. This projection represents the incisor overbite.

of the maxillary central incisor based on the ideal tooth-lip relationship. Draw a horizontal line in the incisor region to indicate the ideal vertical position of the maxillary incisor. In this case, the existing height of the maxilla will be maintained (Fig 3-35b).

Step 2

Place a clean sheet of acetate over the original tracing. Trace all skeletal and soft tissue structures that will not be affected by surgery (Fig 3-35c). Do not trace the bone and teeth of the maxilla below the osteotomy line or the soft tissue inferior to the supratip break of the nose, upper lip, and lower lip. The soft and hard tissues of the mandible are also not traced at this stage. In this case, it is clear that the mandibular incisor is tangent to the line indicating the ideal vertical position of the maxillary incisor. To achieve a normal incisor overbite, the mandibular incisor needs to be rotated to 2 mm above the line. Place a pencil posterior to the condylion, and rotate the prediction tracing clockwise until the incisor is 2 mm above the horizontal line. Now trace the mandibular hard tissue and soft tissue of the chin below the labiomental fold (Fig 3-35d).

Step 3

Move the prediction tracing to the left (the original tracing structures will move to the right), and superimpose the skeletal tissue of the original tracing to establish the best interincisal and molar relationship with the teeth on the prediction tracing (Fig 3-35e). Trace the skeletal tissues as well as the osteotomy line (Fig 3-35f).

Step 4

The soft tissue can now be drawn; bear in mind the soft tissue changes caused by maxillary advancement procedures. Place the prediction tracing over the original tracing to superimpose the structures that did not move. The nose and upper lip changes are now predicted. Draw the soft tissue first in dotted lines until the prediction is satisfactory, then complete the lines of the nose and upper lip (Fig 3-35g). Vermilion (stomion) movement will represent 50% to 75% of the horizontal movement. The nasolabial angle decreases 1 to 4 degrees per 1 mm of advancement. The nasal tip advances 30% (although this is variable) and can be controlled.

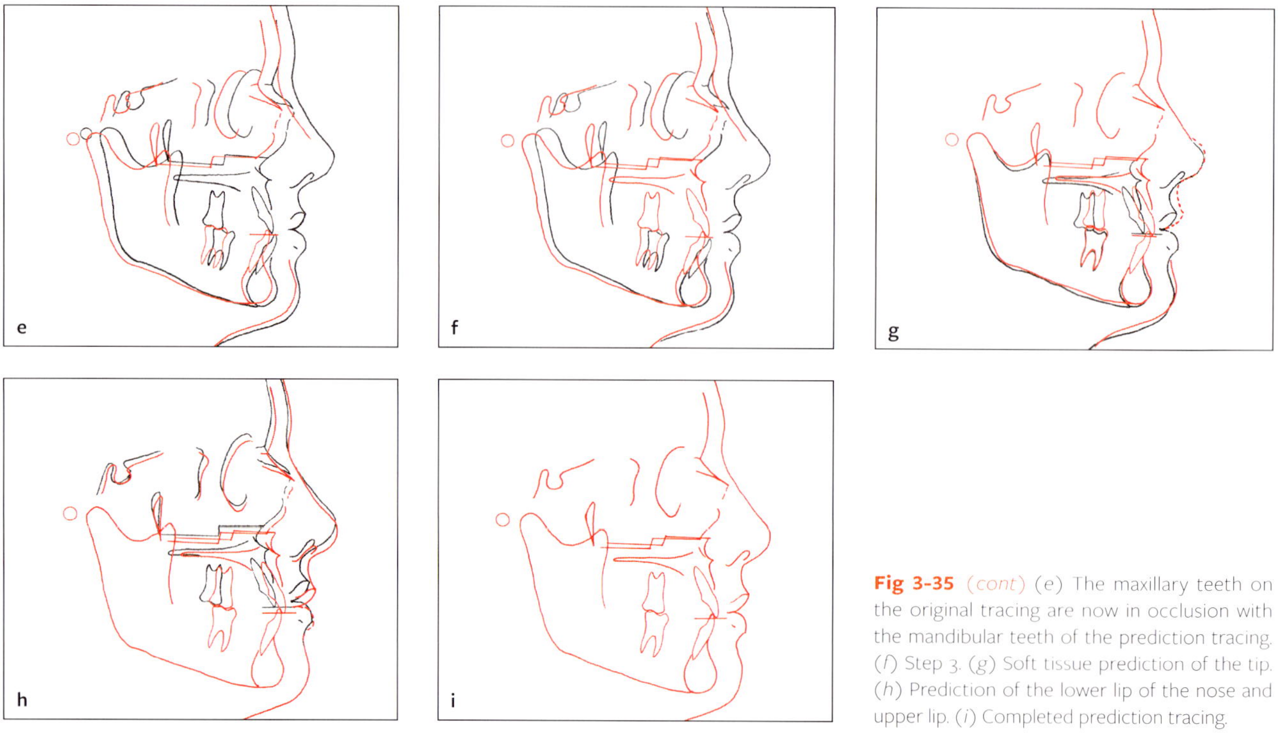

Fig 3-35 *(cont)* (*e*) The maxillary teeth on the original tracing are now in occlusion with the mandibular teeth of the prediction tracing. (*f*) Step 3. (*g*) Soft tissue prediction of the tip. (*h*) Prediction of the lower lip of the nose and upper lip. (*i*) Completed prediction tracing.

To predict the soft tissue change of the lower lip, superimpose the prediction tracing on the original tracing with the mandibular hard tissue and soft tissue of the chin coinciding. The new relationship between the upper and lower lips is evident. The upper lip will tend to push the lower lip down slightly, somewhat everting the lower lip. First draw the predicted change with a dotted line, and then finish the prediction tracing (Fig 3-35h).

Figure 3-35i shows the completed tracing predicting the hard and soft tissue changes. The amount of surgical advancement can be measured by comparing the preoperative and postoperative osteotomy reference lines.

Maxillary superior repositioning

Step 1

The original tracing of a patient requiring superior repositioning of the maxilla for correction of vertical maxillary excess is shown in Fig 3-36a. The radiograph must show the lips in repose and the teeth in centric occlusion. When correcting vertical maxillary excess, the maxillary central incisor–upper lip relationship forms the basis of the development of a visual treatment objective.

Draw a horizontal line on the original tracing with a vertical step that simulates the Le Fort I maxillary osteotomy as close as possible to where the actual osteotomy will be performed on the maxilla. The most important decision of the surgical treatment objective—the final vertical position of the maxillary incisor tip—must now be made. The decision is made with the aid of cephalometric guidelines, knowledge of soft tissue response to maxillary superior repositioning, clinical experience, and artistic sense. The following are a few guidelines to assist in making this decision:

- Maxillary incisor exposure of 1 to 4 mm under the upper lip is considered normal.
- Less maxillary incisor will show under long upper lips, and more maxillary incisor will show under short upper lips.
- Never treat the gummy smile. The smile may expose a larger amount of gingiva than the amount of superior repositioning indicated by the incisor exposure under the upper lip. Treatment of the gummy smile will lead to excessive superior repositioning of the maxilla, resulting in a toothless appearance.
- Superior repositioning of the maxilla combined with maxillary setback undermines soft tissue support of the upper lip and paranasal areas, leading to poor esthetic results.

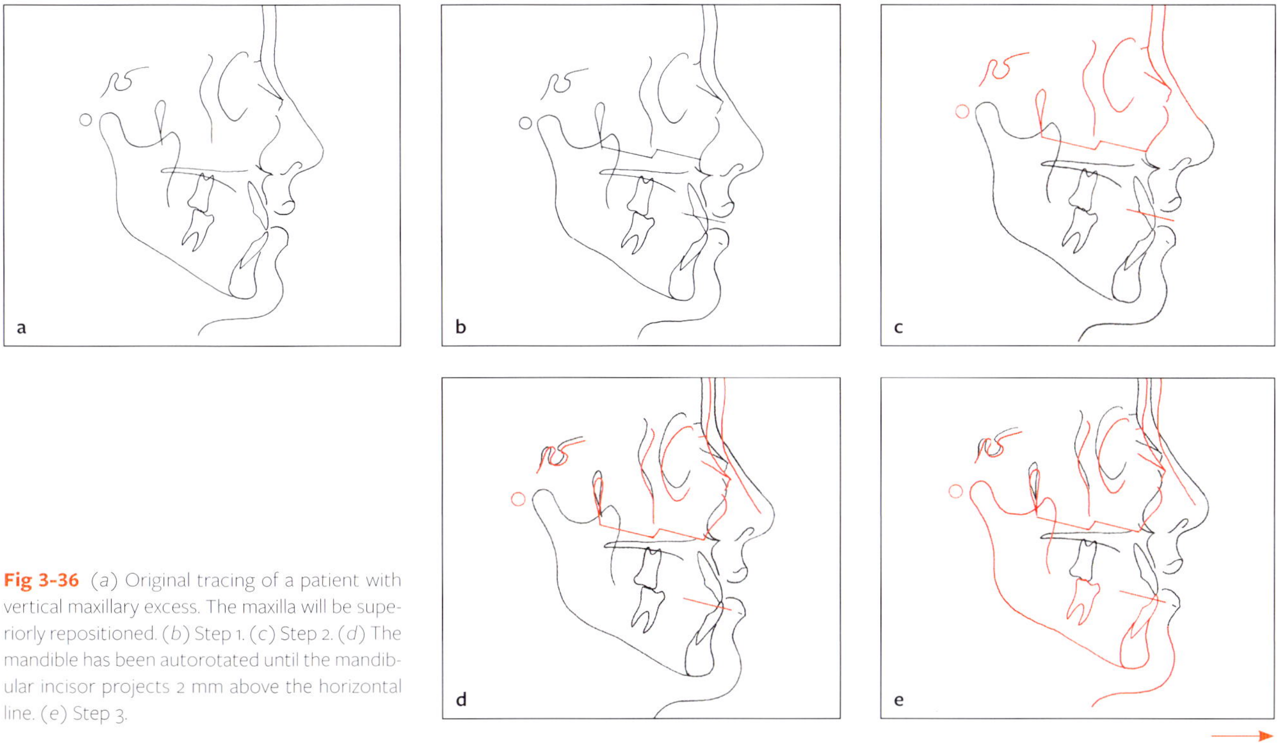

Fig 3-36 (*a*) Original tracing of a patient with vertical maxillary excess. The maxilla will be superiorly repositioned. (*b*) Step 1. (*c*) Step 2. (*d*) The mandible has been autorotated until the mandibular incisor projects 2 mm above the horizontal line. (*e*) Step 3.

- Superior repositioning of the maxilla will lead to upper lip shortening (10% to 20% of the amount of superior repositioning).
- Never treat the interlabial gap. Correction of vertical maxillary excess and establishment of the ideal tooth-lip relationship will create a lip seal in most cases. An interlabial gap of 1 to 3 mm is acceptable and often very attractive. The amount of superior repositioning should not be guided by the interlabial distance.
- The upper lip length, lip thickness, and overall esthetics are also influenced by the surgical technique (see chapter 5).
- Err on the long side rather than the short side in superior repositioning of the maxilla.

Consider these guidelines while drawing a horizontal line on the original tracing to indicate the required vertical position of the maxillary incisor edge (Fig 3-36b). The anteroposterior position of the maxillary incisor will be determined by the mandibular incisors after autorotation.

Step 2

Place the prediction tracing over the original tracing, and trace all skeletal and soft tissue structures that will not be affected by the superior repositioning of the maxilla. In other words, the nasal tip and the maxillary and mandibular hard and soft tissue are not traced (Fig 3-36c).

Step 3

The mandible is now autorotated by placing a pencil just posterior to the condylion and rotating the prediction tracing clockwise until the mandibular incisor tip projects 2 mm above the horizontal line. The amount of incisor above the line represents the amount of overbite (Fig 3-36d). Trace the mandibular hard tissue and soft tissue of the chin below the labiomental fold (Fig 3-36e).

Step 4

Superimpose the mandibular teeth of the prediction tracing on the original tracing to obtain the best incisor and molar relationship. The anteroposterior position of the maxilla is dictated by the mandibular incisor position. The occlusal plane is dictated by the mandibular occlusal plane after autorotation (Fig 3-36f). Trace the maxillary hard tissue as well as the Le Fort I osteotomy reference line (Fig 3-36g).

Step 5

Slide the prediction tracing on the original tracing to superimpose the structures that were not affected by the surgery. The superior repositioning of the maxilla is now

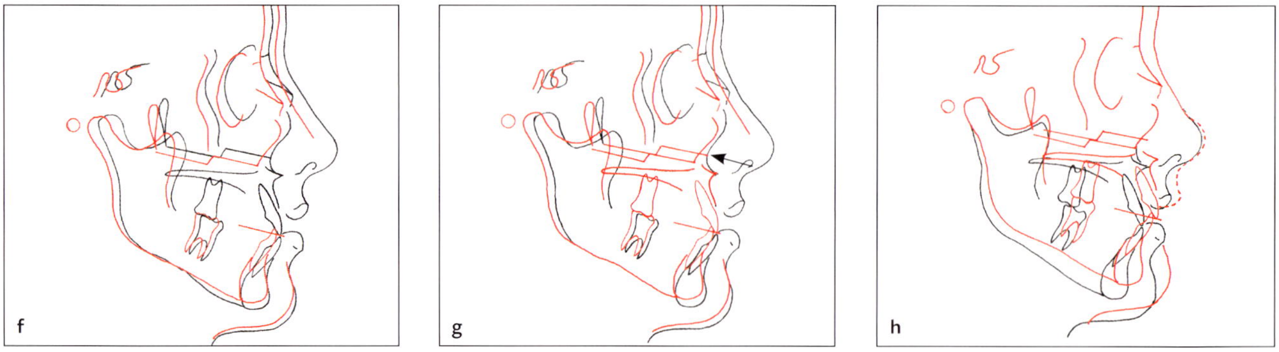

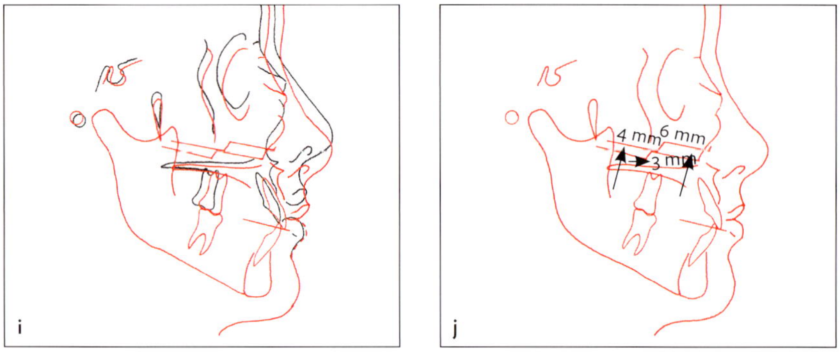

Fig 3-36 (*cont*) (*f*) The mandibular teeth on the prediction tracing now occlude with the maxillary teeth on the original tracing. (*g*) Step 4. The maxillary structures and the osteotomy line are traced to indicate the maxillary repositioning (*arrow*). (*h*) Soft tissue prediction of the nasal tip and upper lip. (*i*) Prediction of lower lip change. (*j*) Completed prediction tracing. The maxilla is superiorly repositioned 4 mm in the posterior area and 6 mm in the anterior area. By following the forward rotation of the mandible, a 3-mm maxillary advancement is necessary.

apparent. The maxillary advancement subsequent to the counterclockwise rotation of the maxilla is also clearly visible. The expected soft tissue changes can be drawn in according to knowledge of soft tissue change in relation to skeletal repositioning. In Le Fort I superior repositioning, the vermilion (stomion) movement represents 10% to 20% of the vertical movement, and the nasolabial angle tends to decrease. In Le Fort I advancement, vermilion (stomion) movement represents 50% to 75% of the horizontal movement. The nasolabial angle decreases 1 to 4 degrees per 1 mm of advancement. The nasal lip turns upward (a change that is variable but controllable).

Draw the predicted soft tissue with a dotted line. When the prediction is satisfactory, the nasal tip and upper lip predictions can be drawn in (Fig 3-36h).

Step 6

Move the prediction tracing to superimpose the mandibular hard tissue structures on the mandibular hard tissue structures of the original tracing. Trace the mandibular soft tissue, bearing in mind that with lip competence now established, the mentalis muscle will relax (the chin soft tissue thickness will increase), and the lower lip will roll back slightly. However, the maxillary incisor may now have an influence on the lower lip, moving it slightly forward. Draw the lip with a dotted line, and when confident about the prediction, finalize it with a solid line (Fig 3-63i).

By measuring the distance between the osteotomy lines on the original tracing and the prediction tracing, the actual skeletal movements can be recorded. The following facts are clear in the case demonstrated here (Fig 3-36j):

- The superior repositioning of the maxilla is less in the posterior area (4 mm) than in the incisor areas (6 mm). This is because a severe anterior open bite is corrected and more superior repositioning was necessary in the molar area to allow for mandibular autorotation.
- The anteroposterior position of the maxilla is determined by the mandibular incisor position after autorotation. As the mandible (the unoperated jaw) is rotated counterclockwise, it is also rotated forward. The maxilla, therefore, has to be advanced (3 mm in this case).

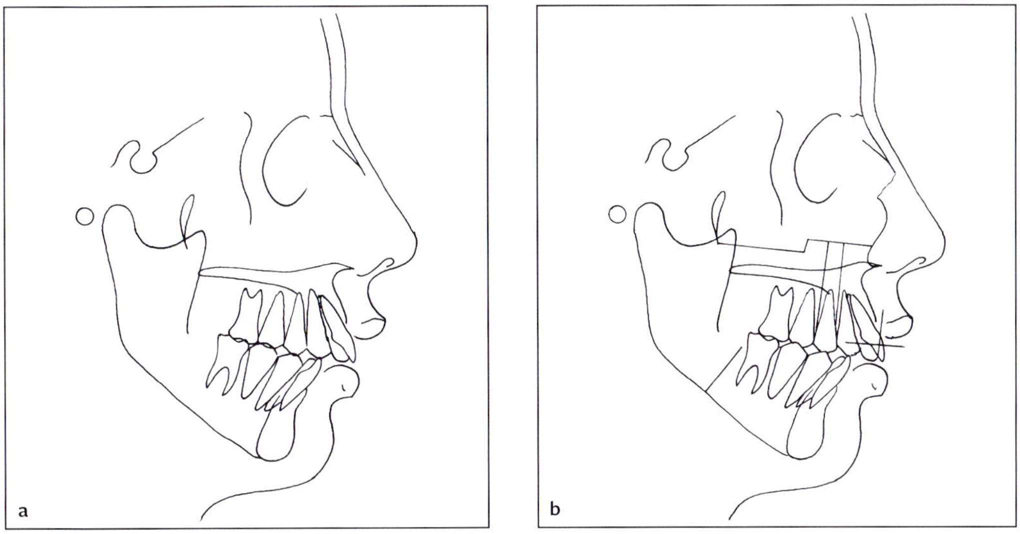

Fig 3-37 (*a*) Original tracing of a patient with vertical maxillary excess, maxillary anteroposterior excess, and mandibular anteroposterior deficiency. The malocclusion is Class II. (*b*) Step 1. The intended osteotomy lines, as well as the required vertical and horizontal positions of the maxillary incisor edge, are drawn on the original tracing. The maxillary first premolars will be removed at surgery and the space closed.

Maxillary segmental superior repositioning with extraction of first premolars and advancement of the mandible

Step 1

Begin the prediction by tracing the original tracing (Fig 3-37a). Draw lines on the original tracing to simulate the osteotomies. A horizontal line with a step simulating the Le Fort I osteotomy is drawn as close as possible to the actual osteotomy on the maxilla. Two vertical lines indicating the limits of the interdental ostectomy are then drawn between the second maxillary premolar and the canine. The first premolars will be removed at the time of surgery and the space closed surgically.

The very important decision—the predicted vertical position of the maxillary incisor—is now made. Guided by the information on the ideal incisor–upper lip relationship discussed elsewhere, a horizontal line is drawn to indicate the vertical position of the maxillary incisor. A vertical line transecting this line, indicating the desired anteroposterior position of the maxillary incisor, is then drawn. The final position of the maxillary incisor tip is indicated by the intersection of these two lines. The fact that surgery will involve both jaws allows the clinician to choose both the final vertical and the final anteroposterior position of the maxillary incisor. Guidelines to assist in the vertical positioning of the incisor have been discussed earlier.

The following guidelines will help the clinician locate the ideal horizontal positioning of the maxillary incisor:

- The maxillary incisors are responsible for upper lip support. Excessive retraction of the anterior maxillary segment will result in loss of lip support and poor esthetic results.
- Retraction of the anterior segment will increase the nasolabial angle and accentuate the nose.
- Lip thickness is often a good indicator of how much retraction of the anterior segment a patient will tolerate before the lip will react to the tooth movement. In general, the thickness of the upper and lower lips is equal.
- Vermilion exposure of the upper lip will decrease after retraction of the anterior maxillary segment.
- Avoid excessive retraction of the anterior teeth. A fuller lip is esthetically more pleasing than a flat, unsupported upper lip.

A vertical line simulating the vertical osteotomy of the bilateral sagittal split osteotomy is drawn on the body of the mandible (Fig 3-37b).

Step 2

Place a clean sheet of acetate over the original tracing, and trace all hard and soft tissue structures that will not

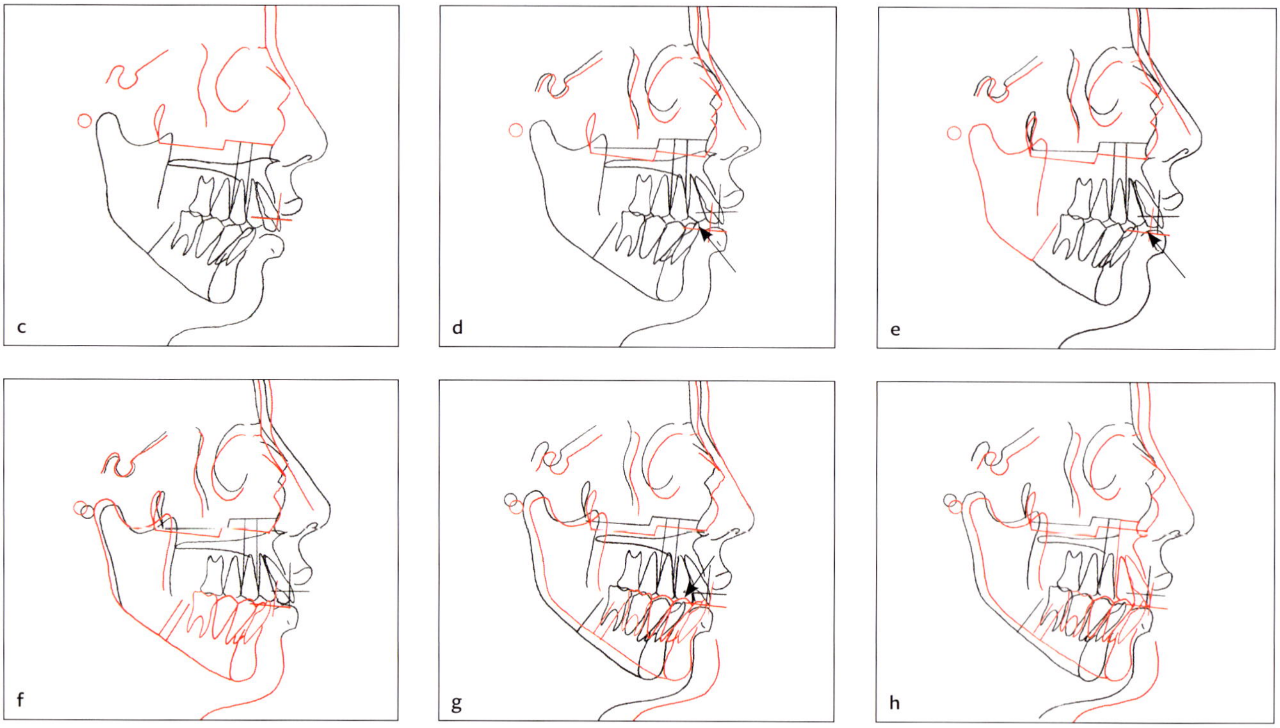

Fig 3-37 *(cont)* (*c*) Step 2. All structures that will not be affected by the surgery are traced in red. (*d*) The mandible is autorotated until the mandibular incisor projects 2 mm above the horizontal line (*arrow*). (*e*) After autorotation of the mandible, the mandibular incisors are still a few millimeters behind the vertical line, indicating the labial surface of the maxillary incisors (*arrow*). The mandible will have to be advanced. (*f*) The mandible is advanced by moving the prediction tracing to the left. (*g*) The teeth of the anterior maxillary segment on the original tracing now fit on the teeth of the mandible on the prediction tracing (*arrow*). (*h*) The maxillary incisor is placed between the mandibular incisor and the vertical line. The labial surface of the maxillary incisor is now tangent to the vertical line.

be affected by the surgery (Fig 3-37c). The maxillary and mandibular skeletal structures, soft tissue of the nose below the supratip break, upper lip, and mandibular soft tissue structures are not traced.

Place a pencil just posterior to the condylion. Rotate the prediction tracing in a clockwise direction until the mandibular incisor projects approximately 2 mm above the horizontal line (the amount of mandibular incisor above the line indicates the desired overbite; Fig 3-37d). Next, trace the skeletal structure of the mandible proximal to the vertical mandibular osteotomy line. The mandibular incisor is now a few millimeters behind the vertical line (Fig 3-37e).

Step 3

Slide the prediction tracing to the left. The original tracing structures will move to the right. Superimpose the prediction tracing so that the mandibular incisor on the original tracing is 1 mm behind the vertical line (the amount of mandibular incisor behind the vertical line indicates the desired overjet; Fig 3-37f). The two vertical osteotomy lines on the mandibular body should be parallel, indicating that no rotational movements of the mandible have taken place. Trace the mandibular skeletal structures distal to the vertical line as well as the soft tissue on the chin below the labiomental fold (pogonion 1:1 response; see Fig 3-37f).

Step 4

Move the prediction tracing so that the teeth in the anterior maxillary segment fit on the teeth in the mandible (which is now autorotated and advanced). The incisor tip position is indicated by the intersection of horizontal and vertical lines drawn as the first step of the tracing, and the maxillary occlusal plane is adapted to the mandibular occlusal plane (Fig 3-37g). Now trace the anterior maxillary skeletal structures, including the vertical (interdental osteotomy) and horizontal (Le Fort I osteotomy) lines on the segment (Fig 3-37h).

Step 5

Slide the prediction tracing to the left. The original tracing structures will move to the right. Position the original trac-

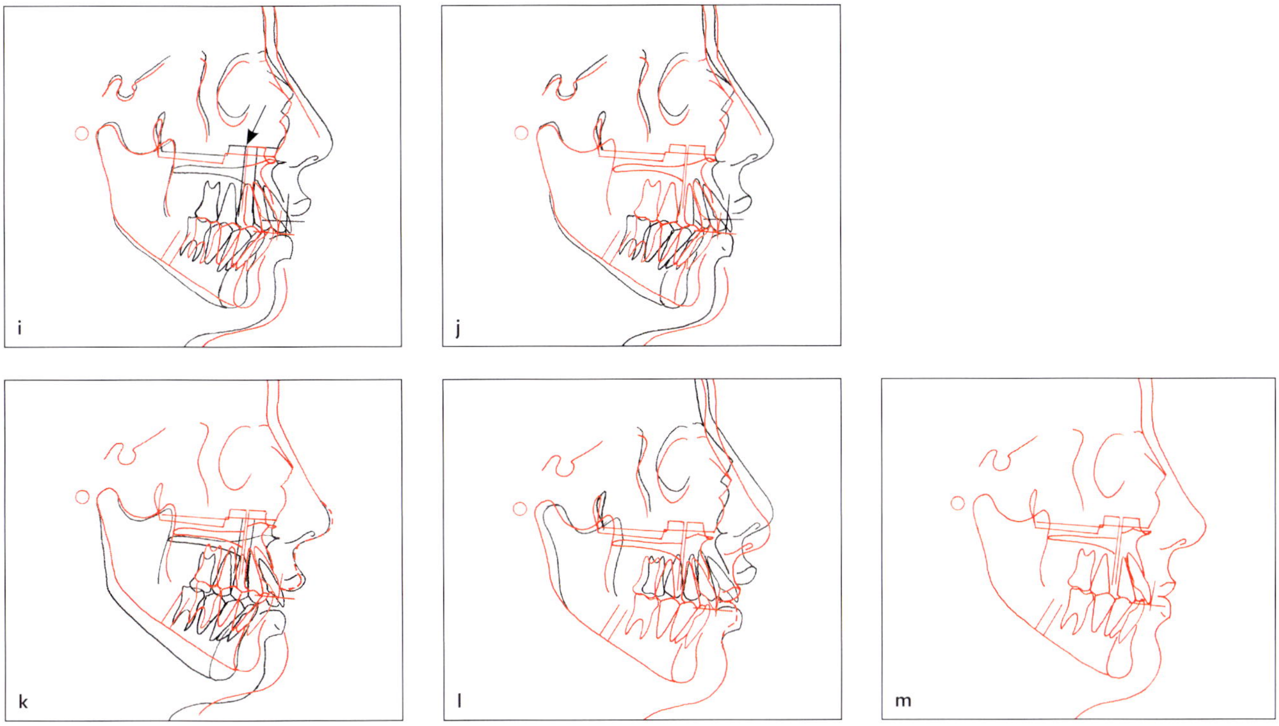

Fig 3-37 *(cont)* (*i*) The posterior maxillary teeth on the original tracing are advanced by sliding the prediction tracing to the left and placed on the posterior mandibular teeth on the prediction tracing. The vertical lines (interdental limits of bone removal) must not overlap and at most can be tangent (*arrow*). (*j*) The interdental osteotomy lines are 1 mm apart, indicating that the interdental ostectomy can be performed safely without damage to the roots of the teeth adjacent to the osteotomy. (*k*) Prediction of the soft tissue of the nasal tip and upper lip. (*l*) Lower lip prediction. (*m*) Completed surgical visual treatment objective.

ing's posterior maxillary teeth (molars and premolars) so that they fit on the mandibular posterior teeth. This should be done realistically, keeping in mind the roots of the teeth adjacent to the extraction socket of the first premolar and interdental ostectomy. The vertical interdental reference lines must touch at most. Further movement will be surgically unrealistic and increase the risk of damage to the adjacent teeth. Again, the mandibular occlusal plane dictates the vertical position of the posterior maxillary segment (Fig 3-37i). Trace the skeletal structures as well as the horizontal osteotomy line of the posterior maxillary segment (Fig 3-37j).

Step 6

Slide the prediction tracing on the original tracing to superimpose the structures that were not affected by the surgery. A vertical and horizontal change is apparent in the relationship of the maxillary incisor and upper lip. The soft tissue change of the nasal tip and upper lip can now be predicted by drawing the soft tissue with dotted lines (Fig 3-37k). As a guide, the vermilion (stomion) will shorten by 10% to 20%, the nasolabial angle change will vary (but tends to increase slightly), and the nasal tip will tip up slightly. Once the clinician is confident with the prediction, the maxillary soft tissue can be drawn in.

Step 7

Move the prediction tracing to superimpose its skeletal and distal mandibular structures on those of the original tracing. Trace the lower lip, using as a guide the known soft tissue response to mandibular advancement procedures (Fig 3-37l). The lower vermilion will decrease by 75% (66% to 100%) of the horizontal movement, the lower lip will curl back, and the labiomental fold will flatten.

Figure 3-37m illustrates the completed surgical visual treatment objective. The hard tissue movements required at surgery can be recorded by measuring the distance between the osteotomy reference lines.

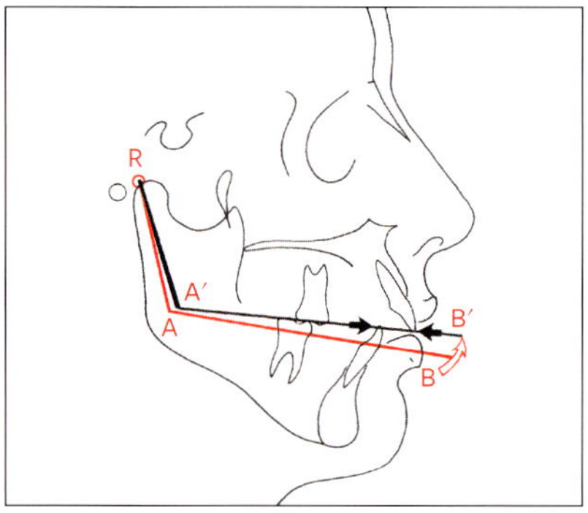

Fig 3-38 The maxilla has been superiorly repositioned and the mandible autorotated around a point (R) at or just posterior to the mandibular condyle. The occlusal plane has changed from A-B to A′-B′. Any anteroposterior corrections will take place along this "new" occlusal plane.

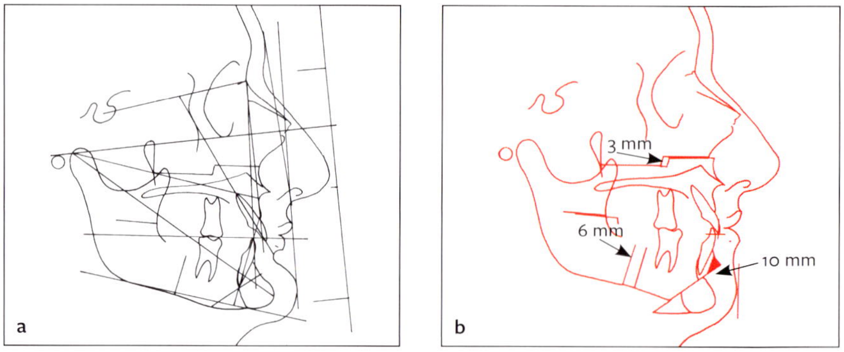

Fig 3-39 (*a*) Presurgical cephalometric analysis of the patient in case 1. (*b*) Surgical prediction tracing according to conventional principles. The surgery involves advancement of both the maxilla and mandible, as well as a large reduction genioplasty necessary to reduce the chin prominence. However, an unesthetic chin contour results from obliteration of the labiomental fold and poor definition of the lower border of the mandible.

Rotation of the maxillomandibular complex

In all the previous prediction tracings, the final occlusal plane was dictated by the mandibular occlusal plane (after autorotation in cases where vertical repositioning of the maxilla occurred). The mandible (and therefore the mandibular occlusal plane) will rotate around a point at or just posterior to the condyle. Any anteroposterior changes will take place along this "new" plane (Fig 3-38). This principle is not adhered to in treatment planning requiring rotation of the maxillomandibular complex and consequent alteration of the occlusal plane.

Case 1: Surgical prediction tracing involving clockwise rotation of the maxillomandibular complex

The presurgical cephalometric analysis of the patient in case 1 is seen in Fig 3-39a. The diagnosis is Class II malocclusion, maxillary anteroposterior deficiency, macrogenia, and mandibular alveolar anteroposterior deficiency.

Figure 3-39b illustrates a conventional surgical prediction involving maxillary advancement, mandibular advancement, and reduction genioplasty. However, it is not possible to achieve both good esthetic chin contour and an acceptable anteroposterior position by means of a reduction genioplasty. The alternative of clockwise rotation of the maxillomandibular complex can be tested by means of a surgical cephalometric prediction.

Step 1

Draw lines on the original tracing representing the intended osteotomies on the maxilla, mandible, and symphysis. Where no vertical change of the chin is indicated, the line is drawn horizontally with the mental nerve and root apices of the mandibular teeth in mind. However, this case requires a vertical increase as well as anteroposterior reduction. The osteotomy line, therefore, should be angulated downward. For accurate measurement, the osteotomy lines should be drawn as close as possible to the anatomical positions where the osteotomies will be performed (Fig 3-39c).

Step 2

Place a piece of acetate over the original tracing, and trace all the structures that will not be altered by the surgery. This will be the prediction tracing (Fig 3-39d). The ideal position of the maxillary incisor edge should be indicated on the prediction tracing by a "box," where the horizontal line indicates the ideal vertical position of the incisor tip and the vertical line indicates the ideal anteroposterior position of the anterior tooth surface relative to the upper lip. The desired anteroposterior position of the chin should also be indicated by a vertical line. Helpful markers for determining this line include the angle of facial convexity and the 0-degree meridian; the clinician's judgment is also paramount (Fig 3-39e).

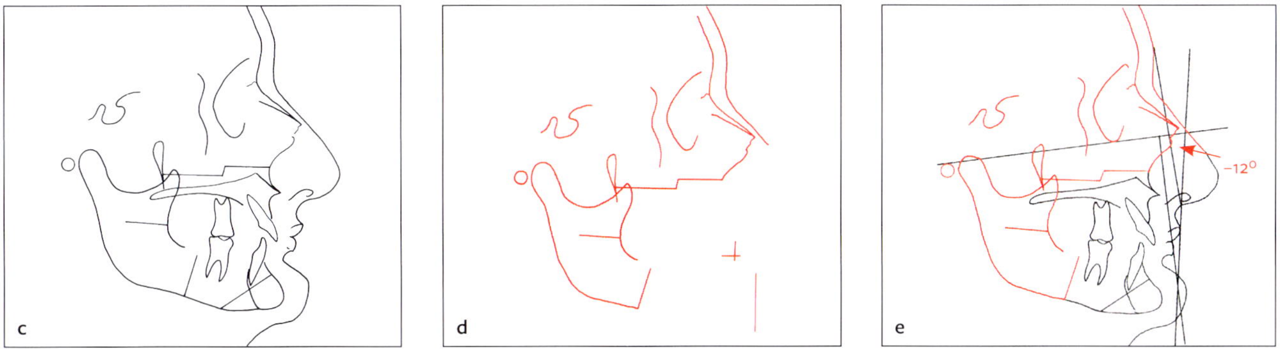

Fig 3-39 *(cont)* (*c*) Original tracing of the patient in case 1. For more accurate measuring, the intended osteotomy lines are drawn as close as possible to the actual anatomical site of the osteotomies. Both the horizontal and vertical osteotomy lines of the sagittal ramus osteotomy are drawn to monitor both horizontal and vertical mandibular movement. (*d*) Prediction tracing. All the hard and soft tissue structures that will not be influenced by the surgery are traced in red. Guidelines for the ideal maxillary incisor position are indicated by a vertical line (indicating the ideal anteroposterior position of the anterior tooth surface) and a horizontal line (indicating the ideal vertical position of the incisor tip), and a vertical line is drawn to indicate the ideal anteroposterior position of the chin. (*e*) In addition to the surgeon's clinical judgment, the facial contour and the 0-degree meridian act as guidelines to establish the ideal anteroposterior position of the chin. →

Step 3

Remove the prediction tracing from the original tracing, and place a new sheet of acetate over the original tracing. Trace the part of the maxilla below the Le Fort I maxillary osteotomy line. Move the acetate (to the left, in this case) to achieve the optimal occlusal relationship between the traced maxillary teeth and the mandibular teeth on the original tracing, and trace the mandibular teeth and the distal part of the mandible anterior to the vertical osteotomy line. Retrace the osteotomy line for the genioplasty at the symphysis (Fig 3-39f). Keep the maxillomandibular complex tracing (Fig 3-39g) in this position on the original tracing.

Step 4

Place the prediction tracing over the original tracing. The maxillomandibular complex tracing can now be moved between the original tracing and the prediction tracing. In this case, the tracing is rotated in a clockwise direction, advancing the maxilla and rotating the mandible posteriorly using the "box" for the maxillary incisor tip and the vertical line for the chin as guidelines. In this case, the clinician should keep in mind that a reduction genioplasty is indicated to correct the macrogenia and increase the vertical height of the symphysis. When a satisfactory position has been achieved, trace the maxillomandibular complex on the prediction tracing. The part of the symphysis below the genioplasty osteotomy line, however, is not traced at this time (Fig 3-39h).

Step 5

Remove the maxillomandibular complex tracing, and superimpose the prediction tracing on the original tracing. Draw the soft tissue prediction using the same principles used for conventional prediction of soft tissue response to hard tissue change (Fig 3-39i). Complete the prediction tracing by tracing the ideal soft tissue of the chin and the required reduction genioplasty (Fig 3-39j). Note that in this instance, a much smaller reduction is indicated than in the conventional prediction (see Fig 3-39b), resulting in better soft tissue chin contour.

Step 6

Evaluate the predicted esthetic and functional results shown on the completed surgical prediction tracing (Fig 3-39k). Changes may be indicated to improve the results. In the case demonstrated here, the magnitude of the chin reduction can be reduced by increasing the rotation of the maxillomandibular complex, keeping in mind the effect of the increased advancement of the maxilla. The surgical prediction tracing, however, should always stay within the limitations of sound surgical technique.

Step 7

Note the point (R) where the Le Fort I osteotomy lines of the original tracing and the prediction tracing cross (see Fig 3-39k). This is the point around which the maxillomandibular complex will be rotated during surgery. The exact

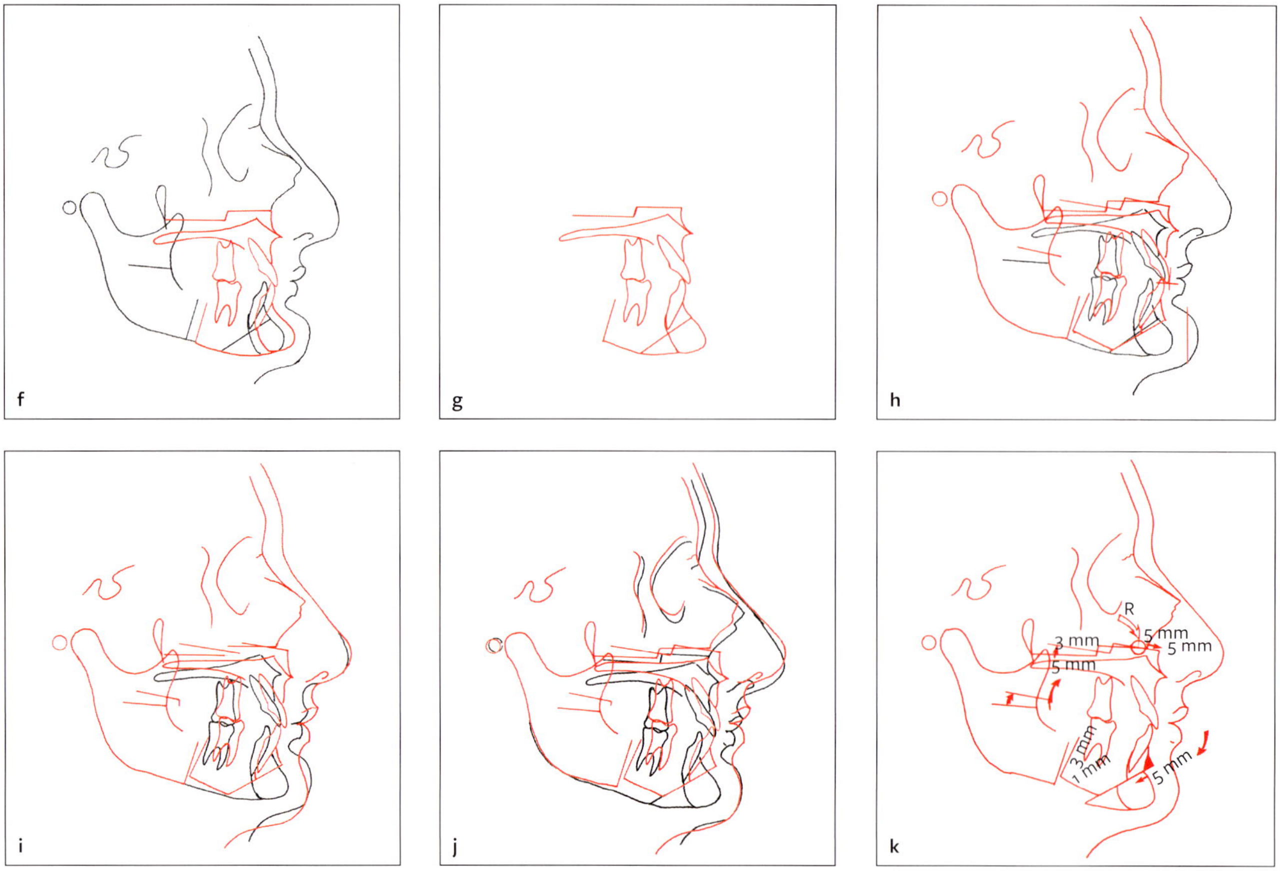

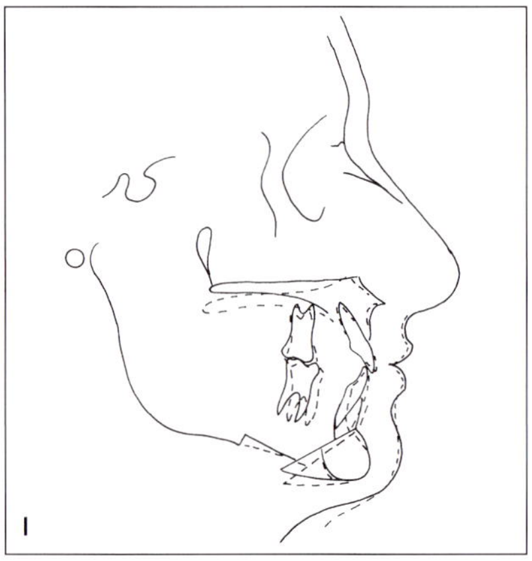

Fig 3-39 (*cont*) (*f*) Maxillomandibular complex tracing developed by first tracing the bone and dentition of the maxilla below the Le Fort I osteotomy line. The tracing is then moved to the left (in this case) to achieve an ideal occlusion between the maxillary teeth of the maxillomandibular complex tracing and the teeth on the original tracing. The mandibular teeth and bone anterior to the vertical osteotomy line are traced. The genioplasty line is also indicated on this tracing. (*g*) Maxillomandibular complex tracing. (*h*) The maxillomandibular complex tracing is placed between the prediction tracing and the original tracing and rotated clockwise, guided by the "box" (indicating the maxillary incisor position) and the vertical line (indicating the chin position). The hard tissue of the maxilla and mandible is traced. (*i*) Prediction tracing superimposed on the original tracing. The expected soft tissue change, including the ideal soft tissue position of the chin, is drawn. (*j*) The prediction tracing is moved to the right to establish the chin reduction required for the predicted soft tissue result. (*k*) Completed surgical prediction tracing for the patient in case 1. The rotation point (R) is located at the point where the Le Fort I osteotomy lines cross—in this case, 5 mm posterior to the piriform rim. (*l*) The composite tracing of the conventional prediction tracing (*dotted lines*) and the prediction tracing involving clockwise rotation of the maxillomandibular complex (*solid lines*) demonstrate the improved soft tissue contour achieved with the latter.

position of the rotation point should be noted and used during the model surgery as well as during the actual surgical procedure. All jaw movements should be measured on the prediction tracing and model surgery and be recorded as in conventional treatment.

A comparison of the prediction tracing of conventional treatment planning and the prediction tracing reflecting clockwise rotation of the maxillomandibular complex shows that the latter yields superior esthetic results (Fig 3-39l).

Case 2: Surgical prediction tracing involving counterclockwise rotation of the maxillomandibular complex

The presurgical cephalometric analysis of the patient in case 2 is shown in Fig 3-40a. The diagnosis is Class II malocclusion, mandibular anteroposterior deficiency, vertical maxillary excess, and microgenia.

Figure 3-40b illustrates the conventional surgical prediction involving maxillary superior repositioning, mandibular autorotation, and mandibular advancement

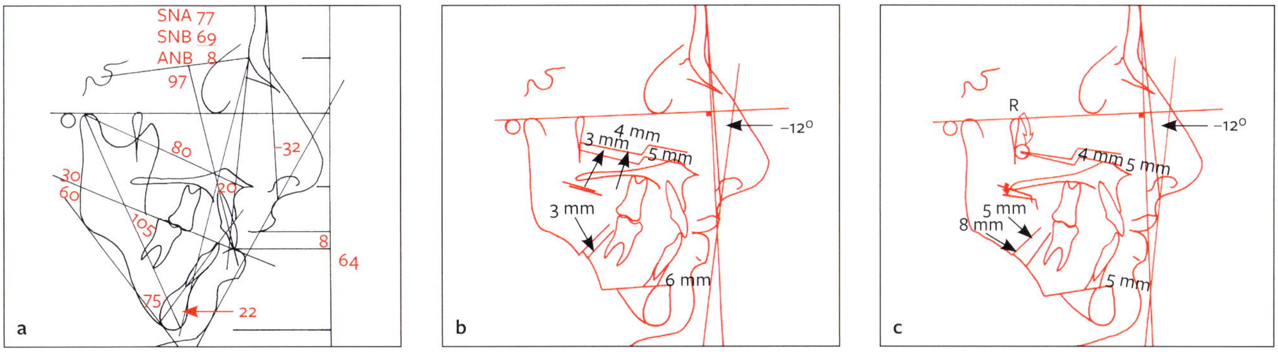

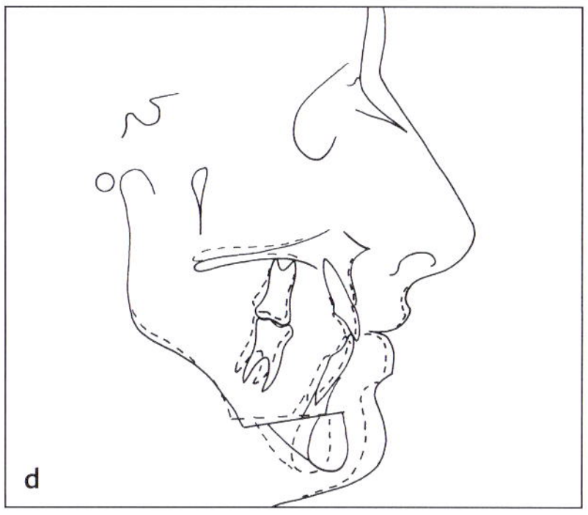

Fig 3-40 (*a*) Presurgical cephalometric analysis of the patient in case 2. (*b*) Surgical prediction tracing according to conventional principles. The surgery involves maxillary superior repositioning. The mandible will autorotate around a point just posterior to the condyle and is then advanced. The chin is advanced by a sliding genioplasty. The profile is still convex, and the chin is positioned too far posteriorly. Any further advancement of the chin through genioplasty, however, will lead to an unesthetic chin contour. (*c*) The surgical prediction tracing demonstrates counterclockwise rotation of the maxillomandibular complex around a point (R) at the posterior nasal spine. The rotation of the maxilla enables the surgeon to advance the mandible farther than is possible with conventional planning. The anteroposterior position of the chin is acceptable and allows good soft tissue contour. (*d*) The difference in results is demonstrated by the composite tracing. The conventional prediction tracing (*dotted lines*) is compared with the prediction tracing using the counterclockwise rotation of the maxillomandibular complex (*solid lines*).

combined with an advancement genioplasty. For an ideal chin position, the chin needs to be advanced more; however, further advancement by genioplasty will cause poor esthetic chin contour. The alternative of counterclockwise rotation of the maxillomandibular complex is tested by means of a surgical prediction tracing. This can lead to an improved esthetic result, as illustrated in Fig 3-40c. Note the rotation point (R), in this case at the posterior nasal spine. The difference in surgical outcome results is demonstrated in a composite tracing in Fig 3-40d.

Immediate Preoperative Model Surgery

The development of CBCT and its application to orthognathic surgery has enabled the clinician to plan corrective surgery accurately in three dimensions. With reductions in the cost of hardware and the radiation dose, 3D imaging has become available for a growing amount of clinicians and is currently a standard tool for diagnosis and treatment planning in several disciplines. Although 3D planning is not an absolute requirement for single-jaw surgery, it has become essential for accurate planning for the correction of craniofacial deformities, facial asymmetries, total TMJ replacement, hemifacial microsomia, and complex rotations of the facial skeleton in three planes. An intermediate surgical splint made by CAD/CAM or 3D printing is the link between the virtual simulation and the surgeon in the operating room.

The author is of the opinion that the basis for any orthognathic surgical planning starts with the examination of the presurgical dental casts and the visualization of the planned occlusion (fit of the teeth). Experience gained from conventional cephalometric analysis and model surgery forms the basis for understanding 3D visual planning.

The primary goal of model surgery is to functionally and spatially simulate the patient's jaws and dental structures as accurately as possible to allow accurate simulation of the intended surgery. The preoperative position of these structures can be measured and recorded. The surgical movement of the jaw(s) or dentoalveolar segments, as indicated by cephalometric prediction tracings, is simulated on the casts, and the specific spatial changes are then recorded. In short, model surgery is the dental cast version of cephalometric prediction of surgical results.

The first step in defining the patient's deformity in three planes of space is to place the dental casts on an anatomical articulator, using a facebow transfer in centric occlusion. The plaster is trimmed to simulate the anatomy of the maxilla and mandible as closely as possible. Reference lines are then drawn on the mounted casts to record their positions in three planes of space. The second step is to determine the desired final position, aided by the cephalometric prediction tracing and clinical

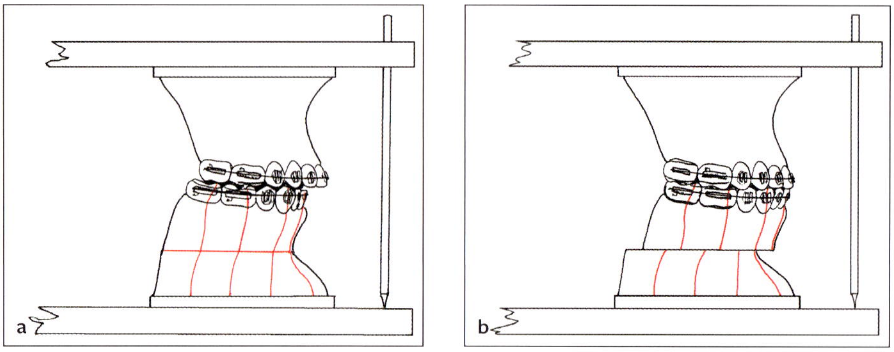

Fig 3-41 (*a*) Surgical repositioning of the mandible should take place along the mandibular occlusal plane. The osteotomy line on the cast should therefore be made parallel to the mandibular occlusal plane to allow the cast to slide along this plane. Clockwise and counterclockwise rotations at the surgical site can be detected and recorded. (*b*) The mandibular cast has been advanced to establish an occlusion. The movements can now be recorded.

data. During the third step, premovement and postmovement measurements are compared. The clinician can now accurately determine what dimensional movements will be necessary to accomplish the intended surgical goals. The surgical options fall into three basic categories: (1) mandibular surgery only, (2) maxillary surgery only, and (3) two-jaw surgery.

Mandibular surgery only

When mandibular surgery alone is contemplated, the mandibular anterior or posterior movement or rotational movements are dictated by the maxillary dentition. The occlusion of the mandible is adapted to that of the maxilla.

For example, in mandibular advancement, model surgery would proceed as follows:

1. Draw a horizontal “osteotomy” line parallel to the mandibular occlusal plane (Fig 3-41a).
2. Draw vertical reference lines from the cusps of the molars, canines, and central incisors to the base of the cast (see Fig 3-41a).
3. Measure the length of the vertical lines, and record the data.
4. Cut the mandibular cast on the horizontal osteotomy line.
5. Advance the cast into the most favorable dental occlusion (Fig 3-41b).
6. Measure anteroposterior vertical and/or rotational movements, and compare them with the premovement data.

Maxillary surgery only

When maxillary surgery alone is contemplated, the mandibular dentition dictates the position of the maxilla. If any vertical changes of the maxilla are planned, the mandible will autorotate, which in turn will affect the anteroposterior position of the maxilla. The anteroposterior position is therefore dictated by the mandible whereas the vertical position can be altered by vertical repositioning of the maxilla. A basic rule is that the postoperative position of the operated jaw is determined by the unoperated jaw, except in the vertical plane when the maxilla is the jaw to be repositioned.

Following are the procedures to be used in the case of maxillary repositioning (advancement in this case):

1. Draw a horizontal osteotomy line as close as possible to where the actual Le Fort I osteotomy will be performed (Fig 3-42a).
2. Draw two horizontal lines, one line 5 mm above the osteotomy line and one line 5 mm below it (the two lines are 10 mm apar; see Fig 3-42a). The lateral walls of the maxilla are not parallel and taper downward. This situation often leads to telescoping, especially of the posterior maxilla, which limits bone contact, accurate surgical positioning, and adequate bone fixation. By measuring the distance between the horizontal lines close to the osteotomy line, a more accurate assessment of the necessary amount of bone removal can be made (Fig 3-42b).
3. Draw vertical lines from the buccal cusps of the teeth to the base of the cast.
4. Measure the length of the vertical lines, and record the data.
5. Cut the cast along the osteotomy line.
6. Perform anteroposterior maxillary repositioning:
   a. Advance the cast into the planned occlusion (Fig 3-42c).
   b. If no vertical changes of the face are contemplated, keep the articulator pin fixed and the vertical height maintained.
   c. Trim the casts to fit into position, if necessary.
   d. Remeasure the vertical and horizontal distances to record the required surgical movement.

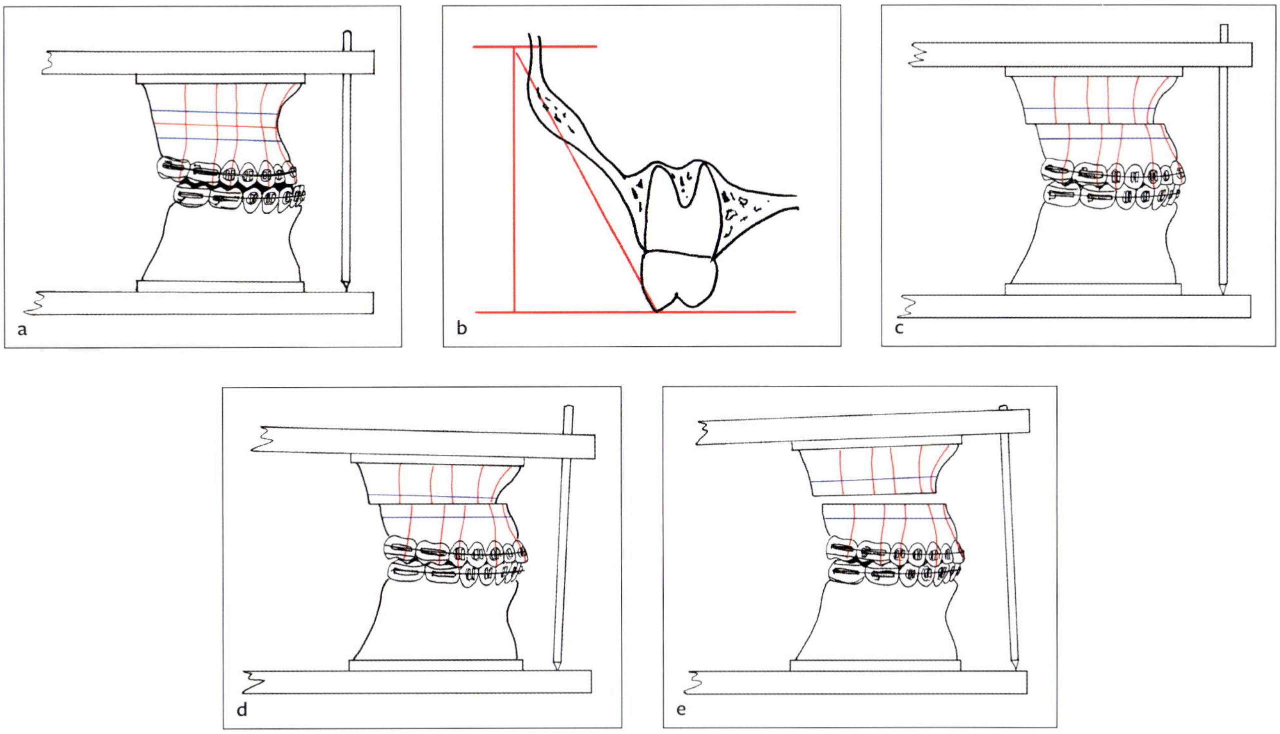

Fig 3-42 (*a*) The osteotomy line is drawn parallel to the occlusal plane. Failure to keep this line parallel to the occlusal plane will lead to vertical lengthening or shortening of the maxilla as it is advanced. For more accurate measurement, trimming of plaster should be limited to between the two lines drawn 5 mm above and 5 mm below the osteotomy line. (*b*) The discrepancy in measuring actual vertical height and measuring the tapering maxillary surface is demonstrated. (*c*) Maxillary cast in the planned position. Surgical changes can be recorded. (*d*) Trim the superior aspect of the cast. Measure the distance from the maxillary incisor tip to the base of the cast to ensure that the required vertical repositioning has been achieved. Measuring the distance between the horizontal lines can establish the exact amount of bone to be removed at the anterior and posterior maxilla. (*e*) Open the articulator until the correct amount of vertical increase has been achieved. (Measure from the incisor tip to the base of the cast.)

Vertical maxillary repositioning

Another example of maxillary surgery only is vertical maxillary repositioning. Following are the procedures to be used for model surgery in such cases:

- Superior repositioning of the maxilla
  1. Loosen the articulating pin to allow free movement.
  2. Trim the cast to allow the necessary superior repositioning.
  3. Place the cast into the planned occlusion, and measure the vertical height from the incisor edge to the base of the cast to ensure that the required vertical reduction has been achieved (Fig 3-42d).
  4. Tighten the articulator pin.
  5. Wax the cast into position.
  6. Remeasure the vertical and horizontal distances, and record the changes required at surgery (see Fig 3-42d).
- Vertical increase of maxillary height (downgrafting)
  1. Loosen the articulating pin to allow free movement.
  2. Place the cast into the planned occlusion.
  3. Open the articulator while monitoring the vertical increase from incisor tip to the base of the cast (Fig 3-42e).
  4. Once the desired vertical increase has been obtained, tighten the articulator pin.
  5. Wax the cast into position.
  6. Remeasure the vertical and horizontal distances, and record the surgical movements (see Fig 3-42e).

Two-jaw surgery

Planning two-jaw surgery involves the most complex combination of procedures; therefore, a systematic approach is essential. After careful clinical, cephalometric, and occlusal analysis, the surgeon faces the following decisions:

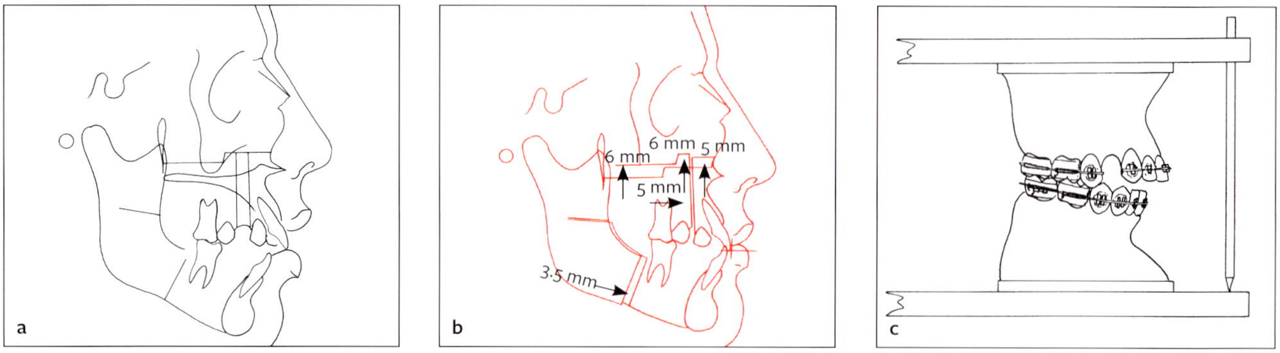

Fig 3-43 (*a*) Preoperative cephalometric tracing. (*b*) Surgical visual treatment objective. The surgical treatment plan consists of a three-piece Le Fort I maxillary osteotomy with 5-mm superior repositioning of the anterior segment, 6-mm superior repositioning of the posterior segment, and 5-mm advancement; expansion of the posterior maxillary segments; and 3.5-mm advancement of the mandible after autorotation. (*c*) Casts articulated in centric occlusion. →

- Position of maxillary incisors. This decision involves the anteroposterior position (lip support), vertical position (tooth-lip relationship), cant of the occlusal plane (transverse and horizontal), and dental midline (facial midline).
- The occlusal plane and the vertical position of the posterior maxilla. This decision is determined by the position of the mandible after autorotation unless either manipulation of the occlusal plane is contemplated or a transverse cant of the mandibular occlusal plane is present and should be corrected.
- Most ideal anteroposterior relationship of the mandible. Once the mandible has been autorotated to the ideal vertical relationship to the new maxillary incisor position, it can be advanced or set back along the new occlusal plane to its most ideal anteroposterior relationship to the maxillary incisor.
- Coordination of anteroposterior changes of the left and right sides of the maxillary arch with the mandibular arch rotations.
- Evaluation of transverse arch discrepancies (arch widths) and their correction (by posterior segmental model surgery) once the mandibular position has been established.

The patient's presurgical situation depicted in the cephalometric tracing shown in Fig 3-43a consisted of the following problem list:

- Class I molar and Class II canine relationships
- Anterior open bite
- Narrow maxillary arch
- Increased overjet
- Interdental space between maxillary canines and second premolars (the first premolars have been removed)
- Mandibular first premolars removed and the spaces closed orthodontically
- Vertical maxillary excess
- Mandibular anteroposterior deficiency

The surgical treatment plan is as follows (Fig 3-43b):

- A three-piece Le Fort I maxillary osteotomy with differential superior repositioning of the anterior and posterior segments to allow the maxilla to autorotate
- Expansion of the posterior maxillary segments
- Closure of the spaces between canines and second premolars
- Advancement of the mandible

Step 1

Articulate the casts on an anatomical articulator in centric occlusion using a facebow recording (Fig 3-43c). Trim the casts to resemble the true anatomy of the maxilla and mandible as closely as possible. Make a duplicate cast of the mandibular dentition. Remove the articulated mandibular cast from the articulator, and articulate the duplicate cast in exactly the same way. Change the casts again, and keep the duplicate cast for use in the construction of an intermediate splint.

Step 2

Draw reference lines:

1. Draw the tooth roots on the casts using the panoramic radiograph as a guide. Pay special attention to the teeth adjacent to the interdental osteotomy (Fig 3-43d).
2. Draw a line high on the maxillary cast and a line low on the mandibular cast parallel to the respective occlusal planes. These lines will serve as references for vertical measurements (Fig 3-43e).

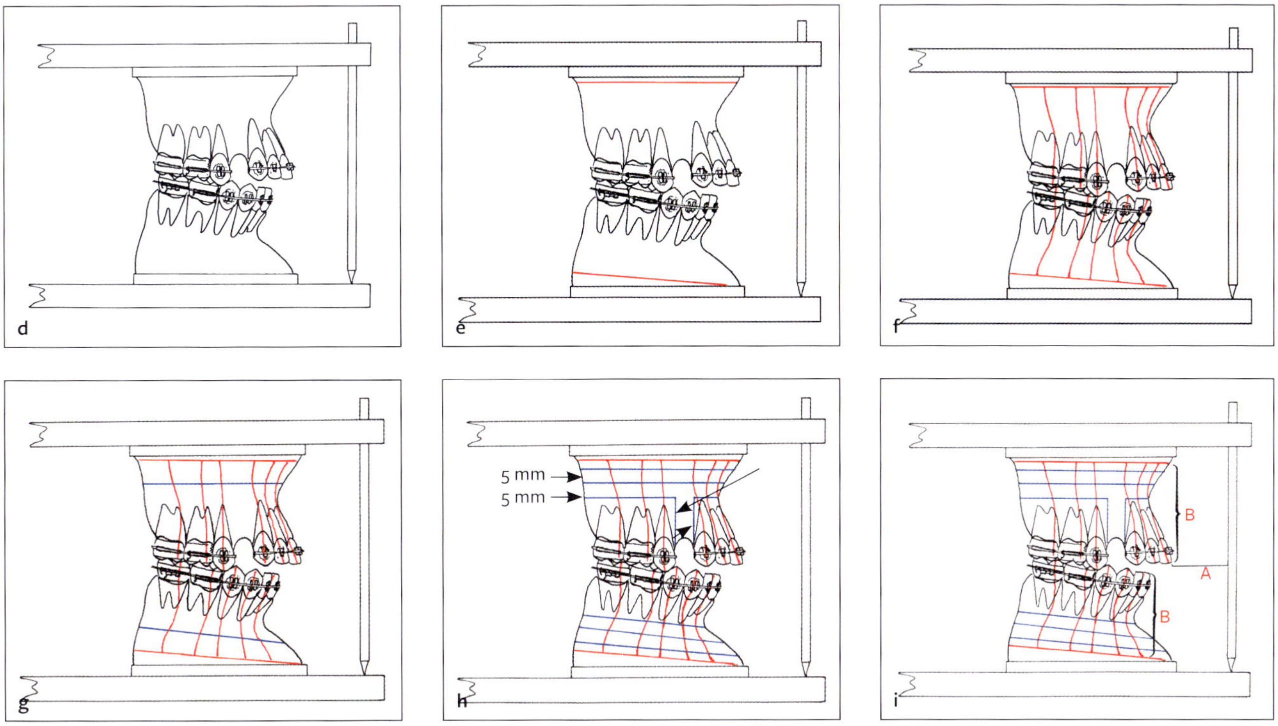

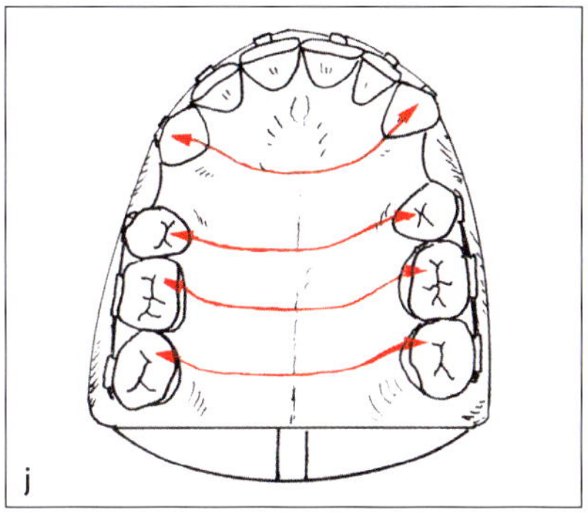

Fig 3-43 (*cont*) (*d*) Draw the roots of the teeth. (*e*) Horizontal lines for vertical measurements. (*f*) Vertical lines to record preoperative heights and measure planned vertical surgical changes. (*g*) Osteotomy lines drawn parallel to the occlusal plane of the maxilla and mandible. (*h*) Horizontal lines equidistant to (5 mm from) the osteotomy lines. The two vertical lines (*arrows*) indicate a safe distance from the roots of the teeth to perform the interdental osteotomy. (*i*) Measurement of the anteroposterior position of maxillary incisors (A) and the vertical distance from the horizontal line to the incisor tips and buccal cusps (B). (*j*) Transverse palatal measurements.

3. Perpendicular to each horizontal line, draw vertical lines to the buccal cusps of the teeth (Fig 3-43f).
4. Draw osteotomy lines representing the actual planes along which surgical movements will take place. It is important, especially on the maxillary cast, to draw the osteotomy line at the same angle and plane at which the actual Le Fort I osteotomy will be performed. The mandibular osteotomy line (a sliding plane) should be parallel to the mandibular occlusal plane (Fig 3-43g).
5. Draw two horizontal lines the same distance (eg, 5 mm) above and below the osteotomy lines. Measure the distance between them (eg, 10 mm; Fig 3-43h; see Fig 3-42b).
6. Draw two vertical lines, one on each side of interdental osteotomies. Measure the distance between these lines (see Fig 3-43h). They should be drawn on a plane so that bone can safely be removed without risk of injury to the roots of the teeth next to the interdental osteotomies. The lines will act as the limits of safe bone removal during model surgery.
7. Measure the distance between the buccal surface of the maxillary incisor and the vertical pin of the articulator (Fig 3-43i).
8. Draw transverse lines on the palatal surface of the maxillary cast from left to right, joining lingual cusps of molars, premolars, and canines. Measure these distances, and record them for use when transverse movements (expansion, narrowing, or differential movement of left and right maxillary segments) are contemplated (Fig 3-43j).
9. Record all the measurements on the cast. Because some of the recorded data may be lost during handling of the articulated casts, these measurements should also be recorded on a separate form.

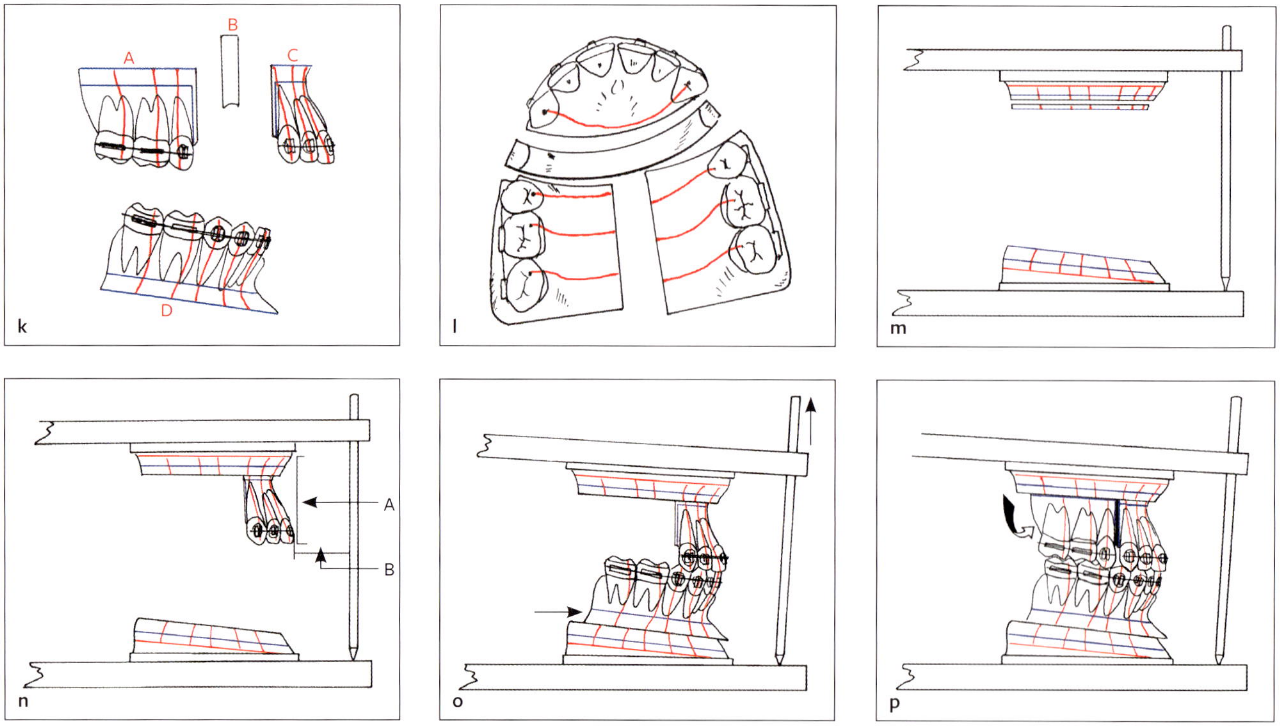

Fig 3-43 *(cont)* (*k*) The cast is cut and interdental bone removed. Posterior maxillary segment (A); removed interdental bone (B); anterior maxillary segment (C); mandibular segment (D). (*l*) Palatal cut separating the posterior segments. (*m*) The base of the maxillary cast is trimmed, but not beyond the parallel line. (*n*) The anterior maxillary segment is waxed into the correct vertical (A) and horizontal (B) positions according to the treatment plan. (*o*) The articulating pin is loosened to allow mandibular autorotation. The mandibular cast is then advanced into the planned anteroposterior position. (*p*) The posterior maxillary segments are trimmed to fit into the occlusion.

Step 3

Using a thin saw, cut the casts along the osteotomy lines. The interdental cuts should not exceed the guiding lines (Fig 3-43k). Also, complete the palatal cut to allow expansion of the posterior segments (Fig 3-43l). The articulator pin should still be tightened. If more than 5 mm of superior repositioning is contemplated, a few millimeters of plaster should be removed from the maxillary cast base (Fig 3-43m).

Step 4

Position the anterior maxillary segment according to the cephalometric visual treatment objective (on which the postoperative anteroposterior and vertical positions of the maxillary central incisor have been planned; see Fig 3-43f). This is done by removing plaster from the plaster segment and using measurements from reference lines and the articulator pin. The segment is then waxed into position (Fig 3-43n).

Step 5

Loosen the vertical pin of the articulator. Place the mandibular cast on the sliding plane and move it anteriorly while altering the vertical position by closing the articulator (autorotation). Ideal incisor and canine relationships are now established, and the mandibular segment is secured to the base with sticky wax (Fig 3-43o).

Step 6

Trim the superior aspect of the posterior maxillary segment, and place the segment into position with the maxillary teeth to fit the mandibular occlusion. If any transverse discrepancies exist, consider a midline palatal osteotomy to facilitate either expansion or narrowing of the posterior maxilla. Trim the cast according to the actual anatomical structures (Fig 3-43p). Unrealistic movements planned during model surgery cause problems during the actual surgery.

Step 7

Measure the vertical and horizontal changes, and record the surgical movements (Fig 3-43q). Transverse changes are measured from the palatal cusps (Fig 3-43r). Replace and tighten the articulator pin.

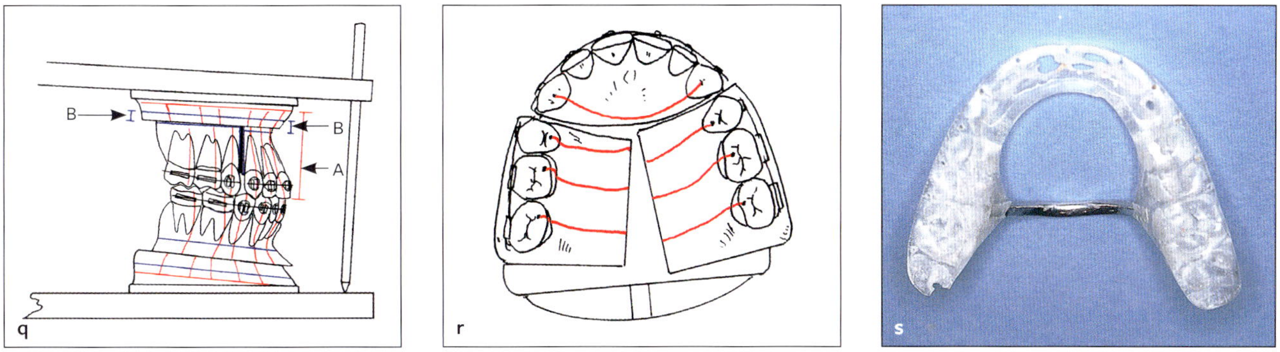

Fig 3-43 *(cont)* (*q*) Vertical changes are measured by remeasuring the vertical lines from the cusps of the teeth to the horizontal lines (A). For accurate measurement of the amount of bone to be removed, the distance between the horizontal lines above and below the osteotomy line is remeasured (B). (*r*) Surgical expansion is measured between the palatal cusps of the teeth. (*s*) Surgical splint reinforced with a palatal bar. (*t*) The duplicate "unoperated" mandibular cast (A) is articulated to establish the relationship between the repositioned maxilla and the unoperated mandible. The intermediate splint is made on these casts.

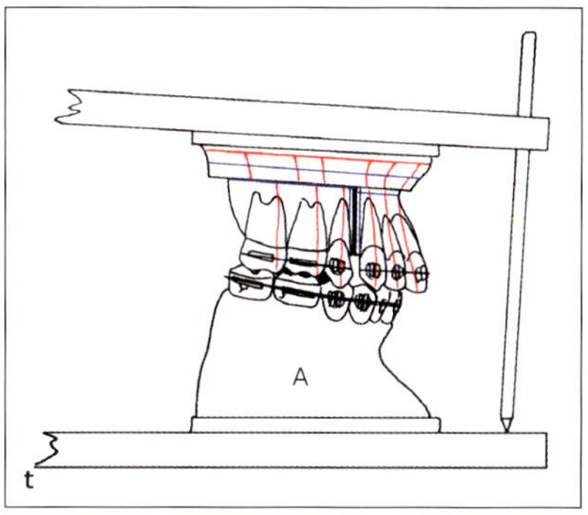

Step 8

The author prefers not to use a final surgical splint. Direct visualization of the occlusal contact during surgery allows for a more accurate bite correction to be established than is possible with use of an acrylic surgical splint. The numerous steps of model surgery and fabrication of a surgical splint leave the process open to imprecision. Even a small error made in the beginning of the fabrication process will be increased in magnitude in each subsequent step, so it is risky to depend totally on a splint for occlusal accuracy during surgery. An imprecise surgical splint will translate into an inaccurate final occlusion that may also compromise the esthetic outcome.

An acrylic splint can now be constructed to secure all the segments in their planned positions during surgery. The occlusal surfaces of the casts are covered with separating solution to prevent acrylic from sticking to the plaster during the curing phase. Mix an adequate amount of self-curing acrylic. Once the acrylic has reached the "dough" stage, mold it into a thin roll long enough to cover the dental arch. The thickness of the roll is critical. If it is too thick, it will be difficult to remove from the cast and will tend to fracture the plaster. If the splint is too thin, however, it could easily fracture at a critical stage of surgery. When a large palatal expansion is contemplated, consider reinforcing the splint with a palatal bar (Fig 3-43s).

Place the acrylic roll on the mandibular occlusal surface. Slowly close the articulator, gently forcing the teeth into the planned occlusion. Trim off any excess acrylic with a sharp knife. Place the articulator into a pressure pot, and allow the acrylic splint to cure under pressure. Once it has cured, remove the splint carefully, and trim and polish it. Make small interdental holes on the buccal side to facilitate intermaxillary wire placement. Some surgeons prefer to keep the splint on the maxilla for some time after surgery. The interdental holes facilitate fixation of the splint to the maxilla only.

Step 9

Remove the mandibular cast from the articulator and replace it with the duplicate cast (see Step 1). An intermediate splint can now be constructed as previously described. This splint will assist in the accurate positioning of the maxilla in relation to the unoperated mandible during surgery (Fig 3-43t). The surgeon may prefer to perform mandibular surgery first. If this is the case, remove the maxillary cast, rearticulate the original maxillary cast, and construct an intermediate splint. This splint will relate the new position of the mandible to the unoperated maxilla.

Virtual Surgical Planning

Steven Sullivan

Virtual surgical planning (VSP) is an increasingly important aspect of oral and maxillofacial surgery, especially orthognathic surgery. It is a tool that combines recent technological advances with traditional surgical procedures. This allows for a more streamlined presurgical workup and improved surgical accuracy.

Advances in technology have improved the surgical planning and efficiency of orthognathic surgery. The actual surgery itself has remained relatively unchanged, but VSP and other innovations have significantly impacted the presurgical workup. Historically, surgeons required lateral cephalometric radiographs and tracings to help predict surgical outcomes, as discussed in the previous section. In the 1970s, it was shown that lateral cephalometric radiographs could be digitized to help with predicting soft tissue outcomes. Early on, there were significant hurdles in the application of digital technology such as difficulties in manipulation and inherent human error. However, with advances in VSP, these difficulties have been minimized.

The CT scan, invented in the early 1970s, was the first of its kind to visualize anatomical structures in a complex, 3D way that had never been done before. The next major advancement in the digital and technological landscape came in 1983 with the invention of 3D printing. Human anatomy was first milled in 1985, leading to the printing of stereolithographic models during the 1990s. However, digital orthognathic surgery planning was largely limited to the academic arena. Although the 1990s saw the commercialization of software that could use 3D imaging for planning and manipulation, even by the end of the decade there had still been very few changes in the way orthognathic surgery was planned because there were significant limitations in actually transferring the 3D virtual plan to the patient. Therefore, surgeons still relied on the traditional orthognathic workup using plaster casts, facebow transfers, and estimation of jaw movements.

In the early 2000s, the first validated system was developed that used 3D virtual imaging for surgical planning, 3D printing, and interocclusal splints that could transfer the virtual plan to the patient. The process was further refined to an all-digital workflow that no longer required plaster casts, but only a CT data set and digital models. Since this time, VSP for orthognathic surgery has become increasingly popular and will hopefully become more affordable.

Traditional orthognathic surgery workups require the fabrication of acrylic splints fabricated on stone casts, which are mounted on semi-adjustable articulators as described in chapter 3. Splint fabrication on stone casts carries inherent risks and error because of the materials being used and processes in which they are made. Though very rare, there have been reports of malposition of up to 5 mm occurring in cases planned this way. Now, these inherent errors can be minimized with CAD/CAM fabrication of splints.

Stone casts of the arches, centric relation records, and imaging are still necessary even with the application of VSP; however, the efficiency is improved by minimizing the amount of laboratory work that is required during the presurgical workup phase. Often, the errors that occur during the presurgical laboratory phase are discovered intraoperatively. However, with VSP, these errors can be identified preoperatively and can be adjusted prior to surgery, thereby reducing operative errors.

Inexperienced surgeons can benefit by using computer-manufactured cutting guides to aid the orientation of the osteotomies. Doing so can help take any uncertainty out of where to place the osteotomy. These cutting guides are fabricated preoperatively during VSP and can help reinforce orientation of the bony segments. Designing these jigs preoperatively can help the surgeon avoid important anatomical structures such as nerves or major vessels. They can guide bony reduction and orient cuts for segmental osteotomies. The surgeon must keep in mind that these additional premanufactured components can add quite significantly to the case costs and could be shifted from the hospital to the patient. Typical plate and screw costs for a two-jaw osteotomy range from $1,200 to $3,000. Adding cutting guides and premanufactured plates can result in costs that can exceed $7,000, with little evidence to suggest there is a discernable difference in clinical outcome.

Surgical simulation also allows the surgeon to precisely determine where osteotomies are to be placed to have the best possible outcome, to avoid important structures, and to enhance the fixation screw locations into areas of high-quality bone. VSP is rapidly becoming the standard of care due to its improved accuracy, ease of presurgical simulation, error identification, and improved intraoperative efficiency.

There have been several studies evaluating the accuracy of orthognathic surgery using VSP and CAD/CAM. It has been found that the accuracy is very good, with errors being under 1 mm for linear measurements and 1 degree for angular measurements. VSP is less accurate, however, when changing the transverse width of the maxilla and when predicting the final chin position when doing genioplasty.

There is a developing consensus that VSP and CAD are more accurate and precise than conventional surgical planning. VSP minimizes the preoperative planning times; however, both types of planning have similar intraoperative times, and intraoperative complications are not decreased with VSP. The differences in clinical accuracy are also small enough to not present a noticeable difference in clinical outcome.

Over the past 25 years, VSP has slowly become the standard for treatment planning in orthognathic surgery and other dentofacial abnormalities. The future of VSP in orthognathic surgery appears promising. Although technology is always changing, the trend toward more accurate planning and user-friendly software will be a great asset for oral maxillofacial surgeons in the future.

VSP workflow

In both VSP and traditional model surgery, a comprehensive physical and radiographic examination is crucial when doing the surgical planning for the correction of dentofacial deformities. Once a treatment plan has been developed, surgical movements are carried out with either traditional model surgery with dental stone casts or virtually using computer programing. Precise surgical splints are fabricated and used to transfer the proposed surgical movements into the operating room.

In order to understand the advantages that VSP offers, one must understand the workflow of traditional model surgery as discussed in the previous sections. Whether using traditional methods or VSP, single-jaw surgery does not require splints to be fabricated from formal model surgery or digital planning. Splints are unnecessary if a stable occlusion can be obtained with tooth-to-tooth contact, so single-jaw surgery will only require a final interocclusal surgical splint if the final occlusion is unusual or unstable. A segmented maxilla will often require a palatal splint to maintain the width change and arch form. Double-jaw surgery will require an intermediate repositioning splint and possibly a palatal splint. When both jaws are being moved, a stable relationship in the intermediate position is essential, so model surgery of digital planning is required.

VSP is very similar to the first appointment with traditional model surgery. Necessary preoperative information is obtained to develop an accurate diagnosis and treatment plan. This includes preoperative photographs, a CT scan, physical measurements, alginate impressions, and a centric relation record. A facebow registration is not necessary for VSP. Traditionally, a crucial aspect of obtaining the CT scan had been verifying that the patient was in a neutral position and in centric relation. There have been multiple ways that have proven effective at obtaining a natural head position. These include taking CT scans with the patient biting on a facebow attached to gyroscope and using a facebow that has numeric values so the pitch, cant, and yaw can be calculated. Thanks to the improvements in CT technology, the process now includes obtaining a CT scan with the patient biting on a centric relation record and then the patient's FH plane is normalized.

The alginate impressions are poured up in die stone similar to traditional model surgery, and the final occlusion will be set. Due to scatter that often distorts the occlusal surfaces of teeth during the CT scan, there must be an accurate method of capturing the occlusal surfaces. This can be done with a CT scan of radiopaque stone or through laser scanning of the die stone casts. The surgeon then will set the final occlusion and provide the virtual planner with the clean preoperative occlusion and final occlusion.

One advantage of having the surgeon set the occlusion by hand with a plaster cast is the appreciation of interdigitation, occlusal nuances, and anatomy by the surgeon. The virtual bite will be merged with the CT scan of the skull by superimposing the digital imaging and communications in medicine (DICOM) data. Once this step is complete, an accurate skeletal and dental depiction of the patient is available (Fig 3-44).

The next step for the surgeon is the planning phase with office-based planning software or via an online meeting between a biomedical engineer and the surgeon. When using an online biomedical engineer, a formulated treatment plan prior to the meeting will expedite the process. This can be accomplished with a traditional acetate tracing or office-based computer software, and those surgical plans become prescriptive in the online meeting. The initial steps in the 3D planning process involve the proper orientation of the 3D rendering of the patient's skeletal and dental anatomy. This is confirmed by the proper alignment of the FH plane. Key anatomical landmarks are now identified and marked for reference, and cephalometric measurements are recorded (Fig 3-45).

The virtual surgery now begins with the surgeon defining and refining the planned osteotomies. With the final occlusion set and the maxilla and mandible coupled, the first movement the surgeon performs is correction of maxillary midline and cant. Anterior-posterior maxillary incisor movements and then vertical maxillary movements follow this (Fig 3-46). Changes in pitch or the occlusal plane can be made to refine the final chin position and to assess the need for genioplasty (Fig 3-47).

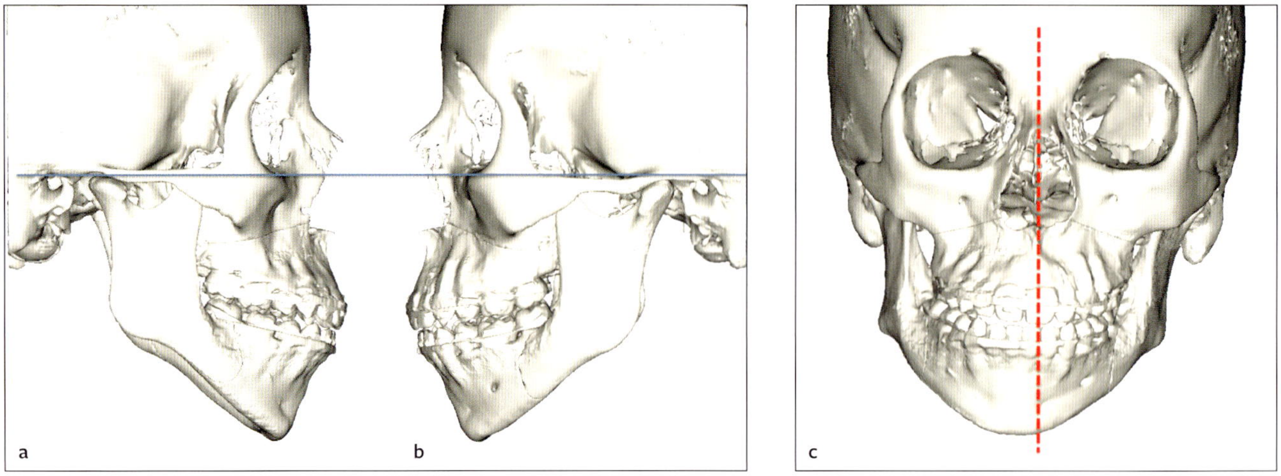

Fig 3-44 (*a*) Right side of reformatted CBCT scan. (*b*) Left side of reformatted CBCT scan. (*c*) Frontal view of reformatted CBCT scan.

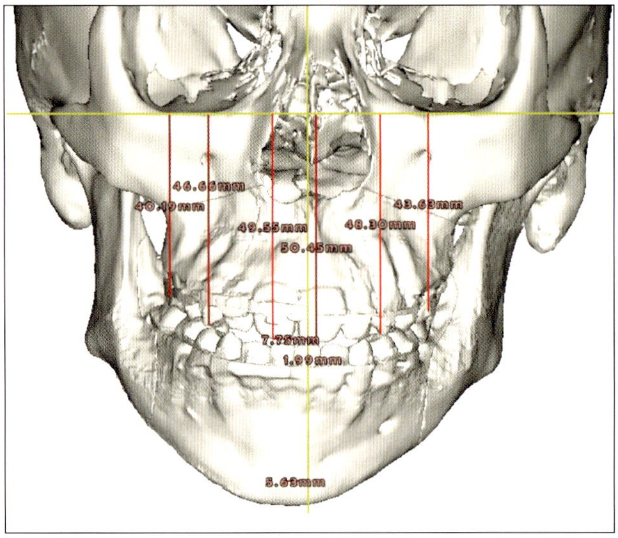

Fig 3-45 Preoperative frontal measurements of specific landmarks used to compare midlines and maxillary cant. The measurements depict a midline discrepancy as well as canting of the maxilla with an elevated right side.

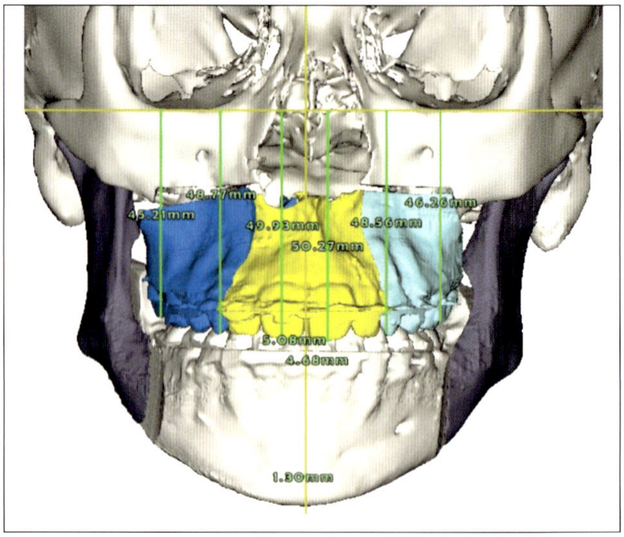

Fig 3-46 Normalized maxillary position following midline and cant correction.

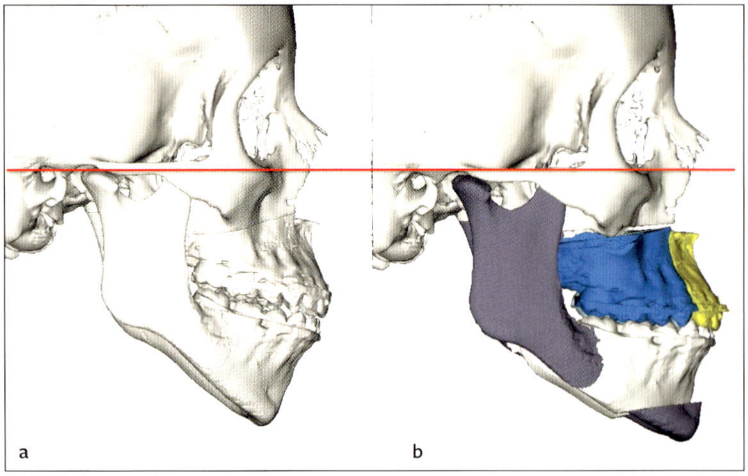

Fig 3-47 (*a*) Lateral view demonstrating high mandibular and occlusal plane prior to pitch correction. (*b*) The planned positions of the maxilla, mandible, and chin following counterclockwise rotation of the maxillomandibular complex, the occlusal plane change, and genioplasty.

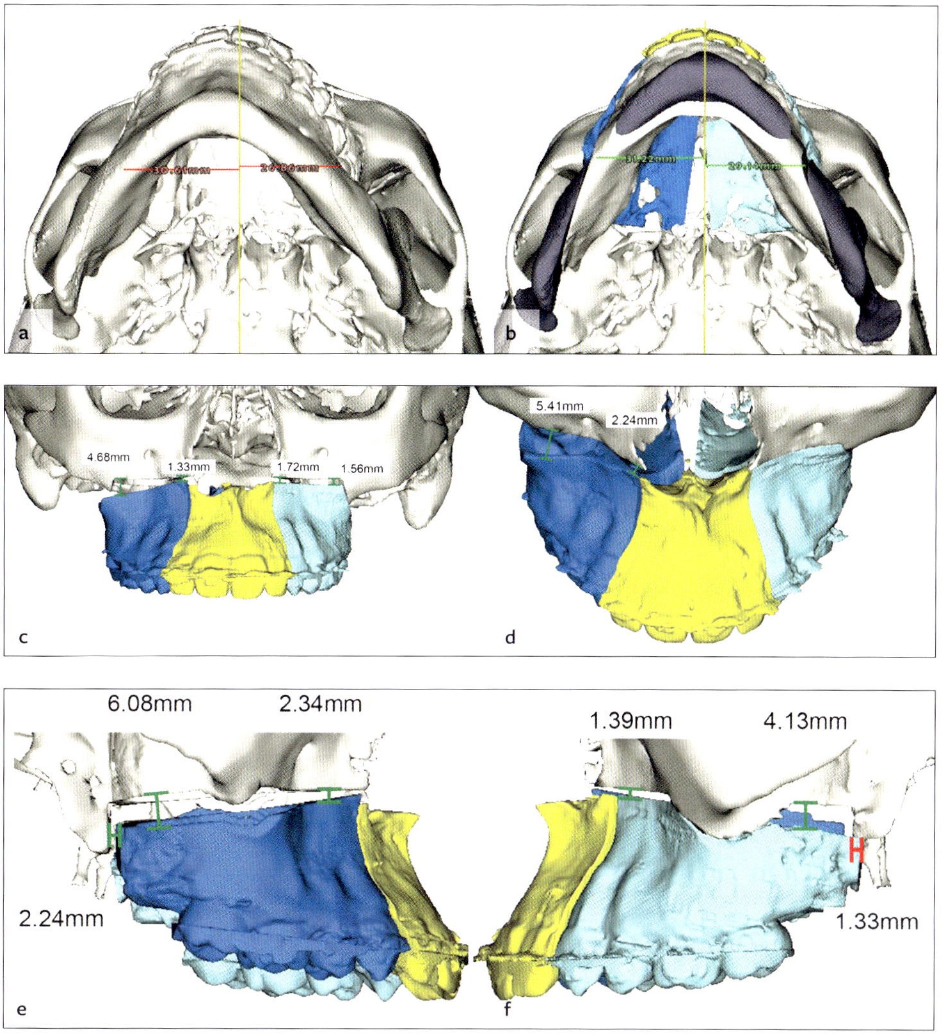

Fig 3-48 (*a*) The presurgical submental vertex view of the mandible demonstrating the significant yaw. (*b*) Submental vertex view of the mandible following correction of midlines, rotation of the maxillomandibular complex, advancement genioplasty, and correction of the yaw. (*c to g*) The defect measurements expected at the time of surgery at various points of the maxilla. Note the maxillary expansion in part *g*.

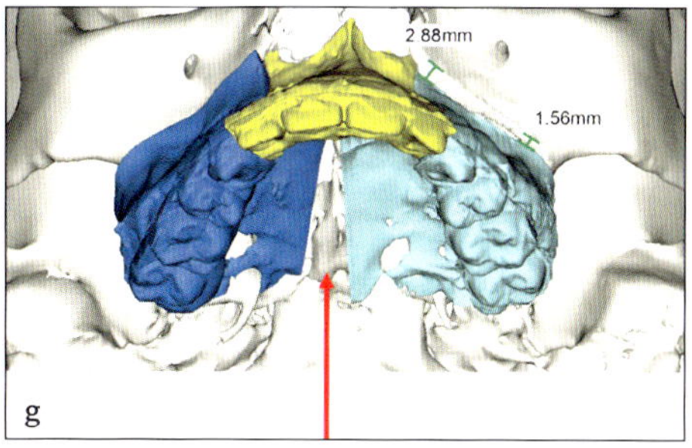

The vertical and sagittal maxillary incisor positions should not be altered with any occlusal plane changes. The final aspect in the planning process is the evaluation of maxillomandibular yaw and proximal segment position, including the presence of interferences, which may impact condylar position during and after application of fixation (Fig 3-48).

The surgeon now has the capability to evaluate the new position of the maxillomandibular complex in every dimension. The software is also able to inform the surgeon of the amount of bony overlap as well as any areas that may require grafting. Another advantage that VSP has over traditional model surgery is that the surgeon can evaluate the proposed position of bony landmarks during VSP—not

Table 3-5 | A summary of 3D surgical changes following virtual planning

	Lateral movement	Advancement or setback	Vertical movement
Maxilla			
ANS	0.56 mm left	0.44 mm setback	0.32 mm down
A-point	0.87 mm left	0.58 mm advancement	0.63 mm down
Central incisors	2.67 mm left	4.05 mm advancement	0.11 mm down
Left canine	1.22 mm left	1.49 mm advancement	0.26 mm down
Right canine	3.68 mm left	3.03 mm advancement	2.11 mm down
Left molar	2.28 mm left	1.63 mm advancement	2.64 mm down
Right molar	0.62 mm right	4.29 mm advancement	5.03 mm down
Mandible			
Central incisors	3.41 mm left	3.24 mm advancement	3.02 mm up
Left molar	2.55 mm left	2.01 mm advancement	2.2 mm down
Right molar	2.52 mm left	2.82 mm advancement	3.84 mm down
B-point	3.83 mm left	6.07 mm advancement	1.94 mm up
Pogonion	5.63 mm left	13.14 mm advancement	1.03 mm up

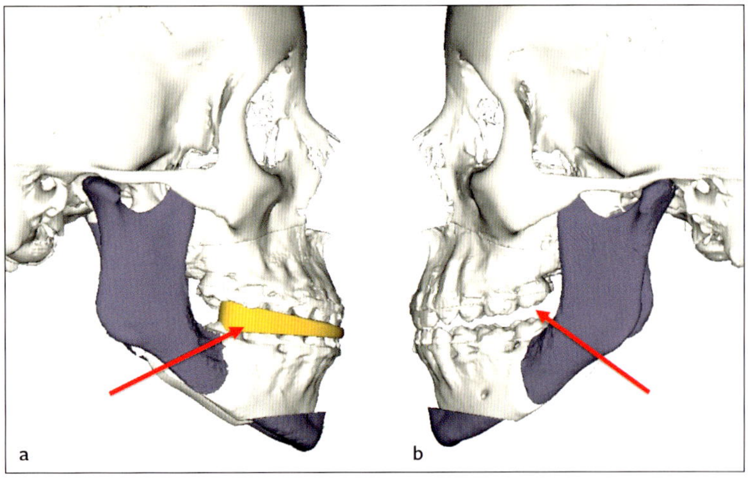

Fig 3-49 (*a*) Intermediate position after mandibular movements with the intermediate splint in place (*arrow*). With the counterclockwise rotation, the splint is thicker in the back in a mandible-first surgery. Conversely, in a maxilla-first surgery, the splint would be significantly thicker in the front, sometimes inhibiting the ability for maxillomandibular fixation. (*b*) Mandibular interim position from the left side showing the magnitude of posterior open bite (*arrow*) and effect of the maxillomandibular advancement with counterclockwise rotation.

just occlusal movements. The surgical plan also charts and records the movements of key landmarks so they can be assessed intraoperatively (Table 3-5).

Once the planned surgical movements are finalized, the surgeon must decide the sequencing of the surgery. Mandibular surgery first tends to be more accurate because it eliminates the influence that an inaccurate bite registration has on the final incisor positions from which the surgery was planned. Mandible-first sequencing is essential with counterclockwise movements because intermediate splint thickness can be quite significant and influence condylar positioning if performed second (Fig. 3-49).

Conversely, with large clockwise maxillomandibular movements, splints can be quite thick if the mandible is

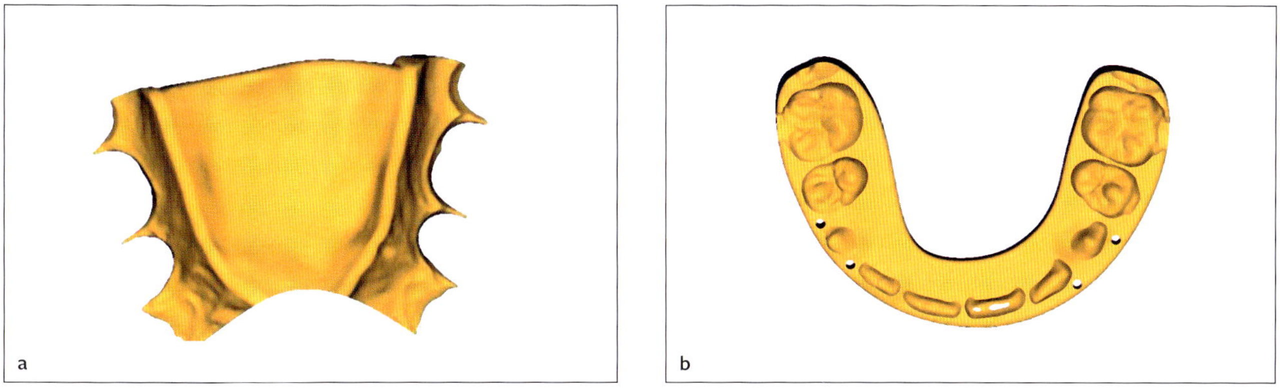

Fig 3-50 Splint designs, from which STL files will be generated for 3D printing. (*a*) Palatal splint. (*b*) Intermediate splint.

operated first. It is imperative that if the maxilla is operated first in either scenario that an extremely accurate preoperative bite registration is obtained. If there are any inaccuracies, the final maxillary position may be altered due to habitual posturing of the mandible because of the malocclusion. This will result in a maxilla that is posterior to the planned position.

Surgical splints are designed through computer programing and then 3D printed (Fig 3-50). Printed splints have a decreased chance of warping when compared with acrylic splints and have been shown to be as accurate as surgeon-fabricated splints using traditional additive methods (if not more accurate).

The previously described VSP workflow is an example of a traditional web-based system in which the surgeon coordinates and conferences with a biomedical engineer who is familiar with the virtual surgical software. With the advent of more user-friendly software and the increased availability of 3D printing technology, there is now an office-based approach. In the office-based workflow, the surgeon and their staff work as the software engineers. They will scan the dental models and merge the accurate occlusal registration with the CT scan. Then it will proceed with the staff or surgeon performing cephalometric analysis, virtual osteotomies, and the virtual surgery to achieve the surgical goal. This workflow can then use an in-house 3D printer or an external laboratory to fabricate the 3D splints.

The increase in popularity of VSP has brought about the question whether or not VSP is more efficient and more cost-effective than traditional model surgery. Multiple studies have tried to address these key questions. Time studies have compared VSP with traditional methods of planning. They have investigated the time spent during the presurgical workup and physical examination, the time spent in the laboratory preparing and performing model surgery, and the time spent during a VSP session and generally found that VSP does save time and ultimately patient costs once the workflow is mastered. The authors feel that it is safe to say that VSP is here to stay and offers many advantages over traditional model surgery, especially when dealing with asymmetries and custom joint replacement with concomitant maxillary procedures.

Recommended Reading

Abramson Z, Susaria SM, Lawler M, Bouchard C, Troulis M, Kaban LB. Three-dimensional computed tomographic airway analysis of patients with obstructive sleep apnea treated by maxillomandibular advancement. J Oral Maxillofac Surg 2011;69:677–686.

Arnett GW, McLaughlin RP. Facial and Dental Planning for Orthodontists and Oral Surgeons. St Louis: Mosby, 2004.

Becker OE, Avelar RL, Göelzer JG, Dolzan Ado N, Haas OL Jr, De Oliveira RB. Pharyngeal airway changes in Class III patients treated with double jaw orthognathic surgery—Maxillary advancement and mandibular setback. J Oral Maxillofac Surg 2012;70:e639–e647.

Butterfield KJ, Marks PG, McLean L, Newton J. Linear and volumetric airway changes after maxillomandibular advancement for obstructive sleep apnea. J Oral Maxillofac Surg 2015;73:1133–1142.

Cossa P, Baccetti T, Franchi L, De Toffol L, McNamara JA Jr. Mandibular changes produced by functional appliances in Class II malocclusions: A systematic review. Am J Orthod Dentofacial Orthop 2006:129: e1–e12.

Epker BN, Stella JP, Fish LC. Dentofacial Deformities: Integrated Orthodontic and Surgical Correction, vol 1. St Louis: Mosby, 1994.

Erickson KL, Bell WH, Goldsmith DH. Analytical model surgery. In: Bell WH (ed). Modern Practice in Orthognathic and Reconstructive Surgery. Philadelphia: Saunders, 1992.

Fish LC, Epker BN. Surgical-orthodontic cephalometric prediction tracing. J Clin Orthod 1980;14:36–52.

Frost DE, Van Sickels JE. Surgical treatment planning. In: Peterson LJ (ed). Principles of Oral and Maxillofacial Surgery, vol 3. Philadelphia: Lippincott, 1992:1307–1332.

Hart PS, McIntyre BP, Kadioglu O, et al. Postsurgical volumetric airway changes in 2-jaw orthognathic surgery patients. Am J Orthod Dentofacial Orthop 2015;147:536–546.

Henzi A. Effects of different orthognathic surgery procedures on pharyngeal airway space: A single center study [thesis]. Zurich: University of Zurich, 2012.

Hernández-Alfaro F, Guijarro-Martínez R, Mareque-Bueno J. Effect of mono- and bimaxillary advancement on pharyngeal airway volume: Cone-beam computed tomography evaluation. J Oral Maxillofac Surg 2011;69:e395–e400.

Hernández-Alfaro F, Guijarro-Martínez R. On a definition of the appropriate timing for surgical intervention in orthognathic surgery. Int J Oral Maxillofac Surg 2014;43:846–855.

Huang CS, Chen YR, Orthodontic principles and guidelines for the surgery-first approach to orthognathic surgery. Int J Maxillafac Surg. 2015;44:1457–1462.

Jacobson A, Sadowsky PL. A visualized treatment objective. J Clin Orthod 1980;14:554–571.

Jeong WE, Choi JW, Kim DY, Lee JY, Kwon SM. Can a surgery-first orthognathic approach reduce the total treatment time? Int J Oral Maxillofac Surg 2017;46:473–482.

Kinnebrew MC, Hoffmann DR, Carlton DM. Projecting the soft-tissue outcome of surgical and orthodontic manipulation of the maxillofacial skeleton. Am J Orthod 1983;84:508–519.

Mansour S, Burstone C, Legan H. An evaluation of soft-tissue changes resulting from Le Fort I maxillary surgery. Am J Orthod 1983;84:37–47.

McCollum AG, Reyneke JP, Wolford LM. An alternative for the correction of the Class II low mandibular plane angle. Oral Surg Oral Med Oral Pathol 1989;67:231–241.

Park JW, Kim NK, Kim JW, Kim MJ, Chang YI. Volumetric, planar, and linear analyses of pharyngeal airway change on computed tomography and cephalometry after mandibular setback surgery. Am J Orthod Dentofacial Orthop 2010;138:292–299.

Perez D, Ellis E 3rd. Implications of sequencing in simultaneous maxillary and mandibular orthognathic surgery. Atlas Oral Maxillofac Surg Clin North Am 2016;24:45–53.

Proffitt WR, Epker BN. Treatment Planning for Dentofacial Deformities in Surgical Correction of Dentofacial Deformities. Philadelphia: Saunders, 1980.

Proffit WR, Phillips C, Douvartzidis N. A comparison of outcomes of orthodontic and surgical-orthodontic treatment of Class II malocclusions in adults. Am J Orthod Dentofacial Orthop 1992;101:556–565.

Radney LJ, Jacobs JD. Soft tissue changes associated with surgical total maxillary intrusion. Am J Orthod 1981;80:191–212.

Reyneke JP. Surgical cephalometric prediction tracing for the alteration of the occlusal plane by means of rotation of the maxillomandibular complex. Int J Adult Orthodon Orthognath Surg 1999;14:55–64.

Reyneke JP. Surgical manipulation of the occlusal plane: New concepts in geometry. Int J Adult Orthodon Orthognath Surg 1998;13:307–316.

Reyneke JP, Evans WG. Surgical manipulation of the occlusal plane. Int J Adult Orthodon Orthognath Surg 1990;5:99–110.

Reyneke JP, McCollum AGH, Evans WG. Towards Greater Acuity in Orthognathic Surgery, ed 3. Johannesburg: University of the Witwatersrand, 1996.

Reyneke JP, Tsakiris P, Kienle F. A simple classification for surgical treatment planning of maxillomandibular asymmetry. Br J Oral Maxillofac Surg 1997;35:349–351.

Reyneke JP. Vertical variation in skeletal open bite: A classification for surgical planning. J Dent Assoc S Afr 1988;43:465–472.

Reyneke JP. Basic guidelines for the surgical correction of mandibular anteroposterior deficiency and excess. Clin Plast Surg 2007;34:501–517.

Rosário HD, de Oliveira BG, Pompeo DD, de Freitas PH, Paranhos LR. Surgical maxillary advancement increases upper airway volume in skeletal Class III patients: A cone beam computed tomography-based study. J Clin Sleep Med 2016:12:1527–1532.

Sarver DM. Esthetic Orthodontic and Orthognathic Surgery. St Louis: Mosby, 1998.

Sarver DM, Weissman SM. Long-term soft tissue response to Le Fort I maxillary superior repositioning. Angle Orthod 1991;61:267–276.

Schendel SA, Eisenfeld J, Bell WH, Epker BN, Mishelevich DJ. The long face syndrome: Vertical maxillary excess. Am J Orthod 1976;70:398–408.

Shin JH, Kim MA, Park IY, Park YH. A 2-year follow-up of changes after bimaxillary surgery in patients with mandibular prognathism: 3-dimensional analysis of pharyngeal airway volume and hyoid bone position. J Oral Maxillofac Surg 2015;73:e1–e9.

Tselnik M, Pogrel MA, Assessment of the pharyngeal airway space after mandibular setback surgery. J Oral Maxillofac Surg 2000;58:282–285.

Wolford LM, Hilliard FW, Dugan DJ. Surgical Treatment Objective: A Systematic Approach to the Prediction Tracing. St Louis: Mosby, 1985.

Woo SJ, Jong WC, Do YK, Jang YL, Soon MK. Can a surgery-first orthognathic approach reduce the total treatment time? Int J Oral Maxillofac Surg 2017;46:473–482.

4

Diagnosis and Treatment of Typical Dentofacial Deformities

This chapter and the following chapter use case studies to demonstrate individual dentofacial problems, combinations of problems, and the nuances involved in treating these patients to achieve optimal results. Patients with similar skeletal, soft tissue, and occlusal characteristics are grouped in description for convenience. Clinicians should remember, however, that each patient has a unique set of dentofacial problems requiring a specific treatment response, and a patient may have more than one deformity.

The following basic deformities and treatment principles for each deformity are discussed: (1) mandibular anteroposterior deficiency, (2) mandibular anteroposterior excess, (3) maxillary anteroposterior deficiency, (4) maxillary anteroposterior excess, (5) maxillary vertical deficiency, and (6) maxillary vertical excess.

Mandibular Anteroposterior Deficiency

Patients with mandibular anteroposterior deficiency and Class II malocclusions are without a doubt the largest single group of surgical orthodontic patients.

Class II, division I malocclusion

Clinical characteristics

Profile view

- Retruded, weak chin
- Deficient mandible that gives the illusion of a large nose
- Short chin-to-throat length
- Obtuse lower lip–chin–throat angle
- Everted lower lip that wedges in behind the incisors
- An upper lip that often appears short, curled, and protrusive
- Acute labiomental fold
- Increased facial contour angle (convex profile)

Frontal view

- Curled lower lip
- Weak chin with the appearance of a double chin
- Deep labiomental fold

Dental characteristics

- Large overjet
- Usually, an increased overbite and an accentuated curve of Spee
- Usually, crowding in the mandibular incisor area
- Tendency for maxillary incisor protrusion and spacing
- Angle Class II malocclusion

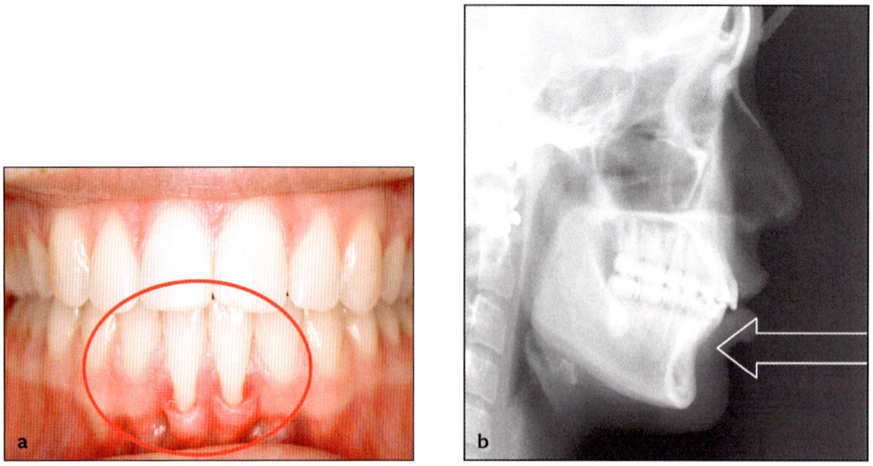

Fig 4-1 (*a*) Severe gingival recession of the mandibular central incisors is evident (*circle*). (*b*) On the lateral cephalometric radiograph, note the excessive proclination of the mandibular incisors beyond the bony base (*arrow*) as a result of dental compensation.

Treatment

Growth modification is not feasible after adolescence. Without surgical correction of the jaw relationship, an orthodontic compromise will consist of the following:

- Correction of excessive overjet
- Retraction of maxillary incisors (with or without extraction of first premolars)
- Proclination of mandibular incisors (limited by the bone thickness in the mandibular symphysis)
- Correction of excessive overbite
- Intrusion of maxillary incisors
- Intrusion of mandibular incisors
- Downward rotation of the mandible by opening the bite

As with most compromised treatment options, this nonsurgical correction may be associated with disadvantages such as questionable stability, a compromised esthetic outcome, increased orthodontic treatment time, and possible periodontal implications because of the proclination of the mandibular incisors (Fig 4-1).

At the beginning of treatment, the clinician must decide whether the treatment approach will be solely orthodontic or orthodontics combined with surgery. Because the orthodontic treatments in the two approaches differ substantially, it does not make sense to tell patients who are beginning orthodontic treatment, "Let's see how the treatment progresses; we may get away without surgery." The clinician should thoroughly discuss each treatment option with the patient (and the family, if applicable) so that an informed treatment decision can be made. It will be prudent to refer the patient for a consultation with the surgeon before commencement of orthodontic treatment. The patient's parents or family should be encouraged to accompany the patient.

Presurgical orthodontics

The basic presurgical orthodontic goals for patients with Class II, division 1 malocclusion are as follows:

- *Align both dental arches.* Both dental arches should be aligned with the teeth in the central trough of bone, establishing harmonious arch forms.
- *Position the incisors in their planned anteroposterior and vertical planes with acceptable cephalometric angulation.* It is extremely important to position the incisors correctly. Incisor position dictates surgical movement to a great extent, and surgical movement in turn dictates esthetic results. On the other hand, the clinician should be cautioned not to over decompensate, which could jeopardize both dental stability and esthetic outcomes.
- *Establish arch compatibility.*

Note particularly the orthodontic goal of properly positioning the maxillary and mandibular incisors presurgically in both anteroposterior and vertical planes of space. The position of the incisors dictates surgical movement, and failure to eliminate dental compensation limits surgical correction. Because of crowding in the incisor area and a severe curve of Spee, it is often necessary to extract two mandibular first premolars. However, extractions in

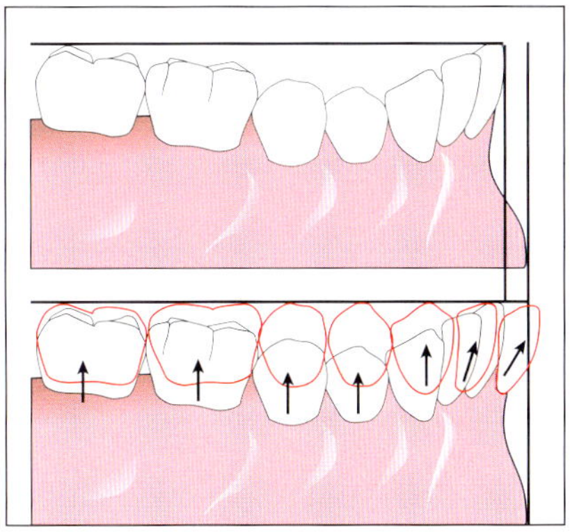

Fig 4-2 Orthodontic leveling of the curve of Spee will increase the anteroposterior arch length. If crowding is present in the incisor area, additional anteroposterior space will be required for arch alignment. Every 1 mm of curve leveling will result in a 0.6- to 1.0-mm increase in arch length.

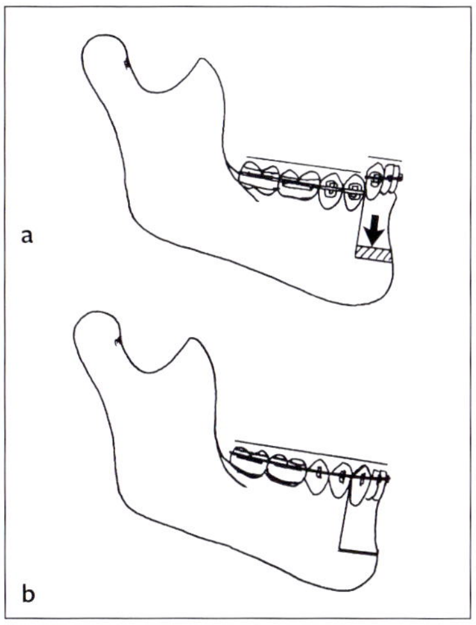

Fig 4-3 The curve of Spee can be leveled surgically by segmental orthodontic alignment of the dental arch (*a*), followed by surgical inferior repositioning of the anterior dentoalveolar segment (*b*).

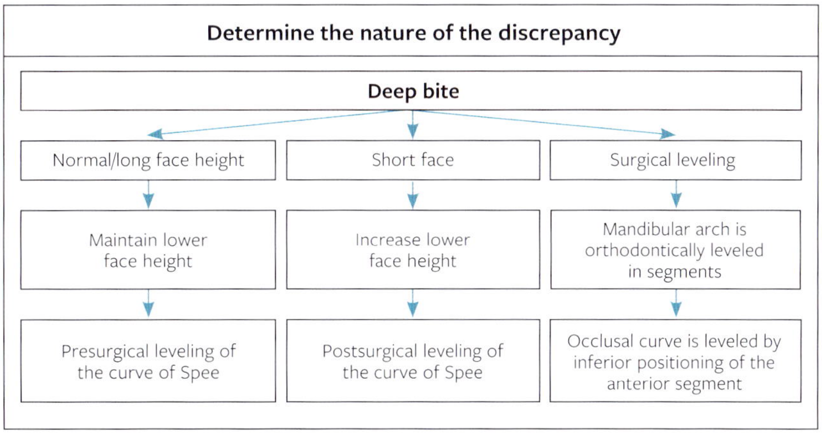

Fig 4-4 Indications for presurgical orthodontic leveling of occlusal curves.

the maxilla are not frequently indicated. If there is some crowding in the maxillary arch, it is often possible to avoid extraction by gaining additional space through expansion of the maxillary arch—an adjustment often needed to accommodate the mandibular arch after surgical advancement. If extraction in the maxilla is deemed necessary, it may be advantageous to extract second premolars to enable minimal retraction of incisors. Retraction of these incisors otherwise would not only limit surgical movement but also have adverse esthetic effects (loss of lip support and increased nasolabial angle).

Patients with a Class II, division 1 malocclusion often have an excessive curve of Spee. It is important not to level the curve routinely before surgery. Patients with short faces often have prominent chins and, from an esthetic point of view, do not tolerate mandibular advancement. In these patients, it is preferable not to level the curve of Spee presurgically. Surgical advancement of the mandible will result in a rotational movement, advancing the mandibular incisors with only minimal advancement of the chin and slight increase in lower facial height (see chapter 3). As a general rule, it is better to level the curve by extrusion of premolars after surgery in patients with short faces. The greater the facial height, the greater the likelihood that leveling should be done presurgically by intrusion of the incisors Because anteroposterior space is needed for leveling and alignment, extractions are more likely to be necessary when a severe curve of Spee is combined with mandibular incisor crowding (Fig 4-2). Surgical leveling of the curve may be considered (Figs 4-3 and 4-4).

Arch compatibility plays an important role in immediate postsurgical stability and gives the surgeon an exact idea of where to position the mandible when a splint is not used during surgery. There are three important aspects of arch compatibility:

1. *Intercanine width is crucial.* If the maxillary intercanine width is insufficient, it will not be possible to advance the mandible into the planned occlusion and anteroposterior position. Because a premature contact may shift the mandible laterally, a rotated canine may make it impossible to correct dental midlines. The use of an acrylic splint at surgery to eliminate this problem does not make sense because the correct intercanine width must be achieved eventually. If the correct intercanine width is achieved before surgery, the surgery will be more accurate, and tooth interdigitation will improve.
2. *The mandibular second molars should be banded and leveled with the first molars.* An overerupted, elevated, often rotated, unbanded second molar frequently causes occlusal interference at surgery (Fig 4-5).
3. *Similar maxillary and mandibular arch forms should be established to prevent possible postsurgical crossbites.* In patients with mandibular deficiency, the maxillary arch is often slightly narrow and will need expansion to accommodate the mandibular arch after advancement. Asymmetric arch forms will also influence the yaw of the jaws.

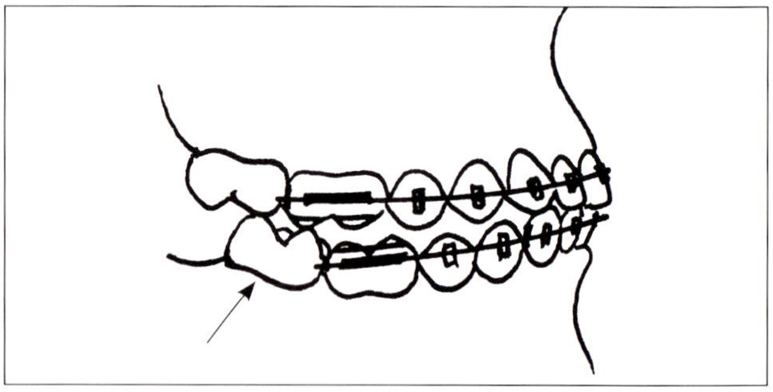

Fig 4-5 Leveling of the mandibular arch should include the second molars. An unbanded molar (*arrow*) often interferes with establishing the planned occlusion at surgery.

Orthodontic mechanics

Crowding in the maxillary arch. When the maxillary arch is crowded and requires tooth extractions, the following approach is recommended:

- Second premolars should be extracted.
- Headgear may be necessary to support the Class III elastics.

Crowding in the mandibular arch. When the mandibular arch is crowded and requires tooth extractions (also see comments on an accentuated curve of Spee), the following methods should be used:

- Extraction of premolars may be required. In patients with crowding, accentuated curve of Spee, and the need for mandibular incisor retraction, the first premolars should be extracted. The second premolars should be extracted when less anteroposterior space is required for the planned mandibular incisor positioning.
- Sectional arch retraction of the mandibular canines is recommended because the anchorage characteristics are excellent.
- Class III mechanics (eg, Class III elastics) may be needed depending on the severity of the mandibular canine malposition, the mandibular incisor position, crowding, and the curve of Spee.

Noncrowding. When minimal crowding or mild spacing between the teeth is present, a nonextraction approach is recommended:

- During the leveling process, the use of Class III mechanics is mandatory.
- As much retraction or uprighting of the mandibular incisor as possible is achieved with the aid of Class III mechanics (eg, J-hooks or Class III elastics and maxillary headgear support).
- Maxillary and mandibular arches are coordinated to fit. When the overjet is not excessive (4 to 5 mm), the patient is asked to move the mandible forward so that the coordination of the maxillary and mandibular arches can be checked. However, the best way of checking coordination is to take rough study casts and hand-simulate the surgical advancement of the mandible. Be sure to coordinate the overjet with the orthodontic prediction tracing.

Surgical treatment

The surgical technique of choice is the bilateral sagittal split ramus osteotomy, which advances the distal (tooth-bearing) segment to maximum dental intercuspation. The position of the maxillary and mandibular incisors controls both the amount the mandible can be advanced as well as the facial height after surgery. Correct condyle positioning during surgery is extremely important (see the discussion of condylar sag in chapter 6, pages 268 to 272).

The chin may still appear deficient after advancement of the mandible, and an advancement genioplasty may be indicated to improve final esthetics. The clinician makes this decision according to the presurgical visual treatment objective.

Light (2.5- to 3.5-oz) Class II elastics are placed after the completion of surgery to override proprioception, guide the teeth into the new occlusion, and establish a solid occlusion. Only two triangular-fashioned vertical elastics are recommended in the canine area. Long Class II elastics should be avoided because elastics cannot move the jaw at this stage, and a surgical mistake (eg, condylar sag or inability to achieve the planned occlusion) cannot be corrected by elastics.

Postsurgical orthodontics

The goals of postsurgical orthodontics are to bring the teeth into final occlusion and maintain them in that position. Treatment usually consists of final leveling of the curve of Spee, correction of minor crossbites, and final closure of small extraction spaces.

Case 1

A 16-year-old girl was referred to the orthodontist for the orthodontic treatment of a Class II malocclusion.

Main complaint

The patient mainly wanted her increased overjet corrected and also thought that her chin appeared too small.

Medical history

Her medical history was noncontributory.

Clinical examination

1. Soft tissue
    - Frontal view (Fig 4-6a)
        - Short, deficient chin
        - Everted lower lip
        - Short lower facial third
    - Profile view (Fig 4-6b)
        - Convex profile
        - Deep labiomental fold
        - Deficient mandible
2. Dental (Fig 4-6c)
    - Class II, division 1 malocclusion
    - Slightly accentuated curve of Spee
    - Slightly narrowed maxillary arch
3. Skeletal (Fig 4-6d)
    - Anteroposteriorly deficient mandible
4. Radiographic
    - Panoramic radiograph
        - Four impacted third molars
    - Cephalometric radiograph
        - Class II, division 1 dental relationship
        - Slight maxillary dental protrusion
        - Mandibular anteroposterior deficiency

Problem list

- Class II malocclusion
- Mandibular anteroposterior deficiency
- Deep bite
- Slightly accentuated curve of Spee
- Narrow maxillary arch
- Slight protrusion of maxillary incisors

Presurgical orthodontics

The surgical removal of impacted third molars preceded presurgical orthodontic treatment, which consisted of the following (Figs 4-6e and 4-6f):

- Maxillary arch: use of lingual orthodontics
    - Slight expansion of the maxillary arch to accommodate the mandibular arch after advancement
    - Slight retraction of maxillary incisors
- Mandibular arch: leveling of the curve of Spee
    - Establishment of a good arch form
    - Use of buccal orthodontics in the mandibular arch

Surgical treatment

The surgical treatment for this patient consisted of a bilateral sagittal split ramus osteotomy to advance the mandible.

Postsurgical orthodontics

The surgery was performed after a 10-month period of orthodontic preparation. The postsurgical orthodontic treatment, which lasted 4 months, involved finalization of the occlusion. After band removal, the patient was given a retainer to wear. Figures 4-6g to 4-6i illustrate the treatment result 8 months after orthodontic band removal.

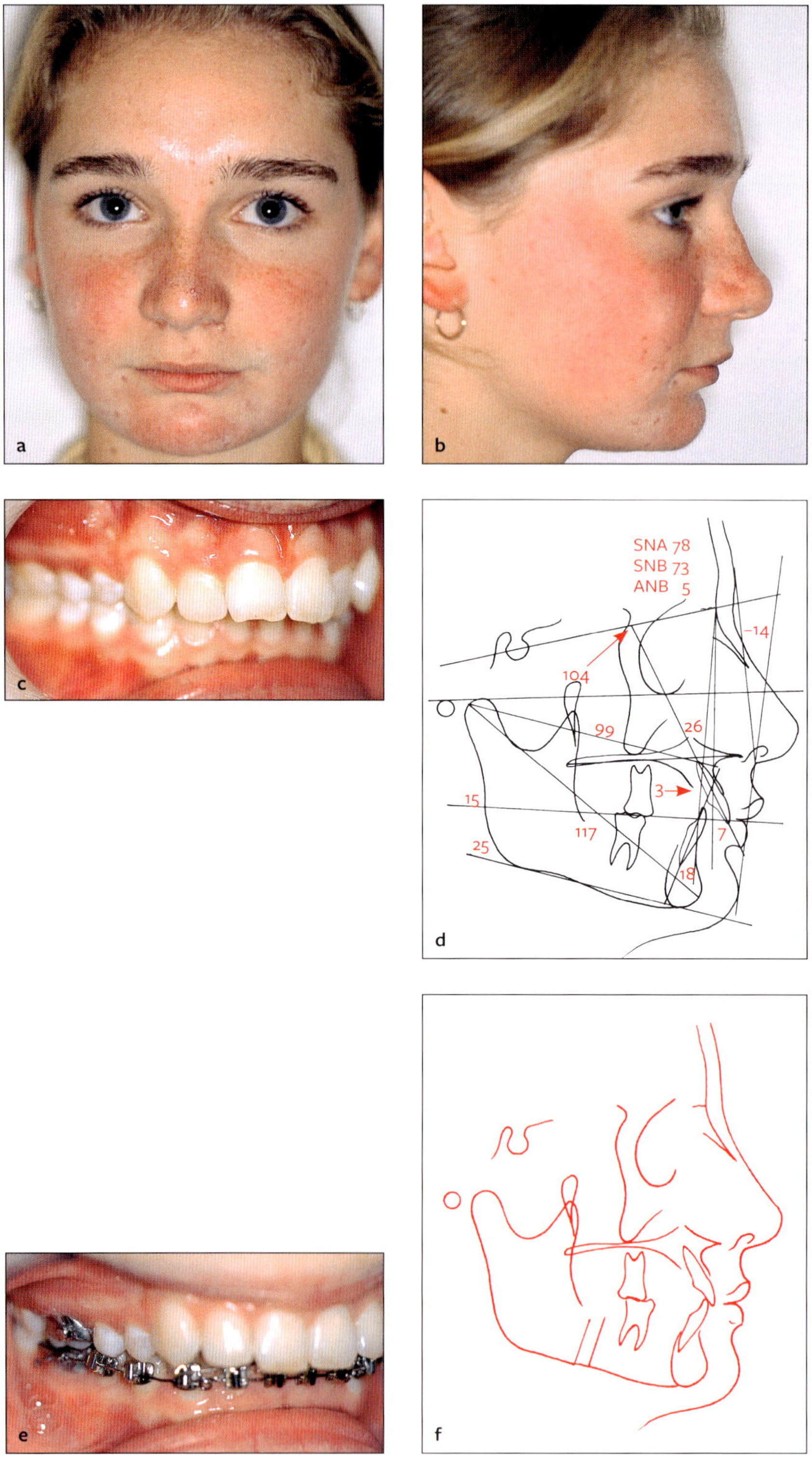

Fig 4-6 Case 1. Pretreatment frontal view (*a*), profile view (*b*), and occlusion (*c*). (*d*) The skeletal, soft tissue, and dental relationships are demonstrated by cephalometric analysis. Increased facial contour angle = −14 degrees; decreased SNB angle = 73 degrees; increased ANB angle = 5 degrees. (*e*) Immediate presurgical occlusion. The patient was treated with lingual orthodontics in the maxilla, and buccal attachments (lingual buttons) were bonded presurgically to assist in intraoperative maxillomandibular fixation and postsurgical elastic control. (*f*) Surgical visual treatment objective indicating that a 6-mm mandibular advancement will be required. The expected soft tissue result is demonstrated. →

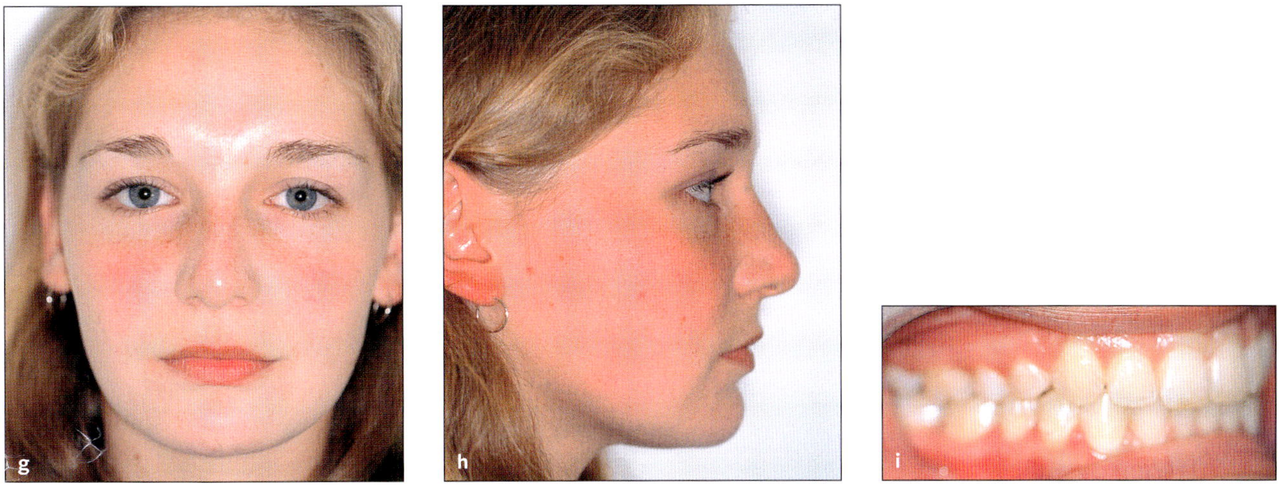

Fig 4-6 *(cont)* Posttreatment results are demonstrated in frontal view (*g*), profile view (*h*), and occlusion (*i*).

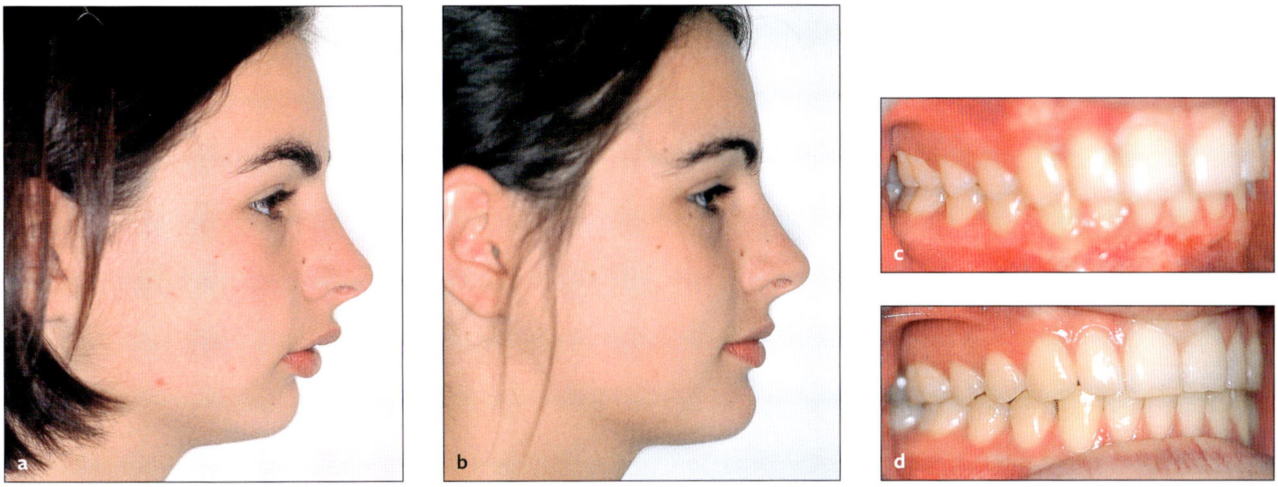

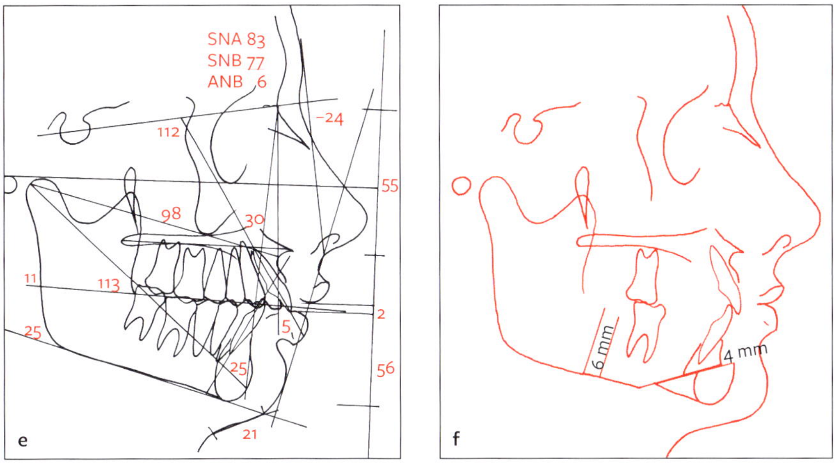

Fig 4-7 Case involving mandibular advancement and genioplasty. (*a*) Preoperative profile view. (*b*) Postoperative profile view. (*c*) Preoperative occlusion. (*d*) Postoperative occlusion. (*e and f*) The cephalometric analysis and surgical prediction tracing demonstrate the esthetic enhancement from a 6-mm advancement of the mandible combined with a 4-mm advancement of the chin.

Because of the general underdevelopment of the mandible, microgenia (chin deficiency) is often found in combination with mandibular anteroposterior deficiency. In patients with this condition, correction requires an augmentation sliding genioplasty in addition to mandibular advancement. However, augmentation genioplasty is not a substitute for mandibular surgery. Figure 4-7 illustrates the improved esthetic result of a patient after both mandibular advancement and augmentation genioplasty.

Class II, division 2 malocclusion

Clinical characteristics

Profile view

- Pronounced "chin button"
- Deep labiomental fold
- Anteroposteriorly deficient and curled lower lip
- Short lower facial height and a mandible that appears square
- Mandibular plane angle that tends to be low

Frontal view

- Appearance of a short face because of decreased vertical height
- Curled lower lip and a deep labiomental fold
- Usually, well-developed elevator muscles of the mandible

Dental characteristics

- Angle Class II, division 2 malocclusion
- Retroclined maxillary central incisors
- Labially flared maxillary lateral incisors
- Deep overbite, which is both skeletal and dental in origin
- Excessive curve of Spee
- Gingival tissue irritation behind the maxillary incisors and sometimes on the labial aspect of the mandibular incisors because of deep bite
- Tendency toward clicking of the temporomandibular joints (TMJs), probably related to the anterior locking effect of the deep bite

Treatment

Presurgical orthodontics

The basic presurgical orthodontic principles apply in Class II, division 2 malocclusion—namely, the need to properly position the maxillary and mandibular incisors (vertically as well as in the anteroposterior plane), the need to level the curve of Spee, and the need to coordinate the dental arches. It is especially important to tip the maxillary incisors labially to create a good arch form, lip support, and a sufficient overjet. In patients with severe deep bite, it may be difficult to level the curve of Spee in the mandibular arch, making it necessary to open the bite with a glass ionomer bite plane cemented to the molars. Surgical leveling by segmental surgery may be considered, in which case segmental orthodontic alignment will be necessary (Fig 4-8).

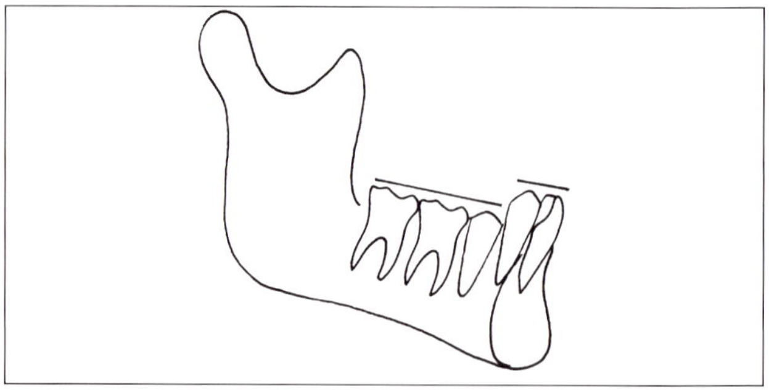

Fig 4-8 When a natural step exists in the mandibular arch, the dental arch may be leveled in segments, followed by surgical leveling. Surgical leveling has two advantages: No additional anteroposterior arch length is required, and orthodontic treatment time is shortened.

In patients with a Class II deep bite malocclusion, postsurgical leveling of the curve of Spee is indicated. Advancement of the mandible before total leveling of the curve will increase the facial height, and because of the rotation of the occlusal plane, the chin will not advance as much as the incisors (Fig 4-9a).

Orthodontic mechanics

Maxillary arch. The maxillary incisors can be leveled and advanced with a curved archwire or a simple flexible archwire followed by a steel round wire with a pronounced inverse occlusal curve. A stabilizing archwire should be fitted as soon as possible. The change in the maxillary incisor position should be reconciled with the arch length and lip support.

Mandibular arch. In the mandibular arch, the teeth should be leveled with the aid of Class III elastics and soft flexible wires, but it is not necessary to completely correct the curve of Spee. This curve correction can be done after surgery, especially if there is a deep overbite and an increase in lower facial height is required. The stabilizing wire should have the curve of Spee bent into it. Presurgically, a deep curve is advantageous because the anterior part of the mandible is advanced downward and forward to create a Class I incisor relationship while the lower anterior facial height is increased (Figs 4-9b to 4-9d).

Surgical treatment

A few surgical options for the correction of the malocclusion and esthetic improvement may be considered:

- Advancement of the mandible by means of a bilateral sagittal split ramus osteotomy.
- Advancement of the mandible by means of a bilateral sagittal split ramus osteotomy combined with a reduction genioplasty to reduce chin prominence. By angling

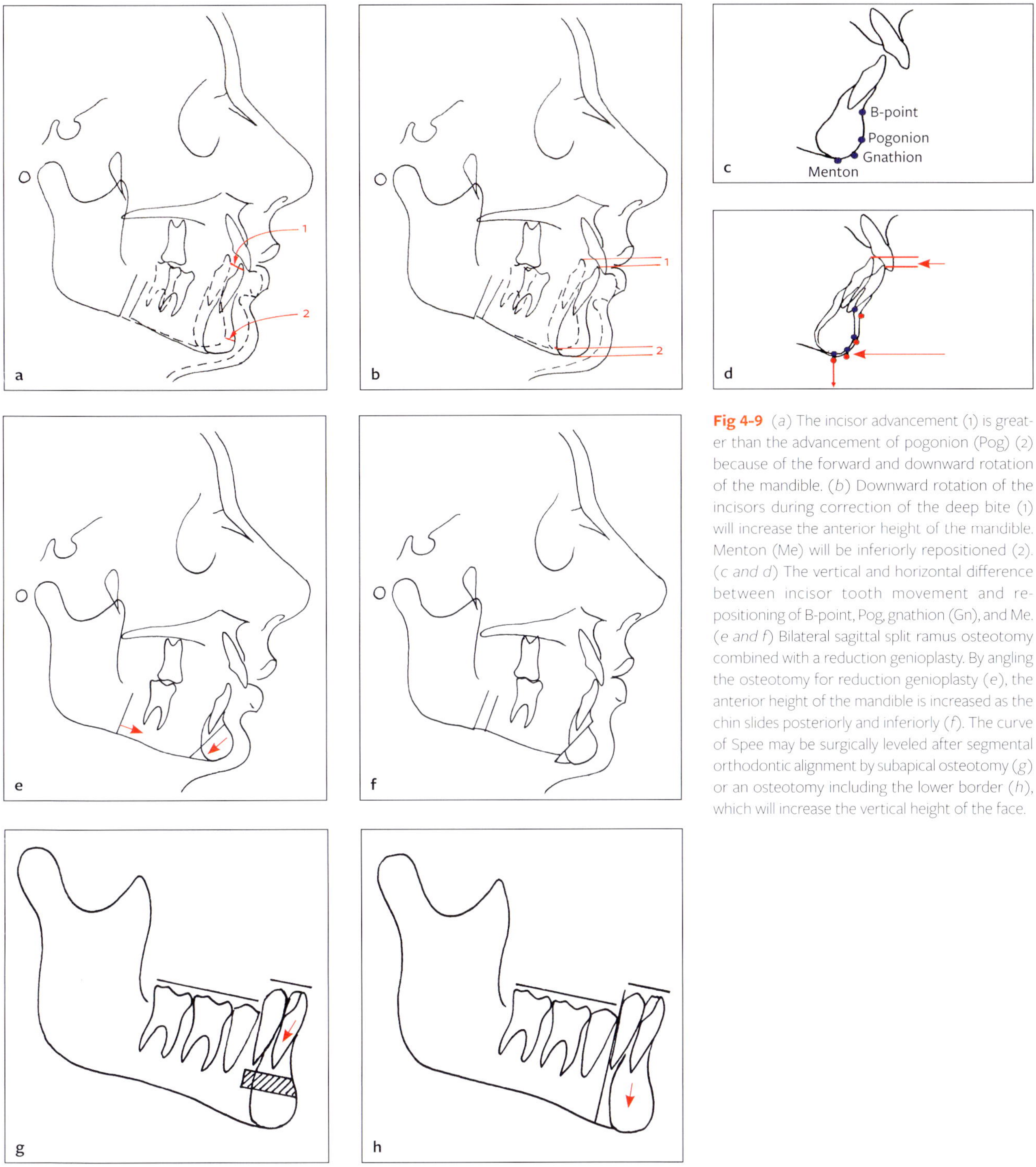

Fig 4-9 (*a*) The incisor advancement (1) is greater than the advancement of pogonion (Pog) (2) because of the forward and downward rotation of the mandible. (*b*) Downward rotation of the incisors during correction of the deep bite (1) will increase the anterior height of the mandible. Menton (Me) will be inferiorly repositioned (2). (*c and d*) The vertical and horizontal difference between incisor tooth movement and repositioning of B-point, Pog, gnathion (Gn), and Me. (*e and f*) Bilateral sagittal split ramus osteotomy combined with a reduction genioplasty. By angling the osteotomy for reduction genioplasty (*e*), the anterior height of the mandible is increased as the chin slides posteriorly and inferiorly (*f*). The curve of Spee may be surgically leveled after segmental orthodontic alignment by subapical osteotomy (*g*) or an osteotomy including the lower border (*h*), which will increase the vertical height of the face.

the osteotomy of the genioplasty, a vertical increase in facial height can be achieved (posterior and inferior slide of the chin). Care should be taken to avoid obliterating the labiomental fold (Figs 4-9e and 4-9f).

- Advancement of the mandible by means of a bilateral sagittal split osteotomy combined with an anterior subapical segmental osteotomy to level the occlusal plane. This procedure will maintain the anterior facial height. The segmental osteotomy may include the body of the mandible, which will increase the height of the face (Figs 4-9g and 4-9h).

- Advancement of the dentoalveolar segment of the mandible by means of a total subapical osteotomy of the mandible. This procedure will maintain the chin position while advancing the lower lip; however, it is not performed often because of an increased likelihood of inferior alveolar nerve damage.
- Rotation of the maxillomandibular complex in patients with a severely low occlusal and mandibular plane angle (see the section "Rotation of the Maxillomandibular Complex" in chapter 5).

The following are a few important points regarding positioning of the mandible during surgery:

- If rigid fixation is used, the incisors are positioned in ideal relationship.
- Keep skeletal midlines correct even if it means a slight dental discrepancy. The orthodontist can correct a mild dental midline discrepancy but not an incorrect skeletal midline.
- There is often a tendency for posterior crossbites, so the crossbites should be kept symmetric. It is much easier to orthodontically correct small bilateral crossbites than a large unilateral crossbite.

Postsurgical orthodontics

After surgery, patients often have a three-point contact occlusion and bilateral open bites with the contact points on the incisors and the second molars (see case 2, Fig 4-10). When a bilateral open bite (created by advancing the mandible where the curve of Spee has not been completely leveled) will be corrected by orthodontic movement of mandibular teeth, the maxillary stabilizing arch is left in place. The mandibular stabilizing archwire is removed and replaced by a working wire, and light up-down or slightly Class II elastics are placed. The elastics serve a dual purpose: (1) to bring the teeth into a solid occlusion, and (2) to "override" the patient's proprioception, which will tend to keep the mandible in maximum intercuspation. Postoperative crossbites can be corrected by through-the-bite elastics. From this point forward, the patient's orthodontic treatment will be routine.

Retainer use for these patients is the same as for patients undergoing routine orthodontic treatment. After 3 to 4 months, retainer use can be reduced to nighttime only. If the teeth are stable, retainer use may be discontinued after a few more months.

Case 2

A 17-year-old adolescent boy was referred to the surgeon by his orthodontist for surgical advancement of his mandible. He started his orthodontic treatment 16 months previously but had not consulted with a surgeon before.

Main complaint

The patient developed an ulcer in his palate as a result of his deep bite.

Clinical examination

1. Soft tissue
   - Frontal view (Fig 4-10a)
     - Short lower facial third
     - Everted lower lip
   - Profile view (Figs 4-10b and 4-10c)
     - Convex profile
     - Deep labiomental fold
   - Everted lower lip
     - Decreased lower facial third
     - His chin appears deficient
2. Dental (Figs 4-10d to 4-10f)
   - Class II, division 1 malocclusion
   - Deep bite
   - Accentuated curve of Spee
   - Increased overjet
3. Skeletal (Fig 4-10g)
   - Mandibular anteroposterior deficiency
   - Macrogenia
4. Radiographic
   - Cephalometric radiograph (see Fig 4-10g)
     - Class II deep bite
     - Mandibular anteroposterior deficiency
     - Macrogenia
     - Accentuated curve of Spee

Problem list

- Class II deep bite malocclusion
- Prominent chin
- Deep labiomental fold
- Labiomental fold superiorly positioned
- Short lower facial third
- Everted lower lip

Presurgical orthodontics

At the surgical consultation, the presurgical orthodontic alignment of his occlusion was completed. Due to his short lower facial third, the orthodontist had not leveled the patient's severe curve of Spee. The intention was that the surgical advancement

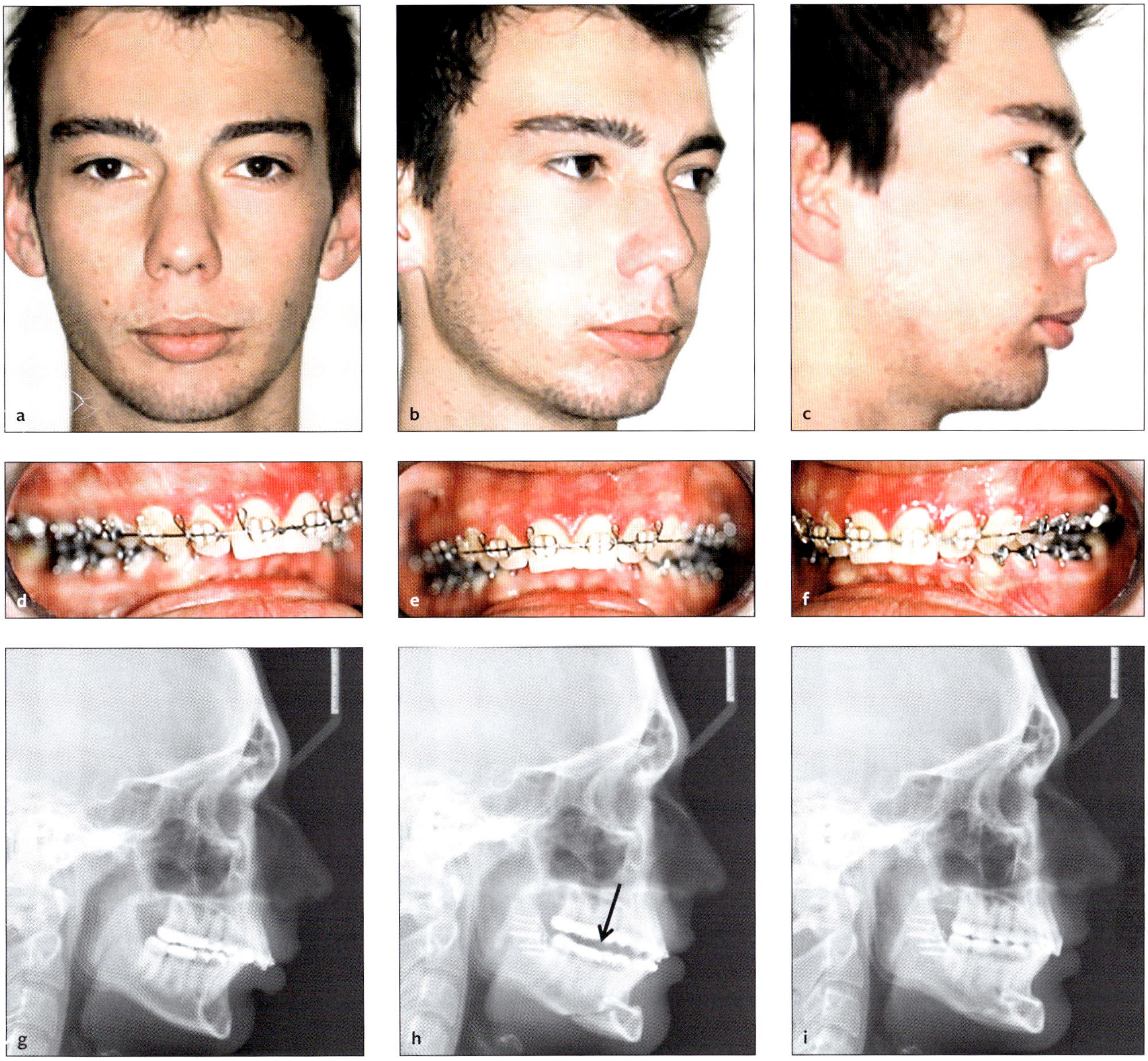

Fig 4-10 Case 2. Pretreatment frontal view (*a*), three-quarter view (*b*), and profile view (*c*). (*d to f*) Presurgical occlusion. (*g*) Presurgical lateral cephalometric radiograph. (*h*) Note the "three point" occlusal contact and bilateral open bites in the immediate postoperative lateral cephalometric radiograph. (*i*) Posttreatment lateral cephalometric radiograph.

of the mandible would allow for an anterior and rotational movement with the incisors being advanced but also moved downward (correcting the deep bite). The chin would move less anteriorly but increase vertically (see Fig 4-9).

Surgical treatment

Surgical advancement of the mandible was completed by means of a bilateral sagittal split ramus osteotomy. The chin shape was corrected with a sliding genioplasty. As a result of the curve of Spee, the postoperative occlusion will end with a "three point" contact: bilateral on the second molars and anterior in the incisor region (Fig 4-10h).

Postsurgical orthodontics

The postoperative bilateral open bites were leveled with a continuous archwire and "up and down" elastics. The orthodontic bands were removed 4 months after surgery and a retainer fitted. The posttreatment results are illustrated in Figs 4-10i to 4-10o.

Case 3

A 16-year-old adolescent girl consulted with the orthodontist about her deep bite and the flat appearance of her maxillary incisors.

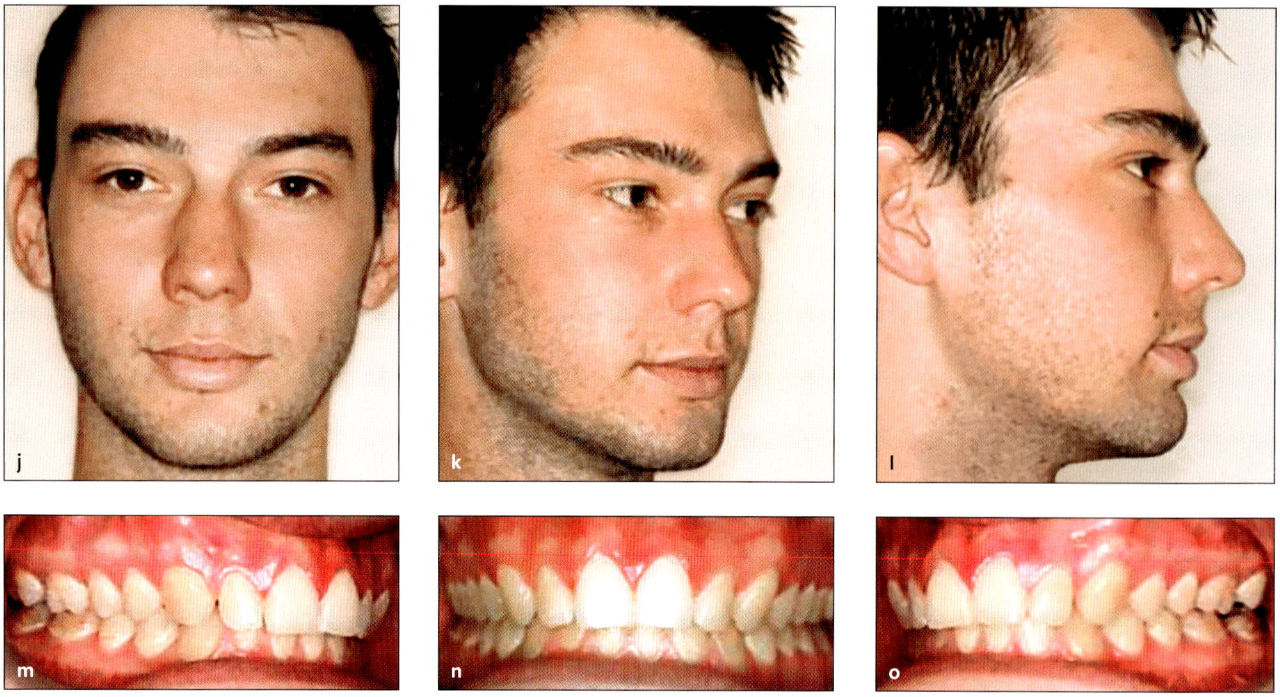

Fig 4-10 (*cont*) (*j to o*) Posttreatment photographs.

Main complaint

The patient's main complaint was a deep bite and the flat appearance of her maxillary incisors.

Medical history

The patient was allergic to penicillin.

Clinical examination

1. Soft tissue
   - Frontal view
     - Vertically short chin
     - Prominent, knobby chin
     - Broad mandible
   - Profile view (Fig 4-11a)
     - Deep labiomental fold
     - Prominent chin
     - Short lower-third facial height
2. Dental (Fig 4-11b)
   - Class II, division 2 malocclusion
   - Deep bite
   - Retroclined maxillary incisors
3. Skeletal (Fig 4-11c)
   - Mandibular anteroposterior deficiency
   - Macrogenia
4. Radiographic
   - Panoramic radiograph
     - Impacted third molars
   - Cephalometric radiograph (see Fig 4-11c)
     - Class II, division 2 malocclusion
     - Deep bite
     - Retroclined maxillary incisors
     - Mandibular anteroposterior deficiency
     - Macrogenia

Problem list

- Class II malocclusion
- Mandibular anteroposterior deficiency
- Deep bite
- Retroclined maxillary incisors
- Prominent chin

Presurgical orthodontics

Maxillary arch

- Improvement of the angulation of the maxillary incisors by labial tipping
- Establishment of a good arch form

Mandibular arch

- Leveling and alignment of the arch and establishment of interarch compatibility

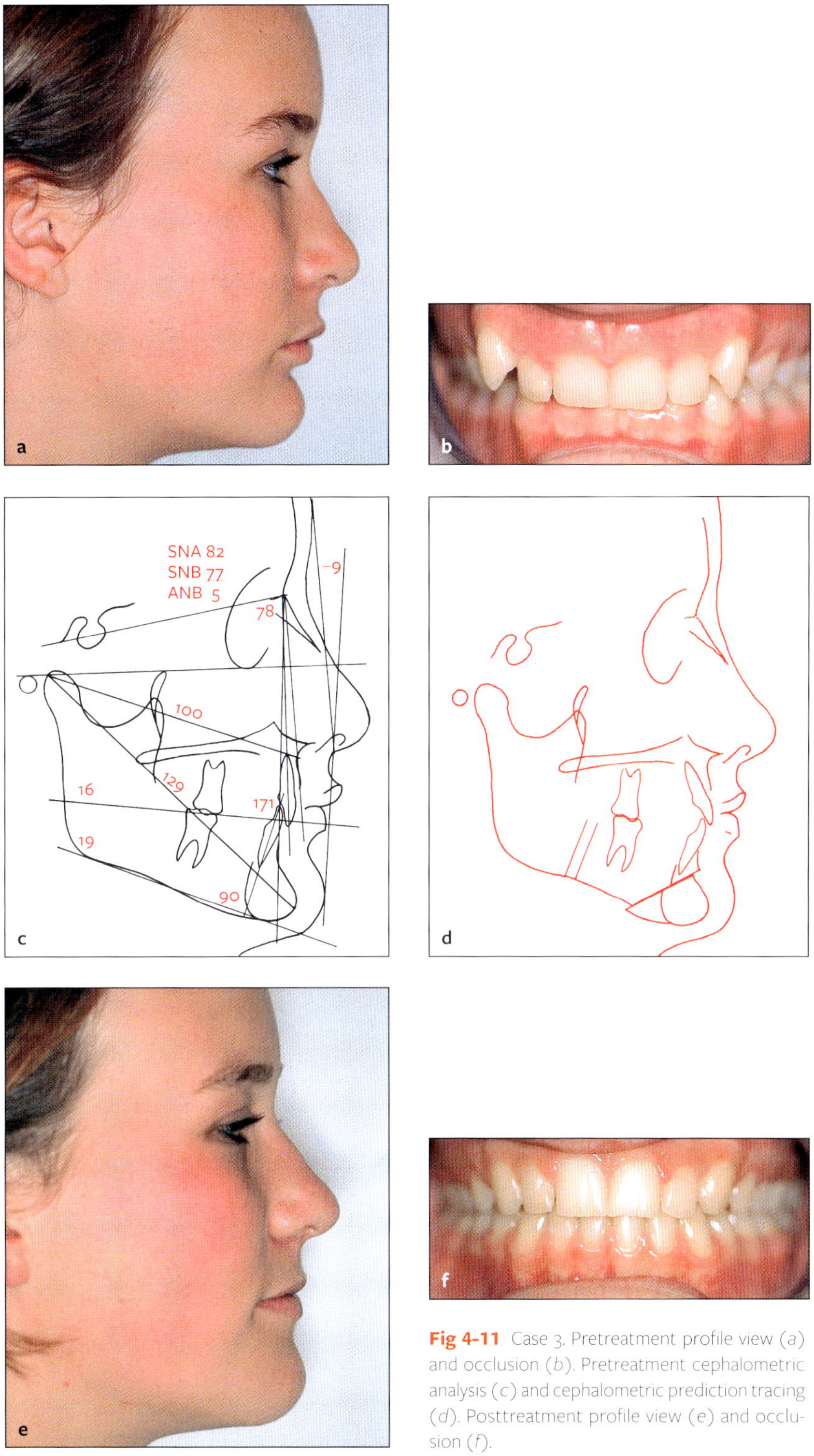

Fig 4-11 Case 3. Pretreatment profile view (*a*) and occlusion (*b*). Pretreatment cephalometric analysis (*c*) and cephalometric prediction tracing (*d*). Posttreatment profile view (*e*) and occlusion (*f*).

Surgical treatment

Advancement of the mandible was accomplished by means of a bilateral sagittal split ramus osteotomy, and the chin was anteroposteriorly reduced using a sliding genioplasty (Fig 4-11d).

Postsurgical orthodontics

The surgery was performed after an 18-month orthodontic preparatory phase, and the orthodontic bands were removed 3 months after surgery. The patient was given a retainer to wear. The posttreatment results are illustrated in Figs 4-11e and 4-11f.

Mandibular Anteroposterior Excess

As early as 1907, Edward Angle suggested that the only way to correct severe Class III malocclusion in adults was to combine surgery and orthodontics. Before the 1970s, most clinicians thought that Class III malocclusions were primarily caused by excessive anteroposterior growth of the mandible, and most of these malocclusions were corrected by mandibular setback procedures. However, later studies indicated that isolated mandibular anteroposterior excess occurs in only 20% to 25% of patients with Class III malocclusions. Some maxillary skeletal anteroposterior deficiency is involved in 75% of patients with Class III malocclusions. Therefore, in patients with Class III malocclusion, the clinician must determine whether one jaw is primarily at fault or the malocclusion is caused by a combination of maxillary deficiency and mandibular excess.

Class III malocclusion

Clinical characteristics

Profile view

- Long chin-throat length with a well-defined inferior border of the mandible
- Protrusive chin resulting in a prominent lower third of the face
- Reduced labiomental fold
- Acute lip-chin-throat angle

Frontal view

- Appearance of a "flat" lower third of the face
- Chin button that is not prominent
- Thin upper lip with reduced vermilion exposure
- Reduced labiomental fold
- Mandible that appears strong
- Asymmetric chin

Dental characteristics

- Often, minimal attached gingival tissue over the mandibular anterior teeth
- Mandibular incisors that are often compensated and lingually inclined (however, some patients have generalized interdental spacing and flared incisors, often combined with an anterior open bite; these characteristics may point to a large tongue)
- Class III malocclusion with anterior and posterior crossbites
- Often, a dental midline discrepancy

Treatment

The timing of treatment for adolescents with Class III malocclusion is important. Many patients with severe Class III dentofacial deformities want definitive treatment as soon as possible, and early treatment may be desirable from a social and psychologic point of view. In patients with particularly severe deformities, early intervention may be attempted to induce growth modification (ie, reverse-pull headgear). However, if surgery is performed before completion of mandibular growth, the malocclusion is likely to recur as a result of growth. The growth of the patient can be evaluated by a study of a hand-wrist radiograph; however, a serial cephalometric radiograph is a more accurate tool for monitoring the growth of the mandible.

Maxillary skeletal maturity is usually achieved at age 14 or 15 years in girls and age 16 years in boys; therefore, when maxillary deficiency is the primary problem, delaying surgery until completion of growth is usually a feasible option. However, mandibular growth may continue until the early 20s. Some patients with severe mandibular excess are not willing to wait and elect to have surgery earlier, recognizing the fact that a second procedure may be necessary later. The decision to proceed with surgery before the completion of growth is complex and should not be made lightly. Case 6 (see page 144) is an example of a patient to whom surgery was offered before the completion of growth.

Presurgical orthodontics

Orthodontic preparation for surgery has five basic goals:

1. Eliminate (or reduce) anterior and posterior dental compensation with guidance from the orthodontic visual treatment objective.
2. Establish appropriate anteroposterior and vertical incisor positions. Improper incisor positions will curtail optimal esthetic correction.
3. Achieve compatible arch forms and intercanine widths, which are essential to make dental midlines compatible during surgery.
4. Manage tooth size discrepancies.
5. Correct the mandibular asymmetries that often accompany mandibular prognathism. If the chin shape is acceptable, the mandibular dental midline should be placed in the middle of the chin. The asymmetry will be corrected during the mandibular setback procedure. It also can be corrected by a genioplasty, if one is indicated, to improve poor chin shape or vertical or anteroposterior chin deformities. Thus, it is not always necessary to orthodontically place the mandibular dental midline in the midline of the chin.

Orthodontic mechanics

Mandibular arch. The following techniques are recommended for orthodontic treatment of the mandibular arch:

- Class III mechanics, including molar tiebacks, are not used when leveling, and the teeth are allowed to level forward. The orthodontic visual treatment objective should be referred to regularly to confirm the extent of incisor decompensation required.
- Upon completion of leveling, Class II elastics may be used to advance the mandibular buccal segments and further procline the mandibular incisors. This movement should be monitored on sequential cephalometric films.
- Arch length discrepancies should be reconciled with the desired mandibular incisor position.
- When decompensating the mandibular incisors, the clinician should bear in mind that patients with mandibular anteroposterior excess often have a very thin, bony symphysis and a small area of attached gingiva in the incisor region. Take care to place the mandibular incisors in the middle trough of the bone.

Maxillary arch. For orthodontic treatment of the maxillary arch, the following approach is recommended:

- High-pull headgear should be applied to the maxillary incisor area nightly. This should be used with Class II mechanics to prevent extrusion of the maxillary incisors when advancing the mandibular dentition.
- Headgear anchorage should aid retraction of the maxillary incisors or merely prevent their proclination during the leveling process.

Surgical treatment

Bilateral sagittal split osteotomy is the procedure of choice, although a transoral vertical ramus osteotomy may be indicated in patients requiring large setback procedures. Correct positioning of the condyle is very important. The surgeon should carefully free the medial pterygoid muscle and the stylomandibular ligament from the medial side of the ramus. Otherwise, the proximal segment will be pushed back by the distal (tooth-bearing) segment, leading to a backward rotation of the ramus. With the return of muscle function, the patient will tend to reposition the mandible forward.

If bicortical screws are used for rigid fixation, positional self-tapping screws are preferred to maintain bone segment positions. With setback procedures, especially where simultaneous correction of asymmetry is required, small intersegmental defects may develop. If these defects are closed by tightening the screws, the torquing effect will displace the condyles laterally (peripheral condylar sag; see the discussion of condylar sag in chapter 6). The incidence of neurosensory morbidity with transoral vertical ramus osteotomy is less than that associated with a bilateral sagittal split ramus osteotomy, but the procedure carries an increased risk of poor condylar control.

On rare occasions, procedures such as body ostectomies or segmental subapical osteotomies are indicated to correct mandibular anteroposterior excess. A genioplasty is often indicated to place the chin in its most esthetic anteroposterior, vertical, and midsagittal positions. The labiomental fold is often obtuse in patients with Class III malocclusion; reduction genioplasty would make this angle more obtuse, causing the chin to appear flat and resulting in an overall poor esthetic result. Chin shape is more important than the anteroposterior position of the soft tissue pogonion (Pog′). A prognathic mandible often is combined with vertical excess and asymmetry of the anterior mandible. In these cases, vertical reduction of the chin, correction of asymmetry, and slight advancement of the chin may be needed to achieve better chin contour.

Postsurgical orthodontics

Postsurgical orthodontics for patients with Class III malocclusion is very similar for all patients. In patients with Class III open bites, the occlusion should be prepared presurgically so that the only postsurgical orthodontic tooth movements required are those with little or no potential to open the bite.

Light (2.5- to 3.5-oz) Class III triangular elastics should be placed in the canine area to override proprioception in the immediate postoperative period. A rectangular archwire should also be placed in the maxilla to prevent molar extrusion.

The clinician should design the retention plan according to the original malocclusion and its possible relapse tendency.

Case 4

A 20-year-old man consulted with an orthodontist who performed an orthodontic assessment and then referred the patient to a surgeon for an opinion regarding the correction of his dentofacial deformity.

Main complaint

The patient felt that his self-confidence was affected by his "large lower jaw" and "flat upper lip." His bite felt uncomfortable, he had a lisping speech defect, and he had difficulty in biting his food.

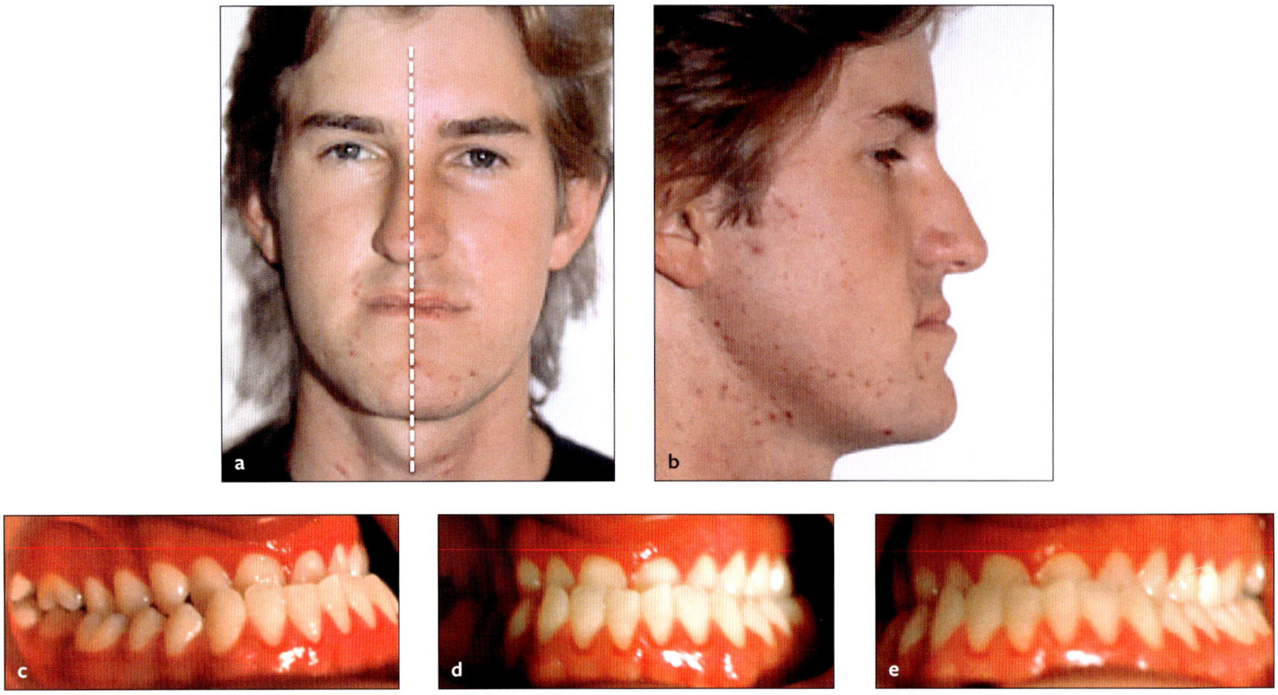

Fig 4-12 Case 4 (*a*) Pretreatment frontal view. (*b*) Profile view. (*c to e*) Pretreatment occlusion. Note the compensated mandibular incisors and mandibular dental midline asymmetry to the left.

Clinical examination

1. Soft tissue
   - Frontal view (Fig 4-12a)
     - Deficient paranasal areas
     - Poor upper lip support
     - Deficient lower lip vermilion
     - Nasal asymmetry to his right side
     - Slight mandibular asymmetry toward the left
   - Profile view (Fig 4-12b)
     - Concave profile
     - Midface deficiency
     - Acute nasolabial angle
     - Prominent nasal dorsum
     - Thin upper lip vermilion
     - Poor upper lip support
     - Concave upper lip
2. Dental (Figs 4-12c to 4-12e)
   - Class III malocclusion
   - Bilateral posterior crossbites
   - Anterior crossbite
   - Relative transverse discrepancy
   - Lower dental midline asymmetric to the left
   - Compensated mandibular incisors
3. Skeletal
   - Class III relationship
   - Maxillary anteroposterior deficiency
   - Mandibular anteroposterior excess
4. Radiographic
   - Panoramic
     - Impacted third molars are present
   - Cephalometric radiograph analysis
     - Class III malocclusion
     - Maxillary anteroposterior deficiency
     - Mandibular anteroposterior excess
     - Lingually inclined lower incisors (compensated)
     - Lack of dental support for the upper lip
     - Decreased facial contour angle

Problem list

- Class III malocclusion
- Compensated occlusion
- Maxillary anteroposterior deficiency
- Mandibular anteroposterior excess
- Asymmetry of his nose

Presurgical orthodontics (**Figs 4-12f to 4-12k**)

- Removal of third molars
- Decompensate the mandibular incisors
- Upright the mandibular posterior teeth
- Level and align both dental arches
- Coordinate the transverse dental relations

Surgical treatment

The maxilla was advanced by means of a Le Fort I osteotomy, while the mandible was set back and the symmetry

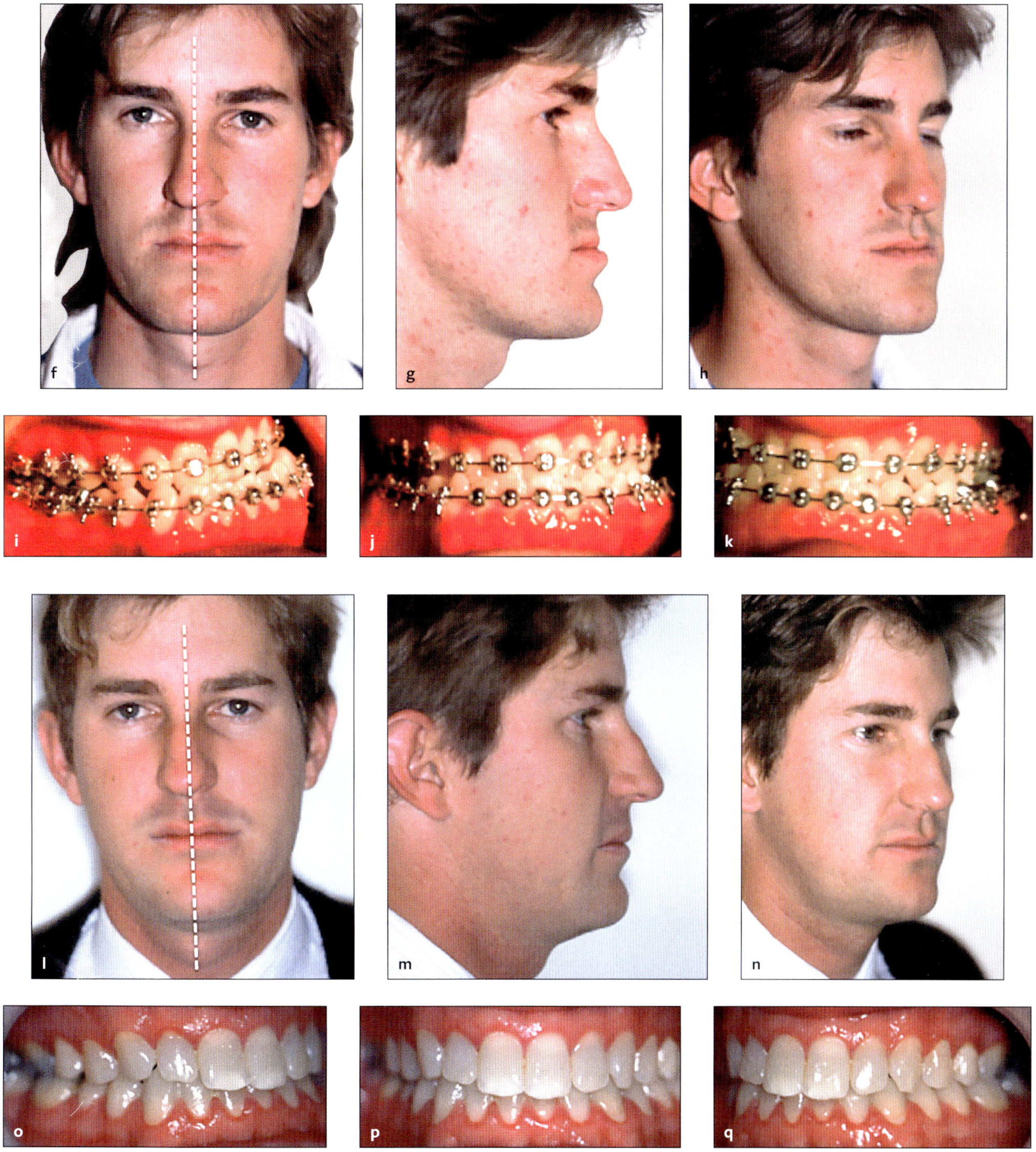

Fig 4-12 *(cont)* (*f*) Immediate presurgical frontal view. (*g*) Profile view. (*h*) Three-quareter view. (*i to k*) Occlusion. (*l to n*) Postreatment views after 6 months. Note the asymmetric nose. (*o to q*) Posttreatment occlusion.

corrected by means of a bilateral sagittal split osteotomy. The anteroposterior discrepancy was corrected by maxillary advancement and mandibular setback. The maxillary advancement was favored to enhance the midface and to not shorten the chin-throat length excessively.

Postsurgical orthodontics

The postsurgical orthodontic treatment consisted of finishing and retention. The long-term posttreatment results are illustrated in Figs 4-12l to 4-12q. The patient required a rhinoplasty for the correction of his nasal asymmetry.

Case 5

This 17-year-old adolescent boy was referred by his orthodontist for an assessment for orthognathic surgical correction of his severe Class III malocclusion.

Main complaint

He had difficulty chewing his food and had a lisping speech defect.

Medical history

The patient was in good health and actively participated in sports.

Clinical examination

1. Soft tissue
   - Frontal view (Fig 4-13a)
     - Flat paranasal areas
     - Mandibular asymmetry to the left
     - Less upper lip vermilion visible
     - His mandible appears prominent
     - Lack of upper lip support
   - Profile view (Fig 4-13b)
     - Concave profile
     - Deficient midface
     - Poor upper lip support
     - Everted lower lip
     - His nose appears relatively prominent
   - Three-quarter view (Fig 4-13c)
     - Flat paranasal areas
     - Prominent mandible
     - Overclosed mandible
     - Poor upper lip support
2. Dental (Fig 4-13d)
   - The mandibular midline is asymmetric to the left
   - Anterior crossbite
   - Accentuated curve of Spee
   - Tendency to posterior crossbites
   - Compensated lower incisors
   - Marginal gingivitis
   - Deep bite
   - Lingually inclined lower posterior teeth
3. Skeletal
   - Mandibular anteroposterior excess
   - Maxillary anteroposterior deficiency
   - Mandibular asymmetry to the left
4. Radiographic (Figs 4-13e and 4-13f)
   - Cephalometric radiograph
     - Class III malocclusion
     - Mandibular anteroposterior excess
     - Maxillary anteroposterior deficiency
     - Maxillary vertical deficiency

Problem list

- Mandibular anteroposterior excess and asymmetry
- Maxillary anteroposterior deficiency
- Class III malocclusion
- Accentuated curve of Spee
- Compensated mandibular incisors
- Tendency to transverse dental arch discrepancy
- Concave profile

Presurgical orthodontics

Maxillary arch

- Level and align the arch in one segment
- Establish arch compatibility with the mandible

Mandibular arch

- Decompensate the incisors
- Upright the posterior teeth
- Level the curve of Spee
- Maintain the lower dental midline in the middle of the chin
- Establish arch compatibility

Surgical treatment

A Le Fort I downsliding maxillary osteotomy was performed to advance the maxilla and increase the vertical dimension. The mandible was set back and mandibular asymmetry corrected by means of a bilateral sagittal ramus osteotomy. The anteroposterior incisor discrepancy (from the lingual surface of the upper incisor to the labial surface of the lower incisors) was 14 mm.

Postsurgical orthodontics

The transverse dental relations were well managed orthodontically, and no surgical correction was required. The final treatment results are demonstrated in Fig 4-13g to 4-13k.

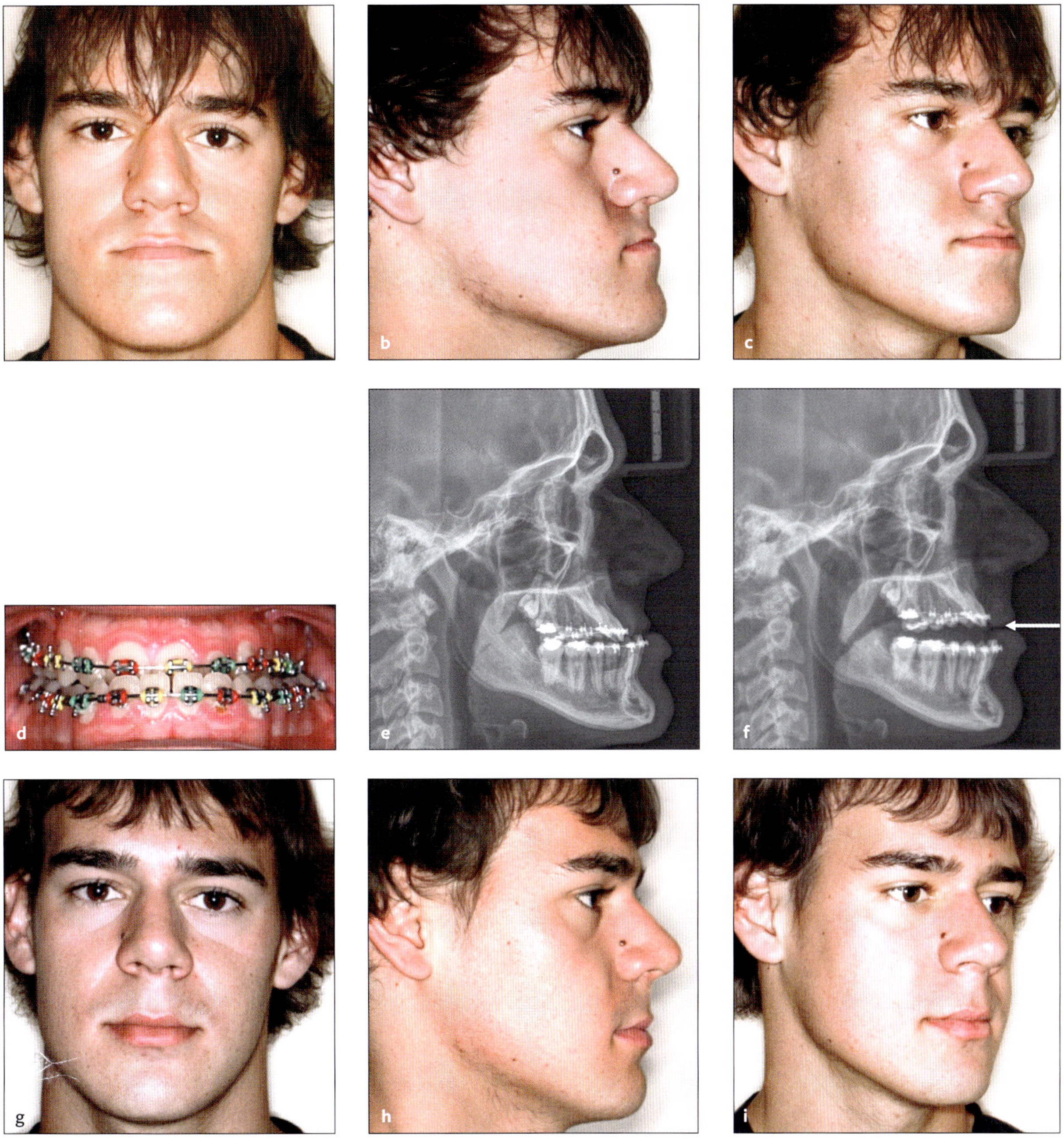

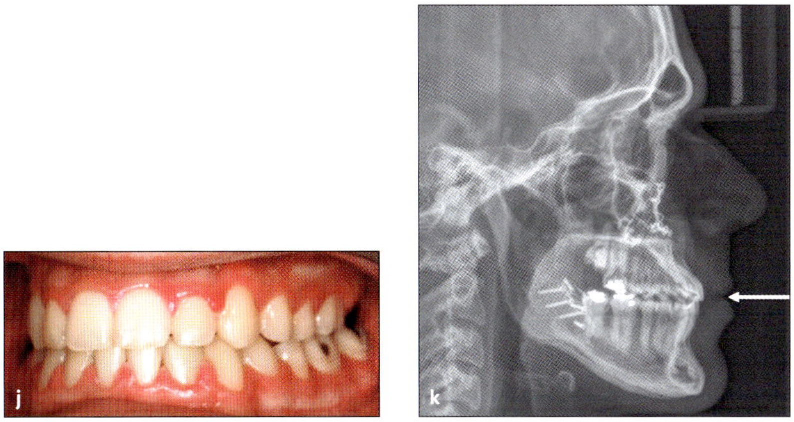

Fig 4-13 Case 5. (*a*) Presurgical frontal view. Note the mandibular asymmetry to the left and closed bite. (*b*) Profile view. (*c*) Three-quarter view. (*d*) Occlusion. Note the asymmetry of the mandibular dental midline. (*e*) Presurgical lateral cephalometric radiograph in centric occlusion. The severe anteroposterior discrepancy and closed bite are demonstrated. (*f*) Lateral cephalometric radiograph with the mandible rotated clockwise until the lips just part. The maxillary incisor/lip relationship indicates the vertical maxillary deficiency (*arrow*). (*g to i*) Posttreatment frontal view, profile view, and three-quarter view. (*j*) Posttreatment occlusion. (*k*) Posttreatment cephalometric radiograph. Note the anteroposterior and vertical increase of the maxilla (tooth/lip relationship).

Continued mandibular growth after surgical correction

Late or continued growth of the mandible after correction of Class III cases is an important factor in postsurgical stability, so the clinician must ensure that facial growth is completed prior to surgical correction. Serial cephalometric and hand-wrist radiographs are helpful in monitoring growth and estimating whether a growing patient has experienced his or her growth spurt.

The surgeon may consider performing surgery before the completion of growth in exceptional cases because "biological interest is not always in the patient's psychological interest" (Enlow, 1990). Ages 12 to 19 years are probably the most formative, and to postpone the correction of severe dentofacial deformities until completion of growth in patients of this age group often is not best for them psychologically. Surgical correction should be offered to these patients with the full understanding of the risk of relapse because of continued growth. Upon the completion of growth, additional surgical correction can be performed. Case 6 illustrates a satisfactory outcome to performing surgery before completion of growth.

Case 6

Main complaint

According to the patient's parents, her facial appearance was burdensome because it affected her schoolwork and social life. She was unhappy and was teased by her peers about her large mandible. She was also concerned about the fact that the unfavorable jaw relationship caused an increasingly severe speech impediment.

Medical history

Her medical history was noncontributory.

Clinical examination

1. Soft tissue
    - Frontal view
        - Increased interlabial distance
        - Unsupported upper lip that appears flat
        - Prominent chin
        - Increased lower facial height
    - Profile view (Fig 4-14a)
        - Mandibular anteroposterior excess
        - Maxillary anteroposterior deficiency
        - "Gummy smile"
        - Increased maxillary incisor exposure
        - Increased lower facial height
        - Concave profile
2. Dental (Fig 4-14b)
    - Class III malocclusion
    - Compensated mandibular incisors
    - Posterior crossbites
    - Canines partially blocked out
3. Skeletal (Fig 4-14c)
    - Maxillary vertical excess
    - Maxillary anteroposterior deficiency
    - Mandibular anteroposterior excess
4. Radiographic (see Fig 4-14c)
    - Hand-wrist radiography
        - Patient still actively growing
    - Cephalometric radiograph
        - Confirms the clinical observations

Problem list

- Vertical maxillary excess
- Maxillary anteroposterior deficiency
- Mandibular anteroposterior excess
- Class III malocclusion
- Blocked-out maxillary canines
- Compensated mandibular incisors
- Patient still actively growing

Presurgical orthodontics

Maxillary arch

- Extraction of both maxillary first premolars
- Arch alignment and closure of the spaces
- Movement of the canines into the arch

Mandibular arch

- Decompensation of the incisors
- Leveling of the curve of Spee
- Establishment of interarch compatibility

The profound vertical and anteroposterior growth during orthodontic treatment is evident when the pretreatment (see Figs 4-14a to 4-14c) and immediate presurgical records (Figs 4-14d to 4-14f) are compared.

Surgical treatment

A Le Fort I osteotomy superiorly repositioned the maxilla 6 mm anteriorly and posteriorly, rotating the maxillomandibular complex slightly clockwise (Fig 4-14g; see the section "Rotation of the Maxillomandibular Complex" in chapter 5) and advancing the maxilla 8 mm.

A bilateral sagittal split ramus osteotomy set the mandible back 12 mm (see Fig 4-14g).

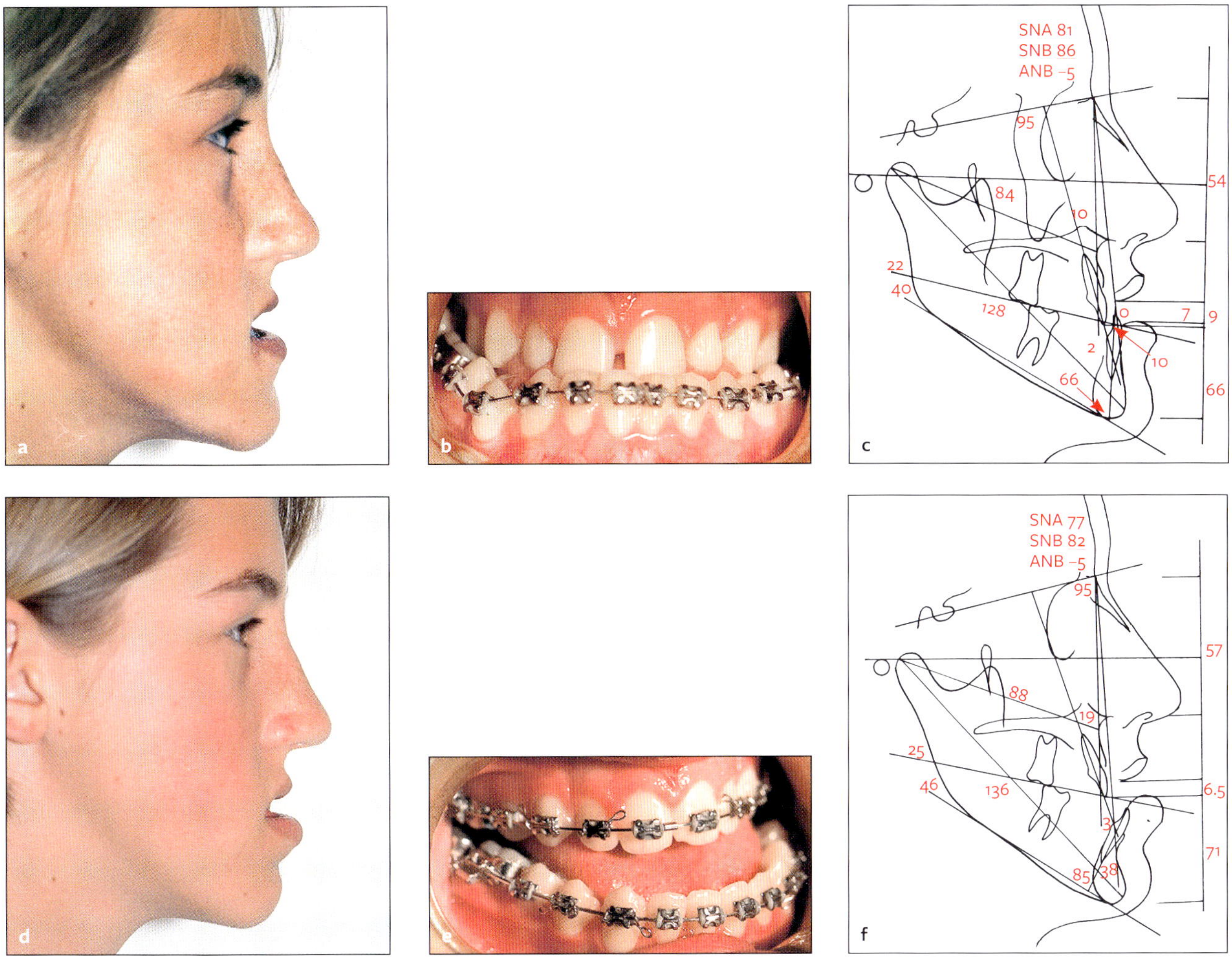

Fig 4-14 Case 6. Pretreatment profile view (*a*), occlusion (*b*), and cephalometric analysis (*c*) 1 week after banding the mandibular arch (age, 12.5 years). Class III skeletal relationship: ANB angle = –5 degrees, mandibular length to maxillary length = 84:128 mm; maxillary vertical excess: interlabial gap = 7 mm, maxillary tooth exposure under the upper lip = 9 mm; compensated mandibular incisors: mandibular incisor to nasion–point B (N-B) = 0 mm and 10 degrees, mandibular incisor to mandibular plane = 66 degrees. Immediate presurgical profile view (*d*), occlusion (*e*), and cephalometric tracing (*f*).

These surgical movements were large. This along with the fact that the surgery was performed on a growing individual made the relapse potential significant in this case.

Postsurgical orthodontics

Postsurgical orthodontic treatment entailed finalization of the occlusion and retention. In cases similar to this one, the postsurgical skeletal change should be accurately monitored and the dentition not compensated for any relapse or further growth. When surgery is performed early and further excessive mandibular growth is expected, the dentition should not be orthodontically compensated for this growth because (1) it will disguise the skeletal growth and (2) the teeth will need to be decompensated again before final surgical correction.

The postoperative results are demonstrated in Figs 4-14h and 4-14i. Postsurgical growth is evident in Figs 4-14j to 4-14l (10 months after surgery) and Figs 4-14m to 4-14o (4 years after surgery). Five years after the initial correction, the clinician decided to perform the final correction. After a short period of orthodontic treatment to slightly decompensate the mandibular incisors (Figs 4-14p to 4-14r), the mandible was set back by means of a bilateral sagittal split osteotomy. The final result is illustrated in Figs 4-14s to 4-14u (1 year after the second surgery). This patient certainly benefited from early surgery, even though a second surgical procedure had to be performed 5 years after the initial correction. The fact that the bicortical screws had to be removed prior to performing the bilateral sagittal split osteotomy made the second surgery challenging. To facilitate this procedure, the use of resorbable fixation at the first surgery was indicated.

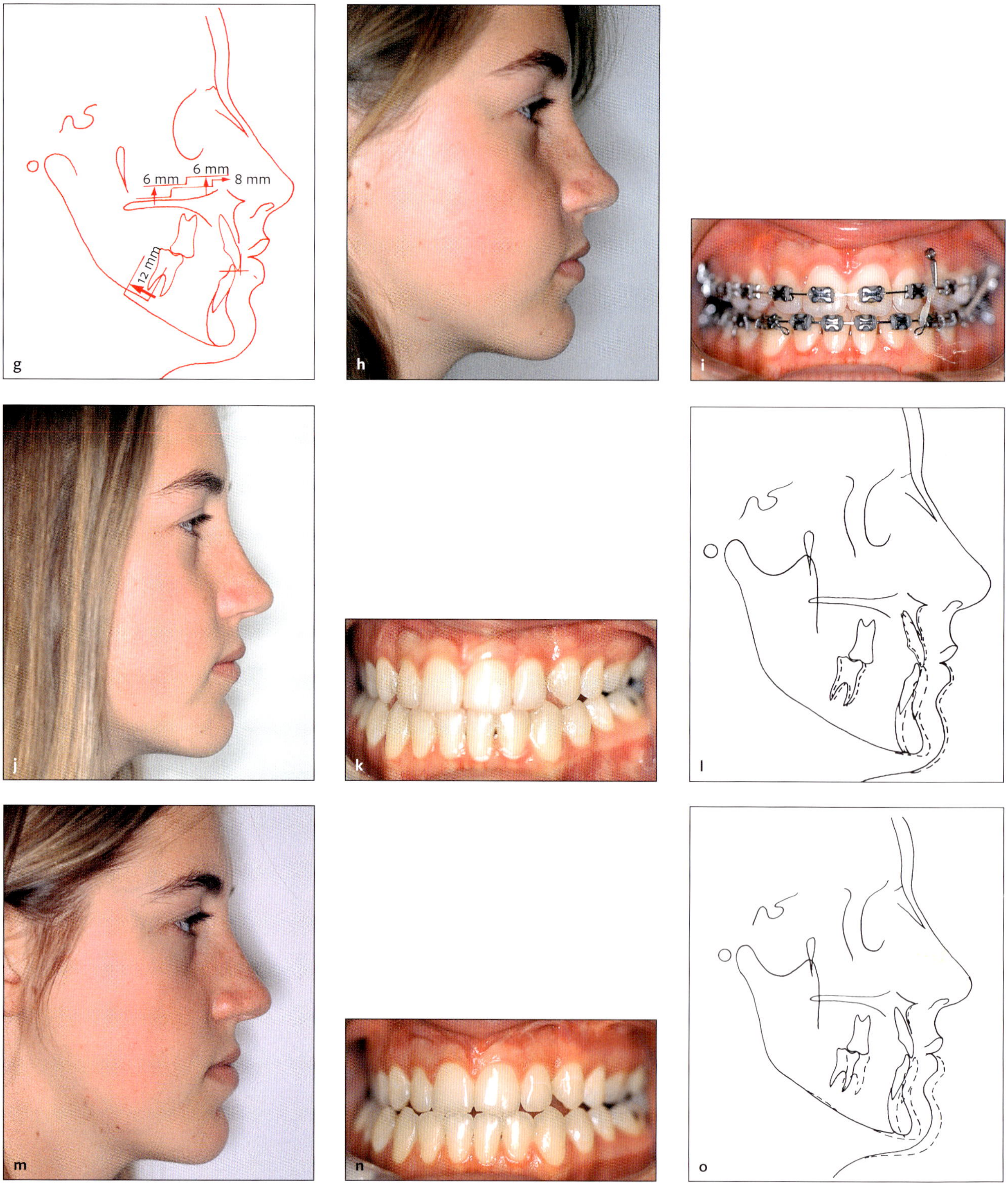

Fig 4-14 *(cont)* Note the profound anteroposterior and vertical growth. Surgical prediction tracing (*g*), immediate postsurgical profile view (*h*), and immediate postsurgical occlusion (*i*). Relapse is evident 10 months after surgery. Profile view (*j*), occlusion (*k*), and cephalometric tracing (*l*) indicating some signs of further mandibular growth. Four years after the initial correction, a Class III malocclusion is present. The maxilla remains stable. Profile view (*m*), occlusion (*n*), and a cephalometric tracing (*o*) illustrate the further growth of the mandible. The decompensation of the mandibular incisors is completed before the second corrective procedure.

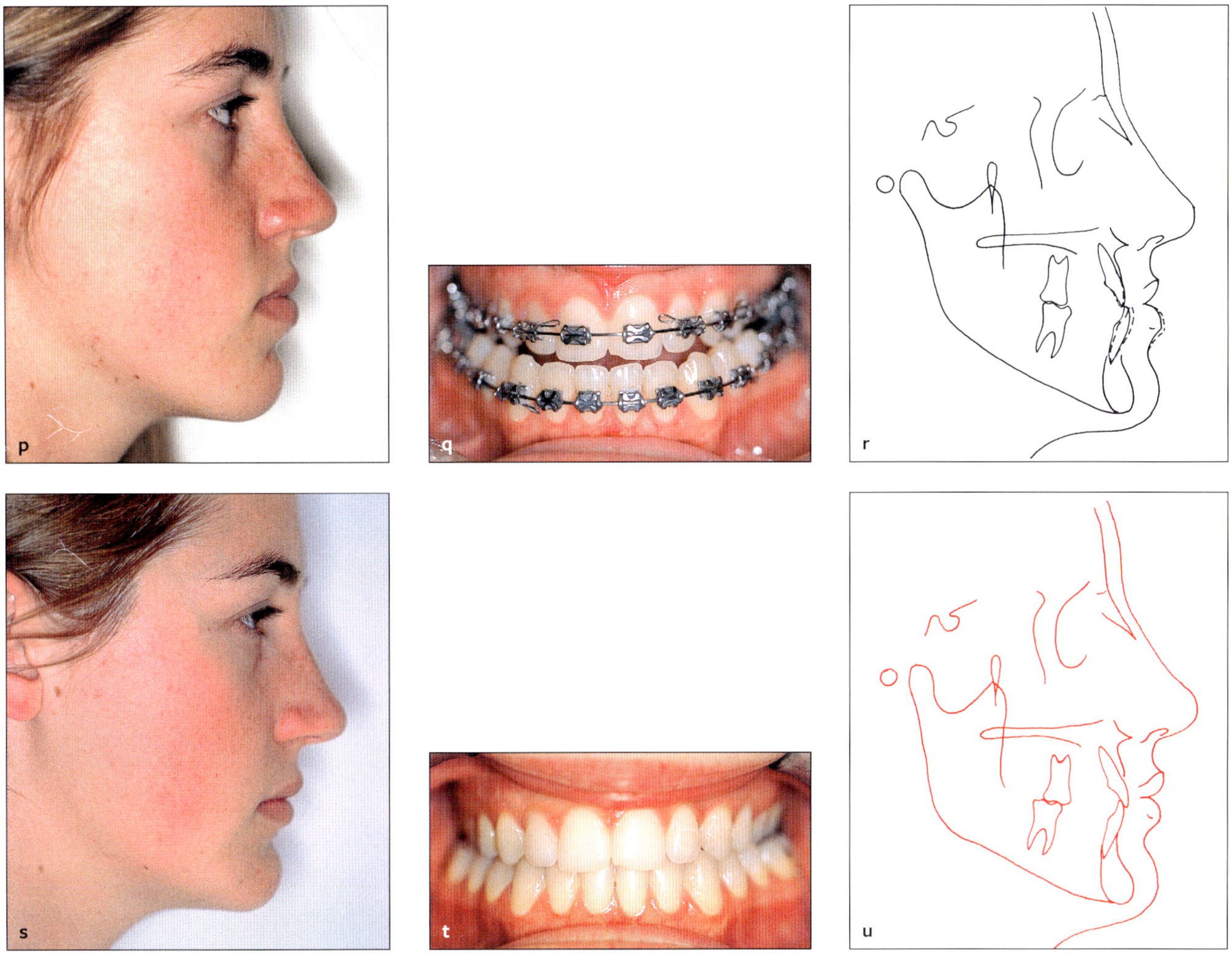

Fig 4-14 *(cont)* Profile view (*p*), occlusion (*q*), and cephalometric tracing (*r*). Posttreatment results are demonstrated in profile view (*s*), occlusion (*t*), and cephalometric tracing (*u*) 1 year after the second surgical procedure.

Maxillary Anteroposterior Deficiency

Maxillary anteroposterior deficiency has often been misdiagnosed as mandibular anteroposterior excess because of the similarity in appearance. Therefore, the clinician must carefully distinguish between the two deformities. In most patients with Class III malocclusion, the deformity is caused by a combination of the two deformities. As many as 75% of patients with Class III malocclusion have some degree of maxillary skeletal deficiency. If there is any doubt about which jaw should undergo surgery, the maxilla should be advanced.

Class III malocclusion

Clinical characteristics

Profile view

- Sunken cheeks
- Chin and lower lip in balance with the nose
- Sunken or flat appearance of the upper lip
- Reduced upper lip length and thin vermilion
- Frequently, an acute nasolabial angle with the columella of the nose oriented more horizontally

Frontal view

- Flat and relatively short upper lip
- Often, a narrow alar base
- Often, sclera seen inferiorly of the iris of the eye

- Sunken cheeks
- Normal to deficient maxillary tooth-to-lip relationship
- Less vermilion exposure of the upper lip
- Paranasal flattening

The relationship of each individual jaw to the cranium can be evaluated clinically by blocking out the mandible and then the maxilla with a hand or card (see Fig 2-23 in chapter 2).

Dental characteristics

- Class III malocclusion
- Often, crowding in the maxillary arch
- Often, small or absent maxillary lateral incisors
- Often, normal inclination of mandibular incisors in comparison with the lingual inclination seen in mandibular anteroposterior excess
- Tendency of the maxillary arch to be narrow and often in lingual crossbite with the mandibular arch

Treatment

Presurgical orthodontics

The treatment of maxillary anteroposterior deficiency has the same basic goals as does the treatment of mandibular anteroposterior excess:

- Eliminate compensations
- Establish ideal incisor position (indicated by the orthodontic visual treatment objective)
- Establish arch compatibility
- Level and align arches

It is important to keep in mind that the transverse discrepancy that often accompanies the maxillary anteroposterior deficiency may have to be corrected by surgical expansion of the maxilla. If this procedure is contemplated, the arch should be aligned accordingly and the roots of the teeth next to the interdental osteotomy should be deviated.

Two-jaw surgery may be indicated in patients with severe Class III malocclusion. Here the orthodontist should adopt the “two-patient” concept, in which the mandibular and maxillary arches are treated independently, almost as if they belong to two different patients; however, the two arches should still be compatible. The objective is to align the maxillary and mandibular incisors in both vertical and anteroposterior planes of space, so the surgeon can achieve optimal skeletal and esthetic correction without the limitations of dental interference.

Patients with maxillary deficiency often have tooth crowding in the maxilla, and retraction of incisors is indicated. Retraction will necessitate extractions, which follow these principles:

- If maximum retraction is necessary or significant crowding is present, removal of maxillary first premolars is indicated.
- If little retraction is necessary and crowding is slight, removal of second premolars is indicated.
- Advancement of mandibular incisors from an upright or lingually tipped position may be limited by lack of attached gingiva and/or a thin alveolar bone and symphysis. Mandibular second premolar extraction may be necessary to provide the required space to manage crowding.
- The most common extraction pattern in patients with Class III malocclusion is extraction of maxillary first premolars and, when extraction in both arches is indicated, extraction of maxillary first premolars and mandibular second premolars (the opposite of Class II malocclusion).

Orthodontic mechanics

Crowding is often present in the maxillary arch and requires tooth extraction. The canines are usually blocked out, which is often the patient’s main complaint before treatment. The decision whether to extract the first or second premolars is influenced by the amount of crowding and required decompensation of the incisors. Presurgically, the maxillary incisors should be placed in good angulation in the central trough of bone. To achieve the best esthetic result, anteroposterior positioning of these teeth should be based on the visual treatment objective. Decompensation of the mandibular incisors is seldom indicated. The mandibular arch should be leveled and aligned to act as the “template” for the maxillary dental arch.

Surgical treatment

The maxilla is advanced by means of a Le Fort I osteotomy. This versatile procedure enables the surgeon to correct discrepancies in the anteroposterior, vertical, and transverse planes. Grafting is recommended for large advancements and expansion of the palate. Various grafting materials are available, including bone harvested from local or distant sites such as the chin or iliac crest; allogeneic freeze-dried bone; and artificial bone substitutes such as hydroxyapatite blocks.

In the past, undesirable soft tissue changes may have occurred, including widening of the alar base, tipping up of the tip of the nose, and an increase in the nasolabial angle. These esthetically unfavorable effects may still occur in patients in whom the nasal morphology is not controlled during surgery. The patient should be informed about the possibility of soft tissue changes. Control of the nose during Le Fort I osteotomy is mandatory and described elsewhere in the text (see the section on Le Fort I maxillary osteotomy in chapter 6).

Postsurgical orthodontics

Postsurgical orthodontic treatment is very similar to that for patients with mandibular setback. A splint is used only when a multi-piece Le Fort I maxillary osteotomy is performed. In two-jaw surgery, an intermediate splint is always used to accurately position the maxilla. The patient will be able to function with the occlusal splint until adequate healing has taken place and active orthodontics can be resumed.

Ligature wires between teeth adjacent to interdental osteotomies should be placed by the surgeon and removed only by the orthodontist during the placement of a continuous archwire.

When surgical expansion has been performed, the transverse dimension should be maintained by an occlusal splint reinforced by a palatal bar. The palatal bar prevents bending of the splint during and after surgery. Once the splint is removed, the orthodontist should place an orthodontic palatal bar and a continuous archwire as soon as possible to further control the transverse dimension.

Case 7

This 17-year-old girl was seen by the orthodontist for alignment of her teeth.

Main complaint

The patient wanted her teeth aligned and her "bad bite" corrected. She also thought that her mandible appeared too prominent.

Medical history

Her medical history was noncontributory.

Clinical examination

1. Soft tissue
   - Frontal view (Fig 4-15a)
     - Flat paranasal areas
     - Lack of upper lip support
     - Relatively small amount of upper lip vermilion exposure
   - Profile view (Fig 4-15b)
     - Concave profile
     - Lack of upper lip support
     - Lower lip ahead of the upper lip
     - Obtuse labiomental fold
     - Acute nasolabial angle
2. Dental (Fig 4-15c)
   - Class III malocclusion
   - Anterior and posterior crossbites (absolute)
   - Compensated mandibular incisors
   - Narrow maxillary dental arch
   - Maxillary dental midline 1.5 mm toward the left
   - Maxillary left first premolar absent
   - Crowding in the maxillary and mandibular arches
3. Skeletal (Fig 4-15d)
   - Maxillary anteroposterior deficiency
   - Maxillary transverse deficiency
   - Vertical excess of the anterior mandible
   - Tendency toward anteroposterior deficiency of the chin
4. Radiographic
   - Panoramic radiograph
     - Maxillary left first premolar absent
     - Four impacted third molars
   - Cephalometric radiograph (see Fig 4-15d)
     - Confirms clinical observations

Problem list

- Class III malocclusion
- Maxillary anteroposterior deficiency
- Maxillary transverse deficiency
- Maxillary dental midline toward the left
- Lingually inclined mandibular incisors
- Anterior mandibular vertical excess

Presurgical orthodontics

Maxillary arch (Figs 4-15e to 4-15g)

- Extraction of the maxillary right first premolar and removal of impacted third molars
- Correction of the dental midline
- Establishment of a good arch form in two segments, from the maxillary right central incisor to second molar and from the maxillary left central incisor to second molar
- Expansion of the arch within the bony base
- Deviation of the roots of the central incisors

Mandibular arch (see Figs 4-15e to 4-15g)

- Extraction of both mandibular second premolars and removal of impacted third molars
- Establishment of a good arch form
- Decompensation of the incisors

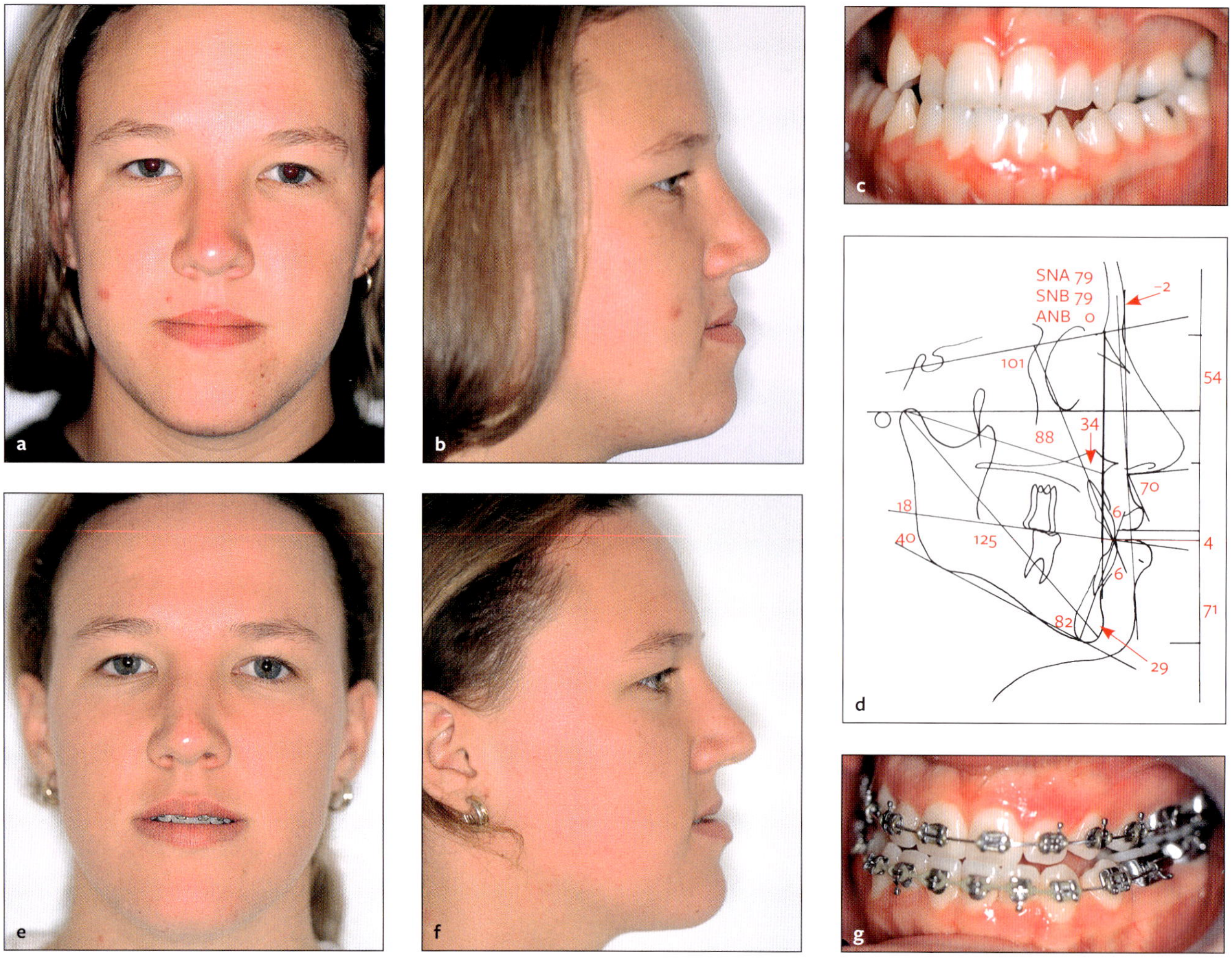

Fig 4-15 Case 7. Pretreatment frontal view (*a*), profile view (*b*), and occlusion (*c*). (*d*) Cephalometric analysis. Class III dental relationship; Class III skeletal relationship; maxillary anteroposterior deficiency: SNA = 79 degrees, ratio of maxillary length to mandibular length = 88:125 mm; increased lower-third facial height: ratio of middle third to lower third = 54:71 mm; increased anterior mandibular height: height = 46 mm, ratio of upper lip to lower lip = 21:46; obtuse labiomental fold; lingually inclined mandibular incisors: mandibular incisor to mandibular plane, 82 degrees; acute nasolabial angle, 70 degrees; concave profile: facial contour angle = –2 degrees. Presurgical frontal view (*e*), profile view (*f*), and occlusion (*g*). Note the orthodontic correction of the dental midlines and the decompensation of the mandibular incisors. →

Surgical treatment

The maxilla was advanced and expanded by means of a two-piece Le Fort I maxillary osteotomy. The interdental osteotomy was performed between the maxillary central incisors. The maxilla was superiorly repositioned to improve the tooth-lip relationship (Fig 4-15h). Finally, genioplasty was performed to reduce the vertical height of the chin and advance the chin slightly.

Postsurgical orthodontics

Postsurgical orthodontics corrected the angulation of the maxillary incisors, controlled the surgical expansion (a palatal bar was placed as soon as possible after surgery), and refined the occlusion. The surgery was performed after a 17-month presurgical period of orthodontics, and the orthodontic bands were removed 4 months after surgery, after which the patient was given a retainer to wear. The treatment results 6 months after band removal are illustrated in Figs 4-15i to 4-15k.

Case 8

Case 8 demonstrates a 22-year-old woman with Class III anterior open bite malocclusion as a result of maxillary anteroposterior and transverse deficiency (Fig 4-16a to 4-16e). She previously had orthodontic treatment in an attempt to compromise her dentition for her skeletal defor-

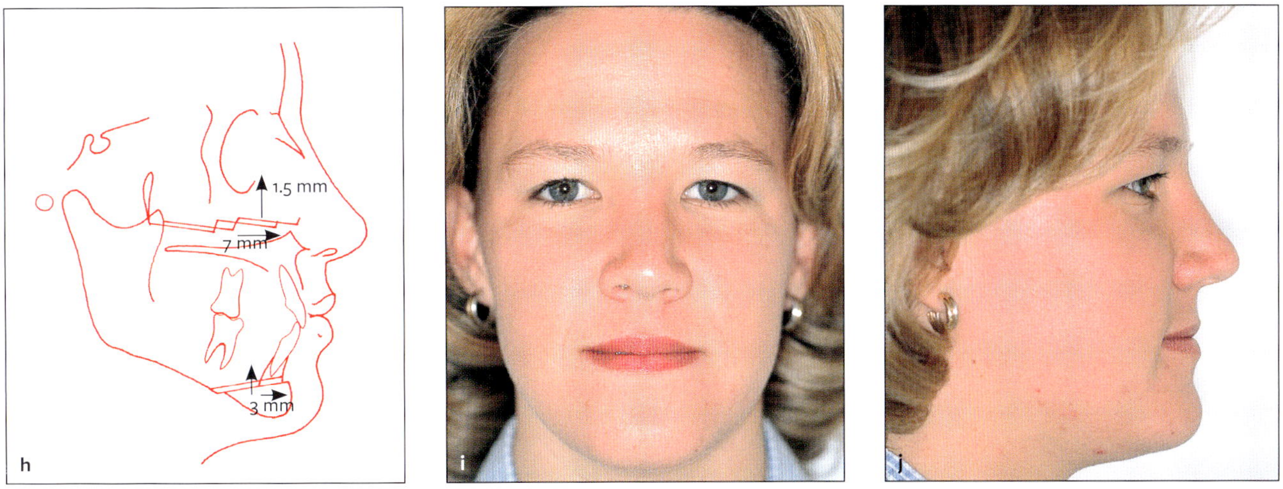

Fig 4-15 *(cont)* (*h*) Surgical visual treatment objective. The surgical plan consists of (1) a Le Fort I maxillary osteotomy advancing the maxilla by 7 mm and superiorly repositioning it by 1.5 mm and (2) a genioplasty with a 3-mm vertical reduction and a 3-mm advancement. Posttreatment results are demonstrated in frontal view (*i*), profile view (*j*), and occlusion (*k*).

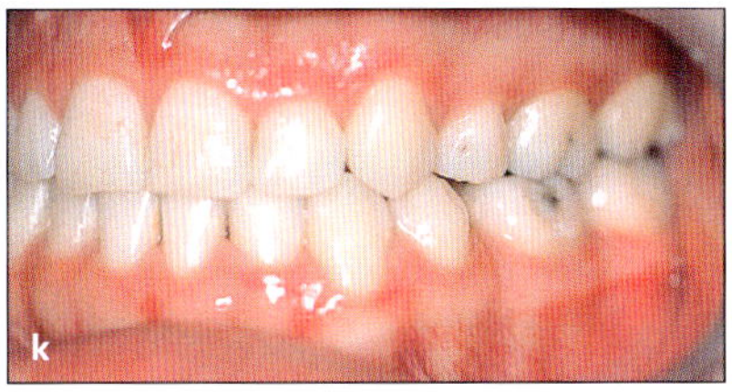

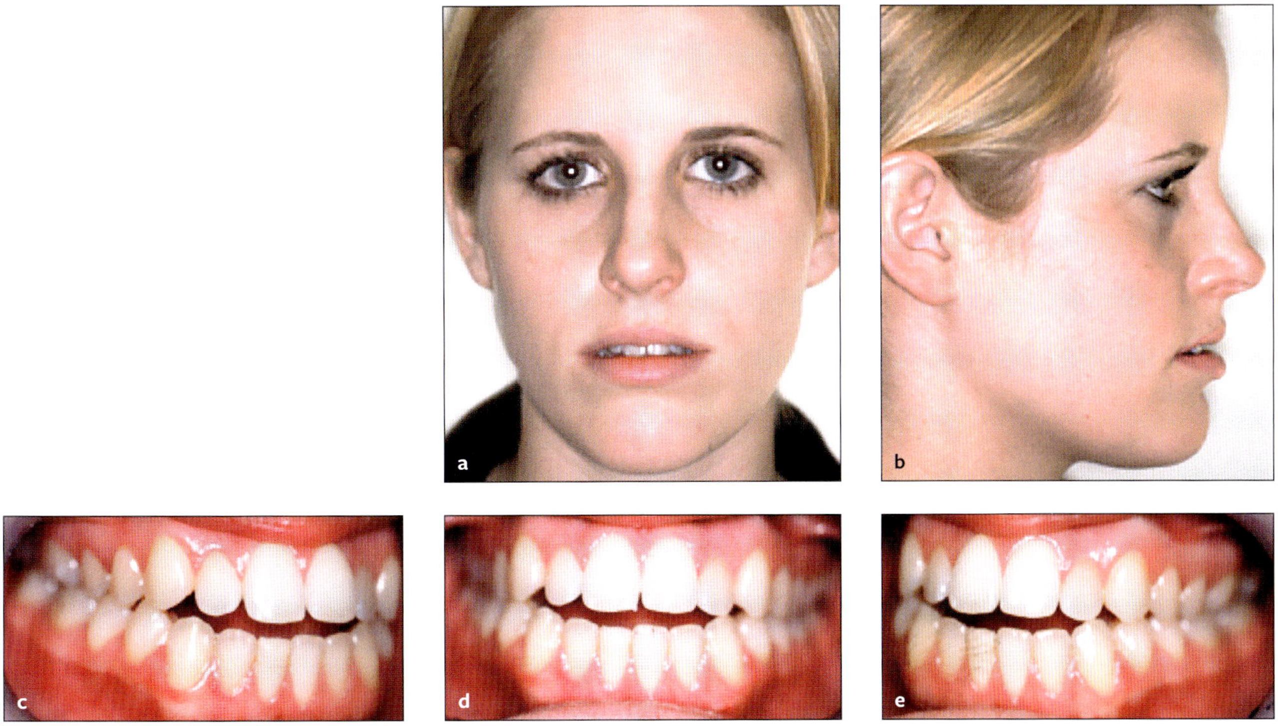

Fig 4-16 Case 8. Maxillary anteroposterior deficiency. (*a*) Pretreatment frontal view. (*b*) Profile view. (*c to e*) Relapsed occlusion. Note the anterior open bite, posterior crossbites, and Class III dental relationship.

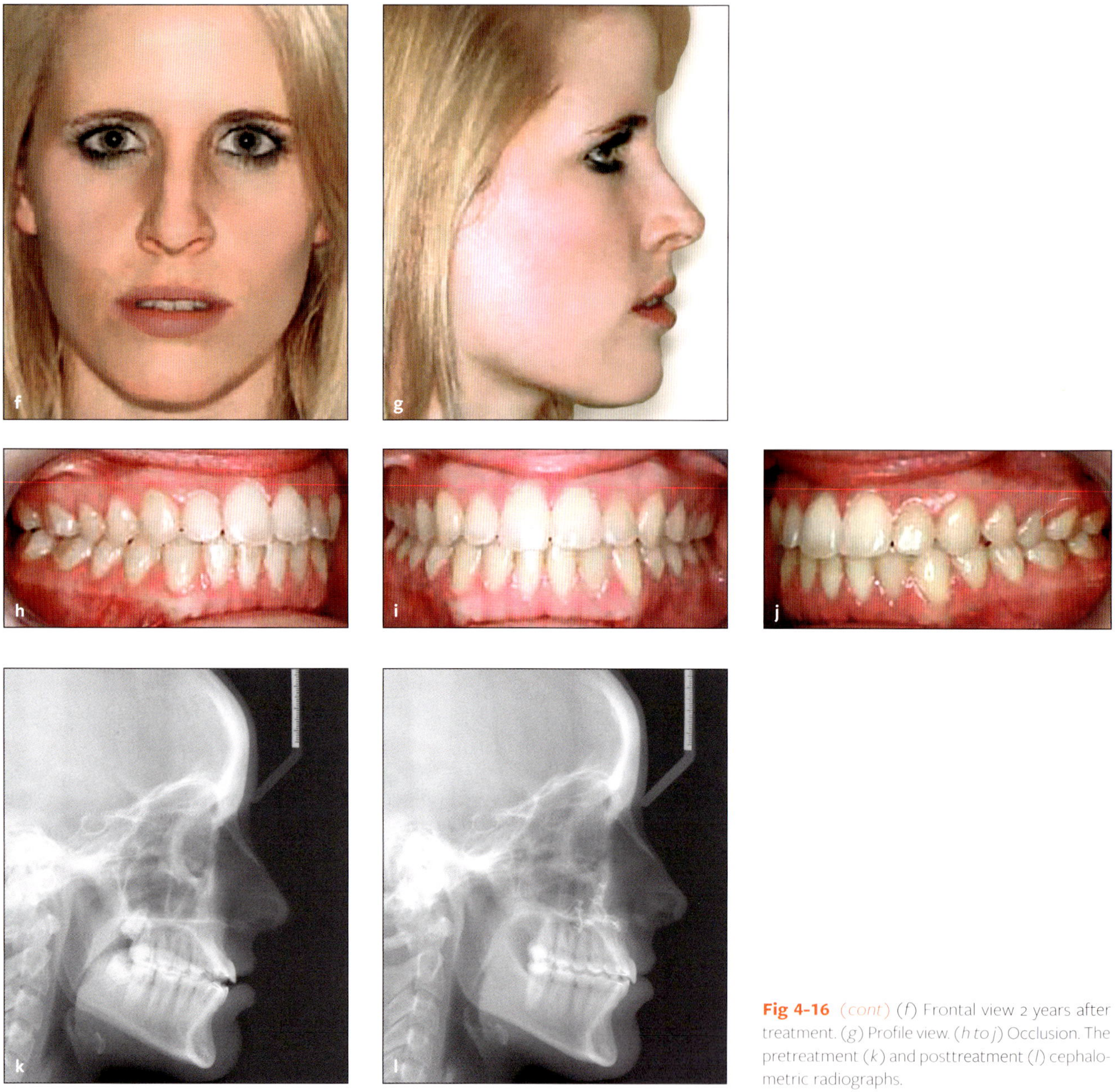

Fig 4-16 *(cont)* (*f*) Frontal view 2 years after treatment. (*g*) Profile view. (*h to j*) Occlusion. The pretreatment (*k*) and posttreatment (*l*) cephalometric radiographs.

mity, but the dentition relapsed. In a second treatment, the orthodontist decompensated the incisors and aligned the maxillary dental arch in three segments. Her maxilla was advanced and expanded by means of a three-piece Le Fort I osteotomy. The esthetic and occlusal changes 2 years after orthodontic debanding are demonstrated in Figs 4-16f to 4-16j. The improved skeletal relationships, soft tissue, and occlusion are illustrated on the pre- and posttreatment cephalometric radiographs (Fig 4-16k and 4-16l).

Case 9

This 18-year-old man was referred by his dentist for the correction of his Class III malocclusion (Fig 4-17a to 4-17c). Following orthodontic decompensation and coordination of his dental arches, his maxilla was advanced by means of a Le Fort I osteotomy. The treatment results are demonstrated in Figs 4-17d to 4-17f.

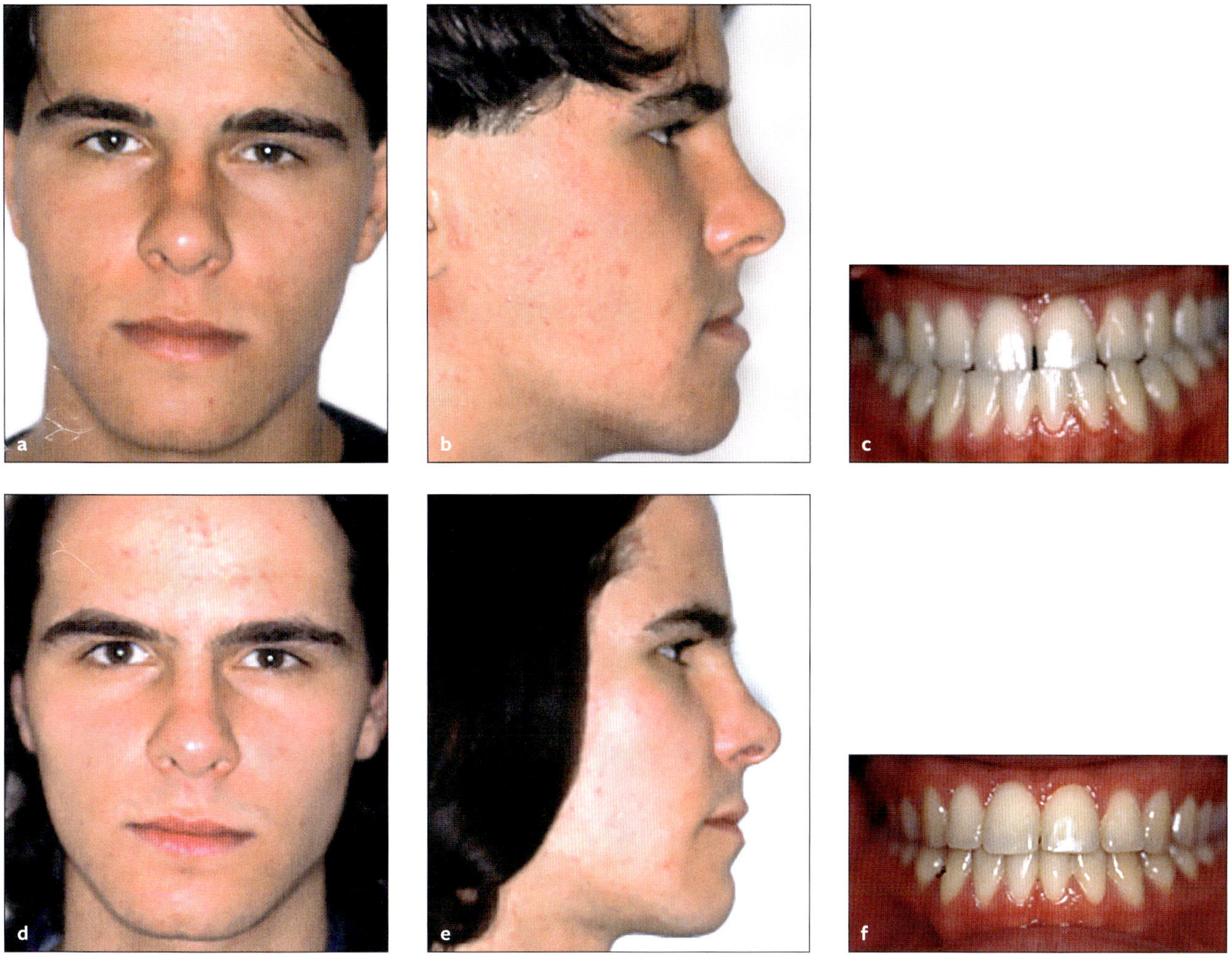

Fig 4-17 Case 9. Maxillary anteroposterior deficiency. The pretreatment frontal view (*a*), profile view (*b*) and occlusion (*c*). (*d to f*) Note the improvement in the nasolabial angle, increased upper lip support, and increased fullness of his midface as well as his occlusion.

Maxillary Anteroposterior Excess

Maxillary anteroposterior excess is certainly not as common as was implied when Class II malocclusions were classified strictly according to the Angle dental classification. According to McNamara (1981), only approximately 10% of a group of 277 patients with Class II malocclusions had true maxillary anteroposterior excess. In the past, anterior maxillary segmental osteotomies were erroneously performed for the correction of Class II mandibular deficiency, resulting in poor esthetic outcomes.

The clinician should carefully differentiate between maxillary anteroposterior excess and mandibular anteroposterior deficiency because of the previously discussed esthetically unfavorable results achieved after the surgical or orthodontic retraction of maxillary incisors in a patient with mandibular anteroposterior deficiency. Of course, maxillary anteroposterior excess can occur in combination with mandibular deficiency (see case 10 later in this section).

Overview

Clinical characteristics

Profile view

- General protrusion of the middle third of the face
- Nose that often appears large and has a dorsal hump
- Prominent infraorbital rims and cheekbones

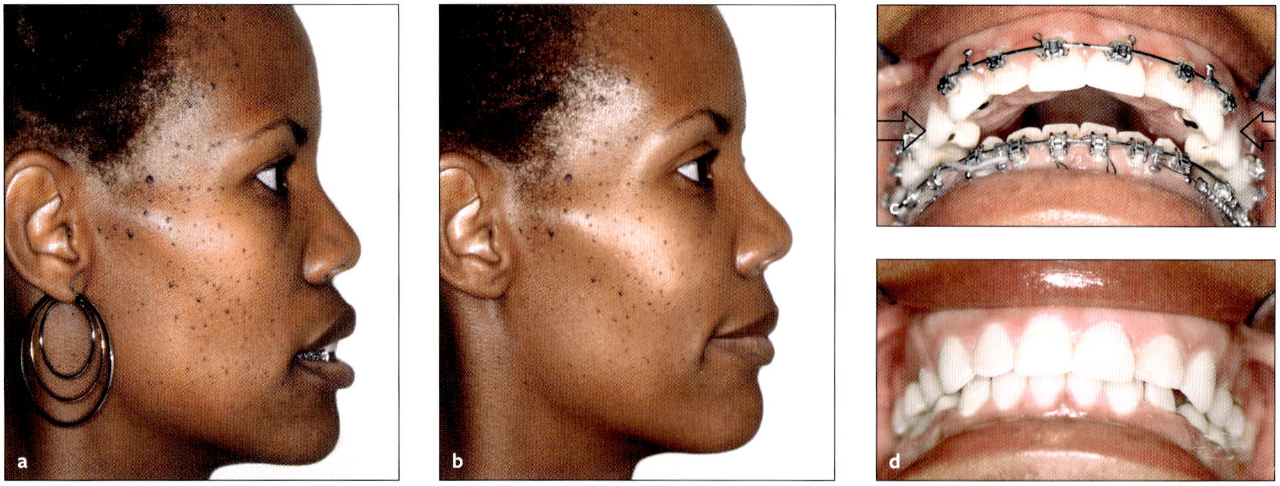

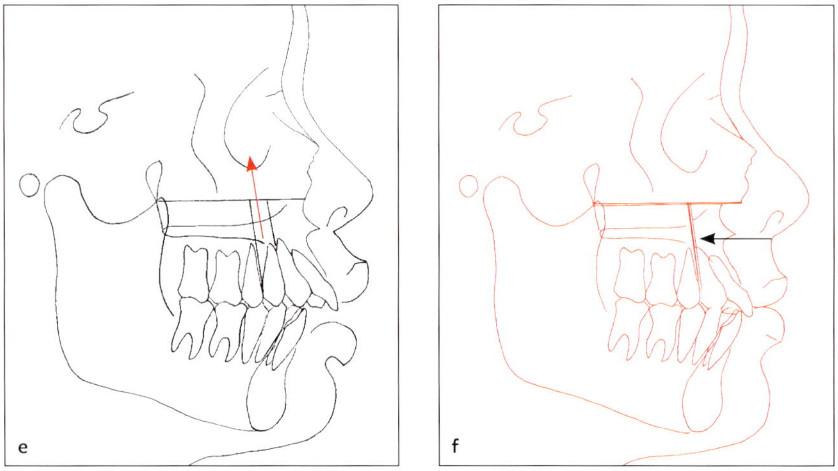

Fig 4-18 (a) The patient's upper lip prominence is evident as a result of maxillary anteroposterior excess. (*b*) Improved lip competence and less prominent upper lip following segmental setback of the anterior maxilla. (*c*) Presurgical occlusion. The maxillary first premolars are not banded and will be removed during surgery. Note the excessive overjet. (*d*) Postoperative occlusion. (*e*) Presurgical cephalometric tracing. Note the first premolar and bone to be removed (*arrow*). The increased overjet is evident. (*f*) The surgical visual treatment objective.

- Upper lip that is often short and everted
- Deep labiomental sulcus because the lower lip curls under the maxillary incisors
- Lip incompetence
- Acute nasolabial angle

Frontal view

- Noticeable prominence of the middle third of the face
- Often, a long lower facial height
- Short, curled upper lip
- Lower lip that is curled under the maxillary incisors

Dental characteristics

- Tendency toward an open bite
- Tendency toward a narrow, constricted maxillary arch
- High, arched palatal vault

Treatment

In the growing child, orthodontic correction is certainly most effective. It usually involves the use of headgear and multibanded fixed appliance therapy. Depending on the severity of deformity and tooth crowding, it also may involve the extraction of four premolars.

In the nongrowing patient, surgery that sets back the total maxilla or anterior maxillary segment hastens treatment and avoids headgear therapy. Total maxillary setback is performed at the Le Fort I level and is seldom indicated and technically difficult.

Surgical treatment

Three surgical techniques for repositioning the anterior maxilla have been described by Wassmund (1935), Cupar (1954), and Wunderer (1963). When posterior movement of the anterior maxillary segment is the main objective, the technique described by Wunderer is the most practical approach.

An anterior segmental osteotomy of the maxilla is often performed as part of a multisegment Le Fort I procedure because patients who need anterior maxillary correction often need additional corrections to the maxilla (eg, superior repositioning and/or expansion of the posterior maxilla).

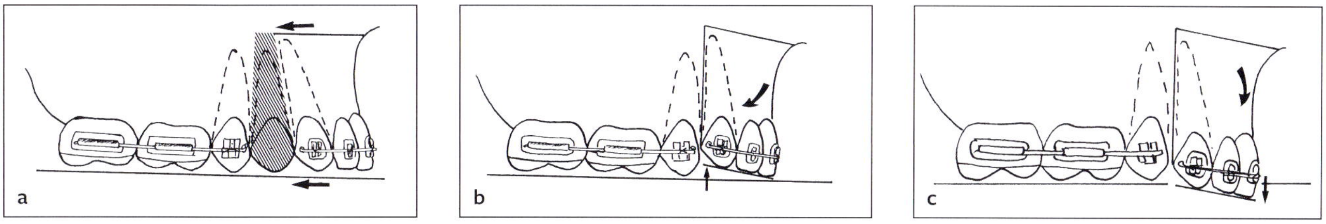

Fig 4-19 Inadequate orthodontic root deviation (*a*) will force the surgeon to either lift the canine superiorly out of the occlusion (*b*) or tip the incisors inferiorly (*c*), increasing the anterior height of the maxilla.

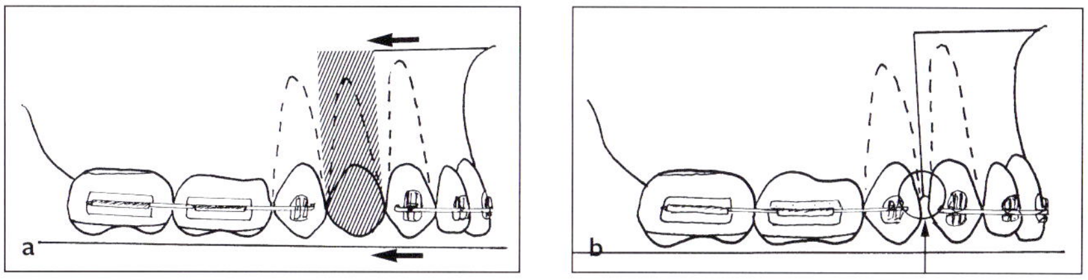

Fig 4-20 (*a*) Adequate orthodontic deviation of the roots of the teeth adjacent to the interdental osteotomy will allow the surgeon to close an interdental space. (*b*) To ensure the integrity of the periodontium, the space should never be completely closed, and a small amount of alveolar bone should always be left intact at the alveolar crest.

The author finds it easier to perform a multi-piece Le Fort I procedure than an anterior segmental osteotomy (Fig 4-18).

In the presurgical phase, the roots of the teeth on either side of the osteotomy cut or ostectomy must be deviated sufficiently. Inadequate deviation of the roots of these teeth will have the following consequences:

- Limit the surgical setback
- Increase the risk of damage to the tooth roots at surgery
- Force the surgeon to rotate the segment, thereby either elevating the canines out of occlusion or tipping the incisors inferiorly (Fig 4-19)

Adequate deviation of the roots allows setback of the anterior maxillary segment. A small area of interproximal bone should be maintained and the crowns of the teeth not forced together (Fig 4-20).

Maxillary setback procedures are seldom indicated. The clinician contemplating such a procedure should consider the esthetic effects carefully before making a final decision.

Clinical cases

Case 10

A 32-year-old woman was referred to the orthodontist by a general practitioner for correction of her protruding teeth.

Main complaint

The patient was self-conscious about her prominent front teeth and was unable to close her lips without strain.

Medical history

Her medical history was noncontributory.

Clinical examination

1. Soft tissue (Figs 4-21a to 4-21c)
   - Frontal view
     - Increased interlabial gap
     - Increased maxillary incisor exposure
     - Everted lower lip
     - Chin that appears narrow
   - Profile view
     - Convex profile
     - Increased interlabial gap
     - Protruding upper and lower lips
     - Deficient chin
2. Dental (Fig 4-21d)
   - Maxillary and mandibular dental protrusion
   - Class II malocclusion
   - Increased incisor overjet
   - Small area of attached gingiva in the mandibular incisor region
   - Gingival recession at the maxillary second premolars
3. Skeletal (Fig 4-21e)
   - Vertical maxillary excess
   - Maxillary anteroposterior excess
   - Mandibular anteroposterior deficiency
   - Microgenia
   - Narrow chin
4. Radiographic
   - Panoramic radiograph
     - Root treated at the maxillary left first molar
   - Cephalometric radiograph (see Fig 4-21e)
     - Confirms the clinical observations

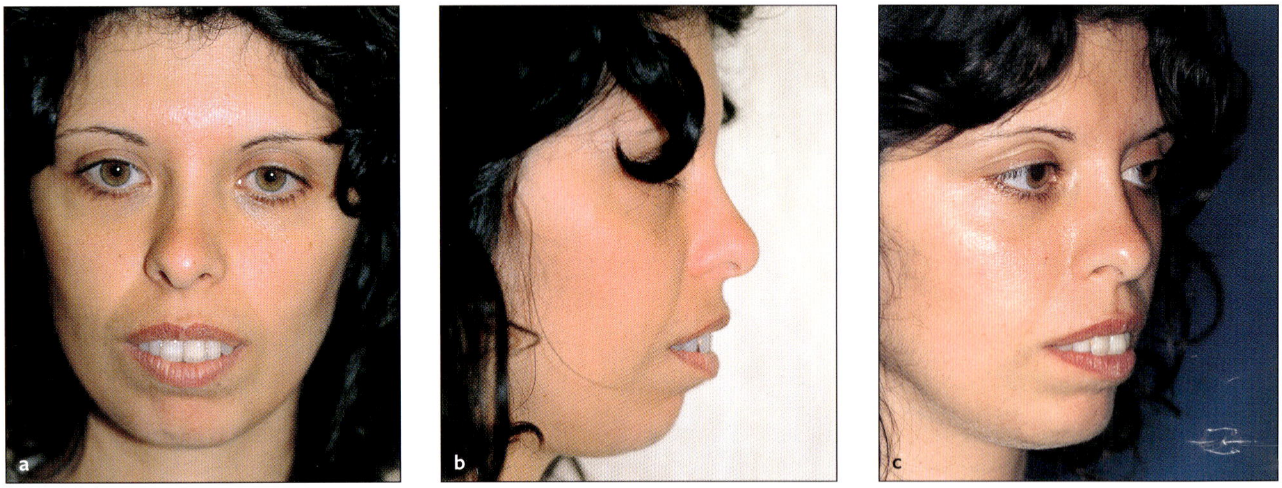

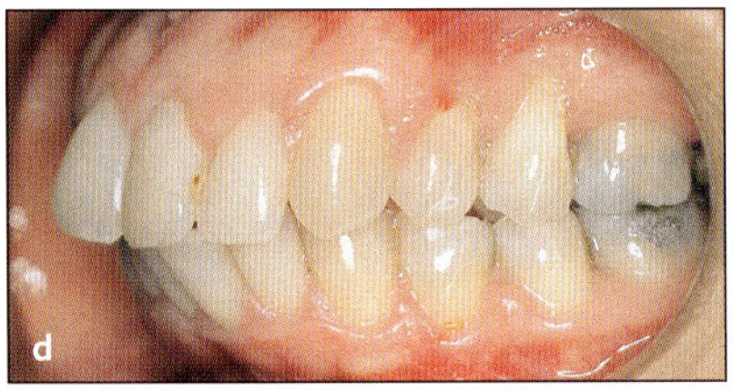

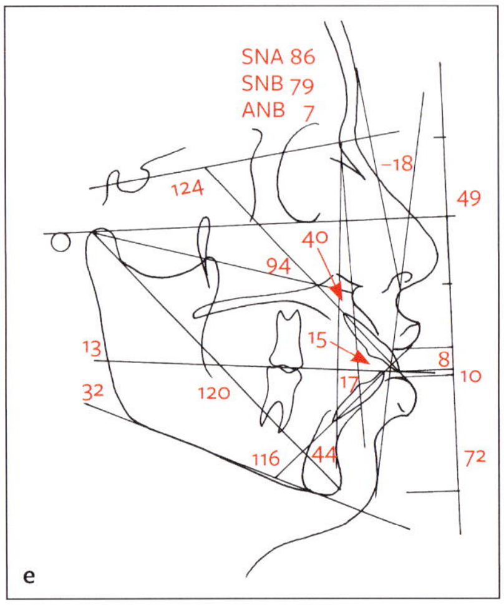

Fig 4-21 Case 10. Pretreatment frontal view (*a*), profile view (*b*), three-quarter view (*c*), and occlusion (*d*). (*e*) Pretreatment cephalometric analysis. Convex profile: facial contour angle = –18 degrees; increased interlabial gap: 10 mm; increased lower-third facial height: ratio of middle facial height to lower facial height = 49:72 mm; maxillary anteroposterior excess: SNA = 86 degrees; maxillary dental protrusion: maxillary incisor to S-N = 124 degrees, maxillary incisor to nasion–point A (N-A) = 15 mm and 40 degrees; mandibular dental protrusion: mandibular incisor to mandibular plane = 116 degrees, mandibular incisor to N-B = 17 mm and 44 degrees. →

Problem list

- Bidental protrusion
- Maxillary anteroposterior excess
- Vertical maxillary excess
- Mandibular anteroposterior deficiency
- Microgenia
- Class II malocclusion

Presurgical orthodontics

Maxillary arch (Figs 4-21f to 4-21i)

- Extraction of both maxillary second premolars
- Retraction of the incisors
- Establishment of a good arch form

Mandibular arch (see Figs 4-21f to 4-21i)

- Extraction of both mandibular first premolars
- Retraction of the incisors
- Leveling of the curve of Spee
- Establishment of interarch compatibility

Surgical treatment

A Le Fort I maxillary osteotomy was performed to superiorly reposition the maxilla with a setback (Fig 4-21j). The mandible was advanced by means of a bilateral sagittal split osteotomy. Finally, a genioplasty was performed to simultaneously advance and widen the chin.

Postsurgical orthodontics

Postsurgical orthodontic treatment completed the interdigitation of the teeth and also involved retention. The surgery was performed 24 months after the commencement of orthodontic treatment, and the orthodontic bands were removed 8 months after surgery. The treatment results are illustrated in Figs 4-21k to 4-21n.

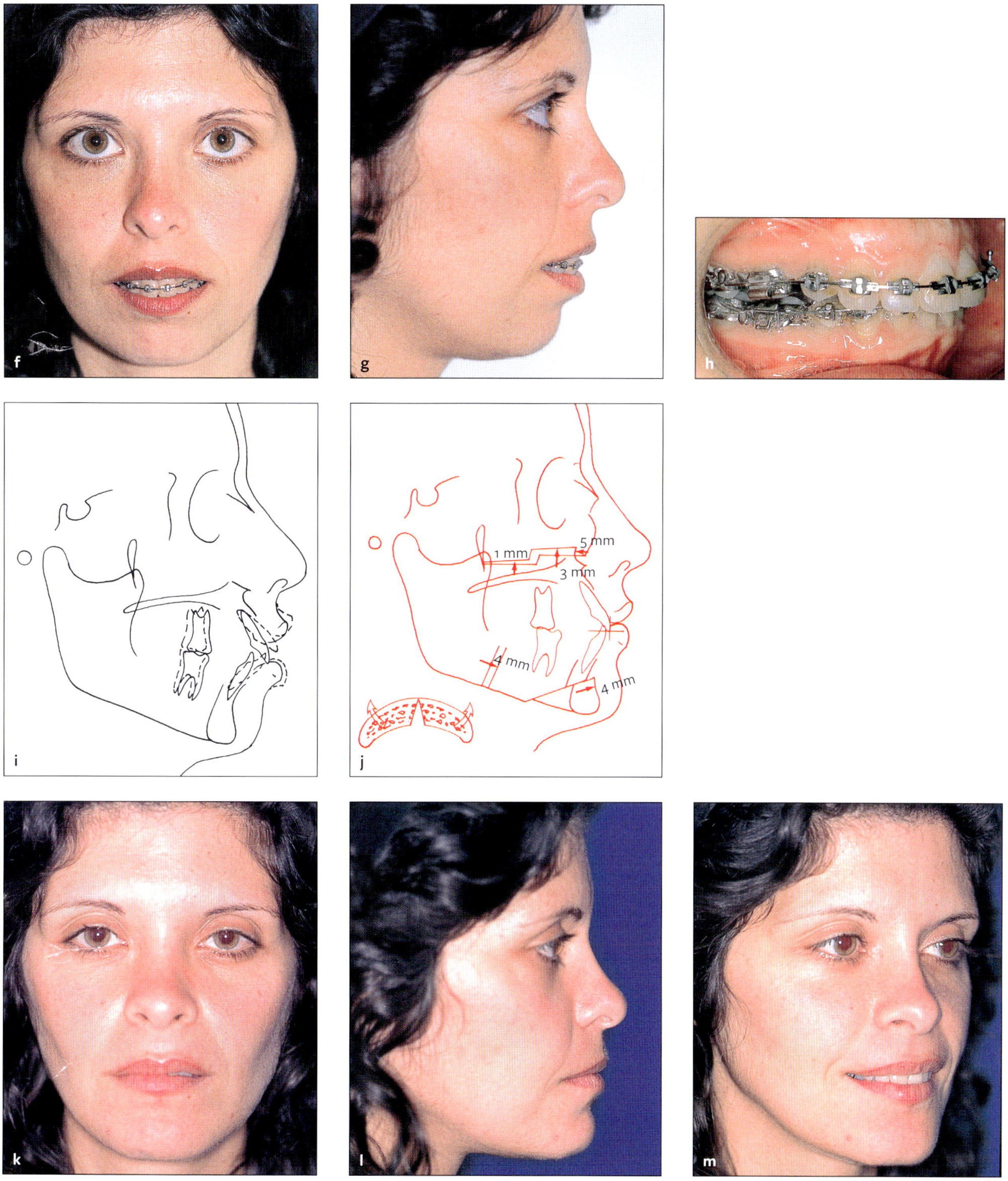

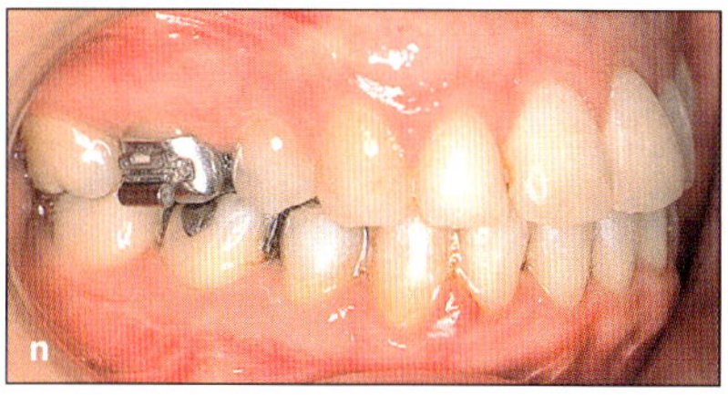

Fig 4-21 *(cont)* Change following orthodontic preparation: (*f*) frontal view, (*g*) profile view, and (*h*) right side of the occlusion. (*i*) Cephalometric analysis of dental change after presurgical orthodontics. (*j*) The surgical correction consisted of a Le Fort I osteotomy to superiorly reposition and set back the maxilla, bilateral sagittal split osteotomy to advance the mandible, and genioplasty to advance and widen the chin (*inset*). Posttreatment results are demonstrated in frontal view (*k*), profile view (*l*), three-quarter view (*m*), and occlusion (*n*).

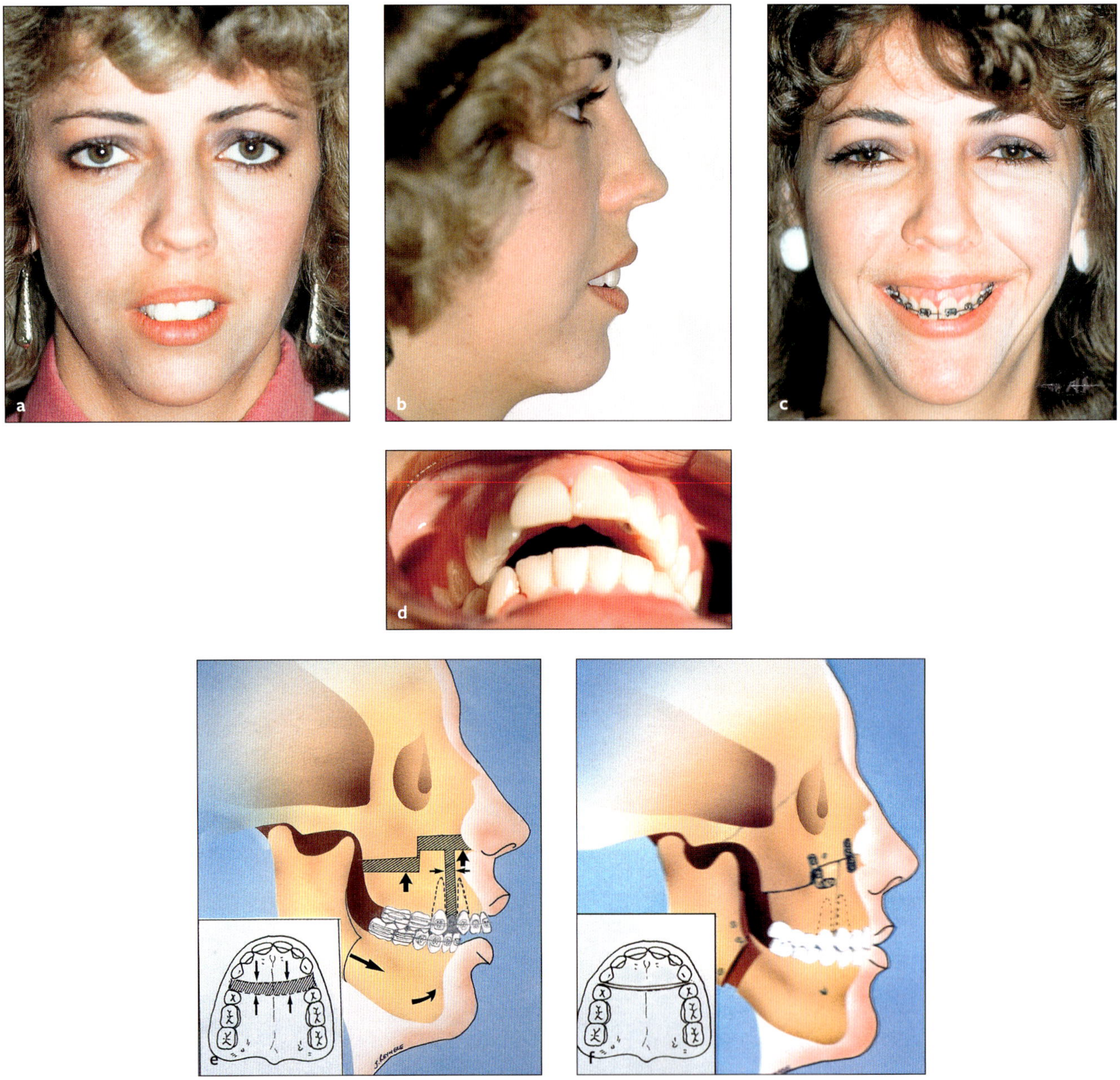

Fig 4-22 Case 11. Pretreatment frontal view (*a*), profile view (*b*), smile (*c*), and occlusion (*d*). The maxillary first premolars were removed and the maxillary arch aligned in three segments. Excessive space was maintained (*e*) and surgically closed by posterior repositioning of the anterior maxillary segments (*f*). The maxilla was superiorly repositioned and the mandible advanced.

Case 11

Case 11 illustrates the anteroposterior and vertical reduction of the maxilla by means of a segmental Le Fort I procedure (Fig 4-22).

Maxillary Vertical Deficiency

Maxillary vertical deficiency is very often associated with maxillary anteroposterior deficiency, in which the maxilla does not develop in a forward and downward direction. It is common in patients with cleft lip and cleft palate, where early surgery often curtails normal development of the maxilla. Because overclosure of the mandible makes patients with maxillary vertical deficiency appear clinically similar to those with mandibular anteroposterior excess, the clinician should differentiate between the two deformities.

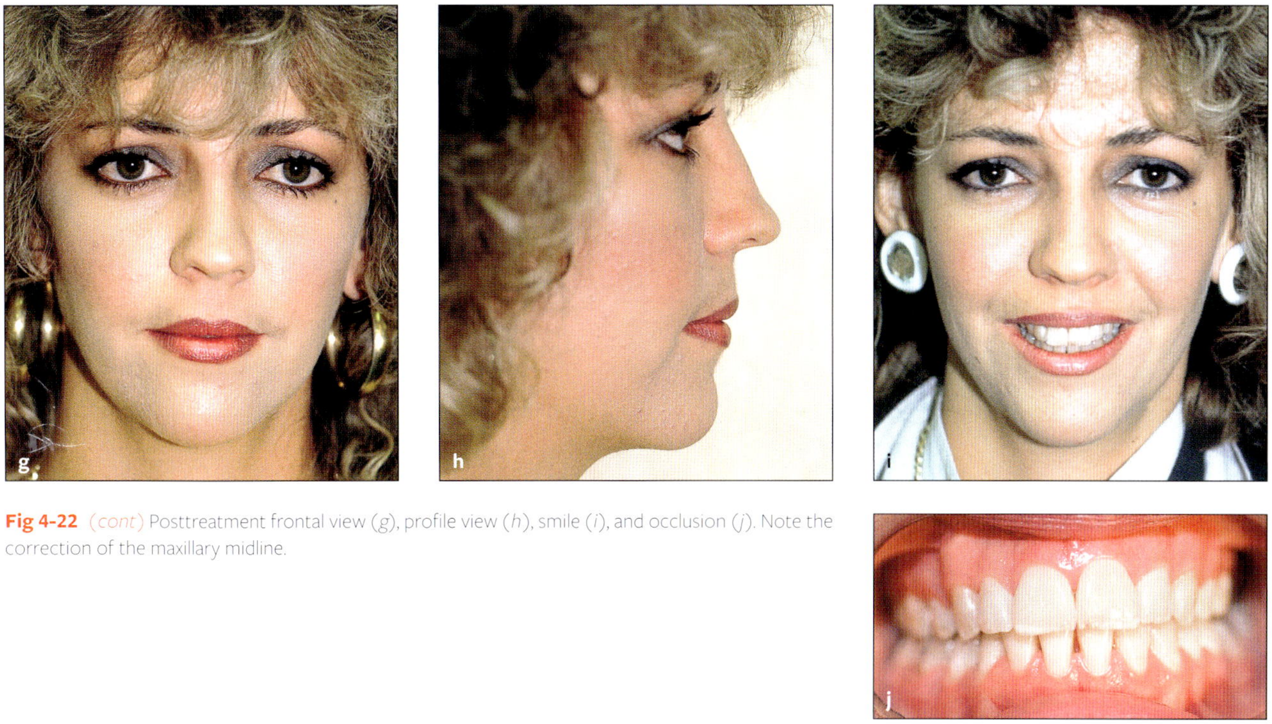

Fig 4-22 *(cont)* Posttreatment frontal view (*g*), profile view (*h*), smile (*i*), and occlusion (*j*). Note the correction of the maxillary midline.

Overview

Clinical characteristics

Profile view

- Lower and middle thirds of the face that are proportionally reduced in height when the patient's teeth are in occlusion
- Acute nasolabial angle
- Appearance of an excessive chin because of overclosure
- Improvement in the profile when the mandible is in the rest position
- Maxillary incisors that are not visible under the upper lip

Frontal view

- Appearance of a short and square face, with strong, exaggerated masseter muscles
- Maxillary incisors that often are not visible with the mouth open, creating an edentulous appearance, and incisors that are only partially exposed when the patient smiles
- When the mandible is closed, corners of the mouth that are turned down and skin folds that are apparent lateral to the oral commissure
- Often, a broad nasal base and large nostrils
- Appearance of an excessive mandible

Dental characteristics

- Heavy musculature and overclosed occlusion that frequently predispose the patient to bruxism and resulting attrition
- Often, increased interocclusal freeway space
- Class III dental relationship

Treatment

The surgical treatment objective for patients with maxillary vertical deficiency is to reposition the maxilla forward and downward. The mandible will rotate clockwise, and the vertical length of the face will increase. Patients with maxillary vertical deficiency invariably have an increased interocclusal freeway space, which should be carefully evaluated. The increase in vertical height achieved by downgrafting the maxilla should be less than the "available" interocclusal freeway space.

The extent of the vertical deficiency can be measured only with the patient's lips in repose and almost touching. Pretreatment cephalometric radiographs should be taken with the mandible in the rest position and the lips barely touching. This positioning can be facilitated by the use of a wax splint. The cephalometric visual treatment objective should be created on a radiograph taken with the mandible rotated open and the lips barely apart. This radiograph will give the surgeon a good indication of (*1*) the required amount of maxillary downgrafting to achieve an ideal lip-tooth relationship and (*2*) the mandibular anteroposterior position following clockwise rotation.

Presurgical orthodontics

The objective in presurgical orthodontic treatment for patients with maxillary vertical deficiency is to (1) level and align the teeth and (2) coordinate the arches. Significant anteroposterior compensations are seldom present, and the incisors can often be left in their original anteroposterior positions. If severe crowding is present, the maxillary and mandibular first premolars are extracted; with mild crowding, the maxillary and mandibular second premolars are extracted. Where larger maxillary advancement is needed in patients with crowding, the first maxillary premolars and second mandibular premolars are extracted to create a large crossbite.

If a transverse deficiency of the maxilla is present, it is best to correct it surgically. The maxillary arch often can be coordinated in two halves to "fit" the mandibular arch and the archwire cut in the center. A stabilizing palatal arch should be placed as soon as possible after surgery, and it should be anticipated presurgically.

Surgical treatment

The maxilla can be repositioned inferiorly by a Le Fort I downgrafting procedure. This procedure was unstable in the past, and as high as a 70% loss of vertical height has been reported; however, rigid fixation has substantially improved the stability of the procedure.

Definitive presurgical planning of the exact amount of maxillary inferior repositioning is critical. The clinician should be guided by both the amount of interocclusal rest space and the maxillary incisor–upper lip relationship.

After the maxilla is mobilized on the Le Fort I level, maxillomandibular fixation is placed. The condyles are seated in the glenoid fossae, and with gentle backward and upward pressure at the mandibular angles, the maxilla is rotated closed until the desired, preplanned interosseous distance is achieved. Four bone plates are placed: two at the zygomatic buttresses and two at the piriform rims.

An interpositioning graft is then placed (or it may be placed before the bone plates). This graft is shaped to fit snugly into the bony defect to prevent displacement into the maxillary sinus. If the transverse dimension of the maxilla is increased by surgical expansion, an acrylic occlusal splint is placed and the palatal bone defect grafted. An interdental wire is inserted between the teeth adjacent to the interdental osteotomy.

Patients with a combination of vertical and anteroposterior deficiency may be candidates for the Le Fort I downsliding osteotomy design. The surgical plan for these patients should include maxillary advancement in addition to correction of the vertical discrepancy. In these patients, the osteotomy is angled to provide an inclined plane that will increase the vertical dimension as the maxilla slides forward. The horizontal length from the piriform rim to the lateral aspect of the zygoma is measured on a lateral cephalogram. This measurement is used to calculate the downward angulation of the osteotomy and the position of the vertical steps.

Postsurgical orthodontics

During the first postsurgical visit, the orthodontist checks the occlusion and instructs the patient to wear appropriate elastics. If surgical expansion of the maxillary arch was performed, the orthodontist should do the following:

- Remove the sectional archwire and replace it with a continuous archwire.
- Place a palatal arch that is carefully adapted to the lingual surface of all teeth distal to the canines.

At first, the orthodontist sees the patient once every 1 to 2 weeks for routine adjustment of archwires and elastics. With good progress, the patient goes to a 4-week adjustment schedule, and postsurgical orthodontic treatment is concluded as previously discussed.

Clinical cases

Case 12

A 15-year-old adolescent girl was referred by her practitioner for the correction of a Class III malocclusion.

Main complaint

The patient said she was unable to bite anything with her front teeth and thought her face appeared too flat.

Medical history

Her medical history was noncontributory.

Clinical examination

1. Soft tissue
    - Frontal view (Figs 4-23a and 4-23b)
    - Paranasal flattening
    - Lack of upper lip support
    - Maxillary incisors barely visible when the patient's lips are apart
    - Mandible appears large
    - Profile view (Fig 4-23c)

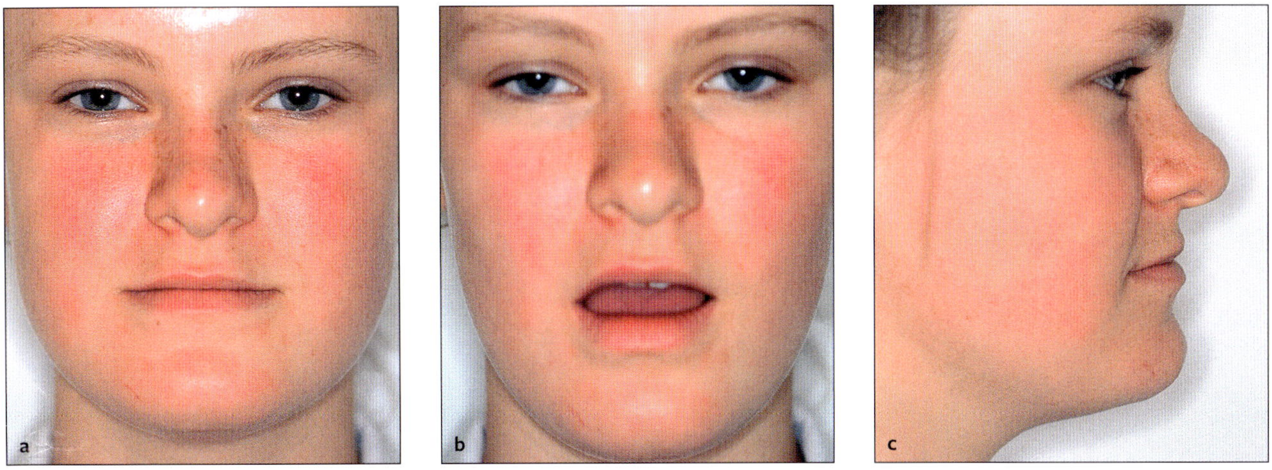

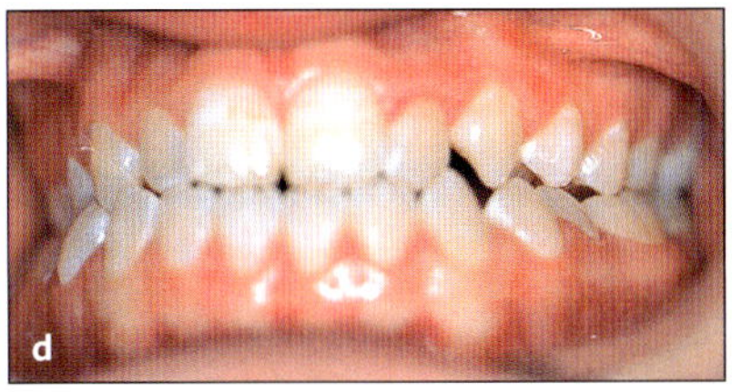

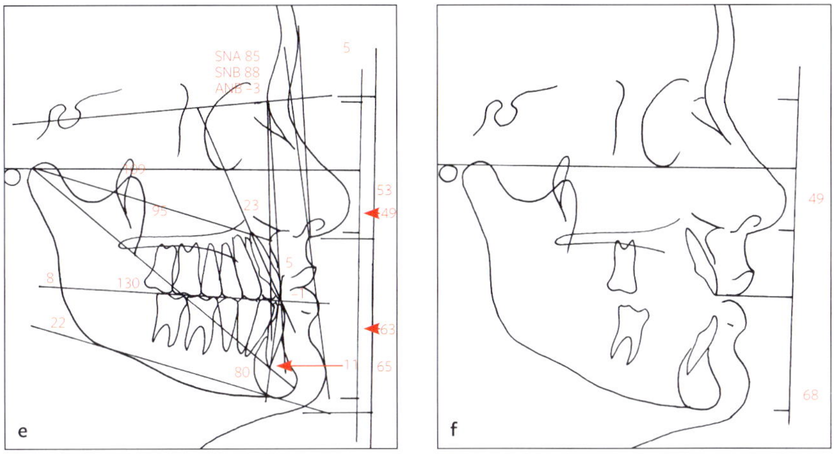

Fig 4-23 Case 12. Pretreatment frontal view (*a*), lips apart (*b*), profile view (*c*), and occlusion (*d*). (*e*) Pretreatment cephalometric analysis. Class III malocclusion; maxillary anteroposterior deficiency; Class III skeletal relationship: ANB = –3 degrees; mandibular incisor compensation: mandibular incisor to mandibular plane = 80 degrees, mandibular incisor to N-B = 11 degrees; concave profile: facial contour angle = 5 degrees. (*f*) Tracing of a pretreatment cephalometric radiograph taken with the patient's mandible rotated clockwise until the lips just part. Note the maxillary incisor–lip relationship. The final vertical position of the maxilla is planned clinically from this tracing.

- Concave profile
- Upper lip that appears flat
- Mandible appears strong and overclosed

2. Dental (Fig 4-23d)
    - Edge-to-edge incisor relationship with an open bite tendency
    - Class III malocclusion
    - Narrow maxillary arch
    - Tendency to posterior crossbites
    - Compensated mandibular incisors
3. Skeletal (Figs 4-23e and 4-23f)
    - Anteroposterior maxillary deficiency
    - Vertical maxillary deficiency
4. Radiographic (see Figs 4-23e and 4-23f)
    - Cephalometric radiograph
        - Confirms the clinical diagnosis of a Class III malocclusion with vertical and anteroposterior maxillary deficiency

Problem list

- Vertical maxillary deficiency
- Anteroposterior maxillary deficiency
- Class III malocclusion
- Anterior open bite
- Narrow maxillary arch

Presurgical orthodontics

Maxillary arch (Fig 4-23g)

- Alignment of the arch
- Expansion of the posterior teeth within the bony limits

Mandibular arch (see Fig 4-23g)

- Decompensation of the incisors
- Establishment of interarch compatibility

Surgical treatment

Surgical treatment involved a Le Fort downsliding osteotomy. The osteotomy is performed at a predetermined angle so that the maxilla will slide downward as it is advanced,

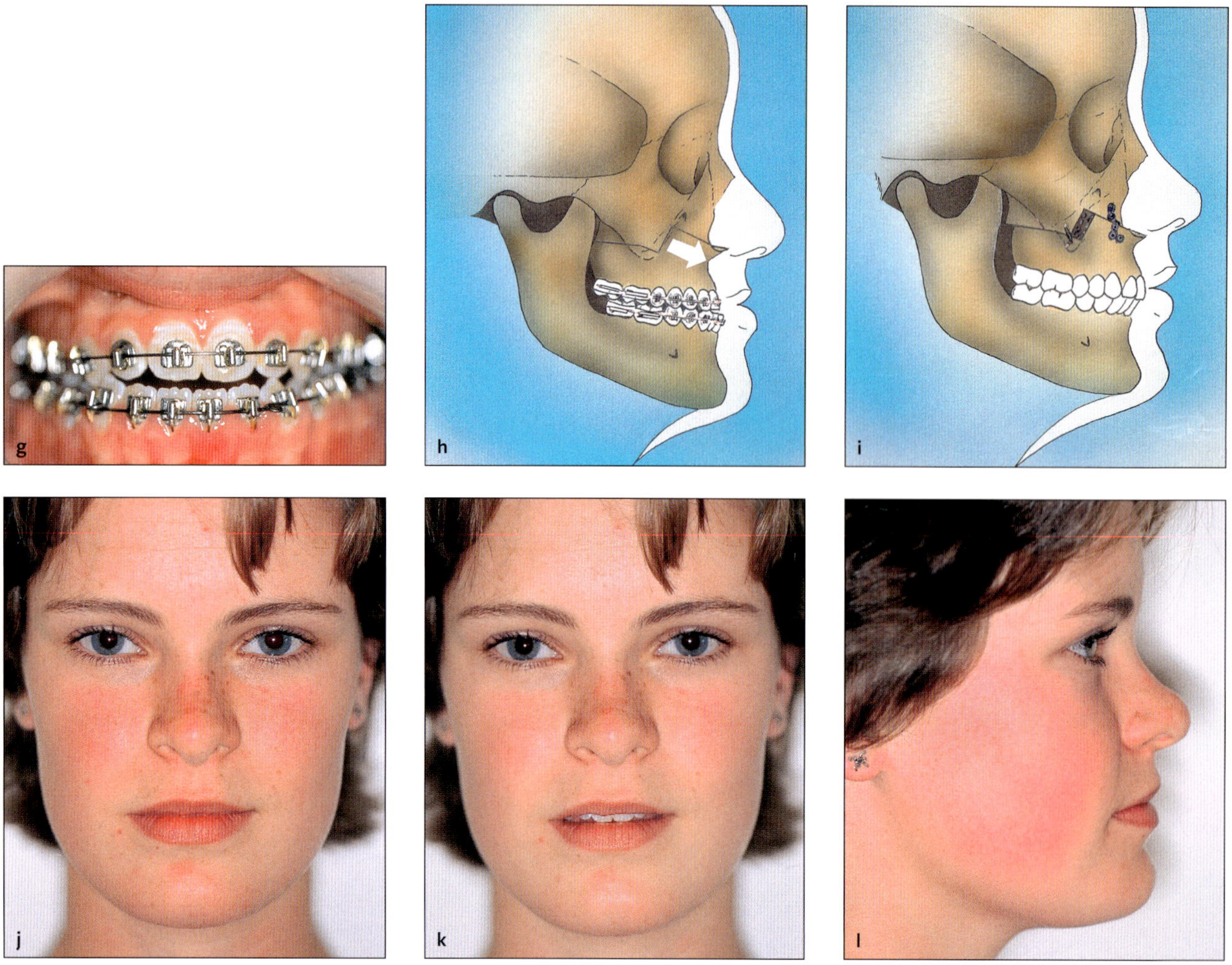

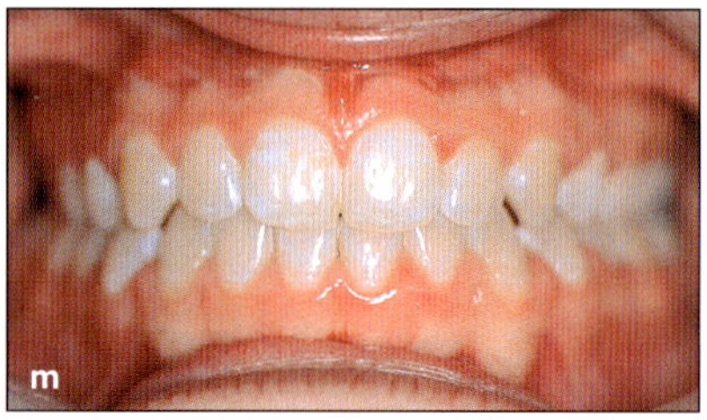

Fig 4-23 *(cont)* (*g*) Immediate presurgical occlusion. (*h*) Surgical plan illustrating the angled Le Fort I osteotomy. (*i*) As the maxilla is advanced, it will slide downward, increasing the vertical height. Posttreatment results are demonstrated in frontal view (*j*), lips apart (*k*), profile view (*l*), and occlusion (*m*).

thus increasing the vertical height while bone contact is maintained (Figs 4-23h to 4-23i).

Postsurgical orthodontics

The postsurgical orthodontic treatment finalized the occlusion and included the use of a retainer. The orthodontic preparation before surgery took 6 months, and the bands were removed 4 months after surgery. Figures 4-23j to 4-23m illustrate the posttreatment results 7 months after surgery.

Case 13

Vertical deficiency of the maxilla is often combined with other dentofacial anomalies that may render treatment planning challenging. This patient presented with a vertically deficient maxilla, a prominent but vertically deficient chin, a Class II malocclusion, and mandibular anteroposterior deficiency. The maxillomandibular complex was rotated clockwise as part of the treatment plan (Fig 4-24). The treatment principles for the rotation of the maxillomandibular complex are discussed in the following chapter.

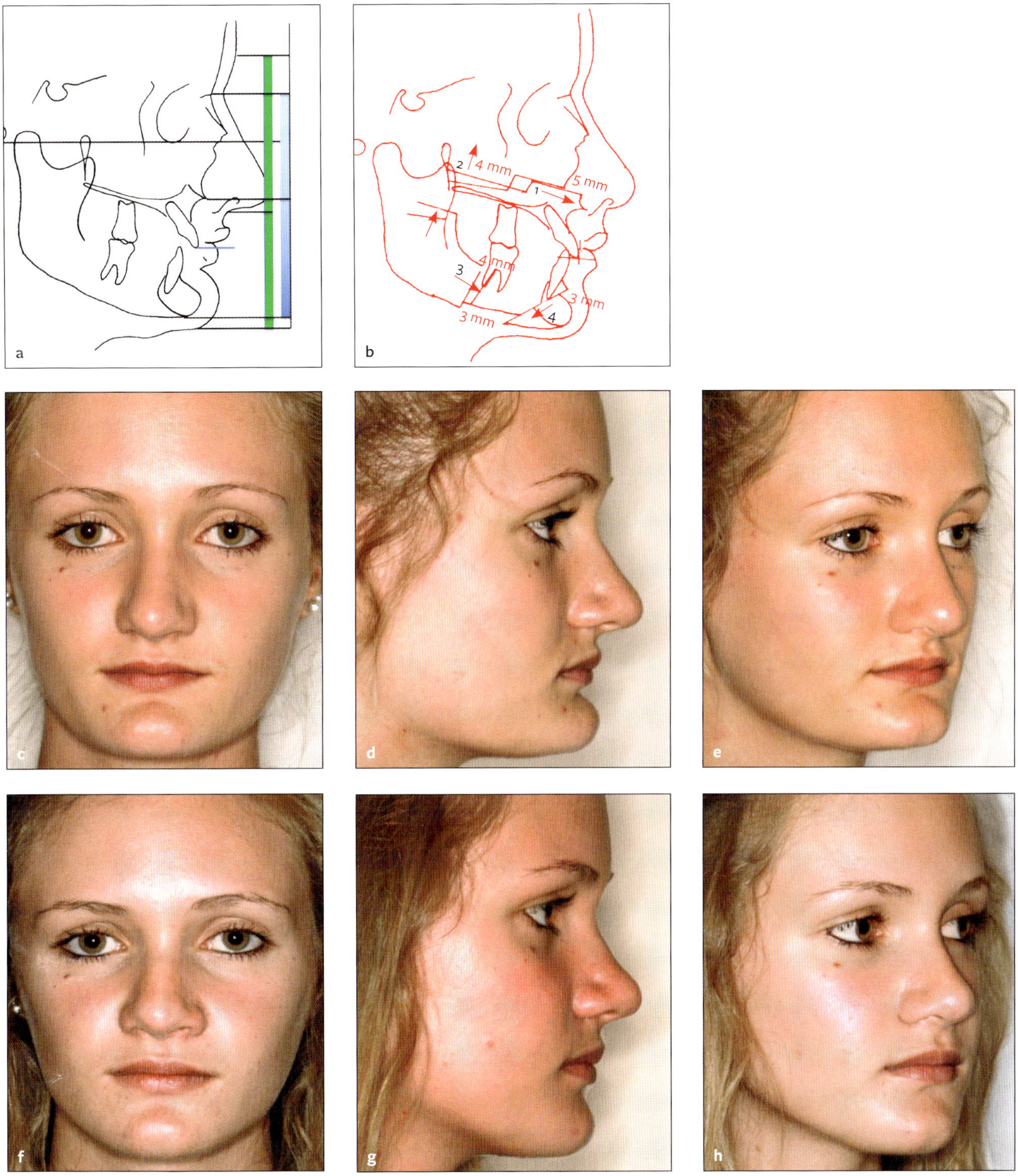

Fig 4-24 Case 13. (*a*) Lateral cephalometric tracing of a patient with a Class II malocclusion. Note the vertical skeletal (*green*) and soft tissue (*blue*) deficiency of the lower facial third. (*b*) The surgical visual prediction. The height of the maxilla is increased by downsliding the anterior maxilla 5 mm (arrow 1), and the posterior maxilla is superiorly repositioned 4 mm (arrow 2) to rotate the maxillomandibular complex clockwise. The mandible followed the rotation and is advanced (arrow 3). The chin contour is improved, and the height of the chin increased by sliding the chin posteriorly and inferiorly (arrow 4). (*c*) Presurgical frontal view. Note the short lower facial third, deficient paranasal areas, and prominent chin. (*d*) Presurgical profile view. Note the straight profile, prominent chin, deep labiomental fold, flat paranasal areas, curled upper lip, deficient lower lip, and relatively prominent nose. (*e*) Presurgical three-quarter view. Several negative esthetic features are apparent: Deep labiomental fold, prominent chin, rounded lower border of the mandible, flat paranasal areas, and a short curled upper lip. (*f*) The postsurgical frontal view. The lower third of the face is increased, the lips fuller, and the chin less prominent. (*g*) Most of the negative esthetic features have improved. (*h*) Dramatic improvement in the vertical facial relations is apparent.

Maxillary Vertical Excess

Approximately 30% of patients seeking treatment have a vertical increase in the lower third of the face. The author's experience shows that the main complaints of patients with vertical maxillary excess are a gummy smile and/or functional problems caused by the anterior open bite, the hallmarks of the long-face deformity.

Overview

Clinical characteristics

Profile view

- Increased total facial height caused by an increased lower facial height
- Mandible that is rotated downward and backward
- Increased interlabial distance (greater than 4 mm)
- Increased maxillary incisor exposure (except in some patients with an open bite)
- Sunken cheeks
- Often, a well-developed, almost excessive, curled lower lip

Frontal view

- Narrow alar base width
- Excessive maxillary incisor exposure (except in some patients with an open bite)
- Increased interlabial distance
- Often, increased vermilion exposure of the lower lip
- Increased lower-third facial height
- Gummy smile
- Depressed paranasal areas with a likelihood of flat cheeks

Dental characteristics

- Often, an anterior bite
- High, arched palate with a large distance between the root apices and the nasal floor
- V-shaped maxilla and teeth often in palatal crossbite
- Mandibular incisors that tend to become more upright and therefore more crowded

Because of the excessive vertical growth of the maxilla, the mandible tends to rotate downward and backward. Patients with maxillary vertical excess therefore often have problems in the anteroposterior plane. Patients with long faces can be described as having a skeletal Class I relationship rotated to Class II or a skeletal Class III relationship rotated to Class I. It can be concluded that excessive vertical growth of the maxilla will make mandibular anteroposterior deficiencies appear worse and mandibular anteroposterior excesses appear improved. Frequently, there is an accentuated curve of Spee caused by overeruption of mandibular incisors, especially in patients without open bites.

There is a tendency for anterior open bites in two-thirds of these patients. The clinician should note that some diagnostic characteristics may be camouflaged in patients with vertical maxillary excess and deep bites (Figs 4-25a to 4-25g). First, because of the deep bite, the lower facial height may not be increased. Second, the maxillary incisors may be excessively exposed under the upper lip; however, this exposure is covered by the lower lip. The combination of the following characteristics may be considered diagnostic for vertical maxillary excess:

- Increased mandibular plane and occlusal plane angle
- Increased interlabial gap
- Increased incisor exposure under the upper lip
- Increased total anterior facial height
- Decreased percentage contribution of upper facial height to total facial height

Treatment

The two most important rules in the treatment of vertical maxillary excess are the following:

1. Never treat the smile.
2. Always plan the treatment with the lips in repose.

There is no alternative to surgery for adult patients with vertical maxillary excess. Attempts to close the open bite by orthodontic extrusion of anterior teeth or intrusion of posterior teeth are not a solution for two reasons: (1) relapse into open bite almost always occurs, and (2) extrusion of the maxillary incisors will worsen the esthetics.

Presurgical orthodontics

As in all surgical orthodontic cases, the approach is to align the teeth presurgically to facilitate the planned surgery so that the teeth will fit into occlusion after surgery. A few guidelines should be considered:

- It is preferable to level the mandibular arch before surgery (in contrast to the approach in patients with short faces).
- Patients with vertical maxillary excess and severe open bites often have an excessive reverse curve in the maxillary arch. For these patients, it is advantageous

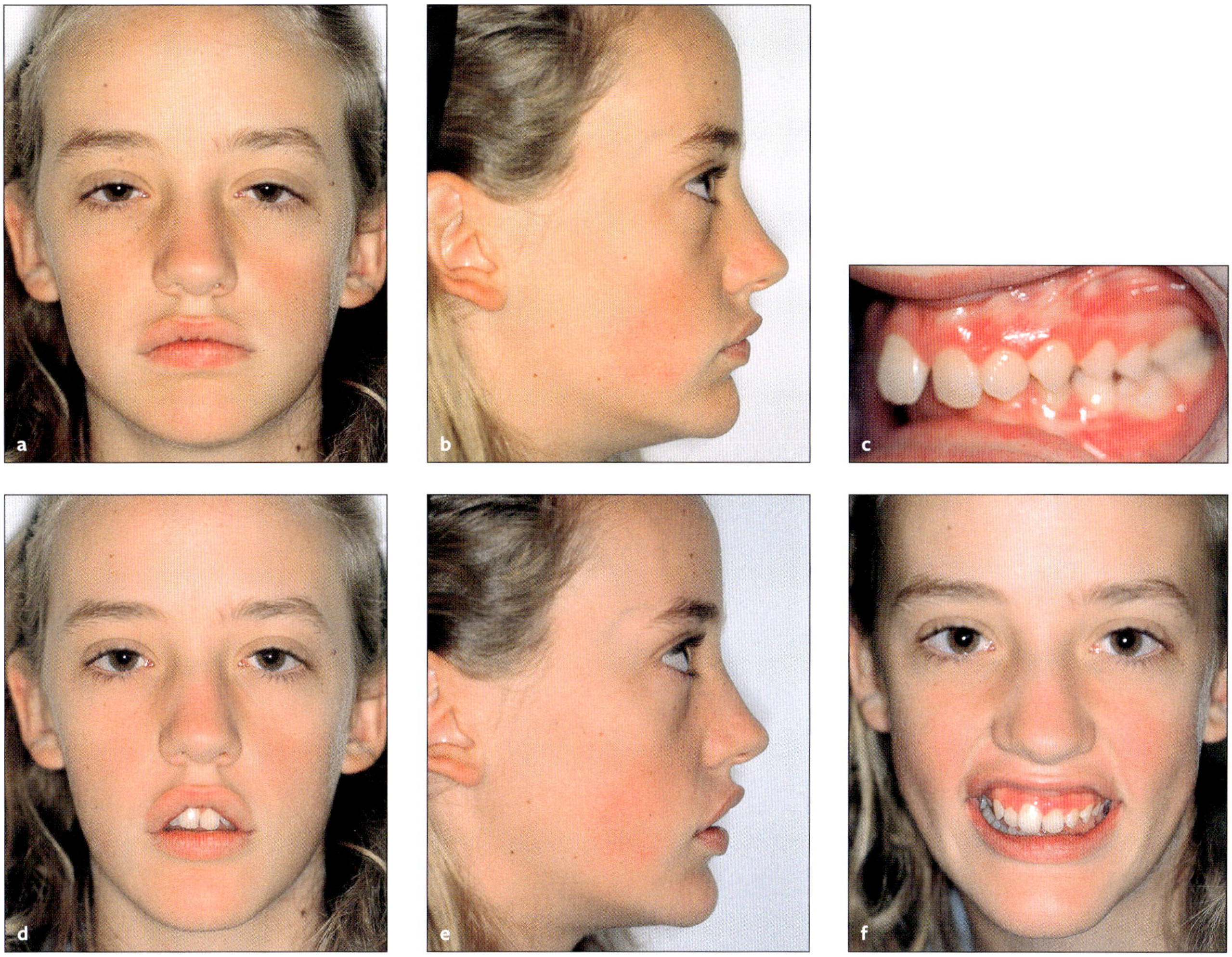

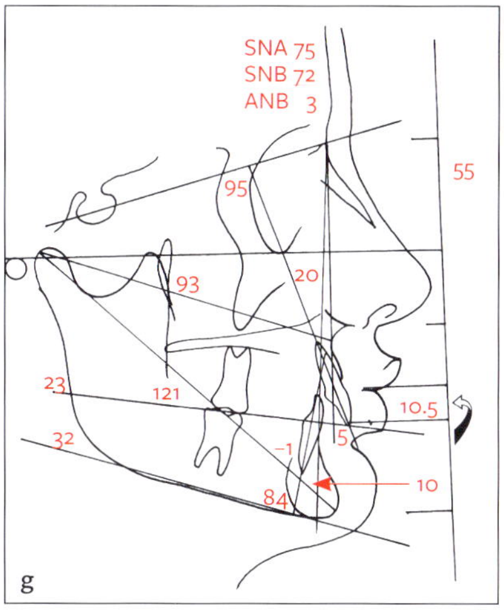

Fig 4-25 Frontal view (*a*) and profile view (*b*) of a patient with a severe Class II deep bite (*c*). The height of the maxilla cannot be assessed because of the overclosed bite. (*d and e*) The vertical excess (excessive tooth exposure under the upper lip) is evident when the mandible is rotated into the correct interincisal overbite. (*f*) Gummy smile. (*g*) Vertical excess (disguised by the deep bite) is demonstrated on the cephalometric tracing.

to level the arch in segments and deviate the roots of the teeth to allow interdental osteotomies. Therefore, level within the segments. Do not attempt to close the open bite; rather, open the bite further.

- A similar principle applies in the decision to expand a narrow maxilla orthodontically. The teeth should not be expanded beyond their bony base. Any relapse of an expanded maxillary arch will tend to open the bite anteriorly. Surgical expansion is recommended, especially in more severely narrowed maxillae and in older patients.

Orthodontic mechanics

Mandibular arch

- Routine orthodontic techniques are used to level, align, close all spaces, and achieve a good arch form.
- Extractions and Class II or Class III mechanics may be necessary depending on the patient.

Maxillary arch

- Teeth adjacent to the proposed interdental osteotomies (eg, between maxillary canines and premolars or between maxillary lateral incisors and canines) are bonded with brackets that will "diverge" the roots away from the surgical site to prevent accidental surgical insult to the roots. For example, a maxillary left canine bracket is placed on the right canine and vice versa. This technique is still applicable if premolars are removed to provide relief from crowding. After surgery is completed, these brackets are removed and the correct brackets bonded to obtain normal root inclination.
- Leveling is accomplished using sectional nickel-titanium alloy (nitinol) wires or similar wires. Stabilization is then undertaken with sectional finishing archwires bent to conform to the arch form for each segment.
- Extraction spaces can be closed by surgically approximating the segments. Keep in mind that interdental spaces should not be totally closed at the time of surgery. A small amount of bone should always be preserved at the tooth margins to prevent periodontal problems.
- If no vertical segmental discrepancies exist, the maxillary arch is leveled with a continuous archwire. Care should be taken that the maxillary incisors are not leveled forward; nightly headgear wear may be required. The maxillary and mandibular arches are coordinated with the aid of study casts.
- Intrusive posterior mechanics, such as palatal bars or high-pull headgear, should be avoided.
- Mandibular molars should be brought upright to encourage bite opening. This situation will accentuate the vertical problem and introduce less chance of relapse.

Surgical treatment

To correct the vertical discrepancy, the maxilla must be superiorly repositioned by a Le Fort I osteotomy. Two critical elements must be considered in the final treatment planning:

1. How far must the maxilla be superiorly repositioned?
2. After straight vertical repositioning of the maxilla, where will the mandible be?

Extent of superior repositioning. The amount of superior repositioning is critical because moving the maxilla too far superiorly is more detrimental to facial esthetics than leaving the vertical excess uncorrected. Consider the following points when planning superior repositioning of the maxilla:

- Patients with short upper lips show more teeth than patients with long upper lips.
- Younger patients tolerate (esthetically and psychologically) more upward movement of the maxilla than do older patients. Remember that the upper lip will lengthen with age.
- Exposure of 30% to 40% of the clinical crowns of the maxillary incisors beneath the upper lip is esthetically pleasing.
- During superior repositioning of the maxilla, the upper lip will shorten. The amount of upper lip shortening is specific to the surgeon and will depend on the individual surgical technique (eg, suturing technique and careful handling of soft tissue during surgery).
- In general, plan for a 4-mm tooth exposure after surgery.
- It is not mandatory to elevate the maxilla until the lips make contact. A few millimeters of lip incompetence is acceptable and, in many instances, attractive.
- Large movements, if not controlled, may lead to widening of the alar base of the nose and tipping up of the nasal tip. Because both effects are controllable, take them into consideration in treatment planning and surgical technique (see the sections on nasal control in chapter 6, pages 295 and 296).
- Moving the maxilla too far superiorly gives poor esthetic results, but moving it posteriorly at the same time yields even worse results.
- Consider the upper lip shape. Patients with an extreme Cupid's bow may have excessive exposure of only the two central incisors. If surgery is planned using the lateral cephalometric radiograph without considering the lip shape, treatment may result in only the tips of the two central incisors being visible under the upper lip. The maxillary incisor exposure should therefore be assessed clinically and not based on the lateral cephalometric radiograph (Figs 4-25h to 4-25j).

Anteroposterior position of the mandible. The mandible will autorotate counterclockwise around a point at the

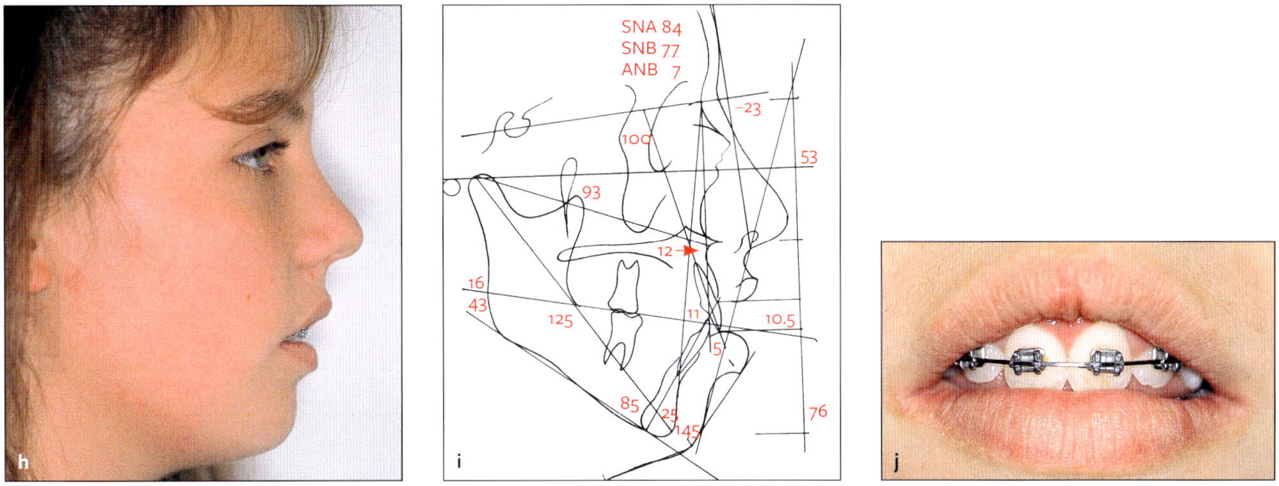

Fig 4-25 (cont) Assessment from a profile view (*h*) and a lateral cephalometric tracing (*i*) reveals an interlabial distance of 10 mm, requiring superior repositioning of the maxilla. If only this view is considered, superior repositioning of at least 6 mm is indicated. (*j*) Because of an accentuated Cupid's bow of the upper lip, the entire crowns of the central incisors are exposed under the upper lip, whereas there is much less exposure of the lateral incisors. If planning of superior repositioning of the maxilla considers only the central incisor exposure, excessive superior repositioning will result in only the tips of the central incisors being visible under the upper lip.

condyle. As a consequence, the mandibular incisors will rotate forward (more so in patients with a high occlusal plane angle). When the extent of maxillary superior repositioning has been decided, the anteroposterior position of the mandibular incisors should be considered. It may be necessary to advance the maxilla slightly to achieve a Class I malocclusion. If the mandible is anteroposteriorly deficient, a maxillary setback may be considered to achieve a Class I malocclusion; however, advancing the mandible is preferable. It is much better to accept the need for two-jaw surgery to achieve a good occlusion than to significantly compromise the esthetics and limit the surgery to one jaw. In patients with Class III malocclusion, the Class III dental relationship will worsen as the mandible is autorotated, necessitating either maxillary advancement or mandibular setback.

Important surgical considerations

- The amount of superior repositioning of the maxilla is critical. Take great care during surgery to accurately position the maxilla in the planned position. An intermediate splint is helpful. The amount of superior repositioning of the maxilla should be evaluated from the frontal view and not the lateral cephalometric radiograph (see Fig 4-18).
- Condyle positioning, again, is critical. The condyle can be displaced by minor bony interferences in the posterior maxilla. With maxillomandibular fixation, this condylar displacement will not be revealed until 6 weeks after surgery, after removal of maxillomandibular fixation. Maxillomandibular fixation is currently seldom indicated and not often used. With rigid internal fixation, incorrect positioning of the condyle can be detected after intraoperative removal of maxillomandibular fixation. The occlusion should be critically evaluated following removal of intraoperative maxillomandibular fixation. If the occlusion differs from the planned occlusion, the cause for the discrepancy should be established. Occurrence of an unplanned and unacceptable occlusion is most often the result of bony interferences at the posterior maxilla. This problem should be corrected by the removal of fixation plates and the elimination of posterior interferences (see the section on intraoperative diagnosis of condylar sag during Le Fort I maxillary osteotomy in chapter 6).
- It is often necessary to surgically expand the posterior maxilla through parasagittal osteotomies in the palate. A bone graft or hydroxyapatite blocks should be grafted into the defect and the segments stabilized by a splint with a palatal bar. Grafting should be used for any expansions greater than 3 mm.
- The piriform rim should be contoured to accommodate the soft tissue of the nose (see the sections on nasal control in chapter 6).
- The bony and cartilaginous septum should be shortened appropriately to prevent warping of the nasal septum during superior repositioning of the maxilla. To centralize the septum, a septum suture may be used to attach the septal cartilage to the base of the nasal spine as it passes through a hole in the nasal spine (see the sections on nasal control in chapter 6).

- Wound closure should be meticulous. A cinch suture can control the alar base width, and V-Y closure can create lip lengthening or control the length of the upper lip. Resuture the perioral muscles, and then carefully suture the mucosa, taking thin bites. Be sure to maintain the soft tissue midline when suturing (see the sections on nasal control in chapter 6).

Postsurgical orthodontics

If a splint is used during surgery, the orthodontist should see the patient immediately after splint removal. Stabilizing archwires are removed and replaced with working archwires, and light (2.5- to 3.5-oz) vertical or slightly Class II elastics are placed.

After surgical expansion, the most important and possibly the most challenging aspect of postsurgical orthodontics is to maintain the transverse dimension of the palate. The expanded dentoalveolar segments must be held in their expanded position during orthodontic finalization. This can be accomplished using either a heavy auxiliary wire in the headgear tubes along with working wires or a transpalatal arch (the latter may be more practical). The dentoalveolar segments do not stabilize until 4 to 6 months after surgery. In general, the postsurgical orthodontic treatment of patients with long faces is often quick because the arches were leveled either before or during surgery.

Clinical case

Case 14

A 16-year-old adolescent boy was referred for surgical correction of vertical maxillary excess and mandibular deficiency. (His mother had the same condition and had been treated 10 years previously by the same surgeon.)

Main complaint

The patient was unhappy about his gummy smile and his inability to create a lip seal without strain.

Medical history

His medical history was noncontributory.

Clinical examination

1. Soft tissue
    - Frontal view (Figs 4-26a and 4-26b)
        - Gummy smile
        - Increased interlabial gap
        - Excessive maxillary incisor exposure under the upper lip
        - Increased lower-third facial height
        - Increased lower lip vermilion exposure
    - Profile view (Fig 4-26c)
        - Convex profile
        - Deficient chin
        - Prominent lower lip
        - Increased lower-third facial height
        - Increased tooth exposure
        - Increased interlabial gap
2. Dental (Fig 4-26d)
    - Class II malocclusion
    - Missing first premolars
3. Skeletal
    - Vertical maxillary excess
    - Mandible rotated clockwise and is relatively deficient
    - Microgenia
4. Radiographic
    - Panoramic radiograph
        - Missing first premolars
    - Cephalometric radiograph (Fig 4-26e)
        - Confirms clinical observations

Problem list

- Vertical maxillary excess
- Microgenia
- Class II malocclusion

Presurgical orthodontics

The presurgical orthodontic treatment was completed by the time of the final referral.

Surgical treatment

A Le Fort I maxillary osteotomy was performed to reposition the maxilla superiorly, the mandible was autorotated counterclockwise into a Class I dental relationship, and a genioplasty was performed to advance the chin (Fig 4-26f).

Postsurgical orthodontics

Postsurgical orthodontic treatment involved completing the interdigitation of the teeth and the wearing of a retainer. The pleasing postsurgical result is demonstrated in Figs 4-26g to 4-26j.

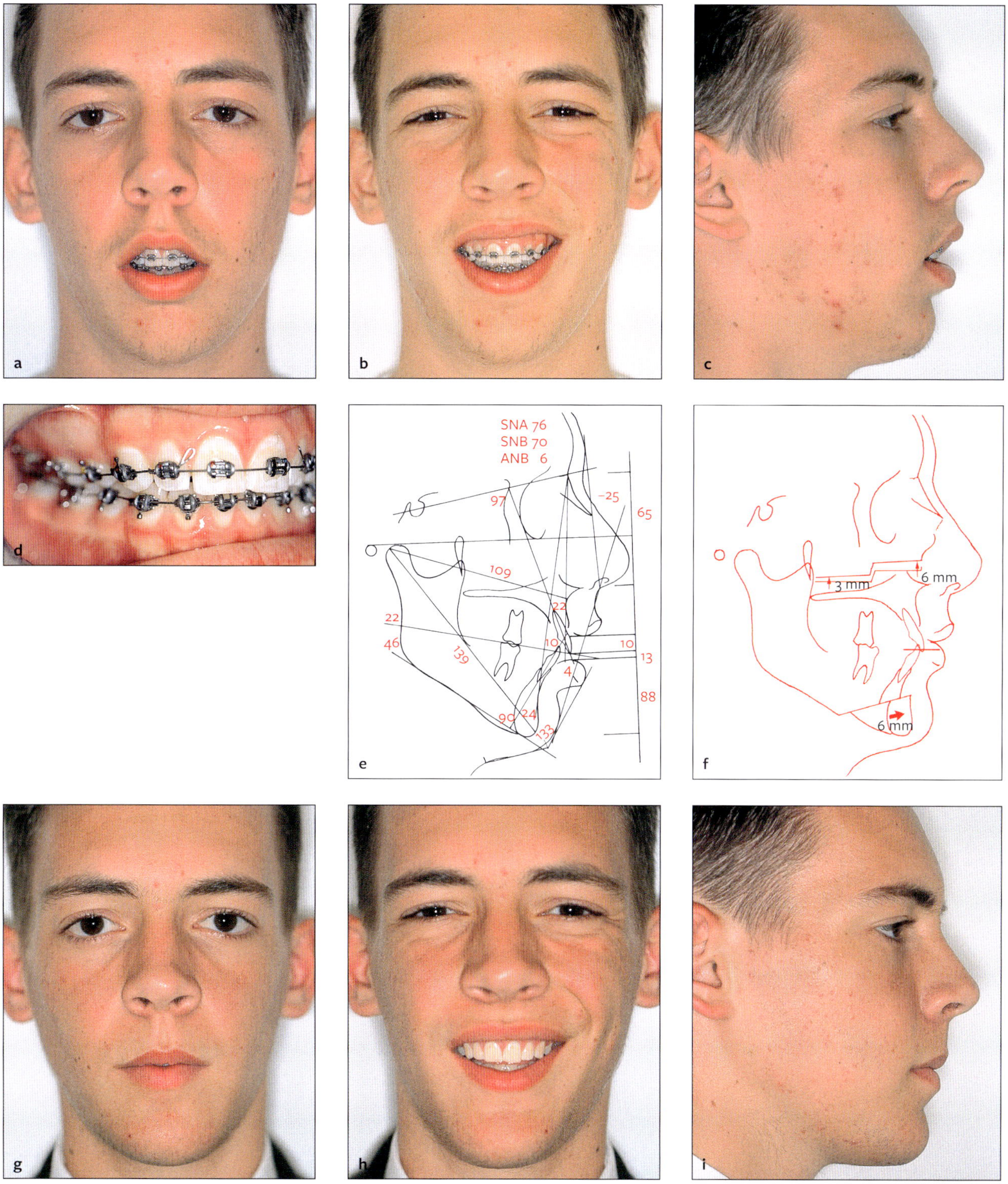

Fig 4-26 Case 14. Presurgical frontal view (*a*), smile (*b*), profile view (*c*), and occlusion (*d*). (*e*) Presurgical cephalometric analysis. Vertical maxillary excess: interlabial gap = 13 mm, maxillary incisor tooth exposure = 10 mm, ratio of middle-third to lower-third height = 65:88 mm; convex profile: facial contour angle = -25 degrees; ratio of normal maxillary to mandibular length relationship: 109:139 mm. (*f*) Surgical cephalometric visual treatment objective. Postsurgical frontal view (*g*), smile (*h*), profile view (*i*), and occlusion (*j*).

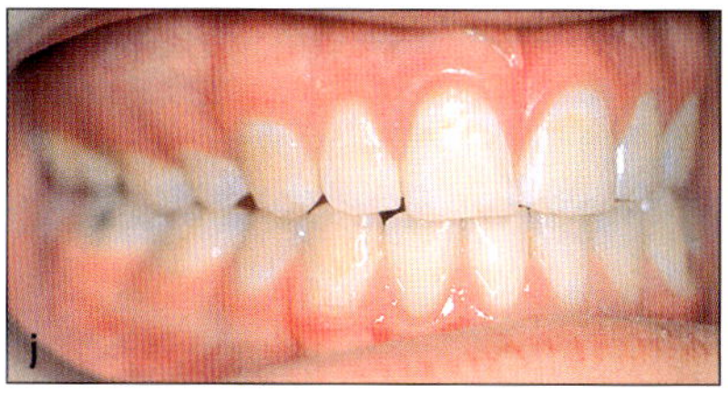

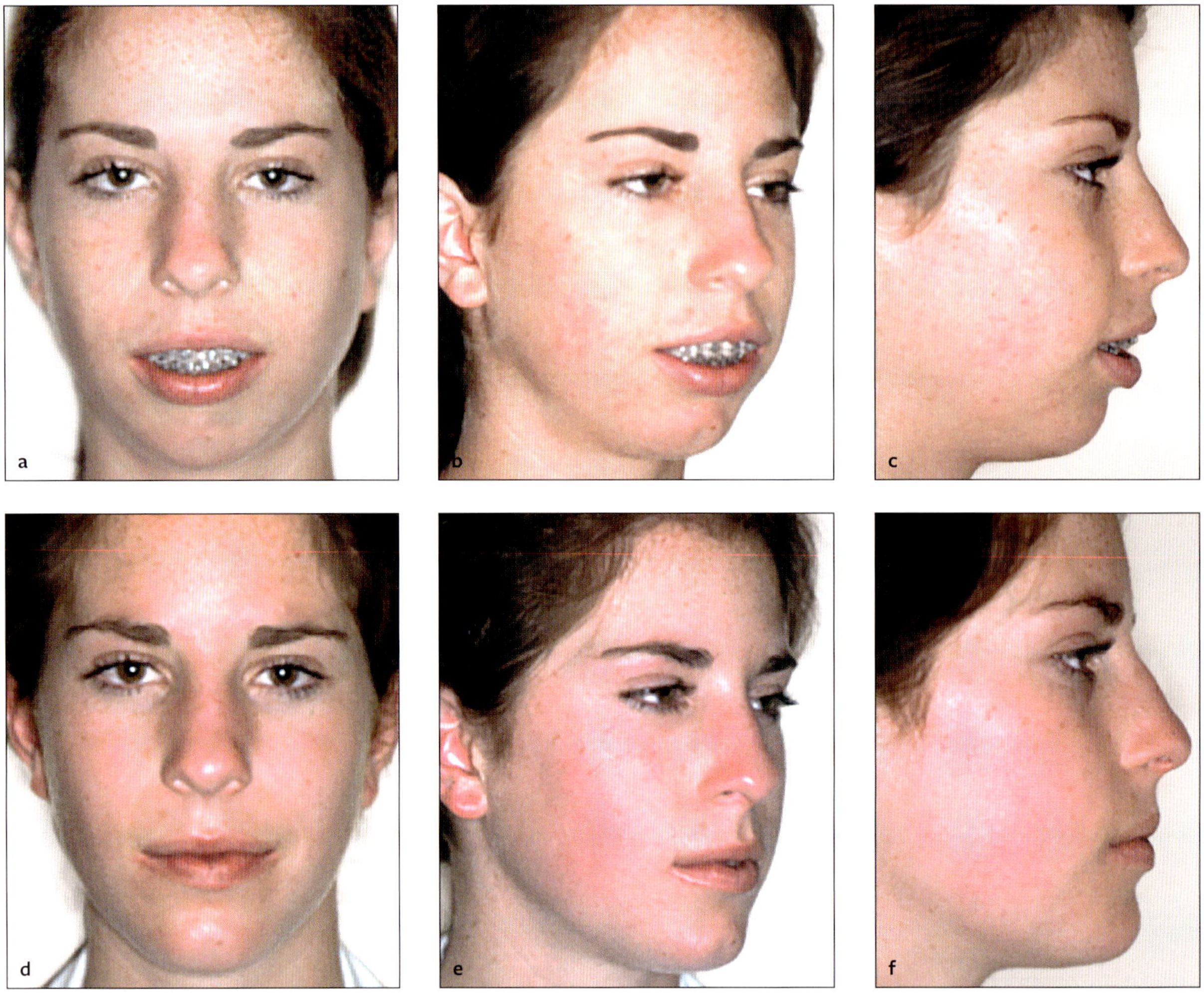

Fig 4-27 Case 15. Vertical maxillary excess. Pretreatment frontal view (*a*), three-quarter view (*b*), and profile view (*c*). Note the typical signs: increased interlabial gap, excessive incisor exposure, convex profile, increased lower facial height, clockwise rotated mandible (also deficient in this case), and everted lower lip. Postoperative frontal view (*d*), three-quarter view (*e*), and profile view (*f*).

Case 15

This case demonstrates the esthetic changes of an 18-year-old woman with vertical maxillary excess, mandibular anteroposterior deficiency, and microgenia (Fig 4-27). Her maxilla was surgically superiorly positioned, her mandible advanced, and her chin advanced. Note the improvements in the following areas:

- Lip competence
- Nasolabial angle
- Upper lip support
- Labiomental fold (the everted lower lip has rotated back)
- Chin shape
- Lip-chin-submental angle
- Chin-throat length
- Chin height
- Facial contour

Recommended Reading

Acebal-Bianco F, Vuylsteke PL, Mommaerts MY, De Clercq CA. Perioperative complications in corrective facial orthopedic surgery: A 5-year retrospective study. J Oral Maxillofac Surg 2000; 58:754–760.

Adlam DM, Yau CK, Banks PA. A retrospective study of the stability of midface osteotomies in cleft lip and palate patients. Br J Maxillofac Surg 1989;27:265–276.

Beukes J, Reyneke JP, Damstra J. Unilateral sagittal split mandibular ramus osteotomy: Indications and geometry. Brit J Oral Maxillofac Surg 2016;54:219–223.

Blæhr TL, Mommaerts MY, Kjellerup AD, Starch-Jensen T. Surgically assisted rapid maxillary expansion with bone-borne versus tooth-borne distraction appliances—A systematic review. Int J Oral Maxillofac Surg 2019;48:492–501.

Booth RP. Reflections on distraction osteogenesis. A surgical distraction or the "future"? Br J Oral Maxillofac Surg 2001;39:179–180.

Bütow KW, van der Walt PJ. The "Stellenbosch"—Triangle analysis of posteroanterior and basilar cephalograms. J Dent Assoc S Afr 1981;36:461–467.

Bütow KW, van der Walt PJ. The use of the triangle analysis for cephalometric analysis in three dimensions. J Maxillofac Surg 1984;12:62–70.

Cupar I. Die chirurgische Behandlung der Form und Stellungs Veränderungen des Oberkiefers. Öst Z Stomatol 1954;51:565–577.

Diner PA, Vasquez MP (eds). Transactions of the International Congress of Cranial and Facial Bone Distraction Osteogenesis. Bologna, Italy: Mondozzi, 1997.

Ellis E 3rd, McNamara JA Jr, Lawrence TM. Components of adult Class II open-bite malocclusion. J Oral Maxillofac Surg 1985;43:92–103.

Ellis E 3rd, McNamara JA Jr. Components of adult Class III open-bite malocclusion. Am J Orthod 1984;86:277–290.

Enlow DH. Facial Growth, ed 3. Philadelphia: Saunders, 1990.

Epker BN. Modifications in the sagittal osteotomy of the mandible. J Oral Surg 1977;35:157–159.

Greulich WW, Pylers I. Radiographic Atlas of Skeletal Development of the Hand and Wrist, ed 2. Stanford, CA: Stanford UP, 1959.

Guerrero CA, Figueroe F, Bell WH, Olmos-Malave Y, Rojas A, Gonzalez M. Surgical orthodontics in mandibular lengthening. In: Guerrero CA (ed). Distraction Osteogenesis of the Facial Skeleton. Hamilton, ON: BC Decker, 2007.

Hamamci N, Basaran G, Sahin S. Nonsurgical correction of an adult skeletal class III and open-bite malocclusion. Angle Orthod 2006;76:527–532.

Houston WJ, James DR, Jones E, Kavvadia S. Le Fort I maxillary osteotomies in cleft palate cases. Surgical changes and stability. J Craniomaxillofac Surg 1989;17:9–15.

Hunsuck EE. A modified intraoral sagittal splitting technic for correction of mandibular prognathism. J Oral Surg 1968;26:250–253.

Ilizarov GA. The principles of the Ilizarov method. 1988. Bull Hosp Jt Dis 1997;56:49–53.

Jacobs JD, Bell WH, Williams CE, Kennedy JW 3rd. Control of the transverse dimension with surgery and orthodontics. Am J Orthod 1980;77(3):284–306.

Koudstaal MJ, Poort LJ, van der Wal KG, Wolvius EB, Prahl-Andersen B, Schulten AJ. Surgically assisted rapid maxillary expansion (SASME): A review of the literature. Int J Oral Maxillofac Surg 2005;34:709–714.

Letzer GM, Kronman JH. A posteroanterior cephalometric evaluation of craniofacial asymmetry. Angle Orthod 1967;37:205–211.

McNamara JA Jr. Components of class II malocclusion in children 8–10 years of age. Angle Orthod 1981;51:177–202.

Mommaerts MY, Lipperns F, Abeloos JV, Neyt LF. Nasal profile changes after maxillary impaction and advancement surgery. J Oral Maxillofac Surg 2000;58:470–474.

O'Ryan F, Schendel S. Nasal anatomy and maxillary surgery. I. Esthetic and anatomic principles. Int J Adult Orthodon Orthognath Surg 1989;4:27–37.

Obwegeser H, Trauner R. Zur Operationstechnik bei der Progenie und anderen Unterkieferanomalien. Dtsch Zahn Mund Kieferheilkd 1955;23:1–26.

Proffit WR, White RP. Surgical-Orthodontic Treatment. St Louis: Mosby, 1992.

Reyneke JP, Masureik CJ. Treatment of maxillary deficiency by a Le Fort I downsliding technique. J Oral Maxillofac Surg 1985;43:914–916.

Reyneke JP. Basic guidelines for the surgical correction of mandibular anteroposterior deficiency and excess. Clin Plast Surg 2007;34:501–517.

Vandersea BA, Ruvo AT, Frost DE. Maxillary transverse deficiency—Surgical alternatives and management. In: Van Sickels JE (ed). Oral and Maxillofacial Surgery of North America, Orthognathics, vol 19. Philadelphia: Saunders, 2007:351–368.

Wagner S, Reyneke JP. The Le Fort I downsliding osteotomy: A study of long-term hard tissue stability. Int J Adult Orthodon Orthognath Surg 2000;15:37–49.

Wassmund M. Lehrbuch der Probleschen Chirurgie des Mundes und der Kiefer, vol 1. Leipzig: Meuser, 1935.

Wunderer S. Erfahrungen mit der operativen Behandlung hochgradiger Prognathien. Dtsch Zahn Mund Kieferheilkd 1963;39:451.

5

Diagnosis and Treatment of Complex Dentofacial Deformities

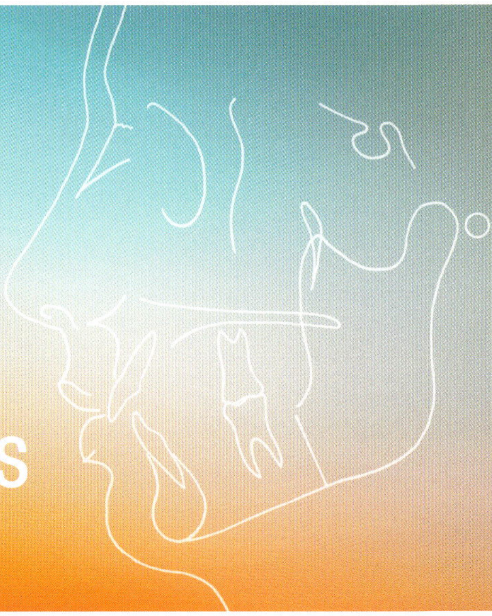

As in chapter 4, this chapter uses case studies to demonstrate individual dentofacial problems, combinations of problems, and the nuances involved in treating these patients to achieve optimal results. Patients with similar skeletal, soft tissue, and occlusal characteristics are grouped in description for convenience. Clinicians should remember, however, that each patient has a unique set of dentofacial problems requiring a specific treatment response, and a patient may have more than one deformity.

The following basic deformities and treatment principles for each deformity are discussed: (1) cases requiring rotation of the maxillomandibular complex, (2) open bite deformities, (3) temporomandibular joint (TMJ) reconstruction and orthognathic surgery, and (4) dentofacial asymmetry.

Rotation of the Maxillomandibular Complex

The correction of most dentofacial deformities requires single-jaw surgery whereby either the maxilla or the mandible is repositioned. The mandible can be surgically advanced or set back, and this horizontal movement should take place along the occlusal plane of the maxilla (ie, the unoperated jaw). Surgical repositioning of the maxilla, either anteriorly or posteriorly (albeit seldom), will also take place along the existing occlusal plane. However, whereas superior repositioning of the maxilla will cause the mandible to rotate counterclockwise, inferior repositioning of the maxilla will result in a clockwise rotation of the mandible. This rotation of the mandibular occlusal plane occurs around a point at or just behind the head of the condyle. To achieve occlusal contact, the maxilla must be aligned along a "new" occlusal plane, which is determined by the extent of the autorotation of the mandible. Hence, it is the position assumed by the mandible that dictates the final anteroposterior cant of the occlusal plane (Fig 5-1).

When corrective treatment requires surgery to both jaws, the same treatment principles as previously discussed will apply and are called *conventional treatment planning*. Most dentofacial deformities can be treated successfully using conventional treatment planning, in which alteration of the occlusal plane is an inevitable consequence of any surgical adjustment to the vertical position of the maxilla with resultant autorotation of the mandible. Any anteroposterior repositioning of the maxilla or mandible must take place along this new occlusal plane (Fig 5-2).

Adhering to conventional treatment principles (especially in patients with high and low occlusal plane angles) may hamper achievement of optimal esthetic results. However, these limitations on the esthetic outcomes can be overcome by rotation of the maxillomandibular complex, also known as alteration or manipulation of the occlusal plane. The alteration in occlusal plane angle should not be considered as an attempt to change or treat an abnormally high or low occlusal plane angle to a more cephalometrically normal angle. The profound effect that the occlusal plane may have on the relationship of the apical bony base of the maxilla to the mandible as well as on the anterior skull base is demonstrated in Fig 5-3. The occlusal plane should therefore always be an import-

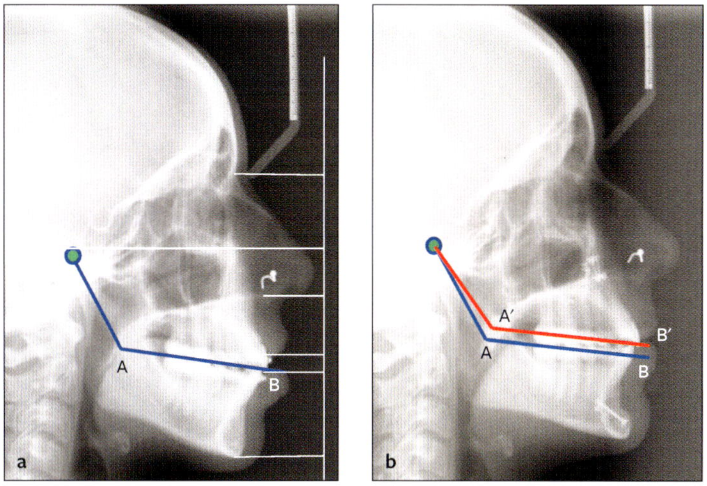

Fig 5-1 (*a*) Lateral cephalometric radiograph of a patient with a Class I occlusion and vertical maxillary excess as indicated by the *white lines*. (*b*) The maxilla has been superiorly repositioned and the occlusal plane rotated from A-B (*blue line*) to A′-B′ (*red line*). The final occlusal plane following superior repositioning of the maxilla is dictated by the occlusal plane of the mandible after autorotation. This rotation took place around a point at the condyle.

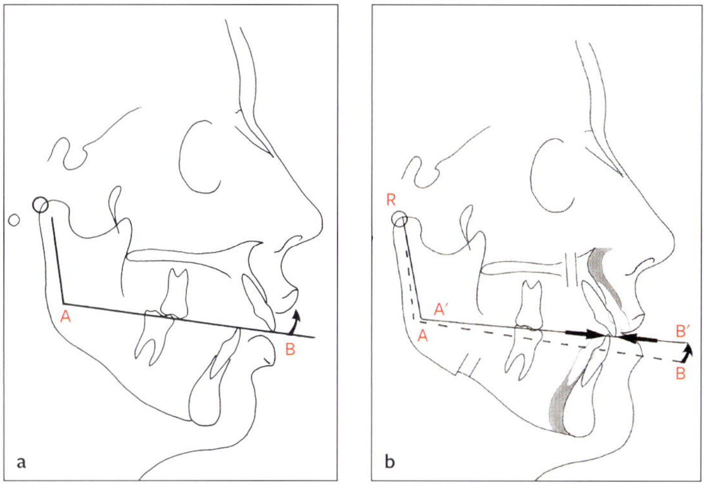

Fig 5-2 (*a*) Lateral cephalometric tracing of a patient with vertical maxillary excess, maxillary anteroposterior excess, and mandibular anteroposterior deficiency. The presurgical occlusal plane is A-B. (*b*) The maxilla is superiorly repositioned and the mandible autorotated around R. The new occlusal plane (A′-B′) has been changed from the presurgical occlusal plane (A-B) by the autorotation of the mandible. The mandible is advanced, and the anterior segment of the maxilla is set back along this plane.

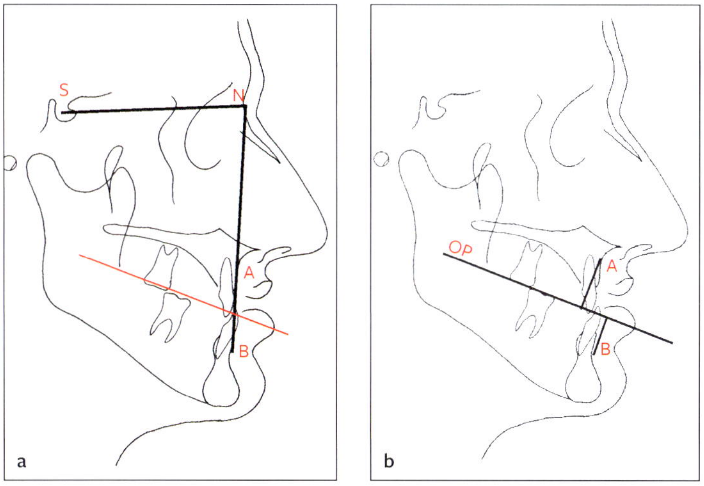

Fig 5-3 (*a*) The Steiner cephalometric analysis of a patient with a Class III malocclusion, high occlusal plane and mandibular plane angles, and vertical maxillary excess. An ANB angle of 0 degrees indicates a mild skeletal Class III relationship between the maxilla and mandible. The relationship is measured relative to the anterior cranial base, and any further vertical growth of the maxilla could result in an increased ANB angle, which would then indicate a normal anteroposterior skeletal relationship. (*b*) A Wits analysis of the same patient expresses the relative relationship of the maxilla to the mandible in relation to the occlusal plane (OP), indicating a severe Class III discrepancy. Any vertical increase in the maxillary height will have no effect on this anteroposterior measurement. S, sella.

ant consideration in orthognathic diagnosis and surgical planning, and various cephalometric analyses should be critically evaluated and compared.

Visualization and planning

Surgical repositioning of the jaws and teeth involves complicated 3D movements of geometrically complex

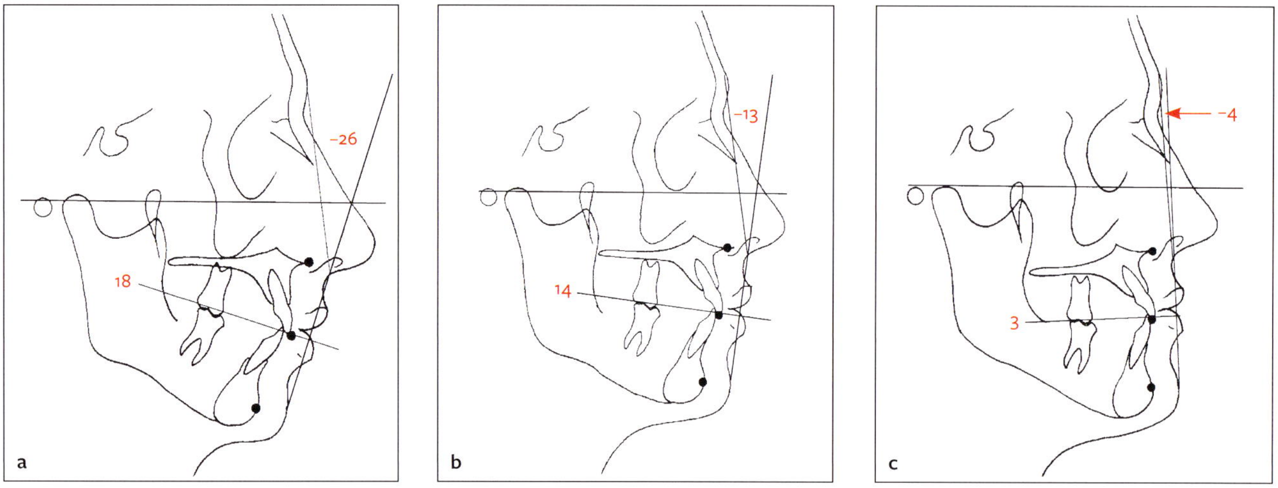

Fig 5-4 In all three patients, the interrelationship among ANS, incisor tip, and Pog is the same. (*a*) Because of the high occlusal plane angle (18 degrees), the profile is convex with a facial contour angle of –26 degrees. (*b*) The facial contour angle is normal (–13 degrees) with a normal occlusal plane angle of 14 degrees. (*c*) A low occlusal plane angle (3 degrees) and facial contour angle of –4 degrees is shown.

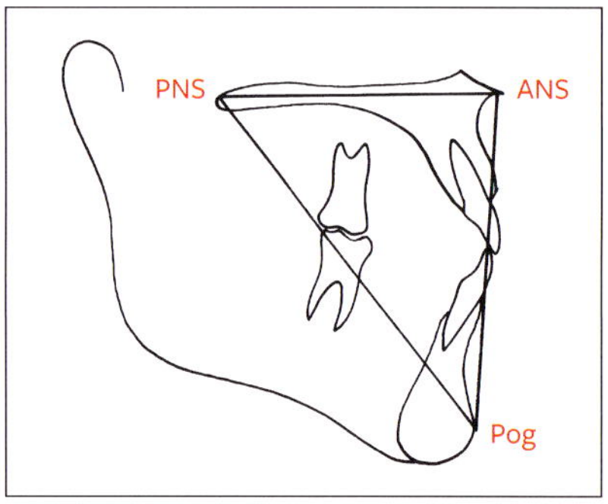

Fig 5-5 A triangle involving the PNS, ANS, and Pog is used to plan the rotation of the maxillomandibular complex.

structures. The diagnostic information gained from the preoperative clinical examination, 3D virtual imaging, study casts, and radiographic evaluation must be carefully integrated to establish the appropriate surgical treatment plan.

When surgery to both jaws is planned and performed, the final horizontal and vertical relationships among the anterior nasal spine (ANS), the maxillary incisor edge, and pogonion (Pog) are key determinants in the esthetic outcome. The horizontal relationship among ANS, incisor edge, and Pog is a consequence of the horizontal skeletal and dental relationship (ie, Class I, II, or III). The vertical relationship among these three key elements is simultaneously influenced by the vertical skeletal and dental pattern: vertical maxillary excess or deficiency, vertical mandibular skeletal excess or deficiency, and deep or open bite malocclusion.

The interrelationship of important soft tissue landmarks such as the subnasale (Sn), upper lip position (Li, and its relation to the maxillary central incisor), and Pog′ are directly dependent on the position of the underlying skeletal and dental structures (ANS, incisor edge, and Pog, respectively).

In some patients, the key hard tissue landmarks may be well related; however, because of hyperdivergency or hypodivergency of the occlusal and mandibular plane, the patient may still have a convex or concave profile. For example, in Fig 5-4, the vertical and anteroposterior interrelationship of ANS, incisor edge, and Pog is identical in each part, but the profiles differ substantially because of the difference of the occlusal plane angle.

Alteration of the occlusal plane should be considered only if conventional treatment planning does not yield satisfactory results. It is extremely difficult to simply "place" or "select" a new occlusal plane without selecting a point around which to rotate the maxillomandibular complex or alter the occlusal plane. It is easier and more accurate, both in planning and in surgery, to rotate the maxillomandibular complex around a preselected point.

The geometry of maxillomandibular complex rotation and the expected effects are simplified and best illustrated by constructing a triangle involving the posterior nasal spine (PNS), ANS, and Pog (Fig 5-5). Any point on the

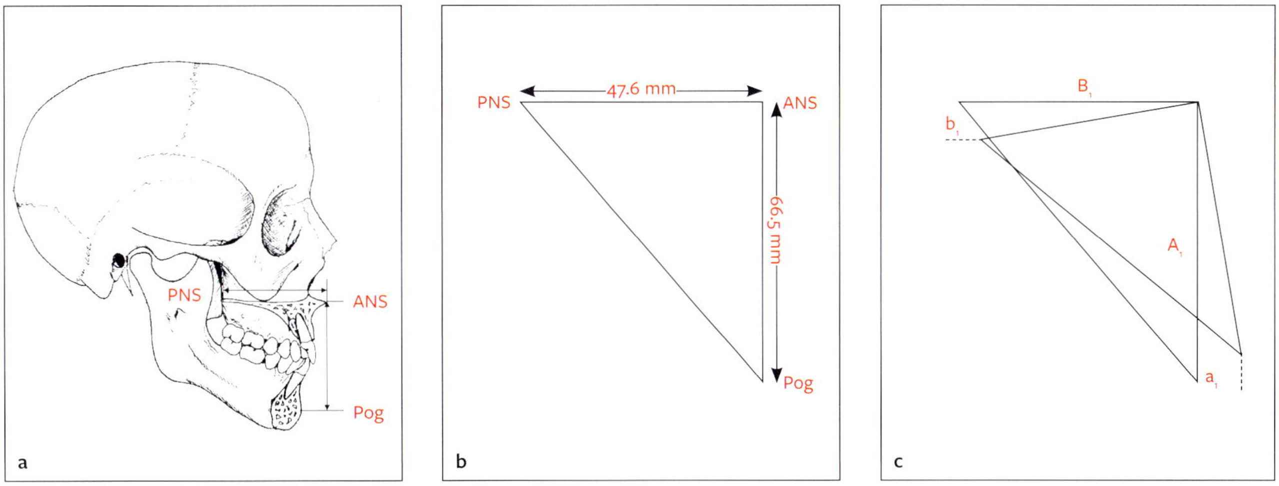

Fig 5-6 (*a*) Forty dry skulls were measured, and the anterior facial height was measured from ANS to Pog and compared with the maxillary length measured from ANS to PNS. (*b*) The anterior facial height (ANS-Pog = 66.5 mm) is longer than the maxillary length (ANS-PNS = 47.6 mm). (*c*) Because the horizontal leg (B_1) is shorter than the vertical leg (A_1) of the triangle, small changes (b_1) will be accentuated (a_1), resulting in a gearing effect.

triangle posterior or inferior to ANS may be chosen as the rotation point. The location of the point and the direction of rotation are dictated by the esthetic requirements of each patient. Opposite esthetic results can be achieved by either clockwise or counterclockwise rotation of the maxillomandibular complex. In addition, the effects can be enhanced by moving the point more anteriorly or posteriorly between ANS and PNS, or inferiorly or superiorly between ANS and Pog. The desired position of the maxillary incisor, paranasal anatomy, and chin prominence will help establish the point of rotation.

The cephalometric tracing (with the constructed maxillomandibular triangle) is used to investigate various soft tissue and hard tissue changes that can be expected by rotating the complex in a clockwise direction (increase in occlusal plane angle) and counterclockwise direction (decrease in occlusal plane angle). The method of developing a surgical visual treatment objective is discussed in chapter 3.

Linear dimensions between ANS and PNS

In a study of 40 dry skulls, Reyneke found that the average maxillary length (ANS to PNS—the horizontal leg of the maxillomandibular triangle) was 47.6 mm and the average facial height (ANS to Pog—the vertical leg of the maxillomandibular triangle) was 66.5 mm (Figs 5-6a and 5-6b) (see Recommended Reading). The fact that the horizontal leg is shorter than the vertical leg will enable the surgeon to use a "gearing" effect when rotating the triangle. Small rotations of the horizontal leg will result in larger changes at the vertical leg (Fig 5-6c). The anterior or posterior movement of Pog (b_1) is greater than the superior or inferior repositioning of the posterior maxilla (a_1) because the height of the lower third of the face (ANS to Pog [B_1]) is greater than the anteroposterior maxillary length (ANS to PNS [A_1]). The ratio of the movements may be expressed as the following:

$$\frac{a_1}{b_1} = \frac{A_1}{B_1}$$

The next section discusses varied dental, skeletal, and soft tissue changes resulting from rotation of the maxillomandibular complex and its esthetic result compared with that of conventional treatment planning, and clinical cases in which this concept is used are demonstrated.

Geometry of the treatment design using the constructed maxillomandibular triangle

Patients with Class III malocclusion who require surgery on both jaws will need maxillary advancement and mandibular setback, which will change the profile from concave (low facial contour angle) to straight (increased facial contour angle). This soft tissue effect will be enhanced by clockwise rotation of the maxillomandibular triangle and limited by counterclockwise rotation. The surgical correction of convex profiles will often require superior repositioning of the maxilla and mandibular advancement, resulting in a straighter profile. The corrective effect will be enhanced by counterclockwise rotation and limited by clockwise rotation of the maxillomandibular complex.

Table 5-1 | Comparison of hard tissue changes based on rotation points and direction

Clinical features	Clockwise at ANS	Counterclockwise at ANS	Clockwise at ZB	Counterclockwise at ZB	Clockwise at PNS	Clockwise at incisor edge
Occlusal plane angle	Increase	Decrease	Decrease	Decrease	Increase	Increase
Maxillary incisor tip	No change	Advance	Inferior, slight retraction	Superior, advance	Inferior	No change
Maxillary incisor angulaltion	Decrease	Increase	Decrease	Increase	Decrease	Decrease
Chin projection	Setback	Advance	Decrease	Increase, superior	Decrease	Decrease
Mandibular plane angle	Increase	Decrease	Increase	Decrease	Increase	Increase
Posterior maxillary height	Decrease	Increase	Decrease	Increase	No change	Decrease
Maxilla at ANS	No change	No change	Inferior	No change	Inferior	Advance

ZB—Zygomatic buttress.

Table 5-2 | Comparison of soft tissue changes based on rotation points and direction

Clinical features	Clockwise at ANS	Counterclockwise at ANS	Clockwise at ZB	Counterclockwise at ZB	Clockwise at PNS	Clockwise at incisor edge
Subnasale	No change	No change	No change	Advance	Slightly inferior	Advance
Upper lip support	Slight decrease	Increase	Slight increase	Increase	No change	No change
Facial contour (convexity)	Increase	Decrease	Increase	Decrease	Increase	Increase
Mandibular promincence	Decrease	Increase	Decrease	Increase	Decrease	Decrease
Nasolabial angle	Increase	Decrease	Increase	Decrease	Increase	Increase
Anterior facial height	No change	No change	Increase	Decrease	Increase	No change
Chin-throat length	Decrease	Increase	Decrease	Increase	Decrease	Decrease
Paranasal fullness	No change	No change	No change	Increase	No change	Increase

ZB—Zygomatic buttress.

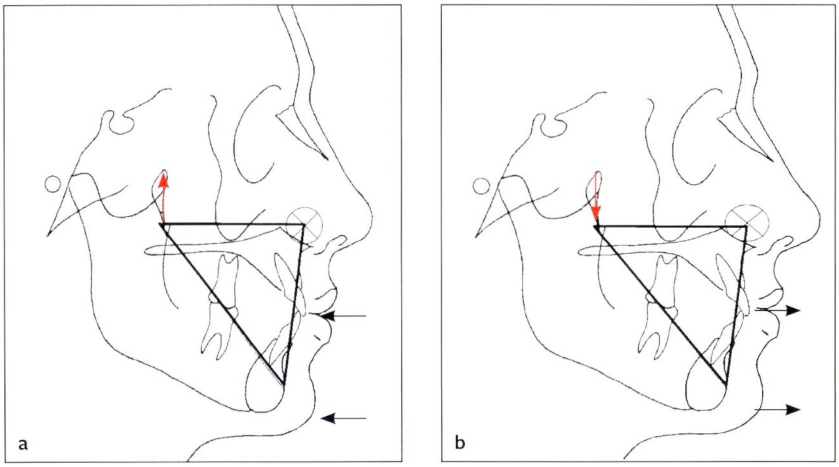

Fig 5-7 (*a*) Clockwise rotation of the maxillomandibular complex (*triangle*) around a point at the ANS. The height of the anterior maxilla is maintained, and the posterior maxilla is superiorly repositioned (*red arrow*). The maxillary incisor and Pog rotate posteriorly (*black arrows*). (*b*) Counterclockwise rotation of the maxillomandibular complex (*triangle*) around a point at the ANS. The posterior maxilla is inferiorly repositioned (*red arrow*). Pog and the maxillary incisor rotate forward and slightly superiorly (*black arrows*).

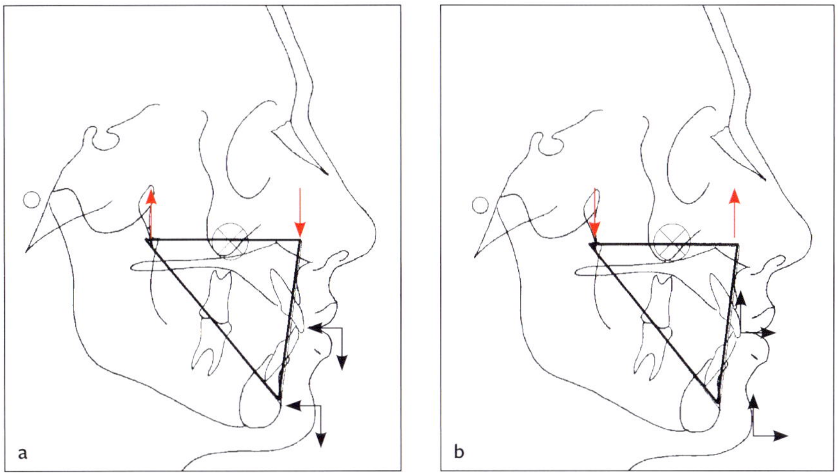

Fig 5-8 (*a*) The maxillomandibular complex (*triangle*) is rotated around a point at the zygomatic buttress in a clockwise direction (*red arrows*). Pog and the maxillary incisor will move backward and downward (*black arrows*). (*b*) The maxillomandibular complex (*triangle*) is rotated around a point at the zygomatic buttress in a counterclockwise direction (*red arrows*). Pog and the maxillary incisor will move forward and upward (*black arrows*).

It should be kept in mind that the convexity or concavity of the facial profile should not be changed by means of an advancement or reduction of the chin by genioplasty in patients with good chin contour. Chin contour is more important than chin projection (position of Pog), and genioplasty is only indicated where chin contour needs to be enhanced. The maxillomandibular triangle should therefore be constructed once the ideal chin contour has been established with Pog in its final position.

Rotation point at ANS

Clockwise rotation

Surgical superior repositioning of PNS as a result of clockwise rotation around a point at ANS will result in the changes depicted in Tables 5-1 and 5-2 (Fig 5-7a).

Counterclockwise rotation

Counterclockwise rotation around a point at ANS will require downgrafting the posterior maxilla and will result in the changes depicted in Tables 5-1 and 5-2 (Fig 5-7b).

Rotation point at the zygomatic buttress

When using rotation points on the horizontal line posterior to the ANS, a vertical component is added to changes.

Clockwise rotation

The hard and soft tissue changes shown in Tables 5-1 and 5-2 can be expected when the maxillomandibular complex is rotated clockwise around a point at the zygomatic buttress (Fig 5-8a).

Counterclockwise rotation

In counterclockwise rotation of the maxillomandibular complex at the zygomatic buttress, the changes depicted in Tables 5-1 and 5-2 can be expected (Fig 5-8b).

Rotation point at PNS

Moving the rotation point more posteriorly will have a more substantial vertical effect on the structures on the vertical leg (incisor edge and Pog) of the triangle.

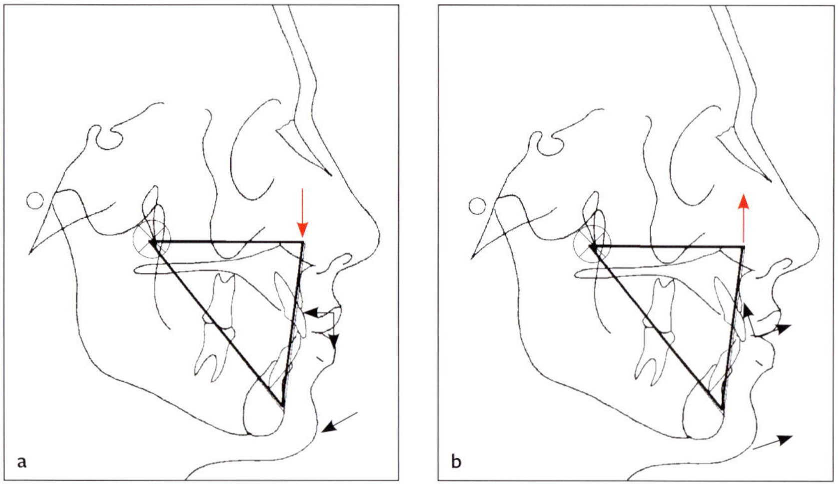

Fig 5-9 (*a*) The maxillomandibular complex (*triangle*) is rotated clockwise around a point at the PNS. The anterior maxilla is moved inferiorly (*red arrow*), the maxillary incisor moves posteriorly with a slight vertical increase (*top black arrows*), and Pog rotates posteriorly and inferiorly (*bottom black arrow*). (*b*) The maxillomandibular complex (*triangle*) is rotated counterclockwise around a point at the PNS. The anterior maxilla is repositioned superiorly (*red arrow*), which advances Pog and the maxillary incisors (*black arrows*).

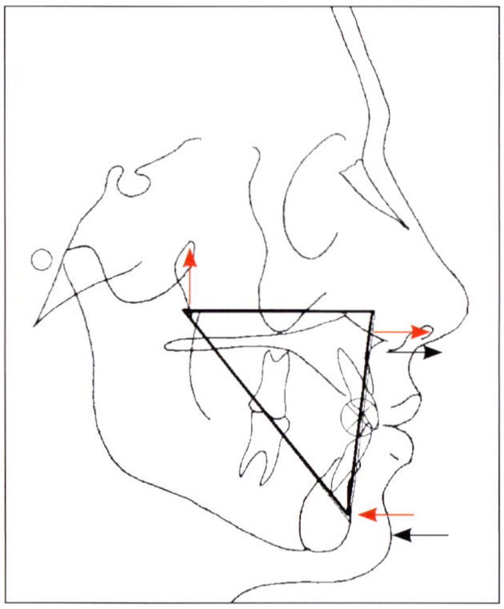

Fig 5-10 Clockwise rotation of the maxillomandibular complex around the maxillary incisor tip. This rotation (*red arrows*) will advance the ANS (*top black arrow*), set Pog back (*bottom black arrow*), and superiorly reposition the PNS. The incisor will become slightly upright. Note that a counterclockwise rotation with a selected rotation point inferior to the ANS is seldom indicated.

Clockwise rotation

This surgical design is often indicated for patients with vertical maxillary deficiency, low mandibular and occlusal plane angles, and short faces. The lower facial height will increase, and the profile will become more convex (Fig 5-9a; see Tables 5-1 and 5-2).

Counterclockwise rotation

This surgical design will enhance the surgical advancement of the mandible and is indicated for patients with vertical maxillary excess, very high occlusal and mandibular plane angles, increased facial convexity, and Class II malocclusion. Ideal esthetic correction may require a large mandibular advancement. However, it may not be possible during the orthodontic preparation to create a sufficient overjet to allow for the required mandibular advancement. In these instances, counterclockwise rotation of the maxillomandibular complex around a point on the horizontal leg and as far as possible posteriorly should be considered (Fig 5-9b).

Rotation at the incisor edge

Clockwise rotation

Clockwise rotation of the maxillomandibular complex around the incisor edge will require the posterior maxilla to be superiorly repositioned and advanced. This rotation will result in the changes depicted in Tables 5-1 and 5-2 (Fig 5-10).

Counterclockwise rotation

Counterclockwise rotation would result in posterior repositioning of the maxilla, which is very rarely indicated, technically difficult, and not recommended.

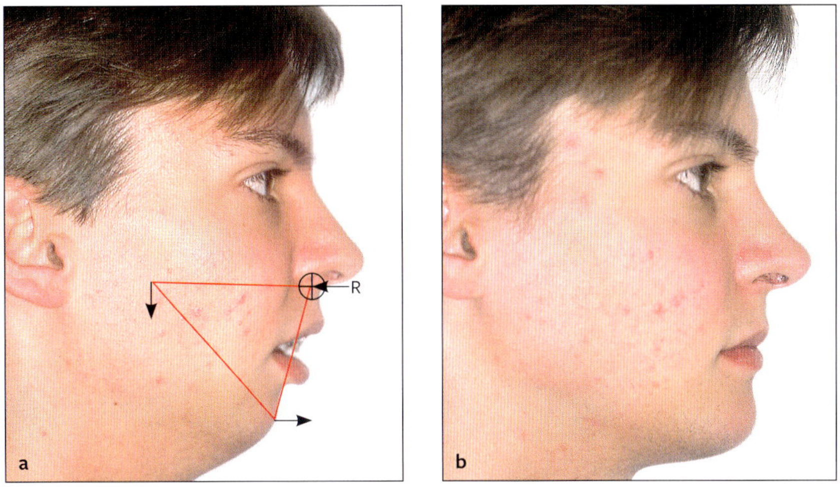

Fig 5-11 (*a*) A patient with a convex profile (facial contour angle of –33 degrees). Surgical correction required superior repositioning of the maxilla combined with mandibular advancement. The maxillomandibular complex (*triangle*) was rotated counterclockwise (*arrows*) around point R. (*b*) Postoperative results. Note the change in profile from convex to straight. This corrective effect was enhanced by the counterclockwise rotation of the maxillomandibular complex; it would have been limited by clockwise rotation.

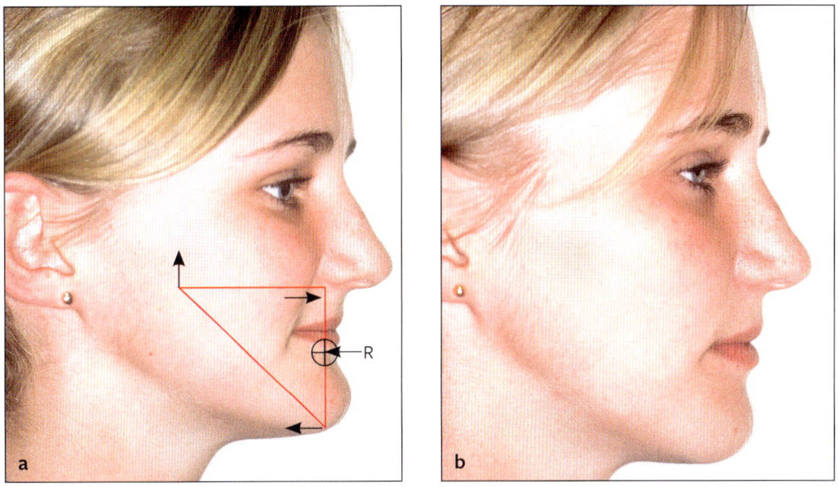

Fig 5-12 (*a*) A patient with a concave profile (facial contour angle of 1 degree). Surgical correction required maxillary advancement and mandibular setback. The maxillomandibular complex (*triangle*) was rotated clockwise (*black arrows*) around point R. (*b*) Postoperative results. Note the change in profile from concave to straight. By rotating the maxillomandibular complex in a clockwise direction (increase of the occlusal plane angle), the corrective effect was enhanced (straighter profile). In contrast, counterclockwise rotation would have limited the effect (less straight profile).

Indications for the rotation of the maxillomandibular complex

A severely convex face, as demonstrated in Fig 5-11a, will require vertical reduction of the maxilla combined with mandibular and chin advancement. This procedure will change the convex profile to a straight one. The corrective measure can be enhanced by counterclockwise rotation of the maxillomandibular complex and can be limited by clockwise rotation. In Fig 5-11b, the substantial change of the profile is demonstrated (note that the chin contour has been maintained). The surgical design has eliminated the need for an excessive advancement of the chin with a genioplasty. The correction of Class III dentofacial deformities will often require maxillary advancement and mandibular setback, and in many instances, this skeletal correction will result in a functional and stable occlusion. It will also change a concave profile to a straighter one and improve esthetics. However, to increase the convexity of the profile or enhance the corrective change, the maxillomandibular complex should be rotated in a clockwise direction. In patients requiring a less convex profile or when the corrective change is limited, the maxillomandibular complex should be rotated in a counterclockwise direction (Fig 5-12).

The surgeon is often required to improve the esthetics of a patient who has a skeletal discrepancy and for whom the occlusion has been orthodontically compromised (see case 1, Fig 5-14). In these instances, the principle of rotation of the maxillomandibular complex should be considered. Figure 5-13 demonstrates the occlusion (compromised Class I) of a situation like this. The first premolars were removed, the maxillary incisors retracted, and the mandibular incisors proclined as compromised treatment for skeletal vertical

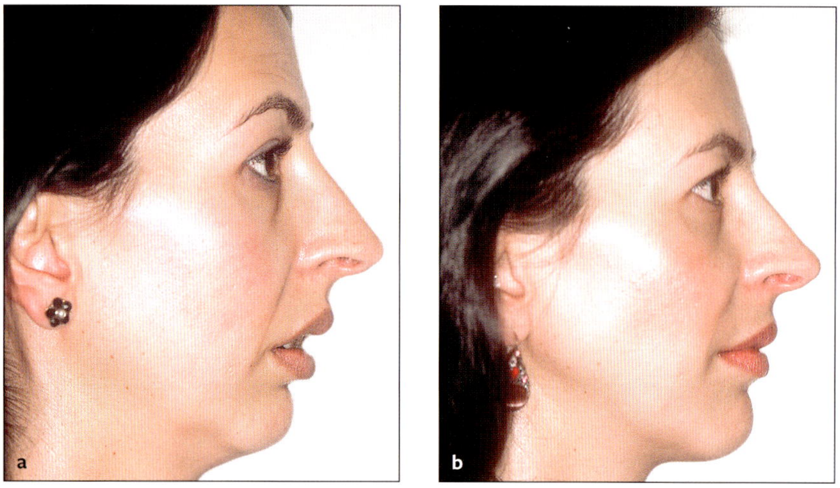

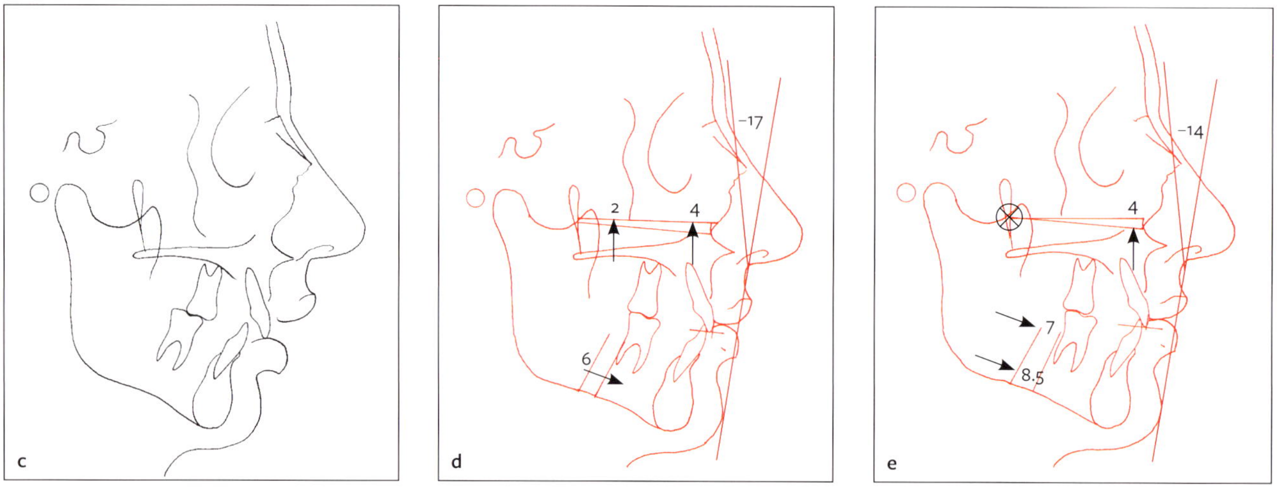

Fig 5-13 (*a*) A patient with a severe convex profile and a compensated occlusion. (*b*) The esthetic correction can be enhanced by counterclockwise rotation of the maxillomandibular complex. (*c*) A cephalometric tracing demonstrates the presurgical soft and hard tissue relations. (*d*) A surgical prediction according to conventional treatment principles. (*e*) The soft and hard tissue prediction following surgical rotation of the maxillomandibular complex around PNS. Note the increased mandibular advancement (6 to 8.5 mm) and improved facial contour angle (17 to 14 degrees) compared with the conventional treatment planning prediction.

maxillary excess and mandibular deficiency. Counterclockwise rotation of the maxillomandibular complex provided a method to correct the severe convexity.

Case 1

The patient in Fig 5-14 was a very unhappy 16-year-old adolescent boy who had undergone 4 years of orthodontic treatment. His dentition was severely compromised for his skeletal vertical maxillary excess and mandibular anteroposterior deficiency, and his facial appearance was very compromised as well. The surgeon had two treatment options:

Option 1

- Extract mandibular first premolars
- Decompensate mandibular incisors
- Improve the angulation of the maxillary incisors
- Surgical superior reposition the maxilla
- Surgically advance the mandible
- Surgically advance the chin

Option 2

- Accept the current occlusion
- Rotate the maxillomandibular complex in a counterclockwise direction
- Use the zygomatic buttress as rotation point
- Advance the chin with a sliding genioplasty

After 4 years of orthodontic treatment, the patient was very reluctant to have further orthodontic treatment, and the author decided to choose the second treatment option. The orthodontic appliances were removed 7 weeks after surgery. The treatment results are illustrated in Figs 5-14d to 5-14f.

For patients requiring superior repositioning of the maxilla for the correction of vertical maxillary excess in combination with rotation of the maxillomandibular complex, the maxilla is first superiorly repositioned on the surgical visual treatment objective, and the maxillomandibular complex is then rotated (see Fig 5-13).

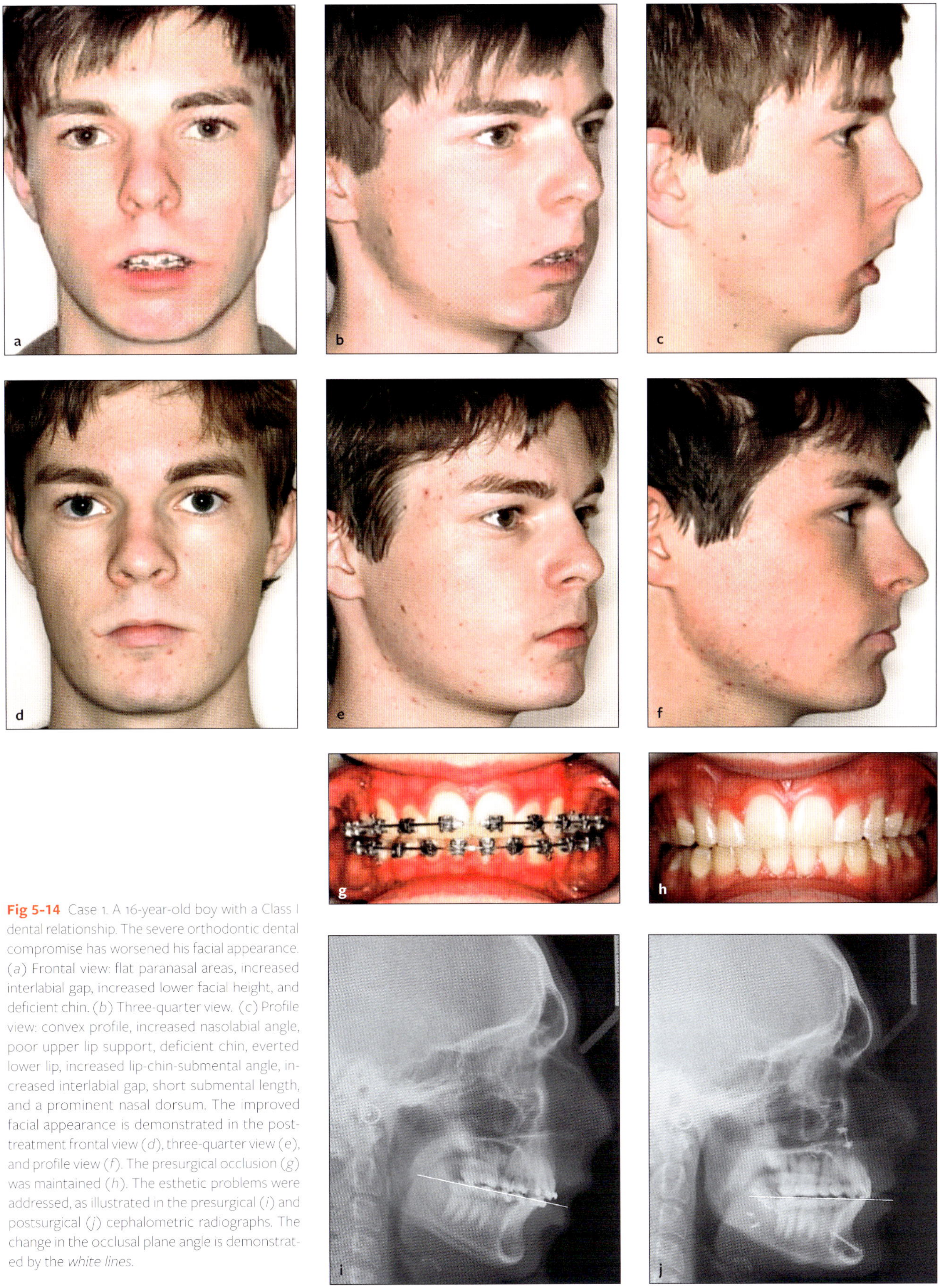

Fig 5-14 Case 1. A 16-year-old boy with a Class I dental relationship. The severe orthodontic dental compromise has worsened his facial appearance. (*a*) Frontal view: flat paranasal areas, increased interlabial gap, increased lower facial height, and deficient chin. (*b*) Three-quarter view. (*c*) Profile view: convex profile, increased nasolabial angle, poor upper lip support, deficient chin, everted lower lip, increased lip-chin-submental angle, increased interlabial gap, short submental length, and a prominent nasal dorsum. The improved facial appearance is demonstrated in the posttreatment frontal view (*d*), three-quarter view (*e*), and profile view (*f*). The presurgical occlusion (*g*) was maintained (*h*). The esthetic problems were addressed, as illustrated in the presurgical (*i*) and postsurgical (*j*) cephalometric radiographs. The change in the occlusal plane angle is demonstrated by the *white lines*.

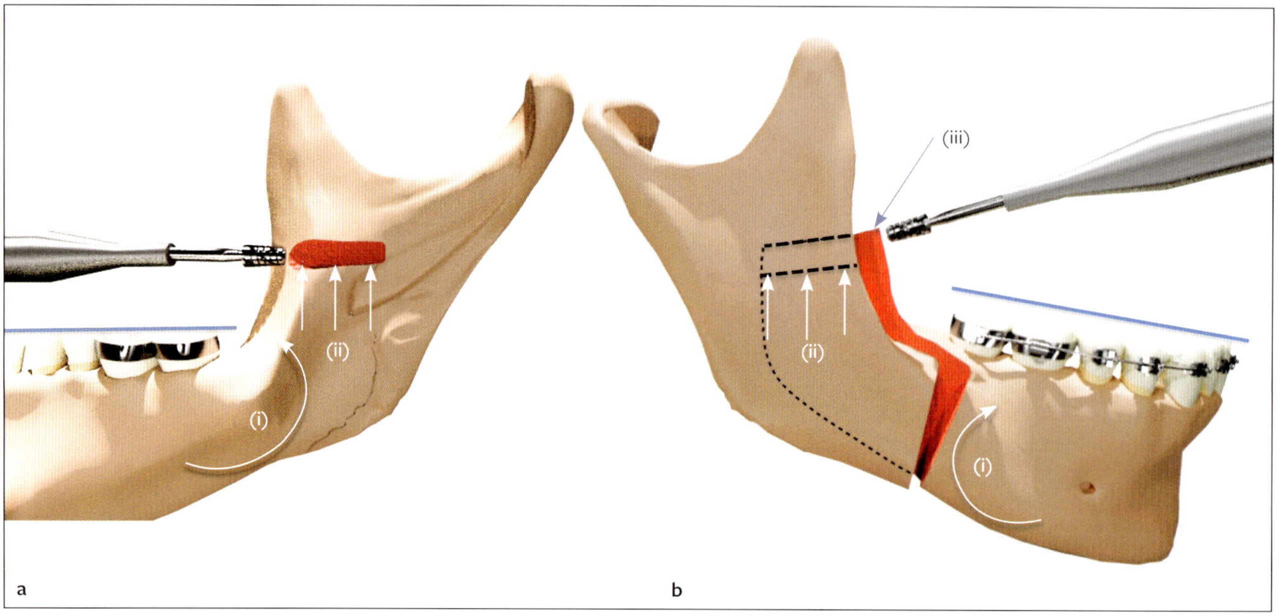

Fig 5-15 (*a*) A lingual view of the mandible in preparation for clockwise rotation of the distal segment (*arrow i*). A segment of bone is removed superior to the horizontal ramus osteotomy on the proximal segment (*arrows ii*) to accommodate the distal segment after superior rotation (*arrow i*). (*b*) A buccal view of the mandible after clockwise rotation of the distal segment (*arrow i*). The distal segment is moved superiorly (*arrows ii*), and the anterior aspect is contoured (*arrow iii*).

In addition to the esthetic objectives, anatomical considerations also influence the selection of the center of rotation and the extent of change of the occlusal cant. Excessive superior repositioning of the PNS (more than 5 to 6 mm) may compromise the nasal airway and is also technically difficult. Where indicated, therefore, it may be necessary to perform a horseshoe-shaped Le Fort I osteotomy to separate the dentoalveolar portions of the maxilla from the palate, which remains attached to the nasal septum. The vertical dimension of the nasal airway is thereby maintained, and the dentoalveolar segments are free to be repositioned.

An excessive change in the occlusal plane angle could affect the balance between the condylar guidance of the articular tubercle (eminentia articularis) and the cuspal angulations responsible for protrusive disclusion. However, the interrelationship and possible effects of changes require further research.

Clockwise rotation of the distal segment of the mandible may lead to segmental interference at the step of the horizontal osteotomy on the medial side of the ramus. This step may need to be contoured (Fig 5-15a) to allow free movement of the segment. The anterior edge of the segment often requires contouring as well (Fig 5-15b). The method for developing a cephalometric prediction tracing involving the rotation of the maxillomandibular complex is discussed in chapter 3.

Clockwise rotation of the maxillomandibular complex around a point posterior to the zygomatic buttress allows vertical lengthening of the anterior facial height.

Case 2

This case demonstrates clockwise rotation of the maxillomandibular complex around the ANS (Fig 5-16).

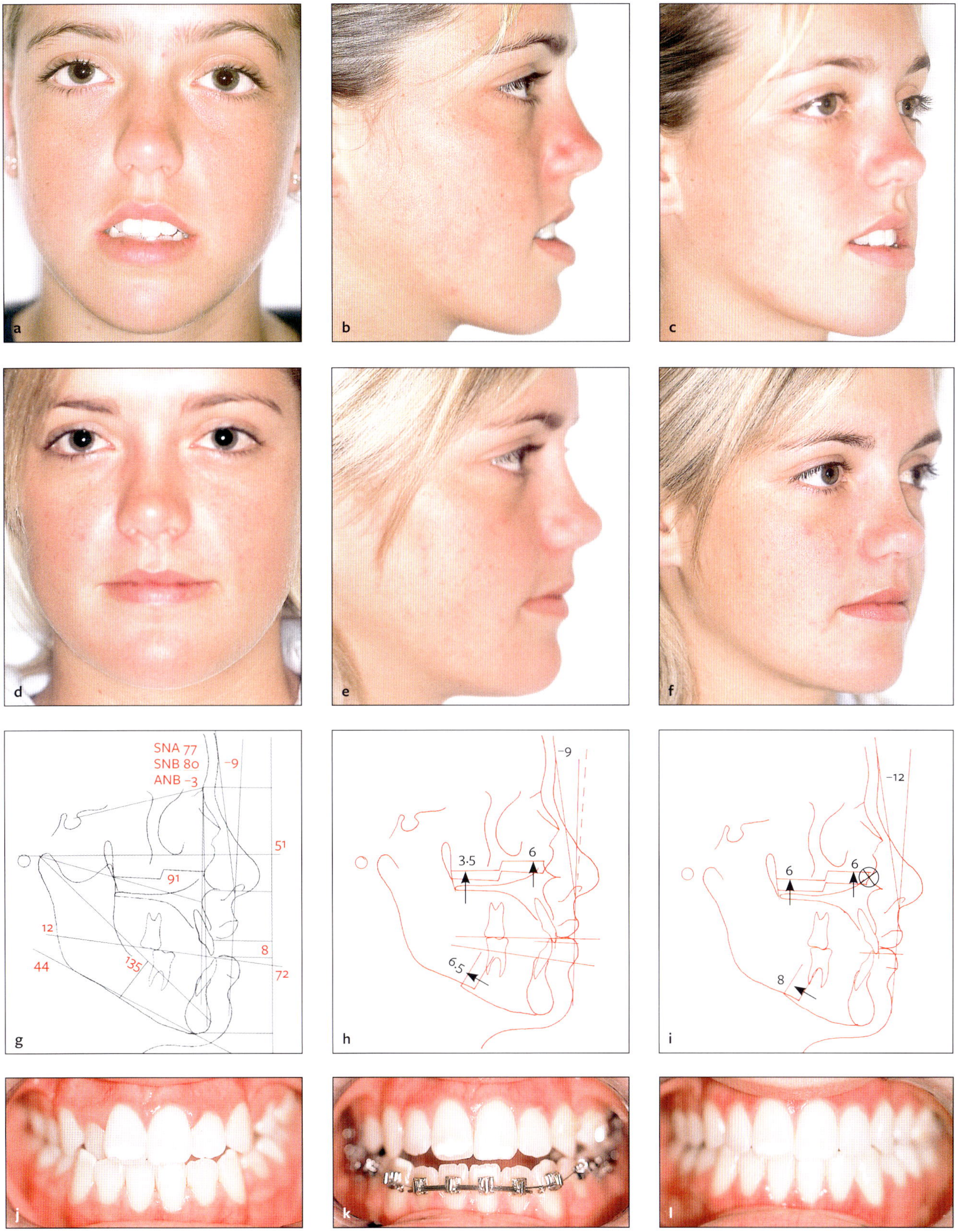

Fig 5-16 Case 2. Presurgical frontal view (*a*), profile view (*b*), and three-quarter view (*c*). Posttreatment frontal view (*d*), profile view (*e*), and three-quarter view (*f*). (*g*) Presurgical cephalometric tracing. Maxillary anteroposterior deficiency: SNA = 77 degrees; mandibular anteroposterior excess: SNB = 80 degrees; Class III skeletal relationship: ANB = −3 degrees; concave profile: facial contour angle = −7 degrees. (*h*) Presurgical visual treatment objective. Conventional treatment planning does not render an esthetically pleasing profile. The facial contour still appears concave (facial contour angle = −9 degrees). (*i*) Clockwise rotation of the maxillomandibular complex at point R enhances the profile change and allows for a more pleasing facial contour angle of −12 degrees. Pretreatment occlusion (*j*), immediate presurgical occlusion (*k*), and postsurgical occlusion (*l*).

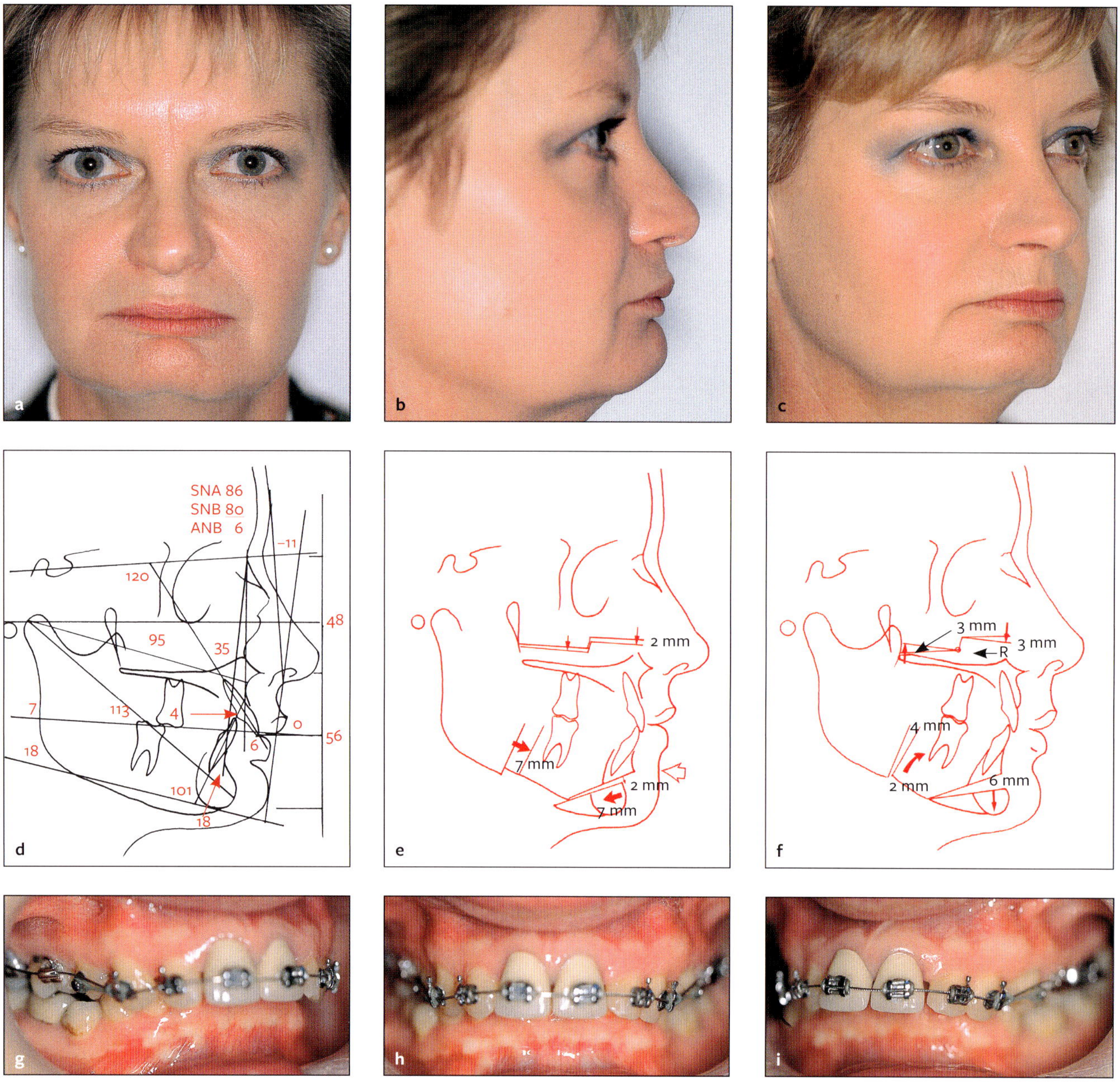

Fig 5-17 Case 3. Pretreatment frontal view (*a*), profile view (*b*), and three-quarter view (*c*). Pretreatment cephalometric analysis (*d*) and surgical plan (*e*). (*f*) The maxillomandibular complex is rotated clockwise around the zygomatic buttress (R). Note the difference between the conventional profiles in *e* and *f*. Pretreatment occlusion from the right (*g*), center (*h*), and left (*i*).

Case 3

In case 3, shown in Fig 5-17, the maxillomandibular complex is rotated clockwise around a point at the zygomatic buttress. Figure 5-17e shows the expected soft tissue result after conventional treatment planning—a flat labiomental curve. The expected soft tissue result after rotation of the maxillomandibular complex is demonstrated in Fig 5-17f.

Case 4

In case 4, rotation of the maxillomandibular complex around a point at the tip of the maxillary incisors is illustrated (Fig 5-18). The treatment is complicated by the fact that the first maxillary premolars were extracted when the patient was young.

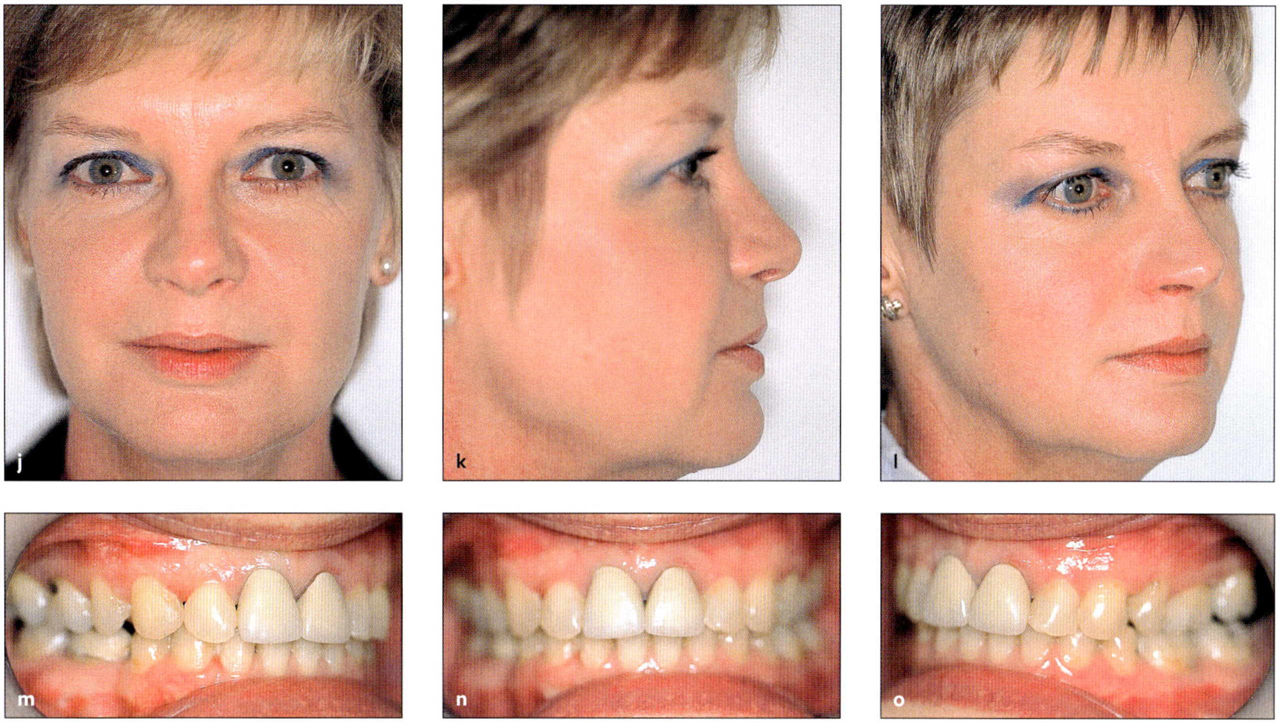

Fig 5-17 *(cont)* Treatment results: frontal view (*j*); profile view (*k*); three-quarter view (*l*); occlusion, right (*m*); occlusion, center (*n*); and occlusion, left (*o*).

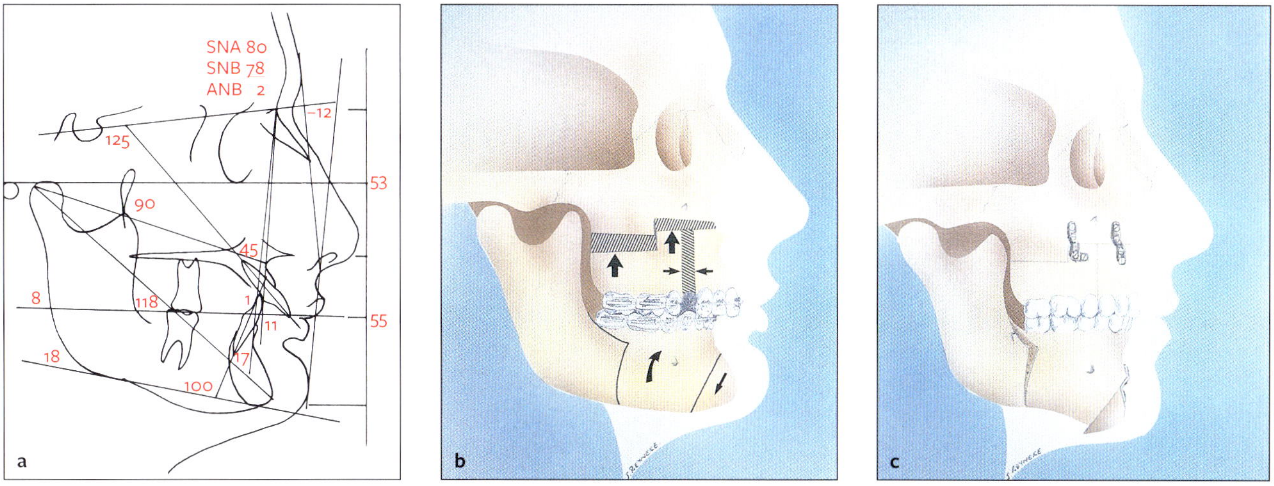

Fig 5-18 Case 4. Pretreatment cephalometric analysis (*a*) and surgical plan (*b and c*). Note that the extraction spaces are closed surgically. →

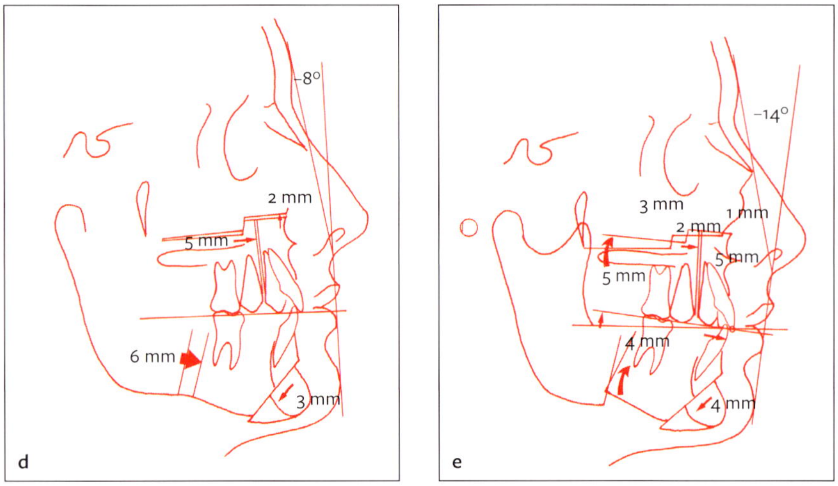

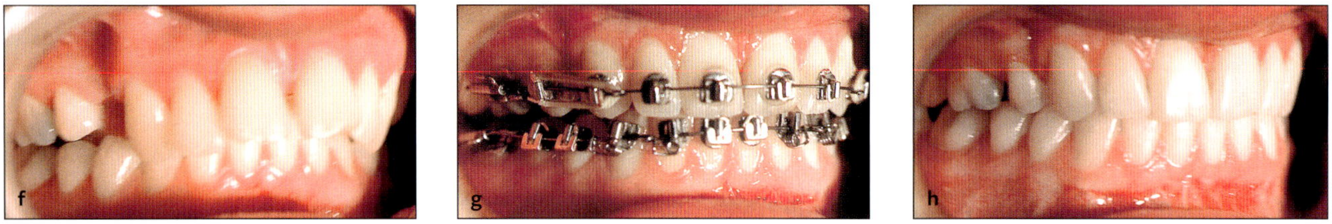

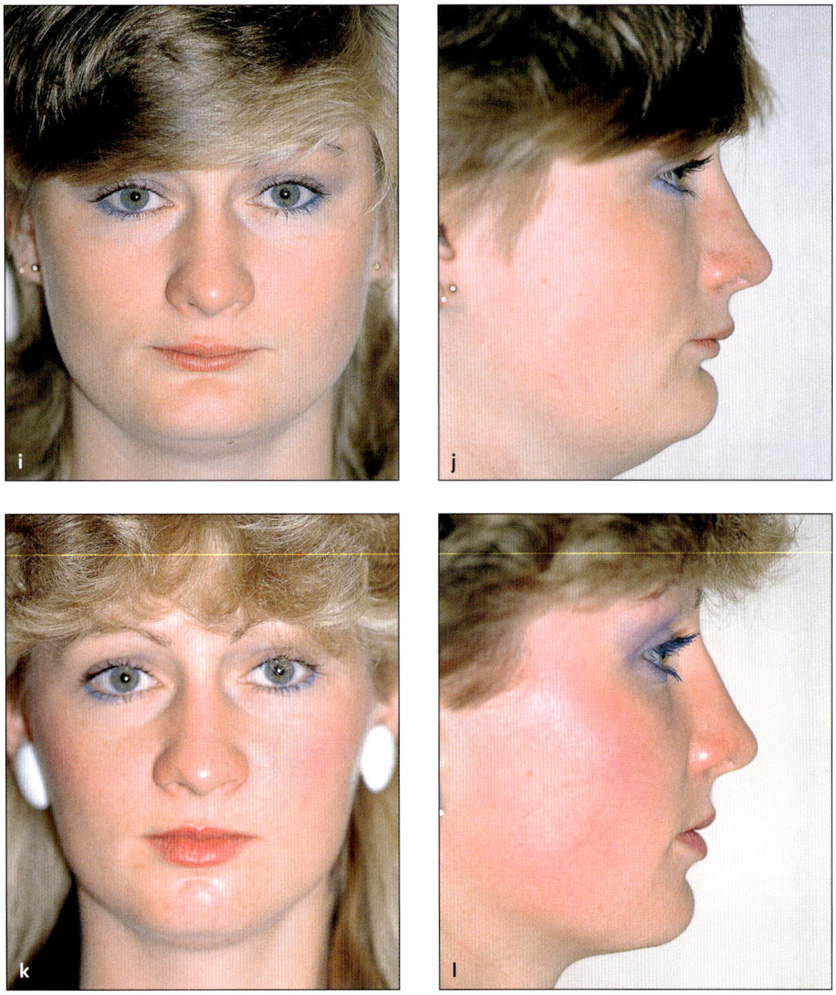

Fig 5-18 *(cont)* (*d*) Surgical prediction tracing done according to conventional treatment planning. Note that the chin appears prominent (facial contour angle is –8 degrees), and further reduction of the chin will obliterate the labiomental curve. (*e*) The maxillomandibular complex is rotated clockwise around the incisor tip, facilitating a more convex profile. Pretreatment occlusion (*f*), presurgical occlusion (*g*), and posttreatment occlusion (*h*). Pretreatment frontal view (*i*), pretreatment profile view (*j*), posttreatment frontal view (*k*), and posttreatment profile view (*l*).

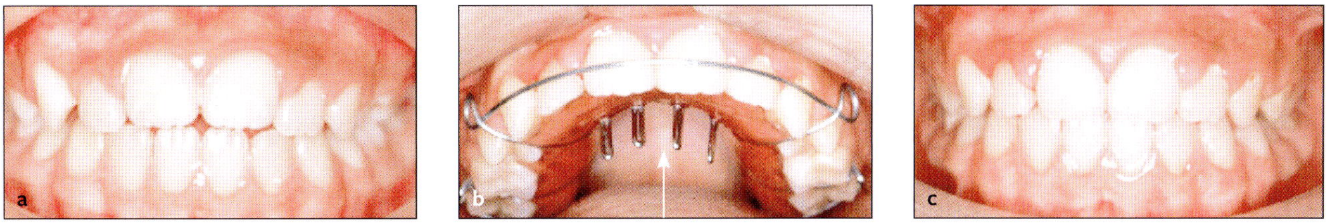

Fig 5-19 (*a*) Malocclusion of a child in mixed dentition: an anterior open bite and tendency to posterior crossbites. (*b*) The removable appliance with crib (*arrow*) to assist in breaking the thumb sucking habit following expansion of the maxillary arch. (*c*) Posttreatment result.

Open Bite Deformities

Open bite dentofacial deformities are some of the most challenging deformities facing surgeons and orthodontists. Diagnosis and formulation of a treatment plan can be difficult because the etiologic factors can be challenging to distinguish. There may be neuromuscular influences, genetic growth factors, and habits. Furthermore, the long-term dental and skeletal stability following treatment are concerns because neuromusculature and/or persistent habits may continue to influence the repositioned jaws and teeth.

The main etiologic factors that should be considered are abnormal sucking habits (eg, thumbsucking), oropharyngeal and/or nasopharyngeal obstruction (eg, enlarged adenoids), or vertical skeletal abnormalities (eg, vertical maxillary excess or shortening of the mandibular ramus). Researchers have developed two philosophies: (1) the morphogenetic theory and (2) the adaptive theory. The *morphogenetic theory* suggests that an anterior open bite may be the result of aberrant genetic control of morphology via growth patterns, whereas the *adaptive philosophy* postulates that a malformation develops secondary to functional aberrations of the oropharyngeal and nasopharyngeal apparatus.

Abnormal sucking habits

Nonnutritive sucking is a normal developmental phenomenon that usually disappears with age. Persistence of the habit beyond the age of 6 years is strongly associated with the development of open bite malocclusion (ie, proclination of the incisors and narrowing of the maxillary arch), although not all children who are thumbsuckers will develop open bites. Control of the sucking habit may lead to spontaneous correction of the malocclusion; however, some patients may need additional orthodontic expansion of the maxillary dental arch (Fig 5-19). When patient response to this treatment is poor, excessive vertical skeletal growth should be suspected (Fig 5-20).

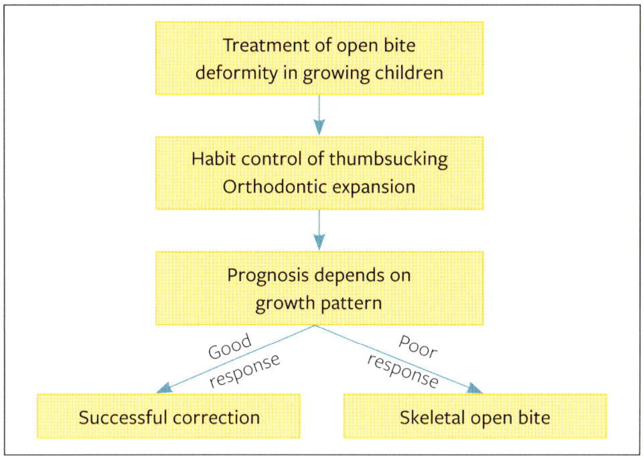

Fig 5-20 Treatment of open bite deformities in growing children.

Oropharyngeal or nasopharyngeal obstruction

There are several factors that may cause oropharyngeal or nasopharyngeal obstruction, such as enlarged adenoids and/or tonsils, allergic rhinitis, obstructive sleep apnea, and deviated nasal septum. The neuromuscular response to these factors has been shown to influence and alter facial and dental structures. However, these morphologic changes may show some recovery following removal of the deleterious impact. Although not all patients respond in the same way to these factors, the neuromuscular responses usually include at least one if not all of the following:

- *Altered mandibular position*. The mandible rotates downward and backward in response to the etiologic factor.
- *Altered tongue posture*. The tongue moves superiorly and anteriorly.
- *Extended head posture*. The cranium and maxilla rotate upward.

There are several implications of these functional adaptations to nasal breathing. First, a change in the direction of mandibular growth from horizontal to vertical results in increased lower facial height. Second, superior and anterior positioning of the tongue has several dental effects, including narrowing of the maxillary arch caused by the unopposed action of the buccinator muscles, retroclination of the maxillary incisors caused by the unopposed actions of the orbicularis oris muscle, and proclination of the mandibular incisors caused by increased tongue pressure. Not all patients respond in the same way to diagnostic factors such as nasopharyngeal obstruction, and in some cases, increased resistance to nasal breathing may be unimportant. Some patients with upper airway obstruction will respond with increased chest activity to overcome the obstruction, and no malocclusion may ensue. The altered head posture (extension or backward rotation) is an attempt to improve breathing. The change in head position has been associated with changes in craniofacial morphology, including increased facial height, mandibular anteroposterior deficiency, and steep mandibular and occlusal plane angle.

Skeletal

Typically, patients with anterior open bite will have increased lower facial height. An open bite dentofacial deformity is basically a vertical condition, and an anterior open bite may develop either as a result of vertical maxillary excess or shortening of the mandibular ramus. Excessive vertical development of the maxilla will result in backward and downward rotation of the mandible, leading to the development of an anterior open bite. Increased vertical development of the maxilla has also been associated with several muscle weakness syndromes. It has been reported that patients with long faces have biting forces below normal; however, the relationship between decreased biting forces, vertical maxillary excess, and anterior open bite is not clear. Shortening of the mandibular ramus may also result in clockwise rotation of the mandible and lead to anterior open bite. A short ramus may be the result of genetic growth predisposition or condylar resorption.

Tongue thrust swallowing and/or abnormal tongue activity during speech has been blamed for the development of anterior open bite malocclusions and poor stability following treatment in the past. Various methods to change swallowing patterns, such as speech therapy and use of a removable appliance with a crib, have been implemented to control the habit and ensure posttreatment stability. Contemporary research has shown, however, that the tongue thrust swallowing pattern is a physiologic response to an anterior open bite rather than the cause of it. The use of a crib in an adult patient is of no value; however, correction of the open bite will eliminate the need to thrust the tongue during swallowing.

An abnormally large tongue or true macroglossia should be differentiated from pseudomacroglossia and then considered as an etiologic factor for open bite. Patients with open bite in whom macroglossia is an etiologic factor will have bimaxillary dental protrusion, diastemas between the incisors, and crenations on the lateral aspects of the tongue (Fig 5-21). An abnormally large tongue does not adjust to the decreased oral volume after surgical correction and plays an important role in postoperative relapse (see case 5, Fig 5-22). However, a normal-sized tongue with forward posturing does adjust to the smaller volume after surgery. Pretreatment tongue thrust swallowing disappears after correction of an open bite because the physiologic necessity for tongue thrust has been eliminated.

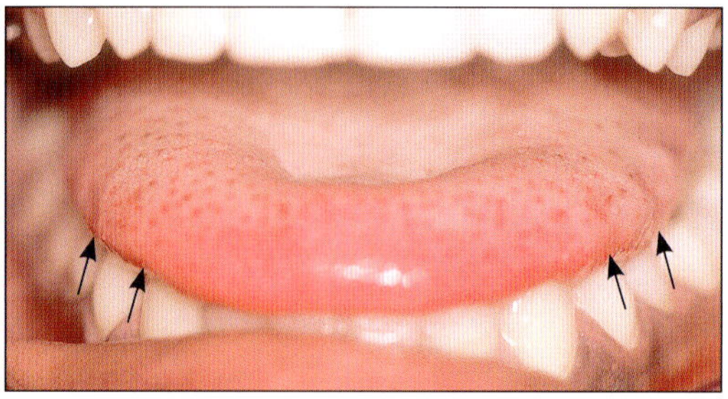

Fig 5-21 Typical crenations on the lateral sides (*arrows*) of a large tongue (macroglossia). Note that the relaxed tongue is covering the occlusal surfaces of the mandibular teeth.

Case 5

A 14-year-old adolescent girl presented with a skeletal Class III anterior open bite malocclusion (Figs 5-22a and 5-22b). The significance of her large tongue was unfortunately not considered in the diagnosis. Her orthodontic treatment in preparation for orthognathic surgery started at the age of 16 years and consisted of leveling and alignment of her dentition, retraction of her mandibular incisors, closing of the interdental diastemas, and coordination of the dental arches (Figs 5-22c and 5-22d). At the age of 18 years, her mandible was set back by means of a bilateral sagittal split osteotomy (BSSO), and the orthodontic appliances were removed 4 months after surgery (Fig 5-22e). Over a period of 6 years, however, there was severe relapse of the results (Figs 5-22f to 5-22h). Figure 5-22i illustrates the dental, skeletal, and soft tissue components of the relapse 6 years after treatment.

The patient returned 15 years after the initial surgery, requesting correction of her malocclusion. The patient's macroglossia was certainly a major etiologic contributor to her relapse. The surgeon therefore decided to correct the open bite by performing a Le Fort I osteotomy, which would create more space for the large tongue; however, it was also planned to surgically reduce the size of the tongue. The cephalometric analysis and the orthodontic and surgical visual treatment objectives for the corrective treatment are illustrated in Figs 5-22j to 5-22l. The treatment plan consisted of

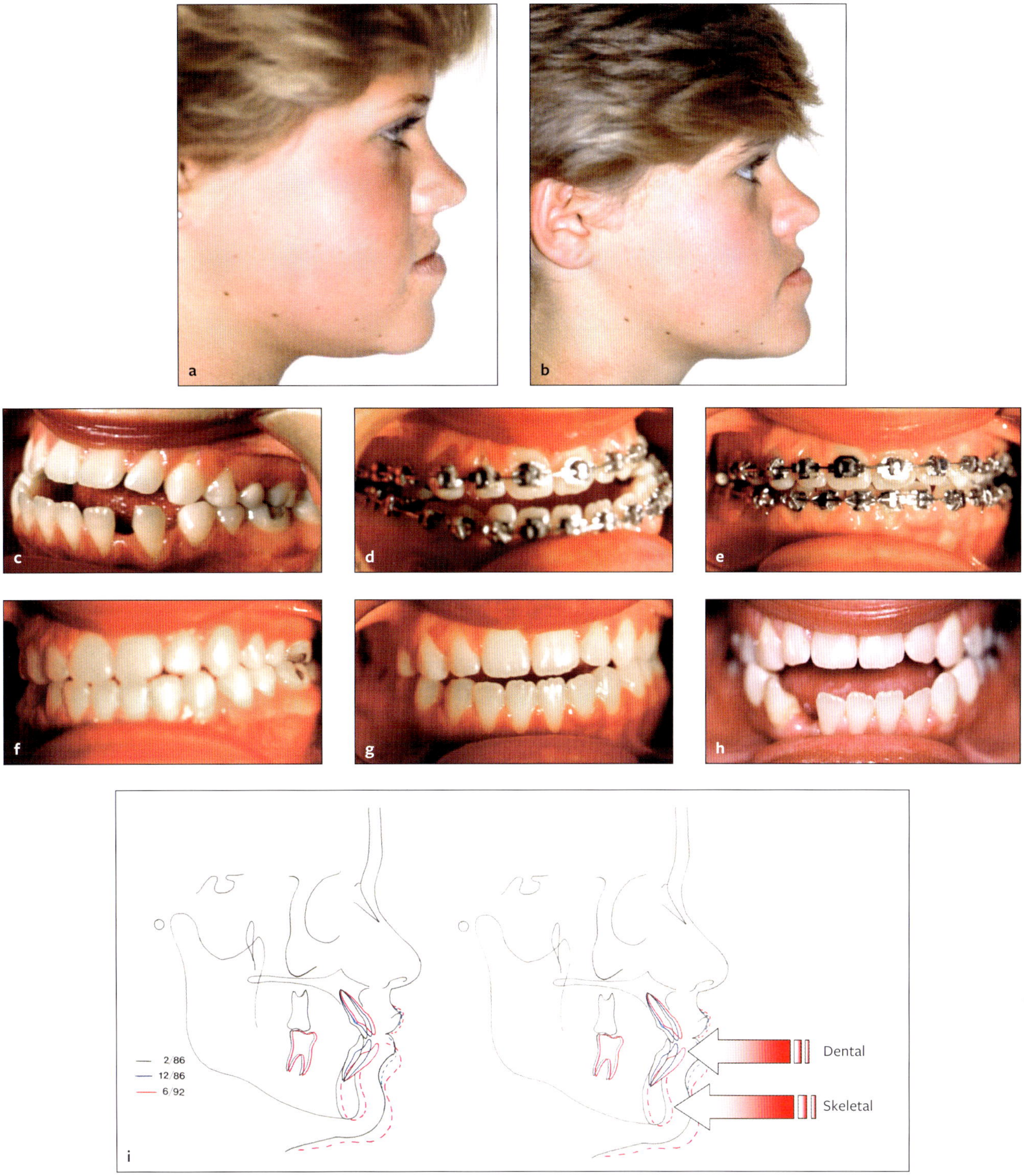

Fig 5-22 Case 5. Profile view at age 14 years (*a*) and 18 years (*b*). Pretreatment occlusion at age 16 years (*c*), presurgical occlusion at age 18 years (*d*), and immediate postsurgical occlusion (*e*). The severe relapse of the occlusion: 1 year after treatment (*f*), 3 years after treatment (*g*), and 6 years after treatment (*h*). (*i*) The cephalometric tracing illustrating the dental, skeletal, and soft tissue relapse: immediately after surgery (*black*), 3 years after surgery (*blue*), and 6 years after surgery (*red*).

orthodontic alignment and coordination of the dental arches followed by a Le Fort I maxillary osteotomy and surgical reduction of her tongue (Figs 5-22m to 5-22o). The pretreatment, presurgical, and 3-years posttreatment occlusions are illustrated in Figs 5-22p to 5-22r. The improved facial esthetic result can be seen in Figs 5-22r and 5-22s.

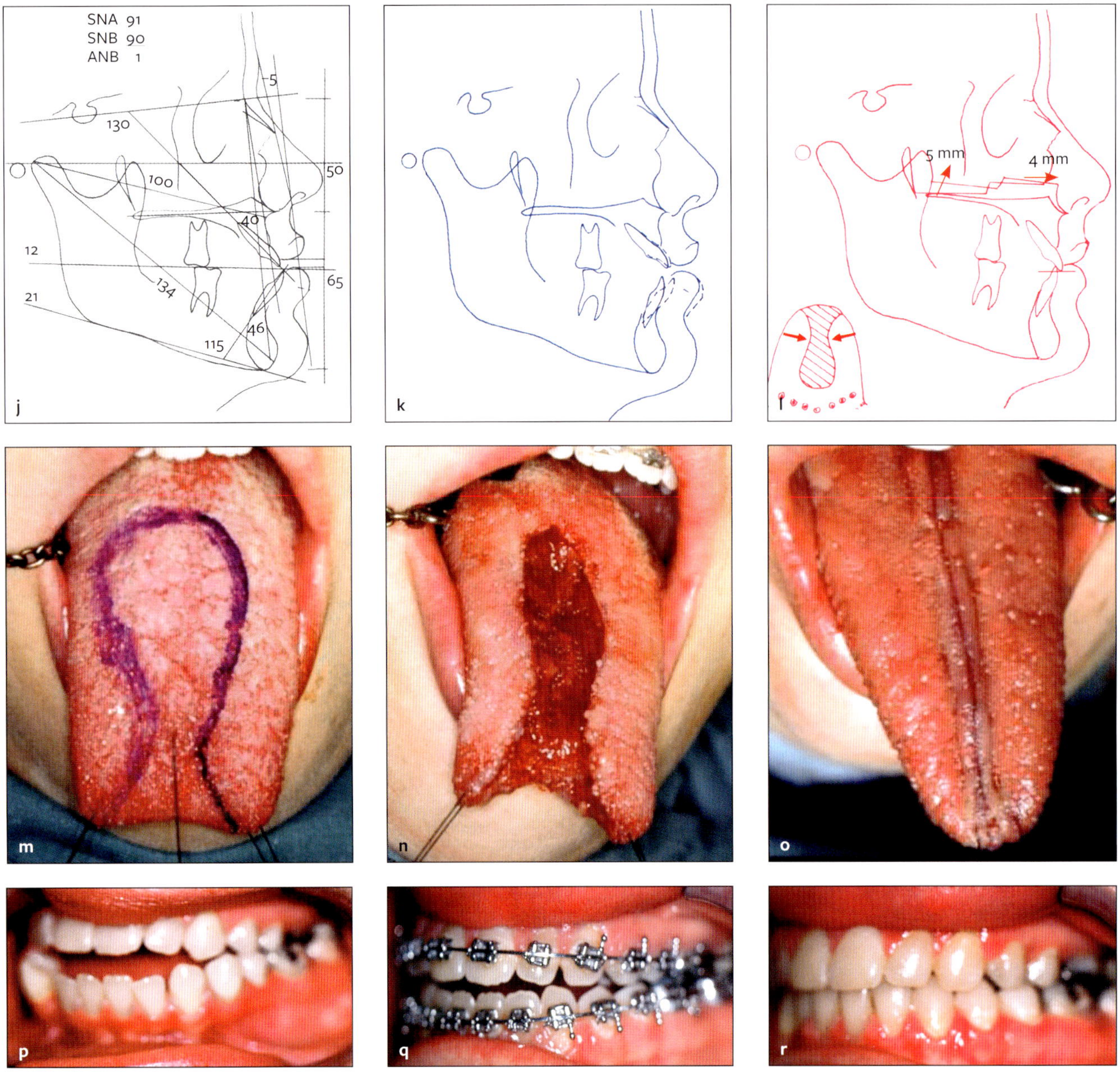

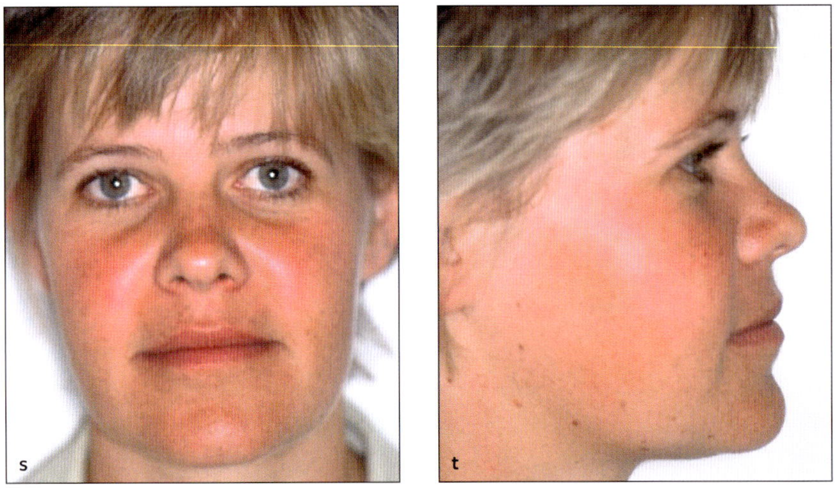

Fig 5-22 *(cont)* (*j*) The cephalometric analysis 15 years after the first surgery. The orthodontic visual treatment objective indicating retraction of the maxillary and mandibular incisors (*k*). The planned Le Fort I maxillary osteotomy with advancement and superior repositioning of the posterior maxilla. The size of the tongue will be reduced at the same time with a keyhole design (*l*). (*m to o*) Keyhole tongue reduction. The occlusion before the second treatment (*p*), immediate presurgical occlusion (*q*), and the occlusion 3 years after final correction (*r*). The frontal view (*s*) and profile view (*t*) 3 years after final correction.

Open bite malocclusion in growing individuals

In young, growing individuals, the major causes of anterior open bite are prolonged thumbsucking (beyond the age of 6 years) and environmental influences. The open bite as a result of thumbsucking is usually limited to the anterior region with a narrow maxillary dental arch, posterior crossbites, and relatively normal facial proportions. The most important corrective measure for these patients is to stop the habit. The posterior crossbites in the mixed dentition can be corrected by maxillary expansion using a removable appliance. The appliance can also assist in habit control with the placement of a crib (see Fig 5-19). If the open bite persists by the time the patient reaches adolescence, with poor response to habit control and maxillary expansion, skeletal factors should be considered.

Mouth breathing as a result of oropharyngeal and nasopharyngeal obstruction of the posterior airway space should always be considered in young patients as a possible etiologic factor in the development of an anterior open bite. Several studies have shown that removal of the cause of the obstruction to normal breathing (eg, enlarged adenoids or tonsils, allergic rhinitis) may decrease the open bite. However, it is important to differentiate between mouth breathing as a result of nasopharyngeal obstruction and mouth breathing as a result of vertical maxillary excess and lip incompetence.

A poor response following removal of an oropharyngeal or nasopharyngeal obstruction is indicative of excessive vertical skeletal growth.

Open bite malocclusion in nongrowing individuals

Orthodontic correction of anterior open bite

Orthodontic correction of skeletal anterior open bite often leads to poor stability and compromised esthetics. However, some patients with anterior open bites can be successfully treated with orthodontics. Orthodontic correction of anterior open bite without surgery usually focuses on three goals: (1) extrusion of maxillary and mandibular incisors, (2) intrusion of posterior teeth, and (3) expansion of the maxillary dental arch. This orthodontic treatment requires the almost exclusive use of vertical mechanics. Extrusion of the incisors may be accomplished in three ways: (1) vertical elastics in the anterior region; (2) a continuous archwire from molar to molar to level the excessive curve of Spee in the maxillary arch; and (3) a continuous archwire from molar to molar to level a reverse curve of Spee in the mandibular arch. Mechanics to intrude the molars may include temporary anchorage devices, bite blocks with repelling magnets, and high-pull headgear and anterior box elastics. Expansion of the maxillary arch in adult patients with skeletal maxillary transverse deficiency usually involves tipping of the molars and questionable stability. For patients in whom the anterior open bite is associated with incisor protrusion (increased incisor angulation), correction of the incisor angulation by tipping the incisors has a relative extrusion effect, thus closing the bite.

Few studies reporting on the orthodontic correction of anterior open bite have addressed pretreatment esthetics and the facial esthetic outcomes. Regardless of the specific mechanics used to achieve tooth movement, stability is often unpredictable and frequently results in compromised esthetics. When initial orthodontic attempts to close an anterior open bite have failed and the patient is referred for surgical correction, the possible instability of the previous orthodontic treatment should be carefully assessed. It would be wise to compare the patient's pretreatment records with the current dental situation. If any unstable tooth movements are suspected, it is recommended that the archwires be segmentalized and the teeth be allowed to relapse before continuation of any further orthodontic or surgical treatment.

Combined surgical and orthodontic correction of anterior open bite

Anterior open bite secondary to vertical maxillary excess: Le Fort I maxillary osteotomy with or without mandibular surgery

The common but variable clinical, dental, and cephalometric features of patients with anterior open bite as a result of vertical maxillary excess are shown and compared with the features of those with open bite as a result of short mandibular rami later in the chapter (see Table 5-4).

Presurgical orthodontics. Orthodontic correction of vertical, transverse, or anteroposterior skeletal conditions should be avoided. Orthodontic tooth movements for the correction of these problems have questionable long-term stability, and relapse might occur after the surgery is completed. An important orthodontic decision to be made is whether the maxillary arch should be aligned in one segment or multiple segments. When a natural step is present in the maxillary arch or surgical expansion is planned, the maxillary arch should be aligned in segments. The use of mechanics to close the bite or expand the posterior teeth beyond the bony base should be avoided. This does not mean that teeth within a segment should not be leveled; correction of incisor angu-

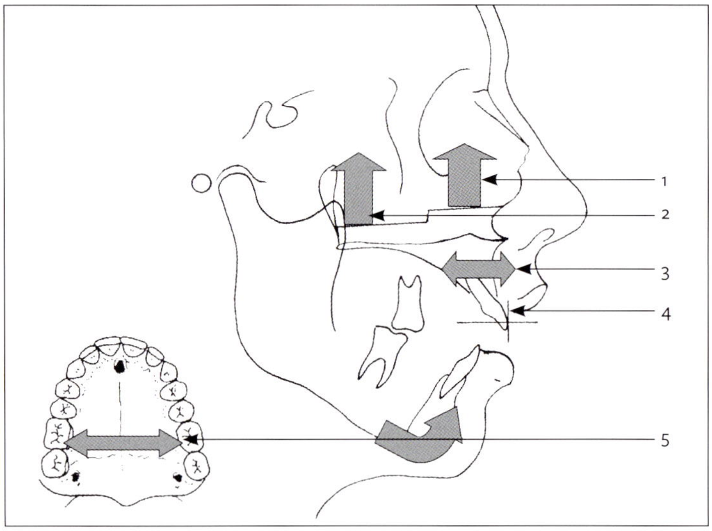

Fig 5-23 The five key factors to be considered when planning correction of an anterior open bite: (1) the amount of superior repositioning of the anterior maxilla to achieve the ideal maxillary incisor–upper lip relationship; (2) the amount of superior repositioning of the posterior maxilla to allow for mandibular autorotation and closure of the anterior open bite; (3) any anteroposterior discrepancy following mandibular autorotation and whether it can be corrected by maxillary surgery (care should be taken not to set the maxilla back for esthetic reasons); (4) the horizontal line indicates the planned vertical location of the mandibular incisor after autorotation; and (5) any maxillary transverse discrepancies to be addressed.

lations may change their height without extrusion. Opening the bite before surgery improves stability because relapse following intrusion will serve to close the bite further after surgery. The need for extraction is indicated by the amount of crowding and the tooth movements required to place the teeth at the correct angulations and in the central trough of bone. If the anterior maxillary segment contains only the four incisors, their angulations can be altered surgically; however, when the canines are included in the segment, surgical correction of the angulation will lift the canines out of the occlusion. Care should be taken to coordinate the arch forms of the segments with the mandibular arch form and to deviate the tooth roots adjacent to the intended interdental osteotomy sites. The mandible will serve as the template for the maxilla, and the mandibular arch should be leveled and the arch form aligned to allow for orthodontic (one-piece maxilla) or surgical (segmental maxillary surgery) coordination.

Surgical treatment. The surgical correction of an anterior open bite as a result of vertical maxillary excess will require superior repositioning of the maxilla by means of a Le Fort I osteotomy. There are five important factors that should be considered during the planning of the treatment (Fig 5-23):

1. *How far should the anterior maxilla be superiorly repositioned?* In most patients, the maxillary incisors require superior repositioning. Whereas in some patients the incisor height should be maintained, in others, inferior repositioning of the anterior maxilla may be required. The final vertical position of the maxillary incisors will be dictated by the incisor-lip relationship (ideal amount of incisor exposure under the upper lip). The final anteroposterior position will be dictated by the required amount of upper lip support. The final vertical and anteroposterior positions of the maxillary incisors are the keys to treatment planning.
2. *How far should the posterior maxilla be superiorly repositioned?* After superior repositioning of the maxilla, the mandible will autorotate to close the anterior open bite. The vertical position of the maxillary molars is dictated by the height of the mandibular molars (mandibular occlusal plane) after mandibular autorotation.
3. *What will be the location of the mandible after autorotation?* Vertical change of the maxilla will always have anteroposterior consequences as a result of rotation of the mandible around the condyle. Following superior repositioning of the maxilla, the mandible will rotate counterclockwise around a point at the condyle. The bite will close anteriorly, and the occlusal relationship will now be either Class I, II, or III. The incisor relationship may be ideal, or an increased overjet or anterior crossbite may be present.
4. *Can the maxilla compensate for the secondary anteroposterior discrepancy that may have developed as a result of the mandibular autorotation (Table 5-3)?* Patients with Class II malocclusion and vertical maxillary excess will end up with Class I malocclusion as a result of the anterior rotation of the mandible. These patients will not require mandibular surgery; however, genioplasty may be indicated to improve the chin contour. The mandible of a patient with a Class I malocclusion will rotate forward into a Class III malocclusion following superior repositioning of the maxilla. Based on esthetic requirements, the clinician must decide whether the Class III

Table 5-3 | Correction of vertical maxillary excess, secondary anteroposterior occlusal problems, and surgical correction

Pretreatment occlusion	Occlusion following vertical correction and autorotation	Correction of secondary anteroposterior problems
Class I	Class III	Mandibular setback or even maxillary setback (seldom). Genioplasty may be indicated.
Class II	Class I	Genioplasty may be indicated.
Super Class II	Class II	Mandibular advancement. Genioplasty may be indicated.
Class III	Super Class III	Maxillary advancement and mandibular setback. Genioplasty may be indicated.

relationship should be corrected by mandibular setback or maxillary advancement. Patients with Class III anterior open bite and vertical maxillary excess will end up with Class III malocclusion with increased severity following vertical correction and mandibular autorotation. A good esthetic outcome in these patients will require advancement and superior repositioning of the maxilla in conjunction with a mandibular setback procedure. Patients who have severe Class II anterior open bite malocclusion will still end up with a Class II malocclusion after autorotation. The correction of the Class II relationship should not be done by maxillary setback because this procedure will often result in poor midface esthetics. Instead, the mandible should be advanced and the maxilla both superiorly repositioned and slightly advanced. The slight advancement has the added technical advantage that the posterior maxilla is moved away from the pterygoid plates, which allows for easy and adequate superior repositioning of the posterior maxilla. In all of these treatment scenarios, the chin contour and position should be evaluated to enhance the esthetic outcome. When considering a genioplasty procedure, two important aspects should be kept in mind: (1) genioplasty is not a substitute for mandibular surgery, and (2) the shape and contour of the chin is more important than the chin position (the anteroposterior position of Pog).

5. *How should transverse occlusal discrepancies be corrected?* An individual with an anterior open bite and skeletal vertical maxillary excess often has a narrow maxillary dental arch and bilateral crossbites. Any transverse occlusal problems should be corrected by orthodontic expansion, surgically assisted orthodontic expansion, or surgical expansion. Skeletal transverse maxillary deficiencies should be corrected by either surgically assisted orthodontic expansion or surgical expansion, whereas pure dental narrowing of the maxillary arch should be corrected by orthodontic expansion. Surgically assisted expansion of the maxillary arch is indicated in patients who would not need any other maxillary procedure, ie, superior repositioning of the maxilla. Surgical expansion by segmental surgery is recommended for patients in whom expansion in addition to surgical superior repositioning of the maxilla is required. Transverse relapse is one of the most common postsurgical complications and inevitably leads to recurrence of the anterior open bite. The problem often stems from poor preoperative diagnosis, inappropriate presurgical orthodontics, poor surgical management, and poor postoperative orthodontic control. When the crossbite is skeletal in nature, compensatory orthodontic dental expansion, headgear, archwires, and through-the-bite elastics should be avoided. These orthodontic methods used on a skeletal crossbite carry a high potential for relapse and may "build" relapse into the surgical result. If the patient was not seen by the surgeon before commencement of treatment, it may be wise to compare pretreatment records with current records before surgery is performed. This knowledge will enable the clinician to establish if any unstable orthodontic tooth movement was performed before surgery. Presurgical orthodontic tipping of the molars may leave the buccal cusps hanging above the occlusal plane and will cause additional surgical complications.

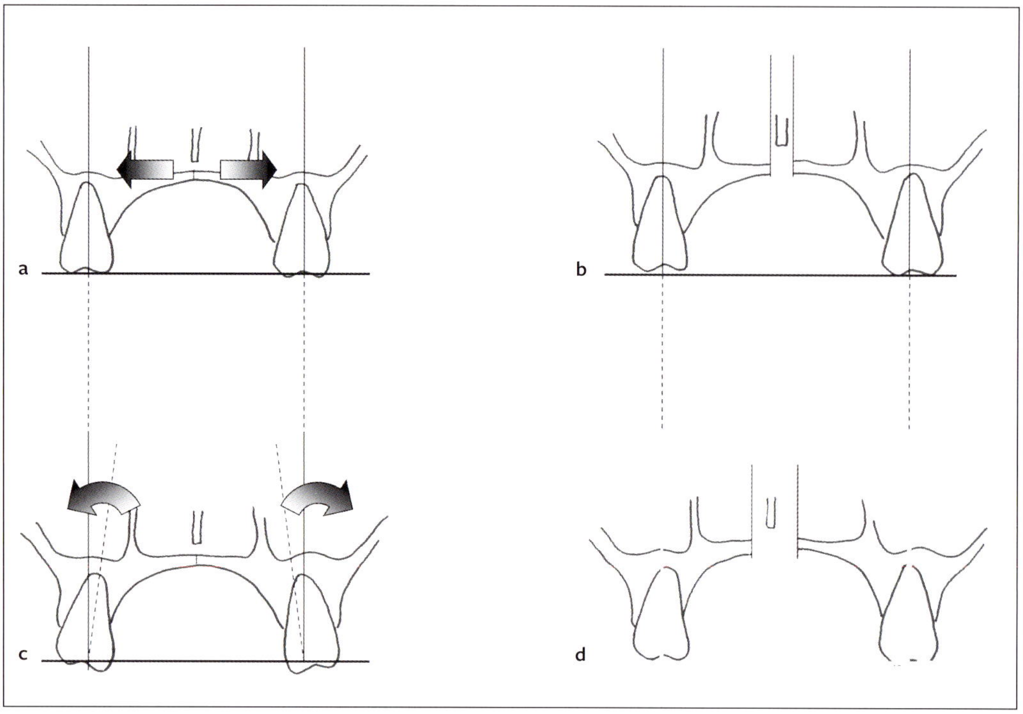

Fig 5-24 (*a*) The molars have been uprighted (*arrows*) and are in the middle trough of bone. (*b*) The intermolar distance has been increased by 5 mm and required 5-mm surgical expansion of the palatal bone. (*c*) The molars have been orthodontically expanded and tipped buccally (*arrows*) with the lingual cusps "hanging." (*d*) A 5-mm intermolar expansion will now require a surgical expansion of 10.5 mm.

Surgical palatal expansion in these patients will involve expansion of the bony base as well as uprighting of the molars. The surgical dental uprighting will add to the amount of skeletal expansion, increasing the potential for relapse (Fig 5-24). Transverse stability following surgical segmental expansion can be enhanced by placing a bone graft in the palatal defect and by using a splint during surgery that is maintained in position for at least 6 weeks afterward. Postoperative stability can be further improved by appropriate postoperative orthodontics. Postoperative orthodontic control should involve placement of a palatal bar, a strong archwire, or both to support the palatal expansion after removal of the splint.

Open bite secondary to short mandibular ramus with a normal condyle: Mandibular surgery

The clinical features of patients with anterior open bite as a result of a short mandibular ramus differ from patients with vertical maxillary excess (Table 5-4). When considering the difference in clinical features in Table 5-4, the clinician should keep in mind that some patients may have developed an open bite as a result of both vertical maxillary excess and short mandibular ramus.

Surgical orthodontics. In general, the same presurgical orthodontic treatment principles as with open bite as a result of vertical maxillary excess should be followed.

Surgical treatment. The anatomical abnormality, esthetic features, and functional correction in these patients demand a different surgical approach. Consideration should be given to closure of the bite with mandibular surgery. This surgical approach will require a counterclockwise rotation of the mandible at the posterior teeth. Historically, this surgical movement of the mandible has been considered unstable. An important factor causing the instability and tendency to relapse is thought to be the increase in posterior mandibular height as a result of the downward rotation of the posterior part of the distal segment and the subsequent stretching of the pterygomandibular sling (Figs 5-25a and 5-25b). When the distal segment of the mandible is rotated counterclockwise during surgery, two muscle groups are stretched: the masseter and medial pterygoid muscles and the suprahyoid muscles. The suprahyoid muscles are stretched even further when the mandible is rotated counterclockwise and advanced at the same time. The original sagittal split

Table 5-4 | **Comparison of open bite as a result of vertical maxillary excess and vertical mandibular ramus deficiency**

	Vertical maxillary excess	Vertical maxillary deficiency
Clinical features		
Facial height	Increased lower facial third	Slightly increased lower facial height
Incisor exposure	Often increased in mandibular incisors	Normal
Interlabial gap	Increased	Normal
Smile line	Gummy	Normal
Nasolabial angle	Obtuse	Normal
Chin	Retrusive	Retrusive
Nasal base	Narrow; tendency for paranasal flattening	Normal
Dental features		
Occlusion	Open bite associated with all types of malocclusion but mostly Class II	Open bite and Class II molar and canine relationship
Arches	V-shaped maxillary arch and U-shapred mandibular arch	Maxillary and mandibular dental arches well shaped
Arch width	Posterior crossbites	Normal dental arch widths
Occlusal curves	Flat or reverse mandibular occlusal curves	Normal occlusal curves but deviated
Cephalometric features		
Facial height	Increased anterior facial height	Slightly increased lower facial height
Mandibular ramus height	Normal mandibular ramus height	Short mandibular ramus height
Mandibular plane angle	Steep mandibular plane angle	Steep mandibular plane angle
Occlusal planes	Deviated occlusal planes often with a step in the maxillary occlusal plane	Deviated occlusal planes
Maxillary height	Increased posterior maxillary height	Normal posterior maxillary height

technique as described by Obwegeser and Trauner in 1955 was further modified several times, first by Hunsuck (1968) and later by Epker (1977). According to the modification, the mandible is split just posterior to the inferior alveolar foramen. By using this technique, counterclockwise rotation of the distal segment would not increase the posterior mandibular height and therefore not interfere with the pterygomassetric sling (Figs 5-25c and 5-25d). As suggested in chapter 6, the medial pterygoid muscle and stylomandibular ligament should be dissected off the medial side of the mandibular angle to ensure free positioning of the proximal segment. The author recommends the correction of an anterior open bite secondary to a short mandibular ramus with a healthy TMJ to be corrected with mandibular surgery (Fig 5-26).

Open bite secondary to short mandibular ramus with an abnormal condyle

The morphology and position of the condyle in the glenoid fossa is altered by any process of bone resorption of the condyle. Resorption of the condyle and subsequent shortening of the mandibular rami will lead to the development of a Class II anterior open bite malocclusion, a convex profile, and mandibular deficiency. Before considering correction of an anterior open bite resulting from condylar resorption, the clinician should differentiate between idiopathic condylar resorption, degenerative joint disease, osteoarthritis, osteonecrosis, traumatic injuries, and rheumatic arthritis with destruction of the condyle. Systemic connective tissue and autoimmune disease also can cause resorption of the condyle.

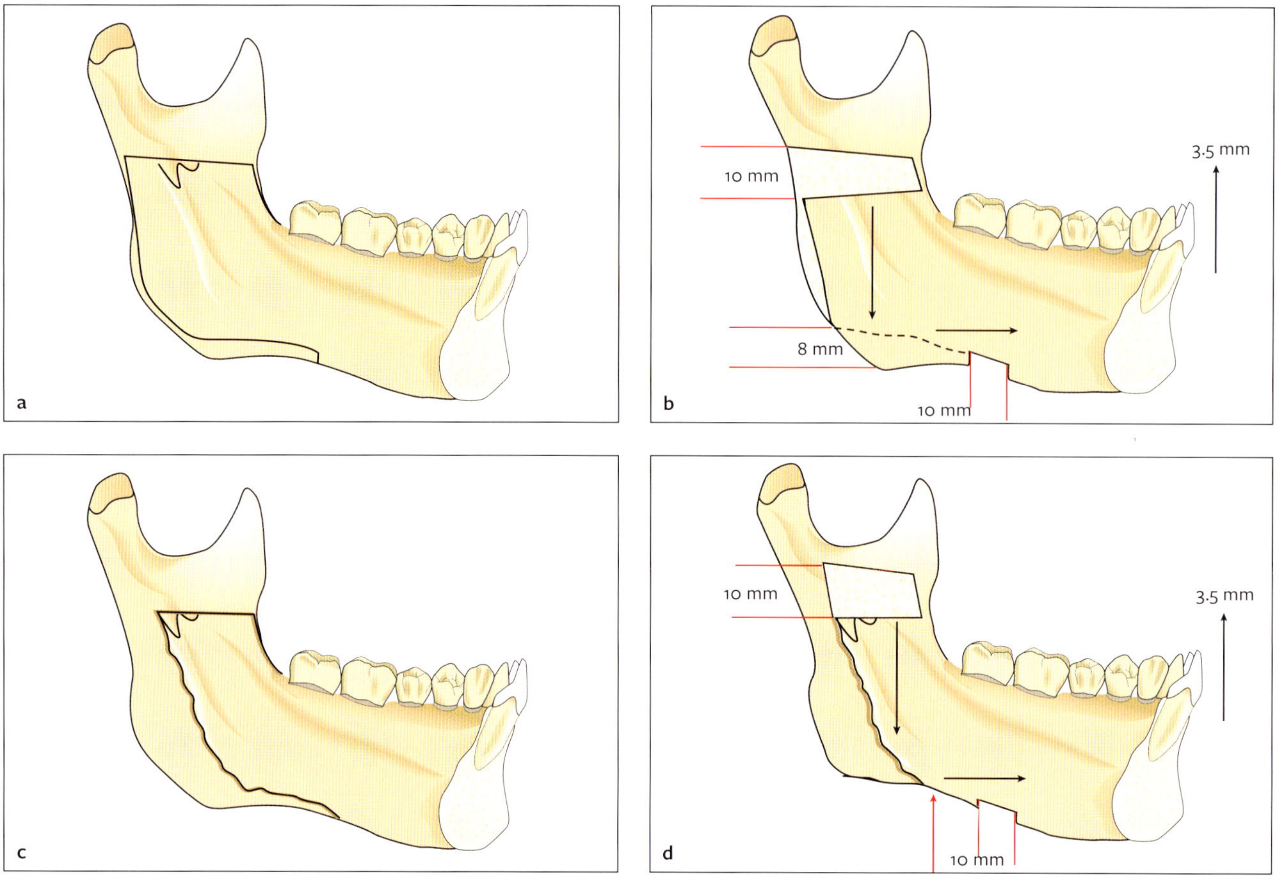

Fig 5-25 (*a*) Medial view of the mandible. The osteotomy design of the sagittal split according to Obwegeser and Trauner in 1955 (*black line*). (*b*) Counterclockwise rotation of 3.5 mm and 10-mm advancement (*arrows*) will result in an 8-mm increase in the posterior mandibular height. (*c*) Modified design of the sagittal split osteotomy on the medial side of the ramus of the mandible (*black line*). (*d*) Counterclockwise rotation of 3.5 mm and 10-mm advancement (*black arrows*) will not increase the height of the ramus (*red arrow*).

Idiopathic condylar resorption (condylysis). This type of condylar resorption may occur in any patient population; however, it is one of the most common TMJ conditions affecting teenage girls. Most of these patients are aged 10 to 16 years and usually have high mandibular plane angles. These patients gradually develop an anterior open bite without pain or hypomobility. The process is usually self-limiting and may last from 6 months to 2 years. Although the specific cause of idiopathic condylar resorption is unknown, the fact that there is a strong predilection for teenage girls in their pubertal growth phase suggests that hormonal mediation may play a role. It is hypothesized that through estrogen mediation and excessive joint loading (eg, parafunction, orthodontic treatment, orthognathic surgery, and trauma), resorption is induced in the subcondylar bone in all three planes of space. Although this condition usually occurs bilaterally, it may occur in only one condyle or at a more rapid rate in one condyle than in the other.

There are three important aspects to consider when planning the correction of the existing deformity: (1) Ensure that the resorptive process has become inactive. Serial cephalometric radiographs are a valuable diagnostic method; however, an alternative method such as radioisotope analysis can be used to detect the presence of resorptive activity in the condyle. (2) Evaluate the articular disc for pathology or displacement. Some surgeons prefer to perform disc repositioning and placement of a Mitek anchor (Johnson & Johnson), when indicated, at the same time as the orthognathic correction. (3) Treat the deformity in such a way that the loads on the condyles are not increased (eg, avoid long Class III elastics during orthodontic treatment).

Osteoarthrosis. Osteoarthrosis of the TMJ is a slow, progressive, degenerative disease that alters the position, morphology, and physiology of all joint structures. It may

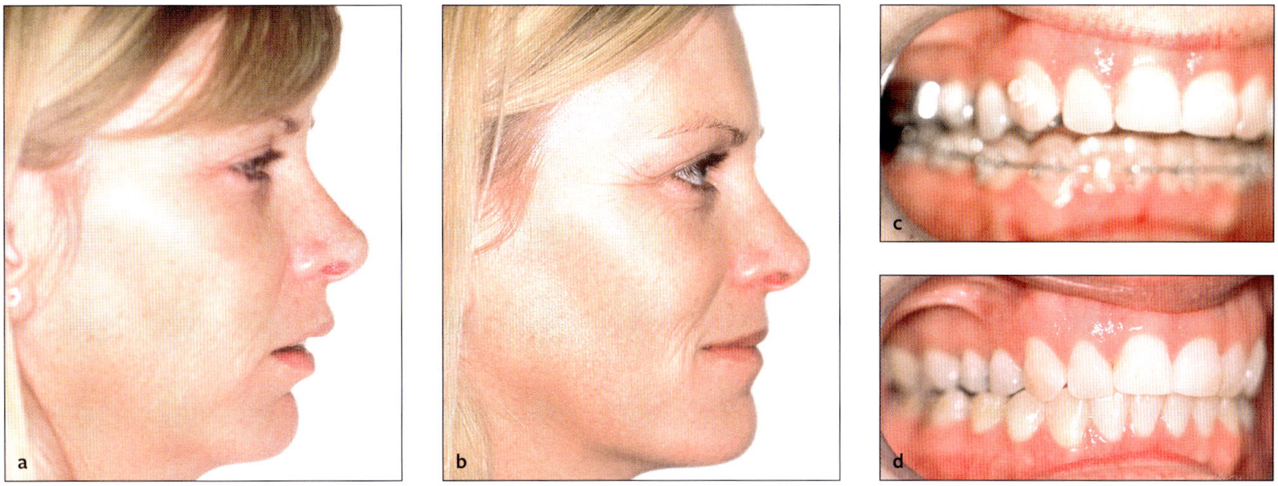

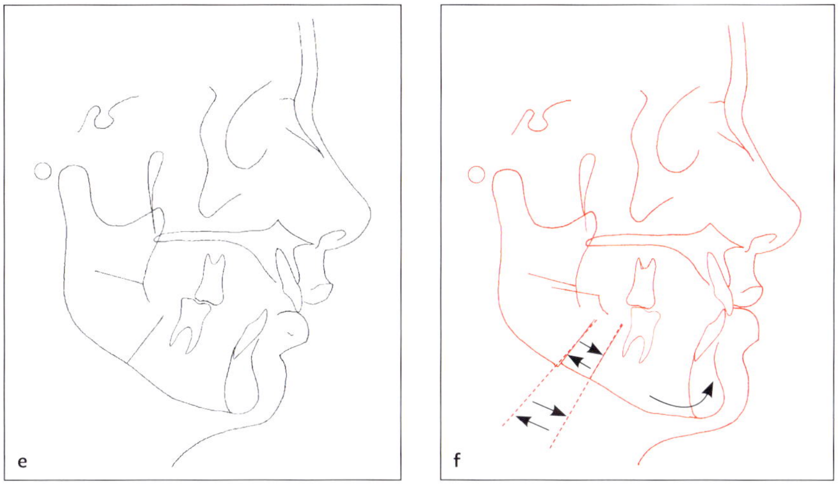

Fig 5-26 (*a*) Profile view of a patient with mandibular anteroposterior deficiency. (*b*) Profile view following mandibular advancement and counterclockwise rotation. (*c*) Presurgical occlusion: Class II anterior open bite. (*d*) Posttreatment occlusion 18 months after band removal. (*e*) Presurgical cephalometric tracing. (*f*) Posttreatment tracing. Note the amount of surgical advancement and counterclockwise rotation (*arrows*).

occur bilaterally or unilaterally, in which instance the mandible will deviate to the affected side. Patients experience chronic pain, clicking, popping, crepitus, myofascial pain, and progressive changes in occlusion and facial appearance. It may be possible to obtain temporary relief of symptoms by conservative partial reconstruction of the joint and orthognathic surgery in some patients whose symptoms have not been present for a long time (less than 4 years). However, for patients who have endured the disease longer and whose condyles are significantly destroyed and articular discs not salvageable, replacement of the joint with an artificial prosthesis would be the procedure of choice.

Treatment planning for combined orthognathic surgery and total joint replacement does not differ from conventional treatment planning. However, there is a limited amount of mandibular advancement that can be obtained with a joint prosthesis. The advancement is limited to an amount of 7 to 8 mm of contact between the ramus and the implant.

Anterior open bite dentofacial deformities are basically vertical problems that develop as a result of excessive vertical growth of the maxilla, vertical deficiency of the mandibular ramus, or both. Although concomitant anteroposterior deformities may also be present in these patients, secondary anteroposterior problems are often present as a result of clockwise rotation of the mandible. The clinician should differentiate between primary and secondary anteroposterior problems, which must be taken into account during treatment planning. Transverse problems, as a result of a narrow maxillary dental arch, should be treated and stability carefully considered because transverse occlusal stability ensures vertical occlusal stability. Figure 5-27 is an algorithm that summarizes the suggested principles of surgical orthodontic correction of anterior open bite dentofacial deformities.

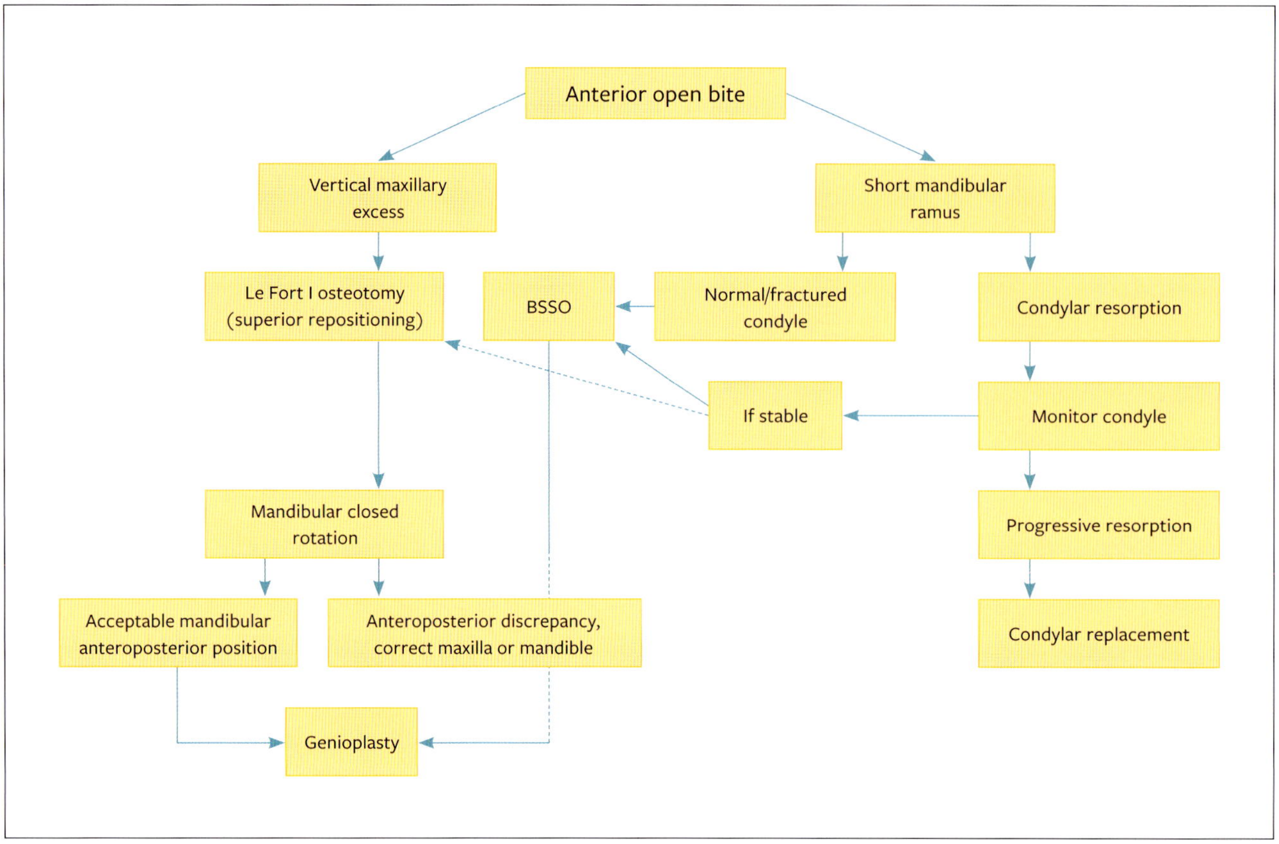

Fig 5-27 Algorithm summarizing the treatment principles of anterior open bites.

General characteristics of Class I open bite

Clinical characteristics

- Vertical maxillary excess, more posterior than anterior
- Mandible rotated clockwise (backward)
- An increased interlabial gap
- Often, increased exposure of maxillary incisors under the upper lip
- Often, transverse maxillary deficiency
- Possibly a skeletal Class III malocclusion rotated to a Class I malocclusion

Orthodontic preparation

Two decisions must be made in orthodontic preparation. The first is to decide between continuous archwire (single-piece) and segmental arch (multi-piece) mechanics. When a dual occlusal plane exists, segmental arch orthodontics is indicated to avoid possible orthodontic extrusion of anterior teeth, which may lead to unpredictable stability (Fig 5-28). Conversely, when a single occlusal plane exists, continuous archwire mechanics is preferred (Fig 5-29).

The second decision is extraction versus nonextraction. The decision to extract teeth is influenced by two factors: (1) crowding and (2) the anteroposterior position of the mandibular incisors. When no mandibular surgery is contemplated (according to the orthodontic and surgical prediction tracings), the final anteroposterior position of the maxilla will be dictated by the anteroposterior position of the mandibular incisors after autorotation of the mandible.

Surgical solutions

Following are surgical solutions to Class I open bites (Fig 5-30):

- Superior repositioning of the maxilla (using segmental or single-piece mechanics): When a preexisting dual occlusal plane is present, segmental orthodontic alignment followed by segmental surgical correction is indicated.

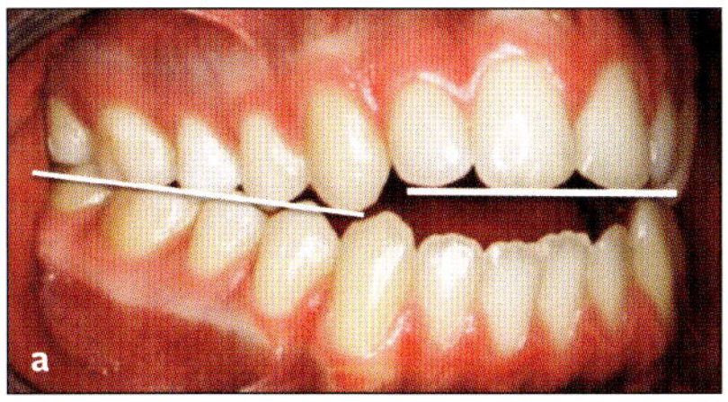

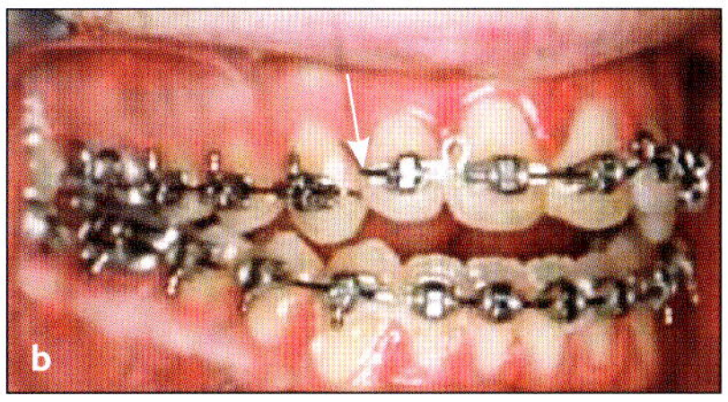

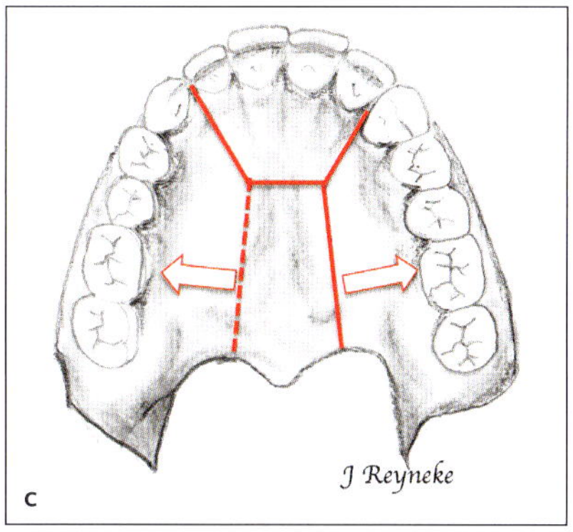

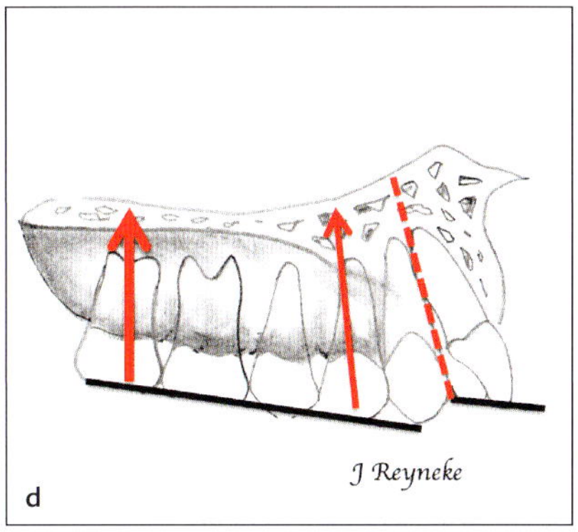

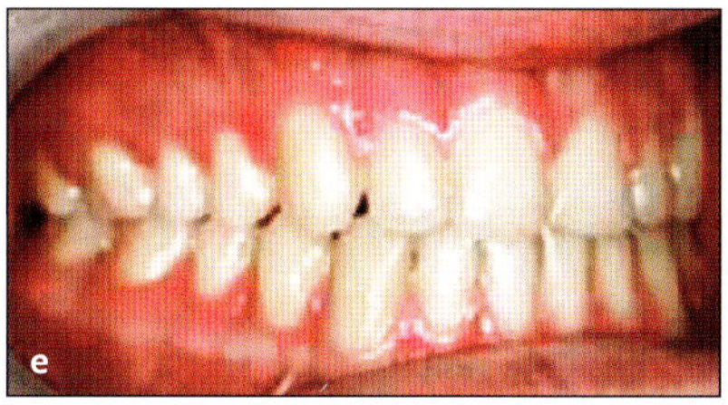

Fig 5-28 (*a*) Dual maxillary occlusal plane. (*b*) The maxillary arch is aligned in three segments, and the segments are aligned to conform to the mandibular arch form. (*c and d*) In this case, the interdental osteotomies (*red lines*) are performed between the lateral incisor and canine teeth to allow for surgical correction of transverse and vertical discrepancies. When the interdental osteotomies are created between the lateral incisors and canines, it allows the surgeon to control the intercanine distance. Unilateral or bilateral palatal osteotomies (*vertical red lines*) are performed lateral to the nasal septum and medial to the greater palatine neurovascular bundle to allow the correction of transverse maxillary discrepancies. If the interdental osteotomies are planned between the canines and premolars, the orthodontist should ensure that the intercanine width is sufficient to accommodate the mandibular arch. (*e*) The posttreatment occlusion.

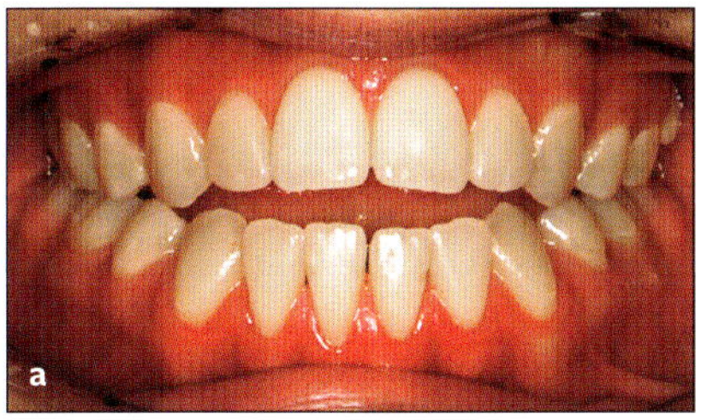

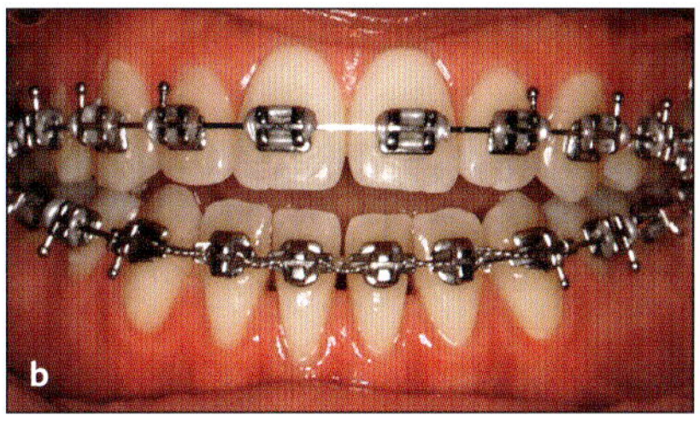

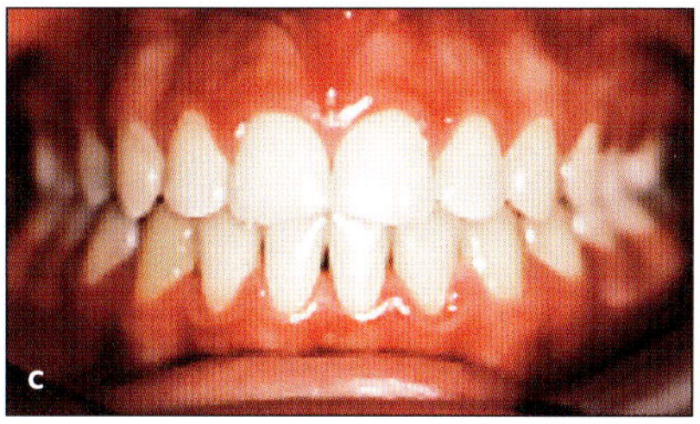

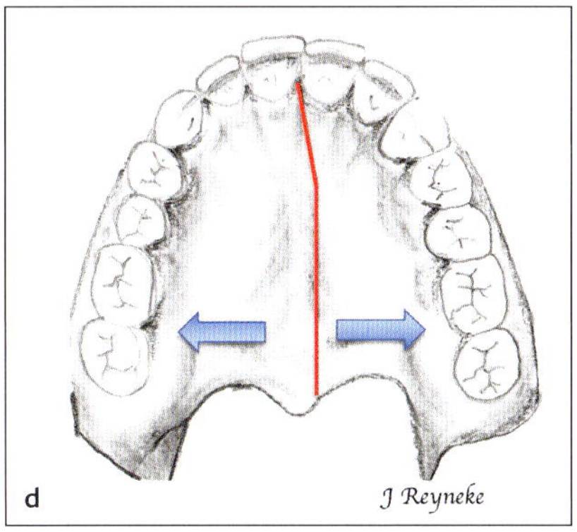

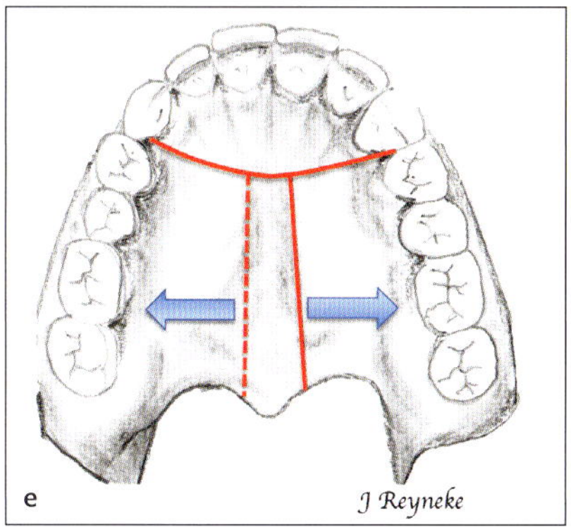

Fig 5-29 (*a*) Single occlusal plane of the maxilla. (*b*) A continuous archwire is used to level the maxillary occlusion on a single plane. Maxillary transverse arch discrepancy is corrected by segmental surgery, and depending on the orthodontic arch alignment, the position of the interdental osteotomy may vary. (*c*) The posttreatment occlusion. (*d*) The interdental osteotomy is planned between the central incisors. (*e*) The interdental osteotomies are planned between the canines and premolars, which will allow for independent transverse repositioning of the posterior segments.

- Surgical expansion of the maxillary buccal segments (segmental surgery): In patients with a dual occlusal plane and transverse maxillary deficiency, a three-piece Le Fort I osteotomy with interdental osteotomies between the lateral incisor and canine is usually performed; single maxillary occlusal plane orthodontic preparation requires a two-piece Le Fort I osteotomy, and depending on the orthodontic preparation of the two segments, the interdental osteotomy is usually performed between the maxillary central incisors or unilaterally between the lateral incisor and canine.
- Autorotation of the mandible: The mandible will autorotate superiorly and anteriorly (the anterior vector is larger in patients with a high occlusal plane angle). Patients

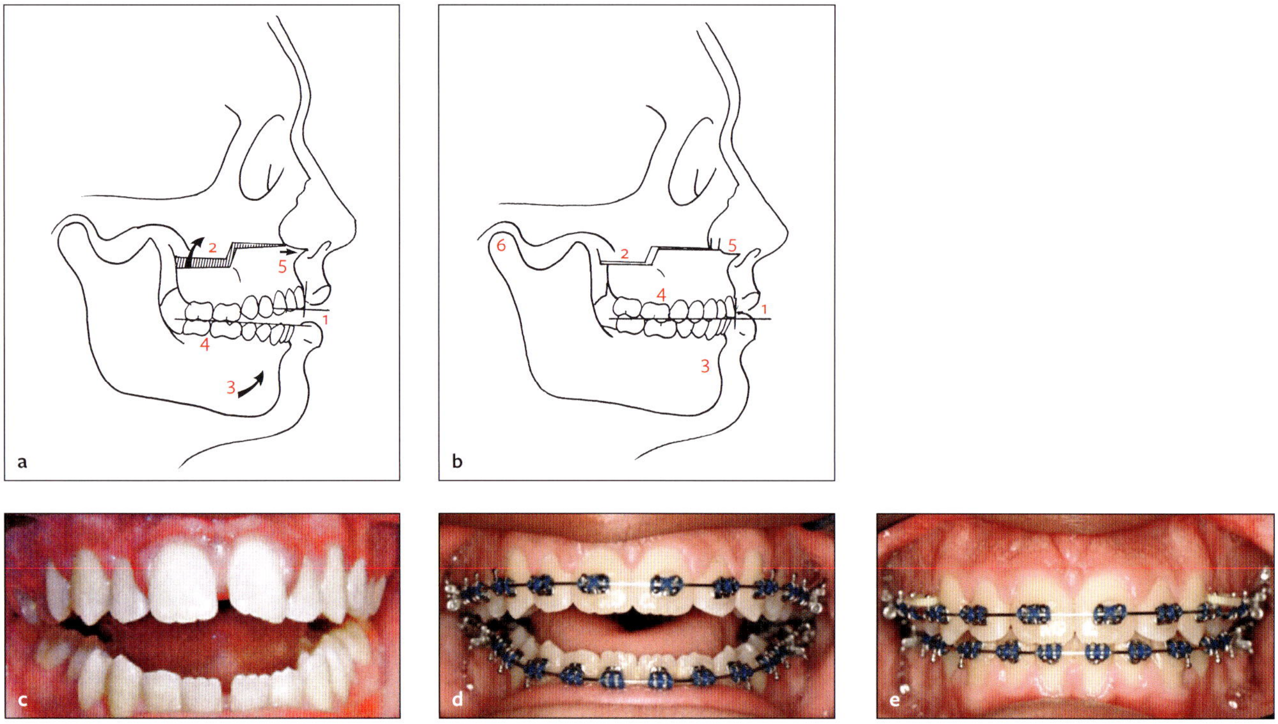

Fig 5-30 (*a*) (1) Maintenance of maxillary incisor–upper lip relationship (anteroposterior and vertical). (2) Superior repositioning of posterior maxilla. (3) Autorotation of mandible. (4) Occlusal plane of mandible, which determines the final occlusal plane. (5) Forward rotation of the ANS. (*b*) (1) Maintenance of ideal maxillary incisor–lip relationship. (2) Posterior maxilla superiorly repositioned. (3) Mandible rotated counterclockwise (rotation around a point at the condyle). (4) Class I malocclusion. (5) ANS advanced. (6) Condyle-fossa relationship maintained. The maxillary arch has one plane (*c*) and is leveled and aligned with a continuous archwire (*d*). (*e*) The occlusion following surgery.

with facial features indicative of maxillary anteroposterior deficiency (large nose, convex nasal dorsum, deficient paranasal anatomy, lack of supratip break, and poor lip support) would benefit from the obligatory maxillary advancement. Those with normal midface esthetics will experience unesthetic changes with isolated superior and anterior repositioning of the maxilla. For these patients, simultaneous mandibular setback is necessary to avoid undesirable maxillary advancement. Finally, the facial esthetics of a small percentage of patients may necessitate more maxillary advancement than is dictated by the mandible after autorotation. For these patients, the clinician should consider additional advancement of the maxilla, which will require simultaneous surgical advancement of the mandible.

The anteroposterior position of the chin is not a primary determining factor in the patients previously discussed. In most of these patients, excessive or deficient chin projection can be corrected by an appropriate genioplasty; however, the shape of the chin and the depth of the labiomental fold should be considered.

In summary, the surgical solutions may include the following:

- Maxillary superior repositioning with or without genioplasty
- Maxillary superior repositioning with mandibular setback, with or without genioplasty
- Maxillary superior repositioning with mandibular advancement, with or without genioplasty
- Possible maxillary superior repositioning in a single piece (more posterior than anterior, as indicated by the mandibular occlusal plane after autorotation) or in segments, allowing differential superior repositioning of the anterior and posterior segments and simultaneous expansion of the buccal segments (again, as dictated by the occlusal plane of the mandible and the mandibular dental arch form)

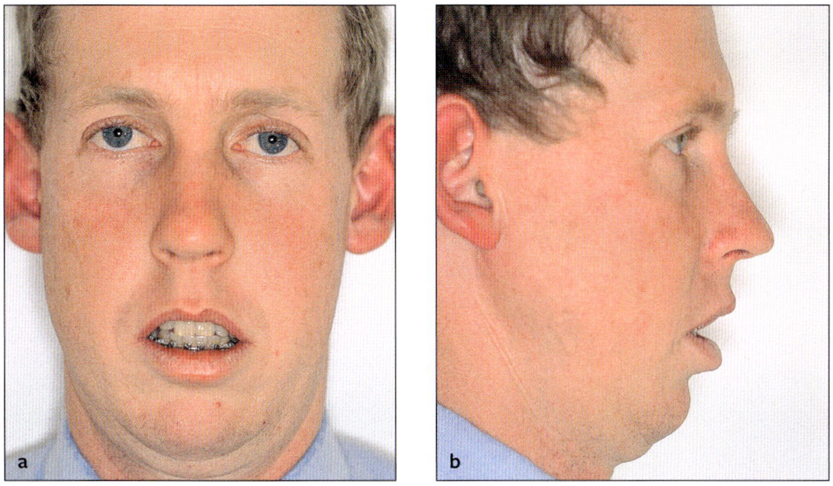

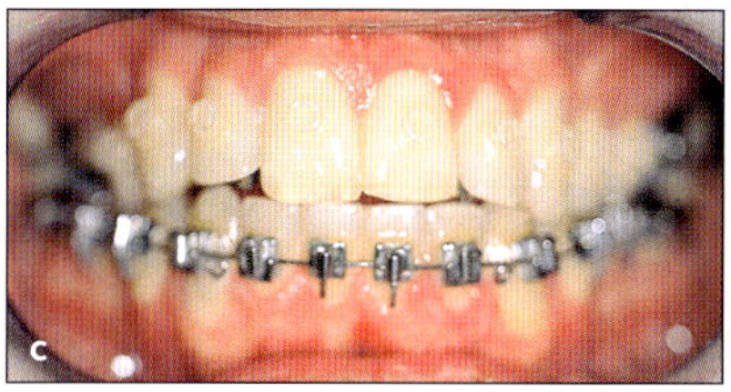

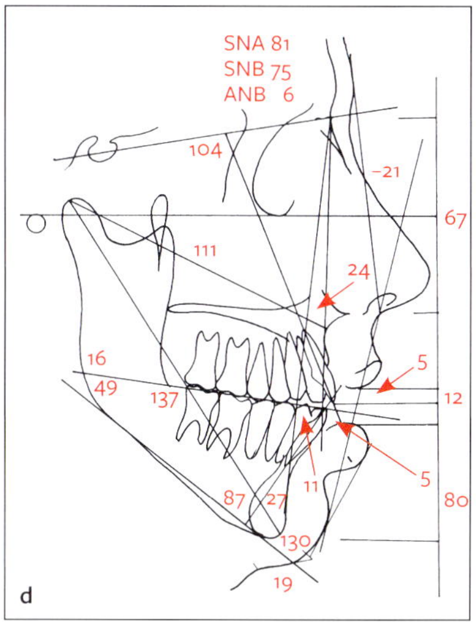

Fig 5-31 Case 6. Presurgical frontal view (*a*), profile view (*b*), and occlusion (*c*). Note the placement of white lingual buttons on the buccal surfaces of the maxillary teeth just prior to surgery. (*d*) Presurgical cephalometric analysis. Posterior vertical maxillary excess: interlabial gap = 12 mm, increased lower facial height: ratio of middle to lower third = 67:80 mm; slight anterior maxillary vertical excess: maxillary incisor exposure = 5 mm; convex profile: facial contour angle = −21 degrees; mandible rotated clockwise because of vertical maxillary excess: mandibular plane = 49 degrees; microgenia: lip-chin-throat angle = 130 degrees, chin-throat length = 19 mm.

Case 6

Case 6 demonstrates correction of a Class I anterior open bite (Fig 5-31).

General characteristics of Class II open bite

Clinical characteristics

- Increased lower facial height
- Recessive chin
- Vertical maxillary excess
- Often, excessive exposure of maxillary incisors
- Increased interlabial gap
- Skeletal Class II relationship
- Transverse maxillary deficiency (posterior crossbite)
- Increased mandibular plane angle
- Possibly a skeletal Class I malocclusion rotated to a Class II malocclusion

Orthodontic preparation

1. Single-piece Le Fort I osteotomy
   - Level, align, and coordinate the maxillary arch, and align the mandibular arch.
   - Do not attempt to close the open bite by expansion of the buccal segments, extrusion of the anterior teeth, or intrusion of the posterior teeth.
   - Expand the buccal segments of teeth only where the teeth are palatally inclined in relation to the basal bone.
2. Segmental Le Fort I osteotomy
   - Level and align the maxillary dental arch in segments.
   - Align the segments to be compatible with the mandibular arch.
   - Deviate the roots at the intended interdental osteotomy areas.
   - Do not attempt to expand or close bites orthodontically.
   - Level and align the mandibular arch.

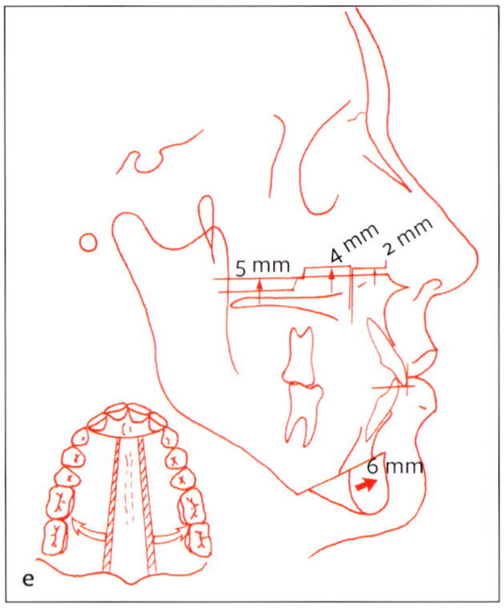

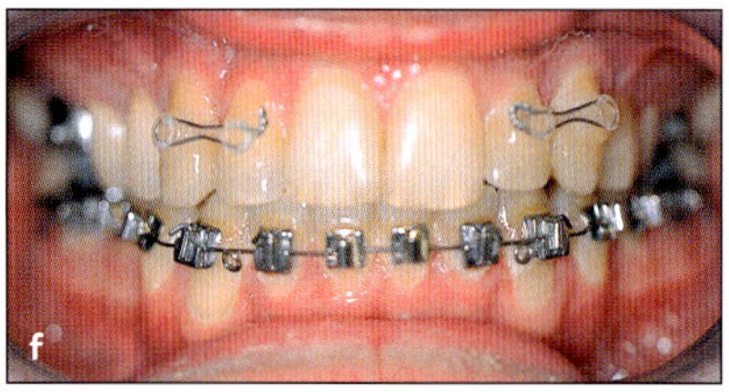

Fig 5-31 *(cont)* (*e*) Surgical cephalometric visual treatment objective—Le Fort I maxillary osteotomy: superior repositioning of posterior maxillary segments (5 mm posterior and 4 mm anterior), superior repositioning of anterior maxillary segment (2 mm), expansion of the posterior segments (inset), counterclockwise autorotation of the mandible, and advancement genioplasty (6 mm). (*f*) Immediate postsurgical occlusion. Note the interdental wires placed around the presurgically placed buccal brackets of the teeth next to the interdental osteotomies. Brackets are placed on all the teeth just prior to surgery to facilitate maxillomandibular fixation during surgery and the placement of elastics after surgery. Posttreatment frontal view (*g*), profile view (*h*), and occlusion (*i*).

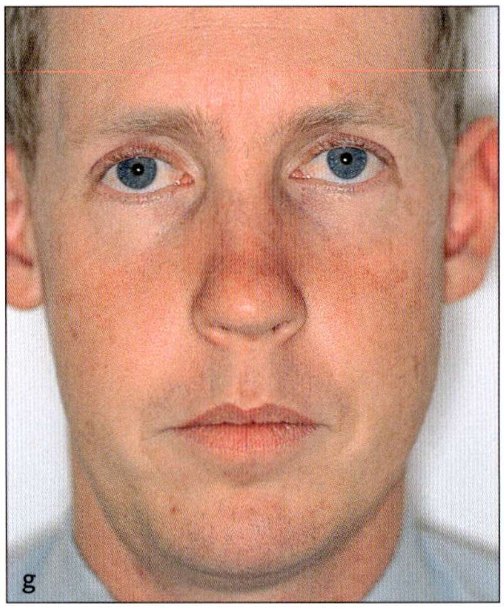

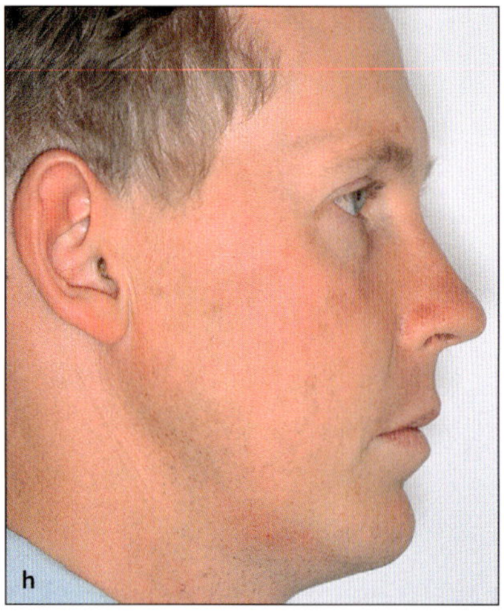

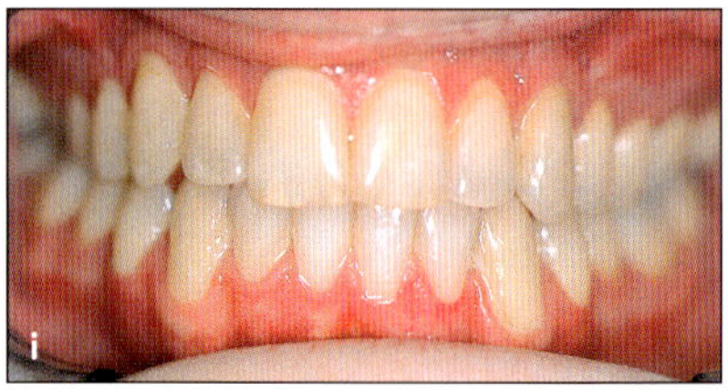

Surgical solutions

Following are surgical solutions to Class II open bites (Fig 5-32):

- Superior repositioning of the maxilla (total or segmental): open bite corrected by repositioning the posterior maxilla (segment) more superiorly than the anterior maxilla
- Surgical expansion of the buccal segments by segmental surgery
- Autorotation of the mandible
- Surgical advancement of the mandible
- Advancement genioplasty

As a consequence of superior repositioning of the maxilla, the mandible will rotate counterclockwise (superiorly and forward) around a point at or just behind the condyle. The forward vector may be sufficient to allow only superior repositioning of the maxilla with no anteroposterior change. Patients with high mandibular plane angles will have more forward rotation of the mandibular incisors than those with low angles.

Patients who do not require mandibular advancement may require slight posterior movement of the maxilla; however, this movement will compromise the facial esthetic results. For patients with normal midface facial esthetics and especially for those with large noses, deficient concave paranasal areas, or obtuse nasolabial angles, maxillary setback should not be attempted. These patients require simultaneous superior repositioning of the maxilla and advancement of the mandible. Mandibular autorotation as a result of maxillary repositioning is demonstrated in Fig 5-33.

Case 7

This 32-year-old woman sought treatment after being told by her general practitioner that she would eventually lose her teeth as a consequence of her open bite.

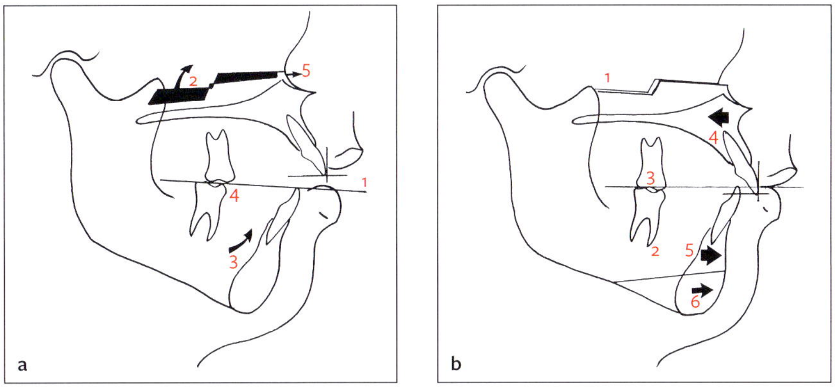

Fig 5-32 (*a*) (1) Maintain maxillary incisor–upper lip relationship (anteroposterior and vertical). (2) Superiorly reposition the posterior maxilla. (3) Mandible will autorotate. (4) The mandibular occlusal plane determines the final occlusal plane. (5) The ANS is rotated forward. (*b*) (1) The posterior maxilla is superiorly repositioned. (2) The mandible has autorotated. (3) There is still a Class II malocclusion with an increased overjet. Options include maxillary setback (seldom used) (4), mandibular advancement (5), and genioplasty advancement (6).

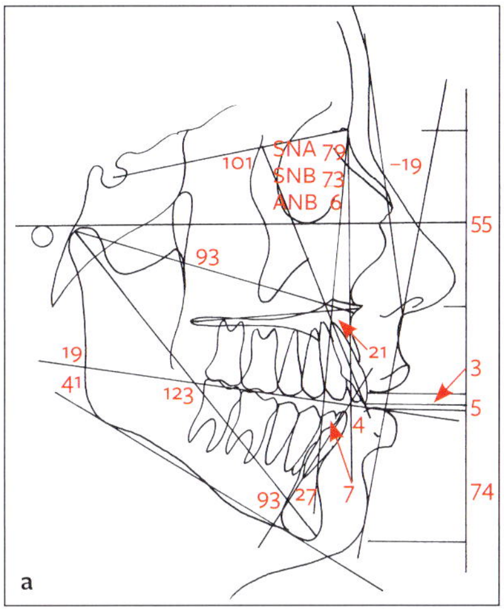

Fig 5-33 (*a*) Lateral cephalometric analysis of a patient with a Class II anterior open bite malocclusion requiring surgical correction. (*b*) On the surgical prediction tracing, the maxilla has been superiorly repositioned and the mandible autorotated around a point at the condyle. The occlusion is still Class II with an increased overjet. The surgeon now has two choices: to set the maxilla back (1) or to advance the mandible (2). (*c*) Prediction tracing illustrating the expected hard and soft tissue changes after maxillary setback. The midface is flattened, the upper lip support is diminished, and the nasolabial angle is increased. (*d*) The maxilla has been superiorly repositioned, and the mandible has autorotated and been advanced on the prediction tracing. A more esthetic result will be achieved with this treatment option.

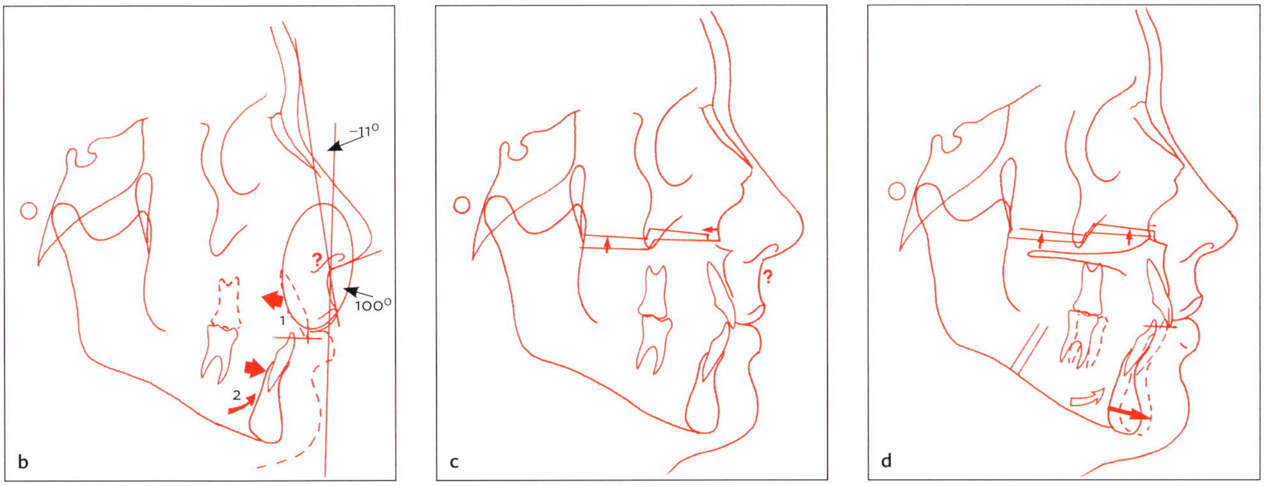

Main complaint

The patient's main complaint was an inability to maintain closure of her mouth and difficulty in chewing, which was sometimes socially embarrassing.

Medical history

The patient had asthma and took medication before physical exercise only.

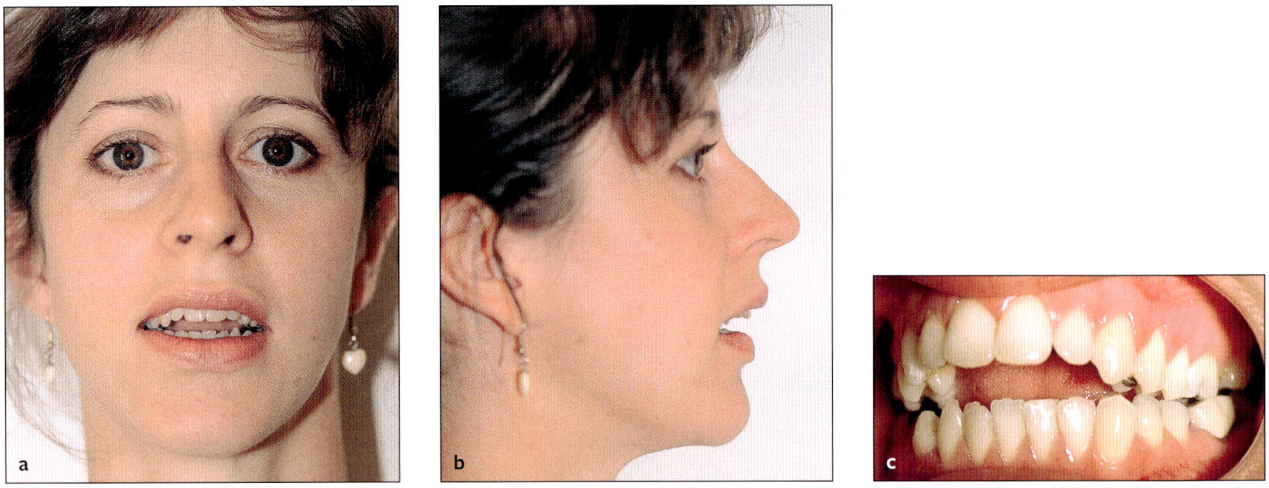

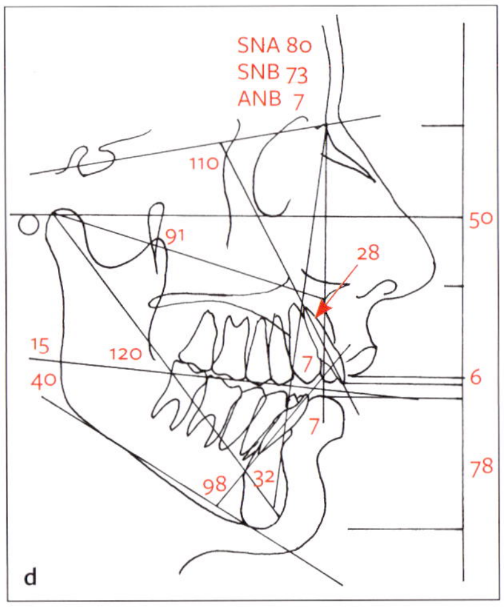

Fig 5-34 Case 7. Pretreatment frontal view (*a*), profile view (*b*), and occlusion (*c*). (*d*) Pretreatment cephalometric analysis. Class II occlusion; anterior open bite; increased interlabial gap: 6 mm; increased lower facial height: ratio of middle third to lower third = 50:78 mm; mandibular anteroposterior deficiency: SNB = 73 degrees; increased mandibular plane angle: 40 degrees; maxillary incisor protrusion: maxillary incisor to S-N = 110 degrees, maxillary incisor to N-A = 28 degrees and 7 mm. The maxillary incisor–upper lip relationship is good (1.5-mm tooth exposure); it is important to maintain this relationship during treatment.

Clinical examination

1. Soft tissue
   - Frontal view (Fig 5-34a)
     - Increased interlabial distance
     - Increased lower facial third height
     - Nasal asymmetry
   - Profile view (Fig 5-34b)
     - Convex profile
     - Increased lower facial third height
     - Increased interlabial distance
     - Mandibular anteroposterior deficiency
     - Protruding upper lip
     - Acute lip-chin-throat angle
2. Dental (Fig 5-34c)
   - Anterior open bite
   - Mandibular left first molar root has been treated but is broken down and has a poor prognosis
   - Narrow maxillary arch
   - Class II malocclusion
   - Tendency for posterior crossbites
   - Maxillary dental protrusion
3. Skeletal (Fig 5-34d)
   - Mandibular anteroposterior deficiency
   - Posterior maxillary vertical excess
   - Transverse maxillary deficiency
4. Radiographic
   - Panoramic radiograph
     - Broken-down crown of the left mandibular first molar (tooth has had root canal treatment)
     - Several restored teeth
   - Cephalometric radiograph
     - Class II malocclusion
     - Mandible rotated clockwise
     - Vertical excess of the posterior maxilla
     - Increased lower facial height
     - Large interlabial gap
     - Ideal upper lip–maxillary incisor relationship (3-mm incisor exposure)

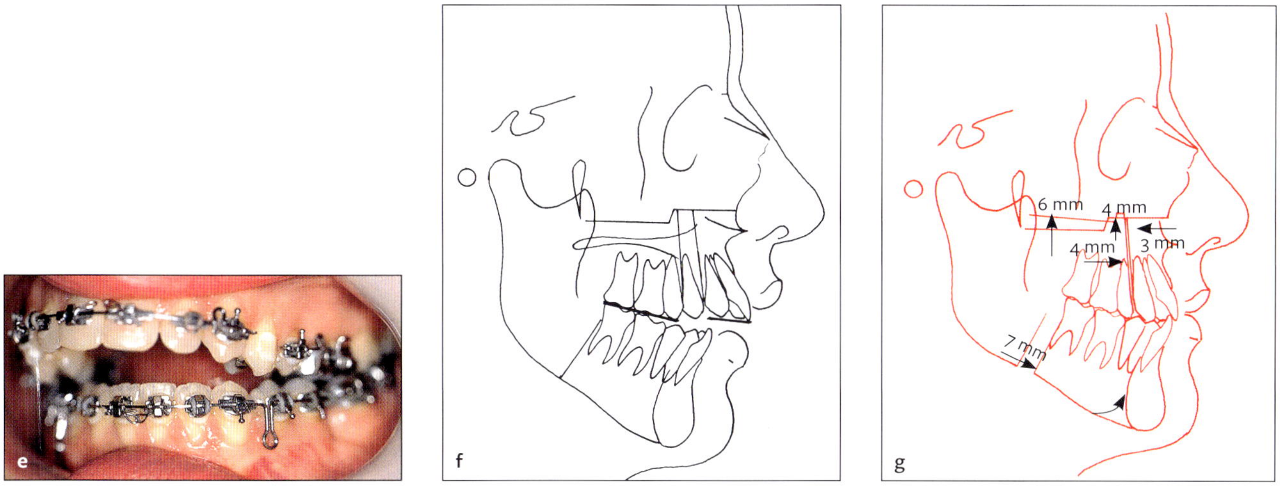

Fig 5-34 *(cont)* (*e*) Immediate presurgical occlusion. Note the segmental orthodontic alignment of the maxillary arch. The first premolars are not banded and will be extracted at surgery. (*f*) Immediate presurgical tracing that plans the extraction of the first premolars, superior repositioning of the posterior maxillary segments, expansion of the maxilla, slight retraction of the anterior maxillary segment, and advancement of the mandible. (*g*) The predicted postsurgical result.

Problem list

- Anterior open bite
- Increased interlabial gap
- Mandibular anteroposterior deficiency
- Maxillary transverse deficiency
- Posterior maxillary vertical excess
- Broken-down left mandibular first molar
- Maxillary dental protrusion

Presurgical orthodontics

Maxillary arch (Fig 5-34e)

- Alignment of the maxillary arch in three segments, from the right second premolar to the right second molar, the right canine to the left canine, and the left second premolar to the left second molar
- Extraction of both first premolars at the time of surgery to allow ideal surgical positioning of the anterior maxillary segment
- Deviation of the roots of both canines and both second premolars to allow surgical closure of the extraction spaces of both first premolars

Mandibular arch (see Fig 5-34e)

- Extraction of the left mandibular first molar
- Closure of the space where the left first molar was extracted
- Leveling and alignment of the arch

Surgical treatment

Both maxillary first premolars were extracted (Figs 5-34f and 5-34g). A three-piece Le Fort I osteotomy was performed with the interdental osteotomy through the extraction sites of the maxillary first premolars. Removal of bone in the extraction spaces allowed surgical closure of the spaces, and a palatal osteotomy allowed expansion of the posterior segments (see Figs 5-34f and 5-34g). The anterior maxillary segment was repositioned; this was critical for two reasons: (1) the vertical upper lip–maxillary incisor relationship had to be maintained, and (2) the segment could not be retracted excessively because that would undermine lip support and increase the labiomental angle. The posterior segment of the maxilla was superiorly repositioned to allow the mandible to autorotate, and the mandible was advanced with a bilateral sagittal split osteotomy (see Figs 5-34f and 5-34g).

Postsurgical orthodontics

Postsurgical orthodontics entailed final closure of extraction spaces, finalization of the occlusion, and retainer wear. Closure of the extraction space of the mandibular left first molar prolonged the orthodontic preparation, and surgery was performed 25 months after commencement of orthodontic treatment. The orthodontic bands were removed 9 months after surgery. The 2-year postsurgical results are illustrated in Figs 5-34h to 5-34j.

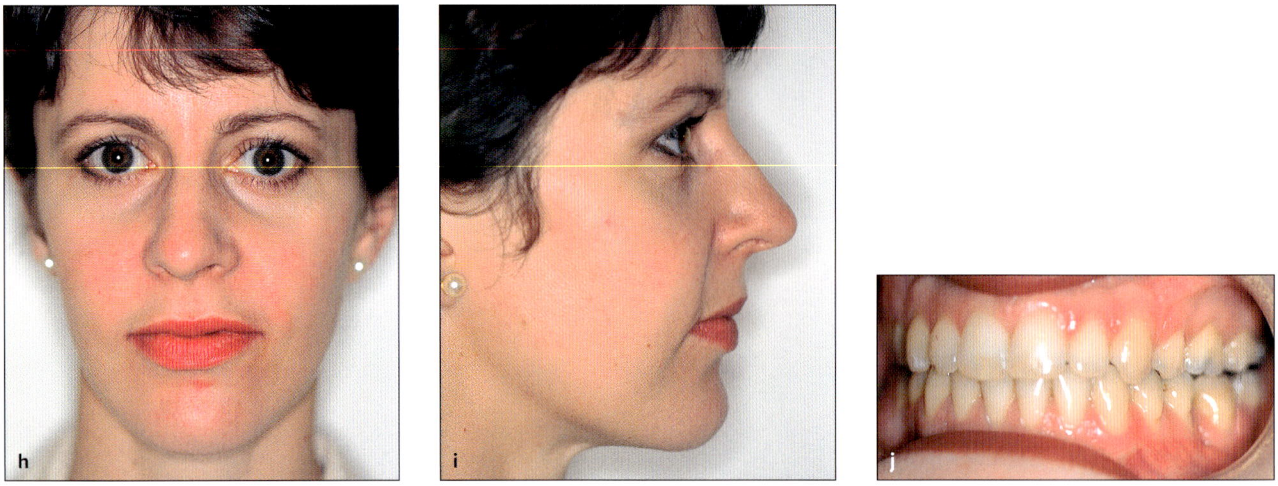

Fig 5-34 (*cont*) Posttreatment frontal view (*h*), profile view (*i*), and occlusion (*j*).

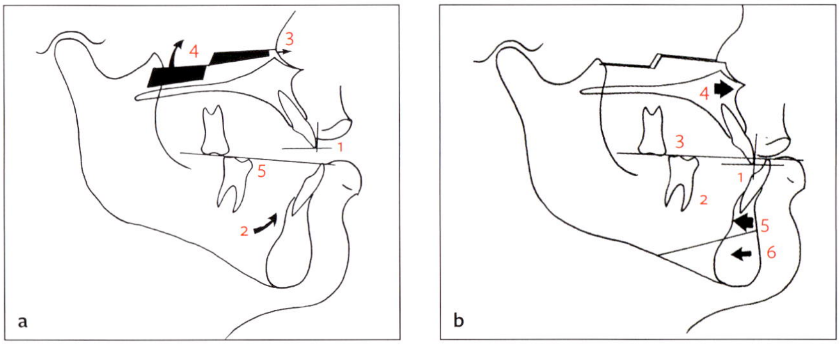

Fig 5-35 (*a*) (1) The maxillary incisor–upper lip relationship is ideal and should be maintained anteroposteriorly and vertically. (2) Autorotation of the mandible. (3) Forward rotation of the ANS. (4) Superior repositioning of the posterior maxilla. (5) Final occlusal plane determined by the mandibular occlusal plane after rotation. (*b*) (1) Ideal maxillary incisor–upper lip relationship. (2) The mandible has autorotated. (3) Occlusion is more Class III with an anterior crossbite. Options include maxillary advancement (4), mandibular setback (5), both options 4 and 5, and/or genioplasty to improve the chin shape (6).

General characteristics of Class III open bite

Clinical characteristics

- Mandibular anteroposterior excess (magnitude of the anteroposterior discrepancy masked by backward rotation of the mandible)
- Maxillary vertical excess (more posterior than anterior)
- Transverse maxillary deficiency
- Posterior crossbites
- Class III malocclusion
- Often, a reverse curve of Spee
- Increased mandibular plane angle
- Clockwise rotation of the mandible improves the Class III relationship, and vertical correction makes it worse

Orthodontic preparation

- Remove any existing dental compensation.
- Where segmental surgery is contemplated, align the maxillary arch in segments, and deviate roots at interdental osteotomy areas.
- Level and align the mandibular arch.

Surgical solutions

Following are surgical solutions to Class III open bite (Fig 5-35):

- Single-piece Le Fort I osteotomy with superior repositioning of the maxilla (more posterior than anterior) to achieve the ideal maxillary incisor–upper lip relationship
- Segmental surgery with differential superior repositioning of the maxilla (the posterior segments more superiorly than the anterior segment)
- Expansion of the buccal segments
- Mandibular setback
- Genioplasty

Comments on Class III open bite

Inferior repositioning of the anterior maxilla and superior repositioning of the posterior maxilla are often indicated. The anterior maxilla often may be vertically deficient in patients with Class III open bite, and the maxillary tooth–lip relationship is an important consideration in planning the final vertical position of the maxilla.

The mandible will autorotate, and the Class III occlusal relationship will worsen.

The anteroposterior discrepancy can be corrected by advancement of the maxilla, mandibular setback, both maxillary advancement and mandibular setback, and/or genioplasty. The treatment of choice depends on the esthetic requirements of the patient.

The cause of the open bite should be determined before treatment planning. Open bites may develop because of deficient eruption of maxillary incisors (anterior), deficient eruption of mandibular incisors (anterior), deficient eruption of maxillary and/or mandibular molars (posterior), or excessive vertical development of the posterior maxilla.

The key element of the analysis is evaluation of the vertical relationship of the maxillary incisors to the relaxed upper lip (keep lip length in mind). Deficient eruption of mandibular incisors with a reverse curve of Spee is often caused by an abnormal size and resting posture of the tongue.

Posterior open bites can develop in three ways:

1. Excessive vertical development on one side, often associated with facial asymmetry (eg, unilateral condylar hyperplasia)
2. Deficient eruption of teeth on one side (eg, impacted teeth) with normal symmetry
3. Bilateral deficient eruption of posterior teeth (eg, cleidocranial dysostosis or large tongue) with normal symmetry

Case 8

This case demonstrates the correction of a Class III anterior open bite. A 19-year-old man was referred to the orthodontist by his general practitioner for the correction of an open bite.

Main complaint

The patient said he was unable to bite properly, and the flat appearance of his midface bothered him.

Medical history

The patient had asthma. He had contracted hepatitis A at age 15 years and recovered satisfactorily.

Clinical examination

1. Soft tissue
   - Frontal view (Fig 5-36a)
     - Deficient paranasal areas
     - Increased interlabial distance
     - Excessive lower lip vermilion exposure
   - Profile view (Fig 5-36b)
     - Concave profile
     - Midface deficiency
     - Everted lower lip
     - Increased interlabial distance
     - Deficient chin
2. Dental (Fig 5-36c)
   - Class III malocclusion
   - Anterior open bite
   - Slightly compensated mandibular incisors
3. Skeletal (Fig 5-36d)
   - Maxillary anteroposterior deficiency
   - Mandibular anteroposterior excess
   - Posterior maxillary vertical excess
   - Microgenia
4. Radiographic
   - Panoramic radiograph
     - Impacted maxillary third molars and partially erupted mandibular third molars
   - Cephalometric radiograph (see Fig 5-36d)
     - Class III malocclusion
     - Class III skeletal relationship
     - Maxillary anteroposterior deficiency
     - Anterior open bite
     - Slightly lingually inclined mandibular incisors
     - Lack of dental support for the upper lip
     - Everted lower lip
     - Mandibular anteroposterior excess
     - Flat chin

Problem list

- Class III anterior open bite malocclusion
- Maxillary anteroposterior excess
- Posterior maxillary vertical excess
- Incisor compensation

Presurgical orthodontics

Maxillary arch (Figs 5-36c to 5-36j)

- Removal of the third molars
- Leveling and alignment of the arch
- Establishment of arch compatibility with the mandible
- No attempt to close the open bite by extrusion of incisors or by intrusion or expansion of posterior teeth

Mandibular arch (see Figs 5-36e to 5-36j)

- Removal of the third molars
- Leveling and alignment of the arch
- Slight decompensation of incisors

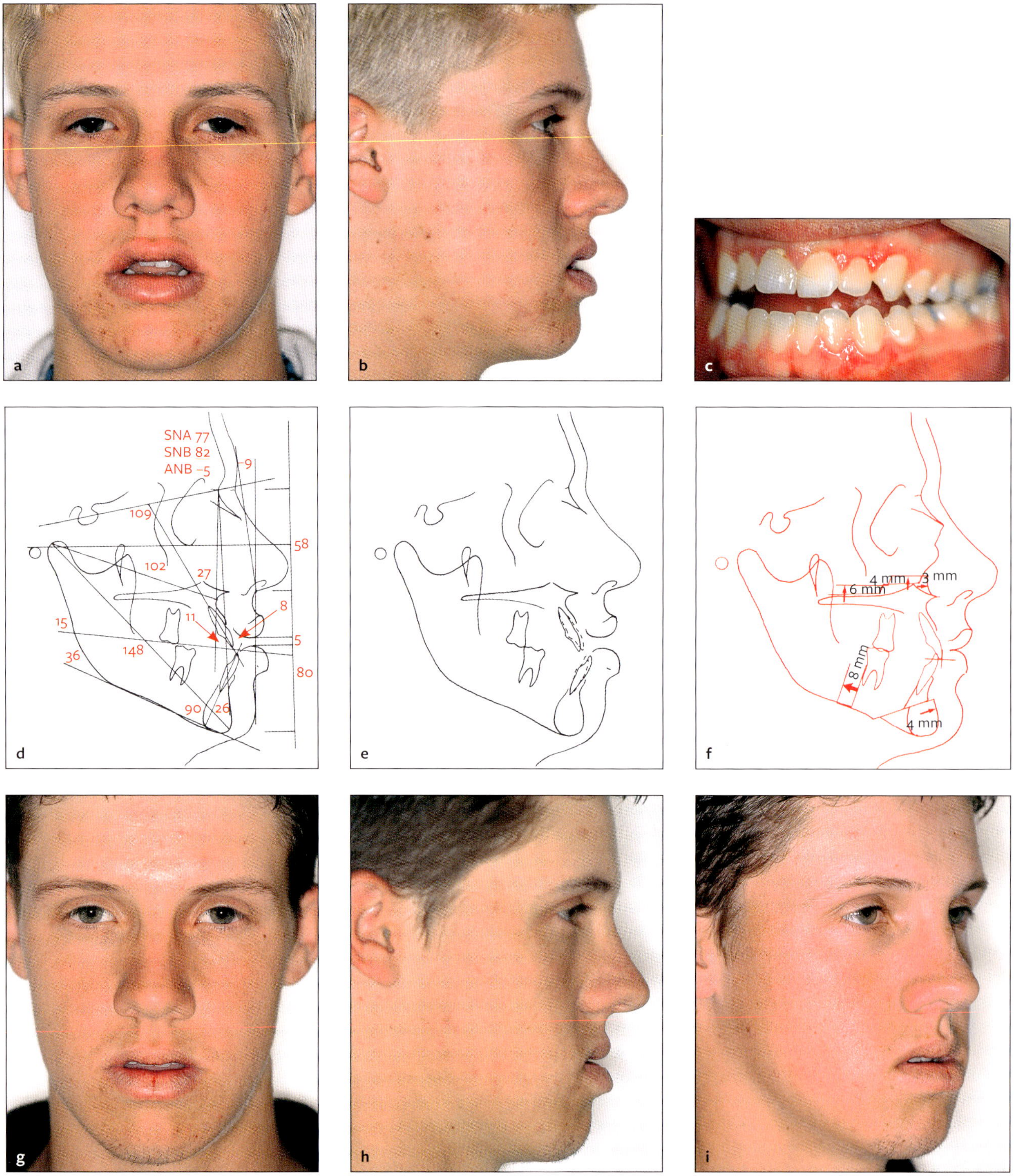

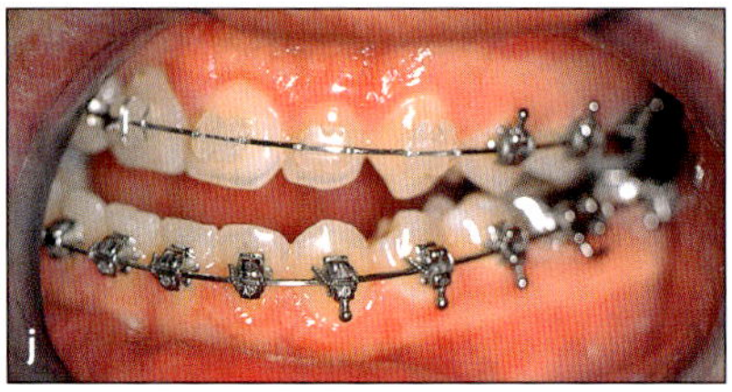

Fig 5-36 Case 8. Pretreatment frontal view (*a*), profile view (*b*), and occlusion (*c*). (*d*) Pretreatment cephalometric analysis. Maxillary anteroposterior deficiency: SNA = 77 degrees; Class III skeletal relationship: ANB = -5 degrees; concave profile: facial contour angle = -9 degrees. (*e*) Orthodontic change: decompensation of the incisors. (*f*) The surgical visual treatment objective includes maxillary superior repositioning with advancement, mandibular setback, and advancement genioplasty. Presurgical frontal view (*g*), profile view (*h*), three-quarter view (*i*), and occlusion (*j*). →

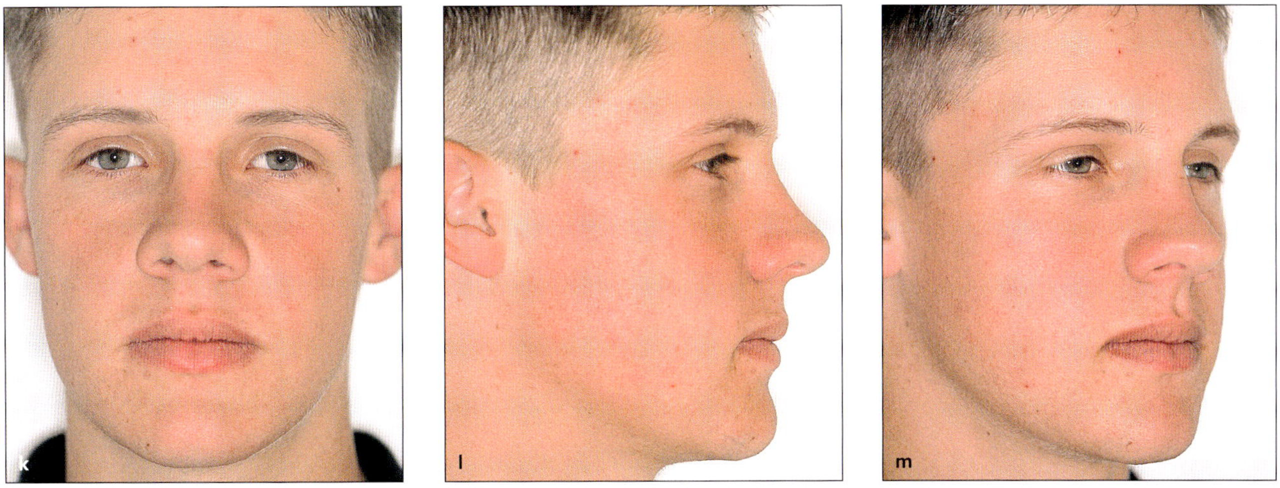

Fig 5-36 *(cont)* Posttreatment results are demonstrated in frontal view (*k*), profile view (*l*), three-quarter view (*m*), and occlusion (*n*).

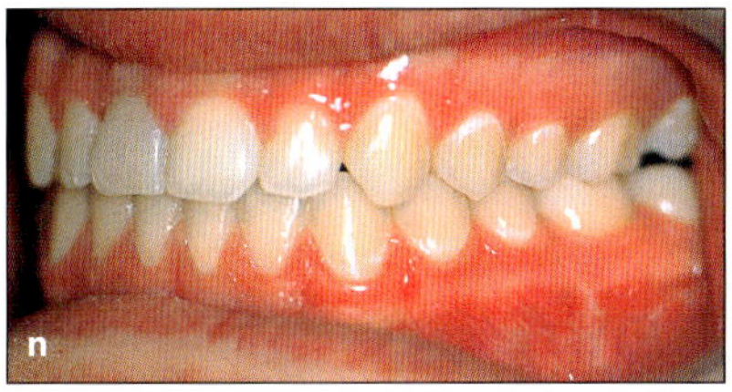

Surgical treatment

A Le Fort I maxillary osteotomy was used to advance the maxilla by 3 mm. At the same time, the maxilla was superiorly repositioned 3 mm anteriorly (to establish the ideal tooth-lip relationship) and 6 mm posteriorly (to allow autorotation of the mandible; see Fig 5-36f).

Because autorotation of the mandible worsened the Class III relationship, the mandible was set back 8 mm with a BSSO. Finally, a 4-mm advancement genioplasty was performed. The advancement of the chin not only enhances the chin shape but also maintains the chin-throat length after mandibular setback.

Postsurgical orthodontics

Postsurgical orthodontic treatment involved finalization of the occlusion and retention. The presurgical orthodontic preparation took 8 months, and the orthodontic bands were removed 3 months after surgery. Figures 5-36k to 5-36n illustrate the treatment result after a total treatment time of 11 months.

Maxillary expansion

The transverse dimension of the maxilla can be increased in four ways: (1) orthodontically through dental tipping; (2) via rapid palatal orthodontic expansion in growing patients; (3) through surgically assisted orthodontic palatal expansion in nongrowing patients; and (4) through surgical expansion by means of segmental surgery. When planning for the correction of transverse maxillary deficiency, the strengths and weaknesses of each applicable option should be understood and considered. The flowchart in Fig 5-37 summarizes the treatment options for transverse arch discrepancies.

Maxillary transverse deficiency usually results in posterior crossbites and has an incidence among the general population of approximately 9.4%. Because the relative transverse dimension between the maxilla and mandible is also influenced by their anteroposterior relationship, Jacobs et al (1980) divided transverse discrepancies into *relative* or *absolute* posterior crossbites. The determination is made when the patient's dental cast is held in central

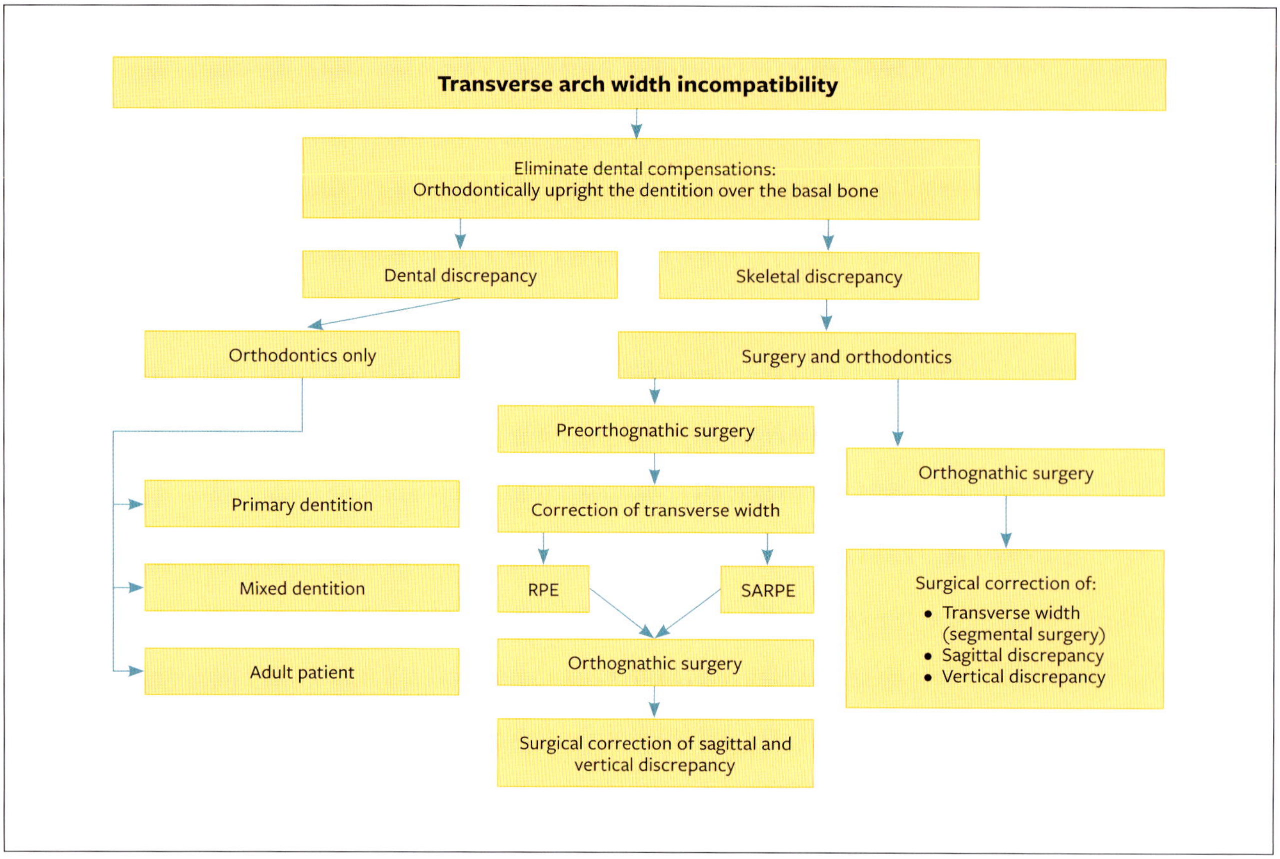

Fig 5-37 This flowchart simplifies the decision-making process in relation to orthodontic dental expansion, rapid maxillary expansion (in adolescents), surgically assisted expansion, and surgical expansion of the maxilla by means of segmental maxillary surgery. It is clear that orthodontic expansion should be reserved when only dental expansion is required. Surgically assisted expansion is indicated when no orthognathic surgery is planned or when severe crowding makes presurgical orthodontic preparation for orthognathic surgery impossible. Existing transverse maxillary deficiency can in most instances be corrected by segmental expansion at the time of definitive orthognathic surgery.

relation and posterior crossbite is evident. The casts are then moved to position the dental arches into a Class I canine relationship. If the crossbite is corrected with the anteroposterior alignment of the arches, it is considered a *relative* transverse discrepancy. If the crossbite still exists following the movement, it is considered an *absolute* transverse discrepancy (Fig 5-38).

An absolute posterior crossbite may occur bilaterally or unilaterally and is often associated with a Class II anterior open bite dentofacial deformity. However, absolute crossbites may also occur in Class I and Class III malocclusions. The etiology of posterior crossbites may be congenital, traumatic, iatrogenic, or developmental. The restricted transverse growth caused by surgical intervention in patients with cleft lip and palate is an example of iatrogenic origin, whereas long-term thumbsucking is a good example of developmental etiology.

The typical clinical findings in a patient with a posterior crossbite are a narrow maxillary dental arch (often with an hourglass-shaped arch form), a high palatal vault, dental crowding often with palatally inclined posterior teeth, an anterior open bite, and a Class II malocclusion. A dental crossbite involving only one or two teeth should be treated orthodontically. However, a crossbite involving more than two teeth is likely skeletal in nature, and a surgical orthodontic approach should be considered.

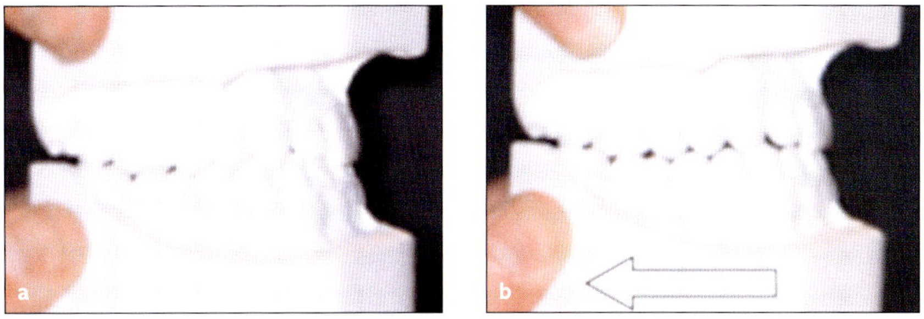

Fig 5-38 Assessment of posterior crossbites on the dental casts. (*a*) In patients with posterior crossbites, the handheld dental casts are repositioned so that the canines are in a Class I relationship. If a crossbite still exists, it should be considered an absolute crossbite and must be addressed during anteroposterior correction of the occlusion. (*b*) However, if the crossbites are corrected by moving the casts (arrow), the crossbites are relative and will be rectified automatically during correction of anteroposterior discrepancies.

Orthodontic expansion

The treatment usually involves dental tipping and is indicated when the skeletal base width is adequate. The required transverse arch dimension can be achieved by moving the teeth buccally using orthodontic forces; however, stability is doubtful after orthodontic tipping of the posterior teeth beyond their bony base. Dental tipping leads to "hanging" of the palatal cusps of the posterior teeth below the occlusal plane and will complicate subsequent surgical expansion. The increased angulation of the molars will require additional surgical expansion of the palate (see Fig 2-24). This action will not only jeopardize the skeletal stability but will also build orthodontic dental relapse into the surgical result.

Rapid palatal expansion

Growth of the maxilla takes place at the suture margins by deposition of new bone from the adjacent cellular layer. The principle of orthopedic expansion of the palate relies on the physiology of normal active growth and elasticity of the new bone at the suture lines. Cellular activity at the suture lines decreases with age, and a wide age range—between 16 and 35 years—before completion of the synostosis has been reported. However, it is generally accepted that rapid palatal expansion without surgical assistance is clinically successful only until the age of 14 to 16 years. As much as 30% to 50% of the gain in the transverse dimension with this method can be lost as a result of relapse, which proves that most of the width is obtained by dental tipping and not skeletal expansion. Orthopedic expansion of the maxilla beyond the age of 16 years has certain disadvantages, including severe pain, pressure necrosis of the palatal soft tissue, dental tipping with no skeletal change, and uncontrolled relapse.

Surgically assisted palatal expansion

This treatment option should be considered in the following situations: (*1*) for the creation of arch length in patients with severe crowding and when extractions are not an option (eg, premolars already removed); (*2*) for patients in whom unilateral maxillary expansion is required; (*3*) where maxillary expansion is the only surgery indicated; and (*4*) for any patient in whom orthodontic expansion has failed and suture resistance must be overcome. The surgical technique involves bilateral osteotomies of the lateral walls of the maxilla carried from the piriform apertures past the zygomatic buttresses. The pterygomaxillary junctures are separated, and the palatal osteotomy is carried forward from the PNS to just posterior to the incisive canal. Two paramedian osteotomies may be performed in patients who require large expansions; this design also prevents unfavorable nasal septum deviation. The distractor may be tooth-borne or bone-borne, and the device should remain in place for at least 8 to 10 weeks following completion of distraction. Relapse occurs following distraction with both appliances; however, the bone-borne appliances prove to be more stable.

Surgical expansion

Surgical expansion can be accomplished by either posterior segmental osteotomies or a Le Fort I osteotomy, segmenting the maxilla in the downfractured position. When a large amount of expansion is required, bilateral palatal osteotomies should be performed. The osteotomy should be made just lateral to the nasal septum where the palatal bone is thin and the mucosa thick. Soft tissue release may be helpful for large expansion and should be performed off the osteotomy line. Care should also be taken to ensure that the nasal mucosa is intact when performing soft tissue release. Perforation of the nasal mucosa as well as the palatal mucosa may result in the development of an oronasal fistula. Grafting and appropriate rigid fixation should be used in palatal expansions of more than 3 mm. Postsur-

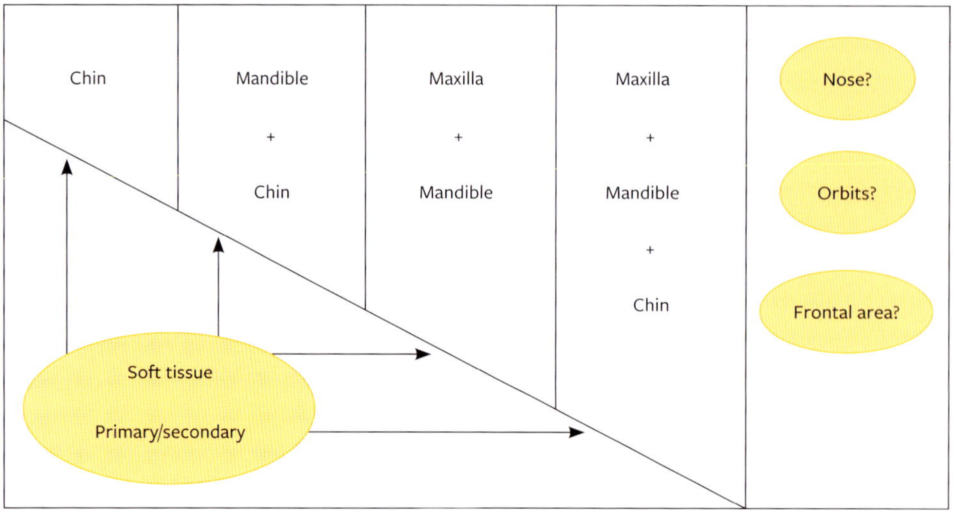

Fig 5-39 Categorization of possible facial asymmetry patterns. This diagram assists in differentiating between the specific areas that may be involved in the asymmetry of the face or a combination of areas influencing the symmetry of the face. When the maxilla is a contributing factor to facial asymmetry, an occlusal cant will play an important role in the correction and should always be considered.

gical orthodontic control of the expanded segments is paramount for optimal postsurgical stability.

Dentofacial Asymmetry

Very few faces are perfectly symmetric. Mild asymmetries of the dental arches and other facial structures are common and often clinically and functionally insignificant. Slight asymmetry of the face is likely of little importance to most patients, but others are very sensitive regarding facial asymmetry. Therefore, the clinician should warn patients that very few faces are perfectly symmetric and that it is impossible to achieve perfect facial symmetry with treatment.

The many causes of facial asymmetry can be classified as congenital, developmental, posttraumatic, or pathologic. Some of the more common abnormalities affecting the face and leading to asymmetry are hemimandibular elongation, unilateral condylar hyperplasia (hemimandibular hyperplasia), hemifacial microsomia (oculoauriculovertebral sequence), TMJ ankylosis, and deformities induced by trauma.

Like all orthognathic patients, individuals with facial asymmetry require a systematic and comprehensive process of examination, diagnosis, and treatment planning, as discussed in chapter 2. Because most facial asymmetries are growth related, special attention should be given to abnormal growth patterns, prolonged growth, and completion of facial growth. During the clinical examination, the clinician should pay special attention to three important factors: (1) the location of the asymmetry, (2) the tissues involved, and (3) the dimensions involved. The asymmetry of the face may be in the chin, mandible, maxilla, nose, orbits, zygoma, frontal areas, or a combination of these structures. Figure 5-39 presents a way to categorize facial symmetry patterns. The diagram should also assist the clinician in differentiating between the specific area and combination of areas of asymmetry. The involvement of other facial structures (eg, nose, orbits, and frontal bone) should be considered, and the soft tissue involvement—either primary or secondary to the skeletal asymmetry—should be evaluated.

The clinician should determine what tissues are causing the asymmetry and whether the involvement is primary or secondary. This information will influence the treatment plan. For example, soft tissue asymmetry caused by mandibular asymmetry will be corrected by the skeletal correction, but the soft tissue deformity seen in hemifacial microsomia often requires further attention to manage the deficient or absent soft tissue.

The dimensions involved in the asymmetry should also be determined. Note that asymmetry of the face seldom involves only one or two dimensions of space, and correction of the asymmetry in one dimension will certainly influence the symmetry in other dimensions. The maxillomandibular complex is a 3D structure (Fig 5-40a). To simplify the determination of the 3D skeletal, dental, and

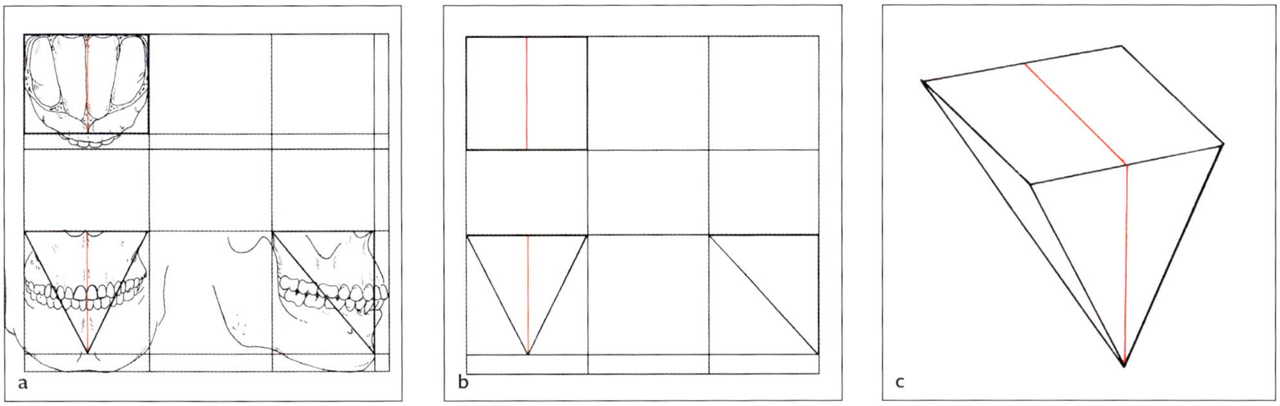

Fig 5-40 (*a*) Diagram of the three dimensions of the maxillomandibular complex. (*b and c*) Constructing a pyramid representing the maxillomandibular complex can assist in visualizing the 3D alterations of the midface and lower face during the correction of facial asymmetry.

soft tissue alteration required for the correction of dentofacial asymmetries, a pyramid can be constructed to represent the maxillomandibular complex (Fig 5-40b). This pyramid helps the clinician visualize and evaluate the various 3D surgical movements (Fig 5-40c). Figure 5-41 shows the effect of unilateral condylar hyperplasia on the spatial position of the prism. The opposite effect is demonstrated in Fig 5-42. In situations of facial asymmetry involving three dimensions, the transverse cant of the occlusal plane obviously differs from anterior to posterior. 3D deformities can be best assessed by combining the data from the lateral, basal, and anteroposterior cephalometric radiographs with articulated dental casts (recorded with a facebow and articulated on an adjustable articulator) and clinical observations. As in the correction of other dentofacial deformities, the anteroposterior vertical and transverse positions of the maxillary incisors play an extremely important role in the final treatment planning (see chapter 2).

Neither presurgical nor postsurgical orthodontic treatment for dentofacial asymmetry differs significantly from the orthodontic treatment in other dentofacial deformities. However, the clinician should consider the following guidelines for presurgical orthodontic treatment in cases with facial asymmetry:

- As in the previously discussed cases of dentofacial deformities, the dentition should not be orthodontically compensated for skeletal disharmony.
- An existing cant of the occlusal plane should not be corrected. However, the dental arch should be leveled, and the orthodontist should ensure that the apical base midline and incisor midlines follow the cant.
- When skeletal asymmetry exists, the dental midlines should not be made to coincide but rather be positioned in the midline of each jaw.
- When facial asymmetry will be corrected by single-jaw surgery, the dental midline of the unoperated jaw should coincide with the facial midline.
- In patients with hemifacial microsomia and TMJ ankylosis in whom a unilateral open bite is created after the ramus height is increased, the height should be maintained while allowing the vertical alveolar growth of the maxilla.

Asymmetry in the adolescent

The two major causes of severe facial asymmetry in children are hemifacial microsomia and early trauma to the mandibular condyle. Both conditions primarily affect the mandible and lead to deficient growth on the affected side. The maxilla is affected secondarily by the inhibition of vertical growth of the alveolar process on the affected side. The basic difference between the two conditions is that in hemifacial microsomia, missing soft and hard tissue structures may affect the growth potential, whereas in ankylosis, all structures are present but underdeveloped because of the lack of function. The basic principle in treating these conditions is to restore and maximize the expression of growth so that the development of both hard and soft tissue structures can be as normal as possible.

Mandibular asymmetry can also develop as a result of excessive growth on one side of the mandible. The clinician should differentiate between hemimandibular elongation and hemimandibular hypertrophy depending on which part of the mandible is involved. Hemimandibular elongation

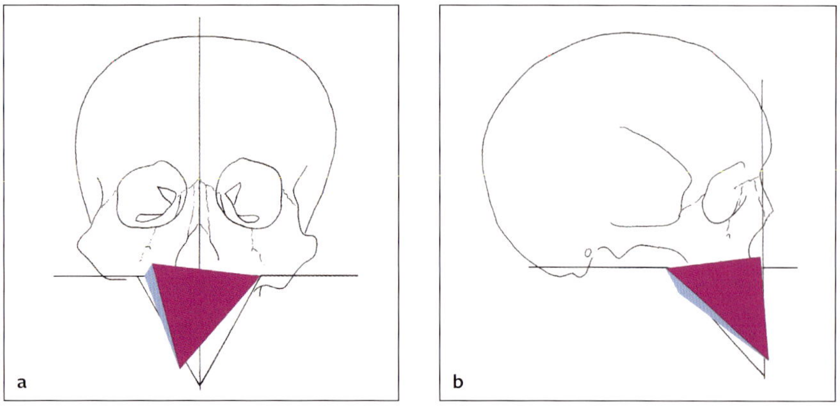

Fig 5-41 Unilateral increase in the height of the left mandibular ramus (eg, condylar hyperplasia) will be followed by the left posterior maxilla. A cant of the base of the prism will develop (more posteriorly than anteriorly), and the apex of the pyramid will rotate forward and to the right. (*a*) Frontal view. (*b*) Lateral view.

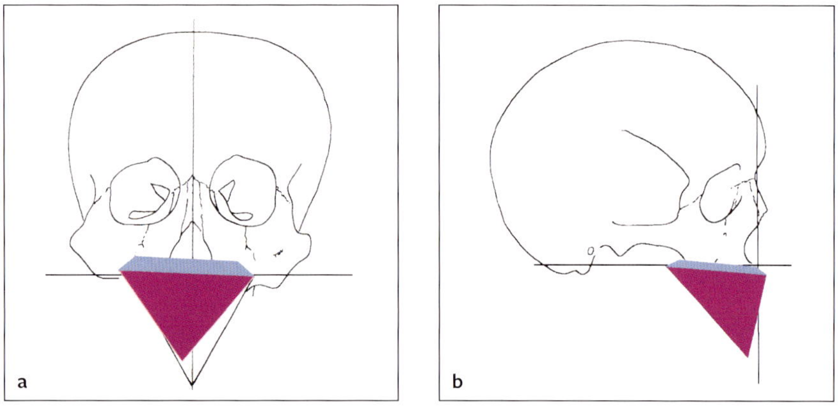

Fig 5-42 Unilateral lack of vertical development of the right mandible will inhibit vertical growth of the right posterior maxilla. The base of the pyramid will cant (more posteriorly than anteriorly), and the apex of the prism will rotate backward and to the right. (*a*) Frontal view. (*b*) Lateral view.

starts during puberty and is caused by rapid enlargement of the body of the mandible. The excessive growth is fast, and the maxilla is not involved; as a result, a unilateral open bite develops on the affected side and a crossbite develops on the nonaffected side. Hemimandibular hypertrophy, or unilateral condylar hyperplasia, is characterized by a diffuse enlargement of the condyle, condylar neck, ramus, and body of the mandible. The excessive growth process is slow and often starts before puberty. Because of the slow growth of the mandible, the maxilla follows, and an occlusal cant develops. Surgical correction should involve surgery to both jaws.

TMJ reconstruction and orthognathic surgery

The form and function of the TMJ can be affected by several conditions, such as the following:

- Severe degenerative joint disease
- Irreparable condylar fracture (trauma)
- Neoplasia requiring resection of joint components
- TMJ ankylosis
- Congenital developmental disorders
- Previously failed TMJ reconstruction

Conditions altering the form, size, and height of the mandibular condyle will inevitably influence TMJ function, occlusion, and facial esthetics (balance) as well as normal facial growth in individuals who are still growing. TMJ reconstruction should therefore form an integral part in the orthognathic treatment planning for patients requiring correction of dentofacial deformities.

The TMJ can be reconstructed by using autogenous bone grafts or alloplastic grafts. For many years, costochondral grafts have been a choice method for reconstructing the TMJ in pediatric patients; however, sternoclavicular grafts and grafts harvested from the iliac crest or calvarium have also been used. Costochondral grafts are favored because these grafts are easy to harvest, they usually fit the native TMJ dimensions, and the cartilaginous section can be adapted to fit the glenoid fossa. Another advantage is its purported ability to provide for growth, matched to the remaining facial skeleton (see case 14, Fig 5-52).

Although the growth potential of a costochondral graft is considered an advantage in growing children, its long-term growth is unpredictable. Unfortunately, complications are common, such as reankylosis in ankylotic patients, unpredictability of overgrowth, resorption of the grafts, and

Box 5-1 | Advantages and disadvantages of alloplastic TMJ replacement

Advantages:

- No postoperative intermaxillary fixation is required.
- The patient can—and actually should—exercise the area immediately after surgery.
- There is no donor site morbidity.
- The surgical time is reduced.
- Existing dentofacial deformities can be corrected at the same time.
- An accurate prosthetic glenoid fossa is created.
- The treatment outcome is more predictable than costochondral graft reconstruction.
- The occurrence of reankylosis is low (heterotopic bone).
- Normal anatomy can be mimicked with a CAD/CAM or patient-matched implant.
- The initial reconstruction of the TMJ in growing individuals does not preclude orthognathic surgical correction either concurrent with the joint replacement or in the future.
- Stable occlusion can be maintained, and there is no remodeling.

Disadvantages:

- The device can be expensive.
- There is no potential for growth.
- There is a risk of postoperative infection.
- Although the risk of reankylosis is lower than with costochondral grafts, it is not entirely eliminated.
- The prosthesis may wear over time (eg, screw loosening, fracturing).

limitation of angle reconstruction. Therefore, prosthetic rehabilitation should seriously be considered for these patients (Box 5-1; see cases 11 and 13, Figs 5-49 and 5-51).

Hemifacial microsomia (oculoauriculovertebral hypoplasia)

Hemifacial microsomia is a progressive asymmetric craniofacial deformity with a wide range of severity. It is the second most common congenital facial anomaly (1 in 5,600 births) after cleft lip and palate and involves the skeletal, soft tissue, and neuromuscular components of the first and second pharyngeal arches. The phenotype may vary from slight mandibular asymmetry to cleft lip and palate, microtia, lateral facial clefts, underdevelopment or absence of the condyle, mandibular ramus, and zygoma combined with several head and neck and other congenital abnormalities.

Although several classifications of the severity of the deformity have been developed that may act as a treatment guide, treatment should not be based on a specific classification. The surgical treatment design and timing of surgical correction for each individual deformity should be carefully planned and based on the individual's morphologic anomalies, function, growth, and psychosocial adjustment. According to Posnick (2014), the basic treatment principles during infancy and early childhood should be based on airway, feeding, vision, hearing, and psychosocial support.

Stages

The treatment can be generally divided into eight stages.

First stage (3 months)
The cleft lip is corrected.

Second stage (9 to 14 months)
The cleft palate is corrected.

Third stage (2 to 5 years)
The cranio-orbital asymmetry is corrected.

Fourth stage (5 years or older)
The zygomatic deformity is corrected.

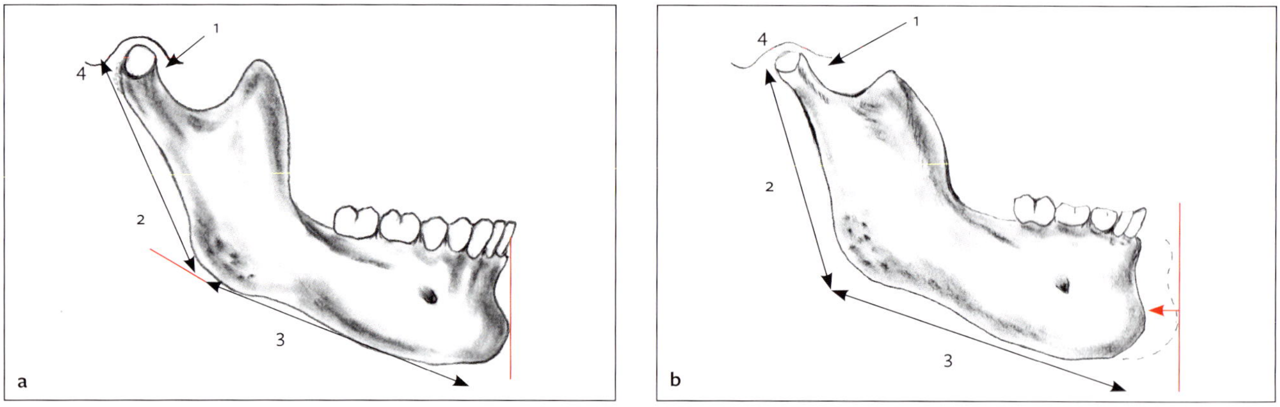

Fig 5-43 (*a*) The lateral view of a mandible with a normal condyle (1), glenoid fossa (4), vertical (2), and anteroposterior (3) relations. (*b*) Kaban Type I mandibular deformity: a "miniature" mandible and TMJ. All structures are present but small, with normal shape and position of the condyle (1) and fossa (4). The ramus is vertically short (2) and the body anteroposteriorly deficient (3).

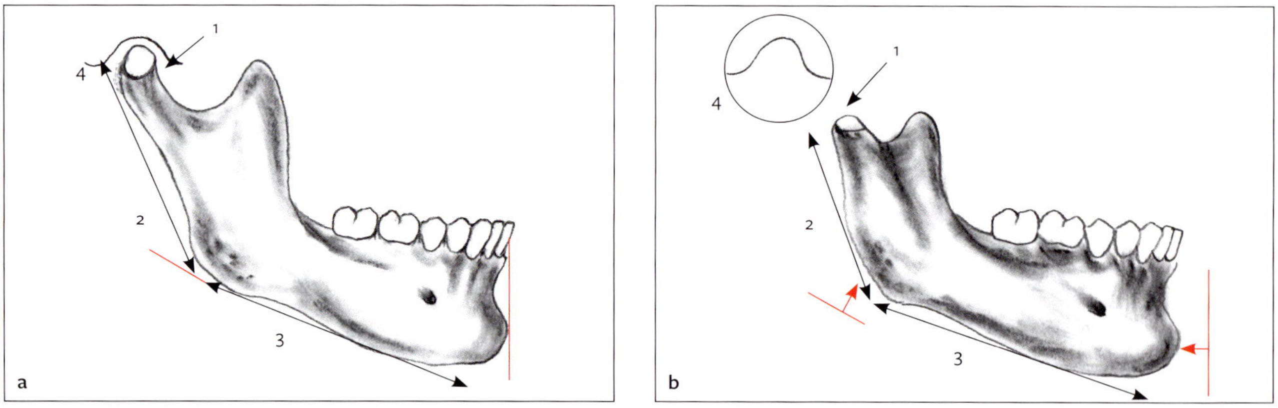

Fig 5-44 (*a*) The lateral view of a mandible with a normal condyle (1), glenoid fossa (4), vertical (2), and anteroposterior (3) relations. (*b*) Kaban Type IIA mandibular skeletal deformity: The condyle (1) and glenoid fossa (4) are hypoplastic while the ramus is vertically short (2, *red arrow*) and the body anteroposteriorly deficient (3, *red arrow*).

Fifth stage (5 to 7 years)
The auricular tags are removed, and in severely deformed cases with unacceptable function and esthetics, the reconstruction of missing bone elements may be considered.

Sixth stage (14 years or older)
Orthognathic surgery for correction of the malocclusion and skeletal asymmetry is performed (see cases 9 to 13, Figs 5-47 to 5-51).

Seventh stage (late teens)
Deficient or absent soft tissue is reconstructed (see cases 9 to 11, Figs 5-47 to 5-49).

Eighth stage (15 years or older)
The deformed or missing ear is reconstructed with the aid of either rib cartilage or an alloplastic frame.

Kaban (1981) has classified the skeletal defects of the mandibular ramus and TMJ as follows:

- *Type I.* All the structures are present with normal shapes, but they are small with a hypoplastic TMJ (Fig 5-43).
- *Type II.* The mandibular ramus is small and deformed with a hypoplastic TMJ.
  - *Type IIA.* The hypoplasia of the TMJ is mild and the position acceptable for symmetric function. The native TMJ usually does not require replacement (Fig 5-44).
  - *Type IIB.* The condyle is hypoplastic and so far medially, anteriorly, and inferiorly displaced that a new joint should be constructed. Normal jaw motion and function are progressively affected while facial asymmetry is obvious (Fig 5-45).

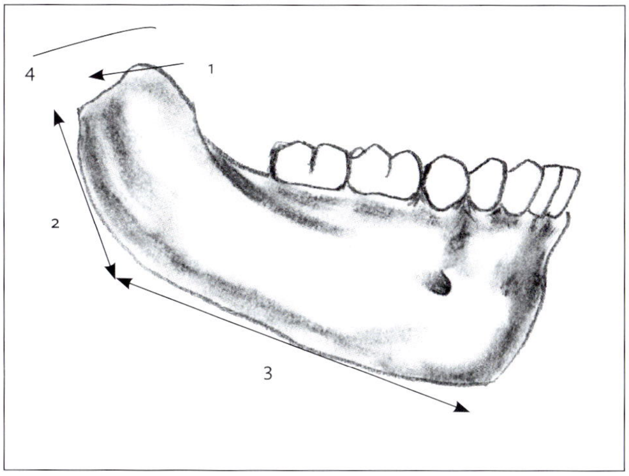

Fig 5-45 Kaban Type IIB mandibular skeletal deformity: The condyle (1) and glenoid fossa (4) are severely hypoplastic. The rudimentary condyle is medially, anteriorly, and inferiorly displaced. The ramus is deformed and vertically deficient (2) while the mandibular body is anteroposteriorly deficient (3). Total TMJ reconstruction is indicated.

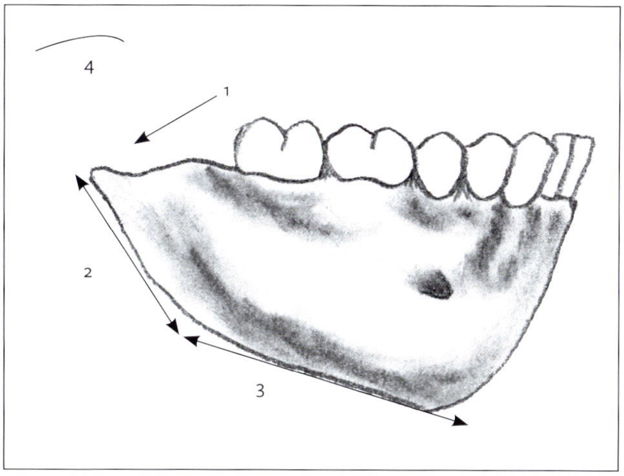

Fig 5-46 Kaban Type III mandibular skeletal deformity: The condyle (1), fossa (4), and ramus (2) are absent while the mandibular body is severely deficient (3). Total TMJ reconstruction is indicated.

- *Type III.* The mandibular ramus, condyle, and TMJ are absent. The glenoid fossa, articular disk, and muscles of mastication are moderately to severely hypoplastic with no translation possible (Fig 5-46).

This section concentrates on the principles of the orthognathic correction of patients with hemifacial microsomia based on mandibular defects. The clinician has several treatment options depending on the age of the patient and the severity of the mandibular deformity.

Treatment options

1. No treatment until completion of growth followed by orthognathic surgery.
2. Distraction of the mandibular ramus and body followed by orthognathic surgery at completion of growth.
3. Costochondral graft followed by orthognathic surgery (if required).
4. Alloplastic joint replacement followed by orthognathic surgery later (if required).
5. Alloplastic joint combined with orthognathic surgery at completion of growth.

Keeping this in mind, the treatment options should be considered based on the classification.

Type I

Clinical signs

- Mandibular condyle is present but deficient
- Articulation is acceptable
- Mandibular ramus body and ramus are short
- Possible occlusal cant
- Lower dental midline displaced to the affected side
- Dental crowding

Treatment options

- No treatment before completion of growth
- Orthognathic surgery (growth completed)

Case 9

A 19-year-old woman presented with Kaban Type I hemifacial microsomia. Apart from the mandibular defects, she had no other deformities associated with the condition. Her treatment was planned in three phases. First, her facial asymmetry was corrected with orthognathic surgery. The posteroanterior cephalometric analysis and treatment planning is demonstrated in Figs 5-47a and 5-47b. The facial changes following orthognathic surgery can be seen in Figs 5-47c to 5-47h. Next, her right mandibular angle was augmented using an alloplastic angle implant (Figs 5-47i to 5-47k). In the third phase, the soft tissue was augmented by using a subdermal fat graft (Figs 5-47l to 5-47o). The treatment outcome is demonstrated in Figs 4-37p to 5-37s.

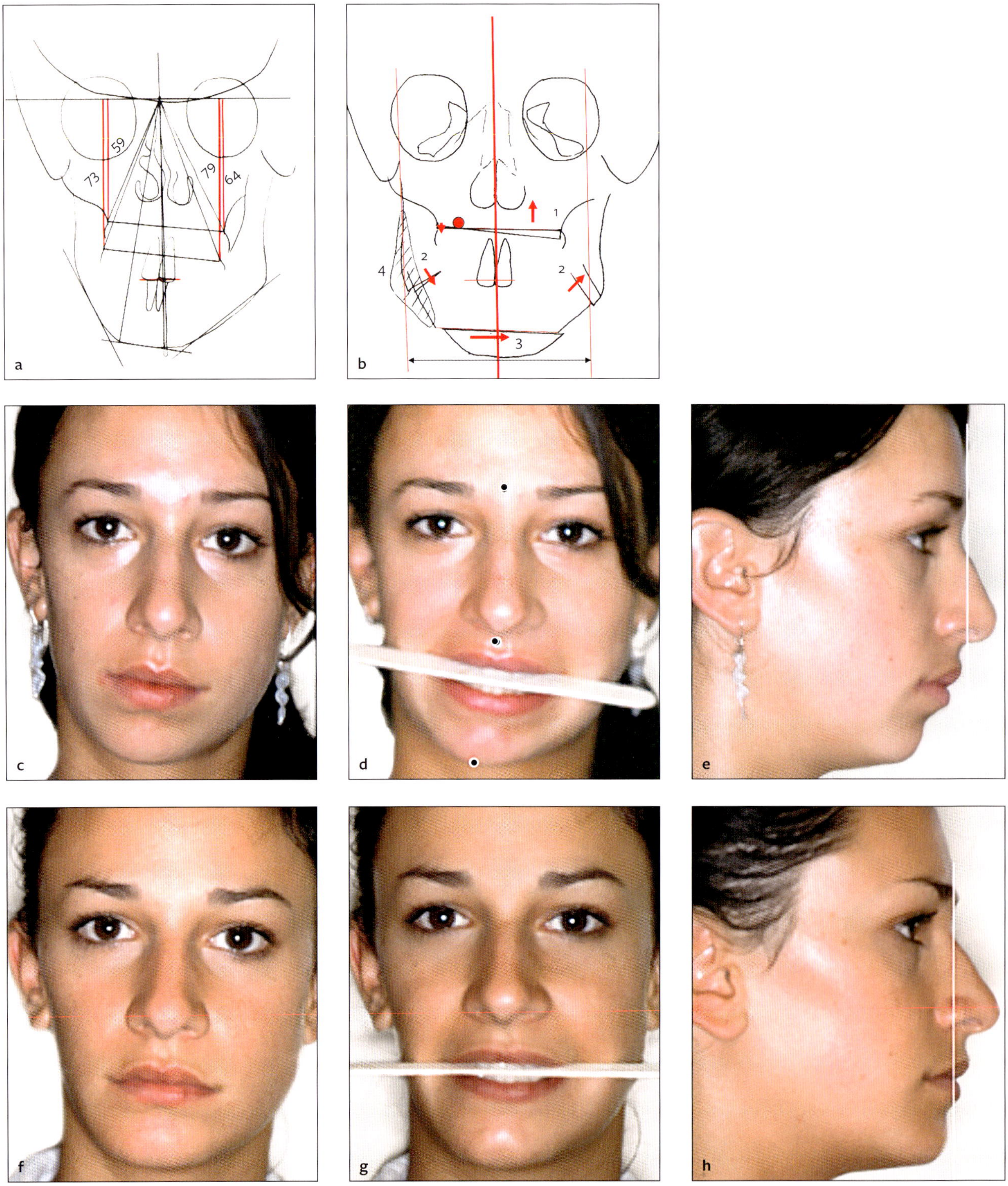

Fig 5-47 Case 9. This patient presented with Kaban Type I hemifacial microsomia. (*a*) Posteroanterior cephalometric analysis. Note the transverse cant of the occlusal plane and mandibular asymmetry. (*b*) The posteroanterior cephalometric visual treatment objective. The occlusal cant is corrected with a Le Fort I maxillary osteotomy (*arrows*). The *red dot* indicates and the rotation point (1). The mandibular asymmetry is corrected with a bilateral sagittal split osteotomy (2). A genioplasty is planned to finalize the mandibular asymmetry (3). Augmentation of the mandibular angle deficiency was planned using an alloplastic angle implant (4). The facial asymmetry (*c*) and occlusal cant (*d*) are evident in in the frontal view, while the convex profile is well demonstrated in profile view (*e*). (*f to h*) The esthetics have improved following the orthognathic surgery. →

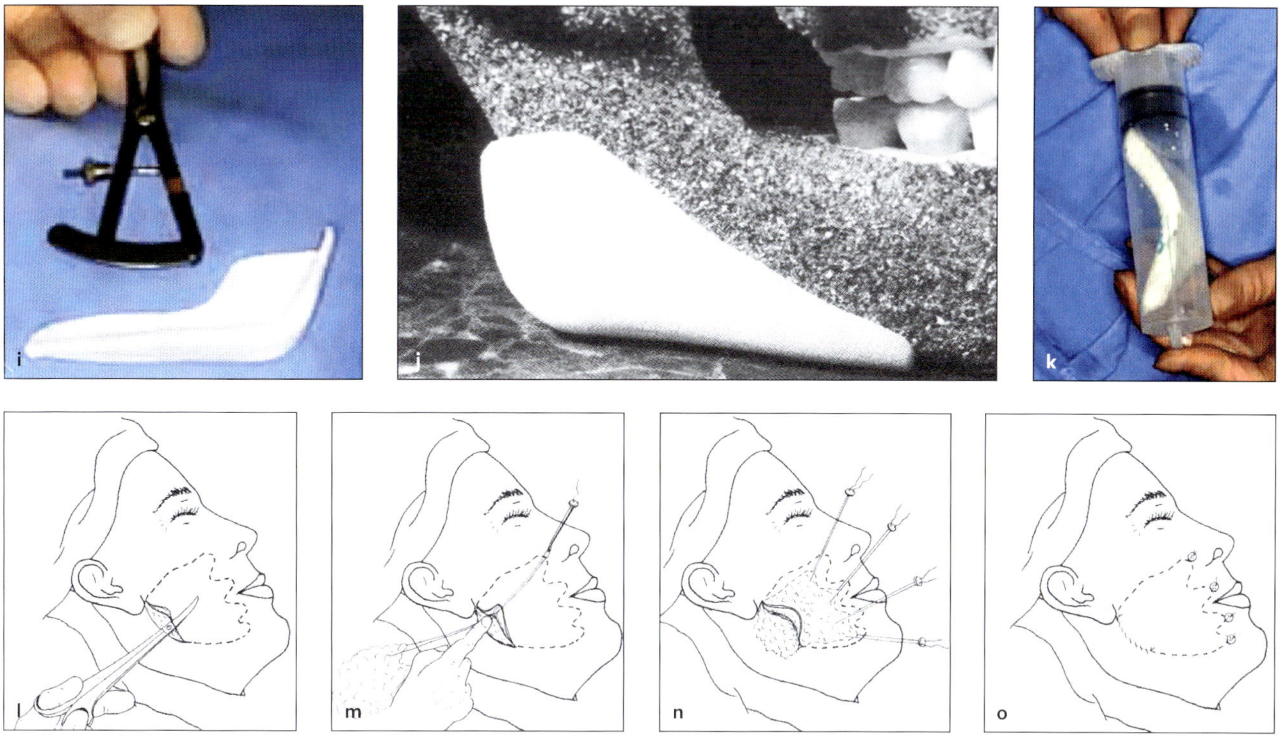

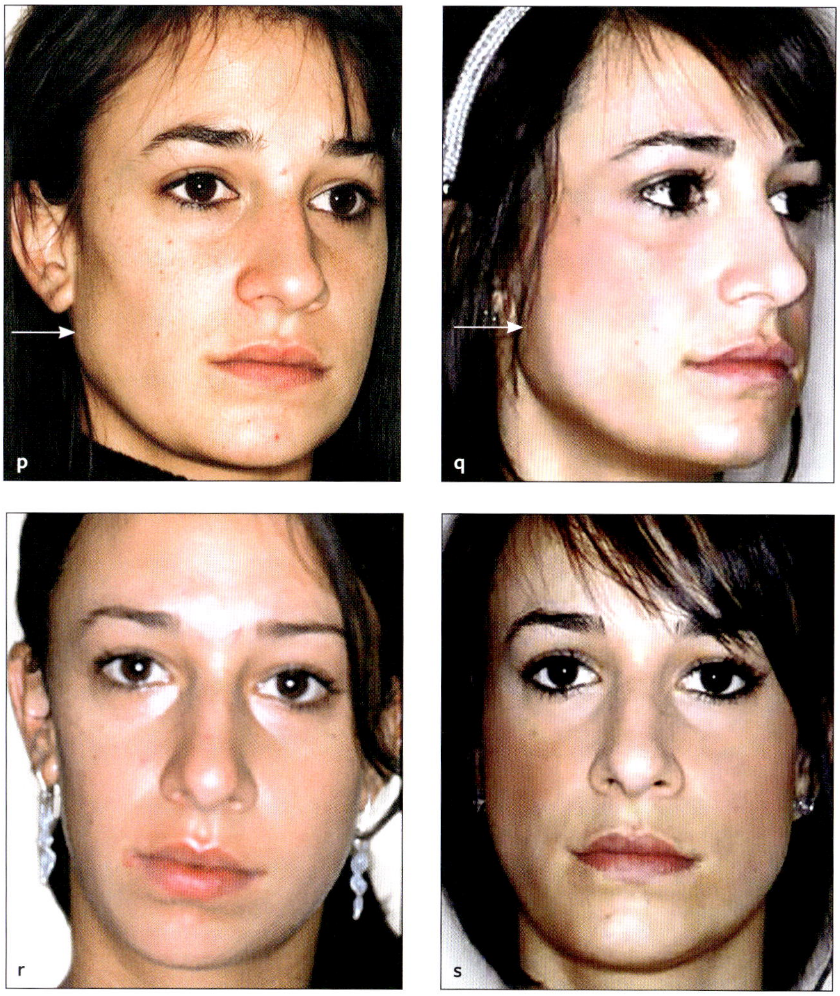

Fig 5-47 *(cont)* The relative size of the prosthesis (*i*) and planned position on the right angle (*j*). The implant is impregnated with an antibiotic solution by creating a vacuum in a 50-mL syringe filled with the solution (*k*). (*l to o*) Placement of a subdermal fat graft. The area requiring augmentation is marked on the face, and a soft tissue pocket is created through a postmandibular incision in the superficial muscular aponeurotic system (SMAS) layer indicated by the markings (*l*). The fat is harvested from the buttock to a size that will fit the defect. Long black silk sutures are then inserted through the distal ends of the implant (*m*). The graft is the pulled through the incision with an awl to the anterior end of the dissection (*n*). Sterilized shirt buttons are attached to the ends and tied to maintain the graft in position (*o*). (*p*) Soft tissue deficiency before fat augmentation (*arrow*). (*q*) Result after augmentation (*arrow*). (*r*) Pretreatment frontal view. (*s*) Posttreatment frontal view.

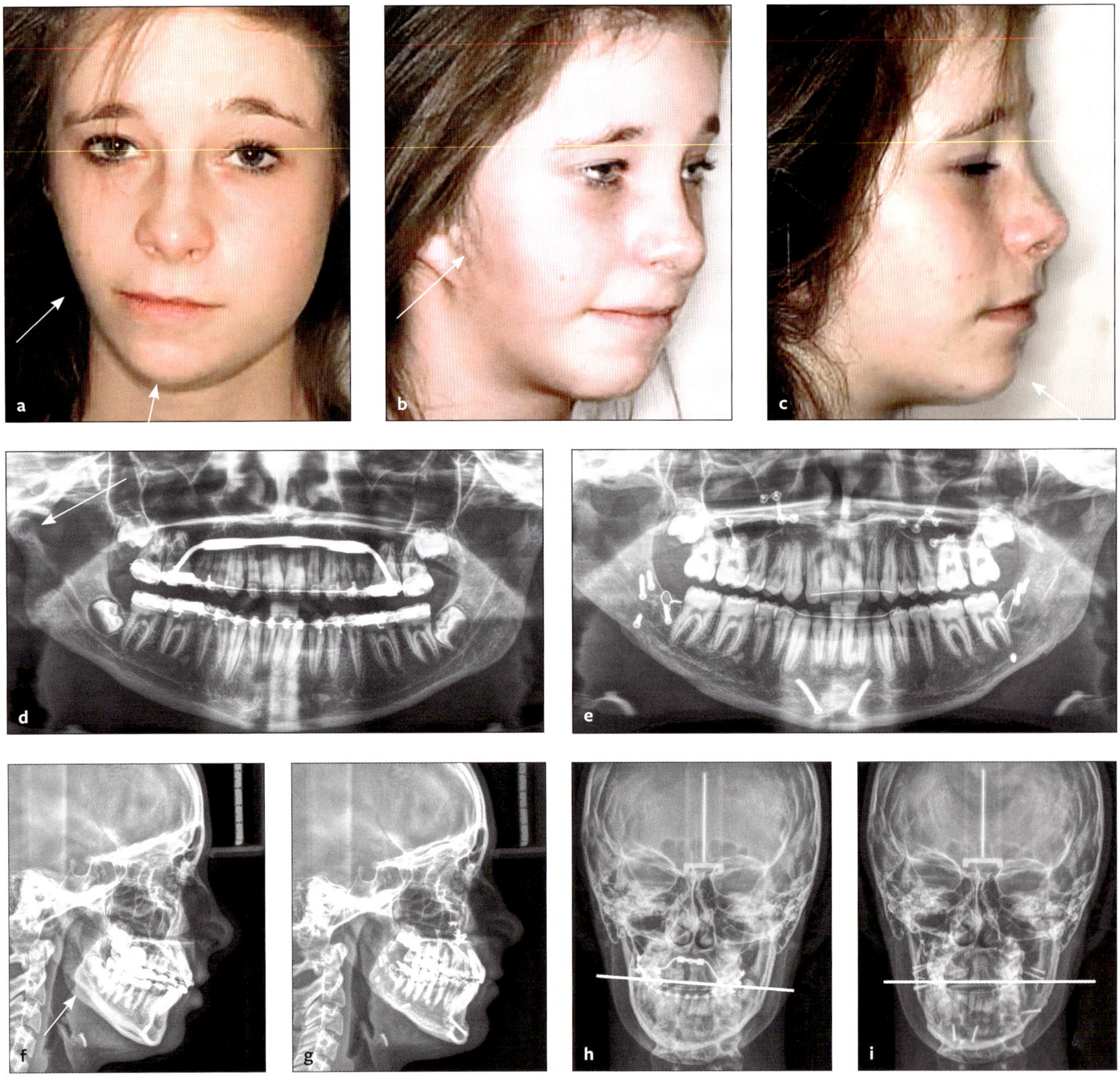

Fig 5-48 Case 10. (*a*) Presurgical frontal view. Note the asymmetry and mandibular deficiency. (*b*) The preauricular cartilaginous tags were removed at an earlier age (*arrow*). (*c*) The patient's profile is convex. (*d*) Presurgical panoramic radiograph. Note the small condyle and mandibular ramus on the right side. (*e*) Postsurgical panoramic radiograph. (*f*) Presurgical lateral cephalometric radiograph. Note the short mandibular ramus on the affected side (*arrow*). (*g*) Postsurgical cephalometric radiograph. A Le Fort maxillary osteotomy corrected the transverse occlusal cant, a bilateral sagittal split osteotomy corrected the mandibular asymmetry and deficiency, and a genioplasty corrected the microgenia and chin asymmetry. (*h*) Presurgical posteroanterior cephalogram. (*i*) Postoperative posteroanterior cephalogram. Note the correction of the transverse occlusal cant and facial asymmetry. →

Case 10

This adolescent girl presented with Kaban Type I hemifacial microsomia. Her orthodontic treatment started at age 15 years, and her orthognathic surgery was performed at age 17 years. Her facial asymmetry involving hard and soft tissue is evident in Figs 5-48a to 5-48c. The surgery was performed in two phases: (1) orthognathic surgery for the correction of her skeletal deformities, followed by (2) augmentation of her soft tissue deficiency with a subdermal fat graft. The postsurgical changes are demonstrated in the panoramic, lateral, and posteroanterior cephalometric radiographs (Figs 5-48d to 5-48i). Her facial symmetry, profile balance, and occlusion improved following orthognathic surgery (Figs 5-48j to 5-48r), but the right mandibular angle defect caused by the deficient masseter muscle is evident. The final treatment outcome is demonstrated in Figs 5-48s to 5-48u.

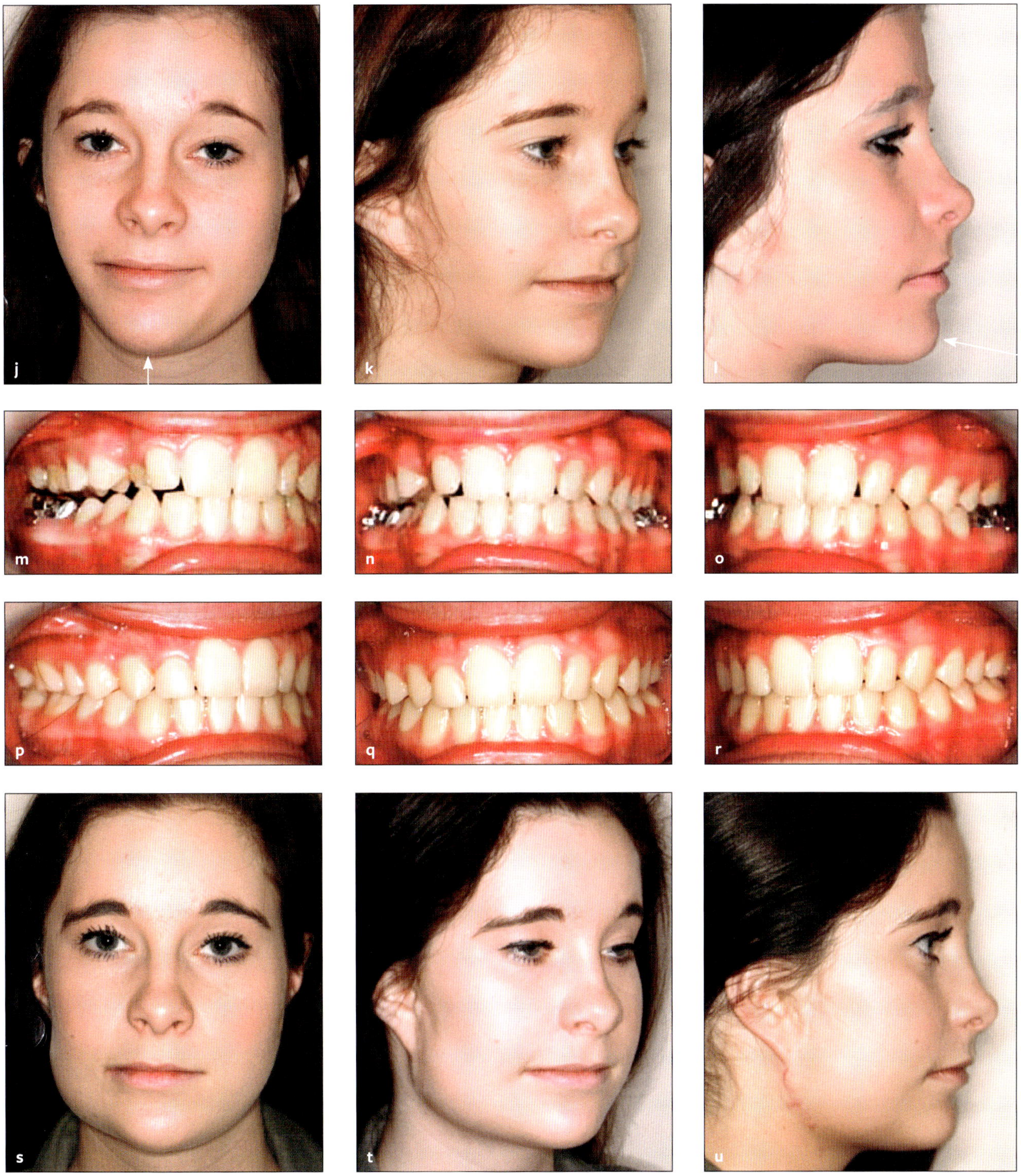

Fig 5-48 *(cont)* The improved esthetic result following the orthognathic surgery is illustrated in the frontal (*j*), three-quarter (*k*), and profile views (*l*). (*m to o*) Presurgical occlusion. (*p to r*) Posttreatment occlusion. Soft tissue augmentation is demonstrated 6 weeks following the subdermal fat graft in the frontal view (*s*), three-quarter view (*t*), and profile view (*u*). The overcorrected soft tissue defect is expected to conform to an esthetic contour after 12 to 18 weeks.

Type IIA

Clinical signs

- Moderate degree of hypoplasia of the glenoid fossa, condyle, and ramus.
- The masticatory muscles have variable degree of hypoplasia.
- Retrognathia with chin asymmetric to the ipsilateral side.
- Often, a Class II occlusion on the affected side with asymmetric dental midlines.
- Moderate maxillary occlusal cant.

Treatment options

- No treatment before completion of growth.
- Distraction of the deficient elements.
- Orthognathic surgery (growth completed).

Type IIB

Clinical signs

- The condyle is severely deficient and medially displaced.
- The masticatory muscles are moderately to severely deficient.
- The facial asymmetry is excessive.
- Cant in the maxillary occlusal plane.
- Lower dental midline is displaced to the ipsilateral side.
- Posterior crossbites.
- Cases are functionally similar to Type III cases.

Treatment options

- *Distraction of the deficient elements.* The author is not in favor of distraction in these patients. The 2D distraction vector is inaccurate, and the absence of the glenoid fossa makes docking questionable.
- *Reconstruction of the TMJ with a costochondral graft.* Due to the unpredictability regarding growth potential (graft resorption, no growth, or graft overgrowth), the indications for TMJ reconstruction by means of costochondral grafts are limited. An additional disadvantage is the poorly developed glenoid fossa, making stable positioning of the proximal graft doubtful.
- *Distraction of the affected side.* This may be indicated following costochondral grafting and poor growth of the graft and should be considered overcorrection.
- *Reconstruction of the TMJ with a patient-matched graft.* The graft has no growth potential if used in the adolescent patient, so overcorrection should be considered. When an alloplastic TMJ graft is used in a growing individual, it does not preclude mandibular advancement by means of a sagittal split osteotomy at a later stage.

Case 11

This 8-year-old girl was referred by her orthodontist for a consultation regarding her facial asymmetry. The clinical diagnosis of hemifacial microsomia Kaban Type IIB was made.

Main complaint

The patient's parents were concerned about their daughter's obvious facial asymmetry and mentioned that her appearance had been affecting her schooling and social behavior.

Medical history

The patient's dentist noticed the asymmetric development of her occlusion and referred her to an orthodontist. The severely deficient left mandibular condyle was noted on the panoramic radiograph, and the deviation of her mandible was evident.

Clinical examination

1. Soft tissue
   - Frontal view (Fig 5-49a)
     - Severe mandibular asymmetry to the left
     - Her chin appears deficient
     - The left ear is slightly smaller than the right ear
   - Profile view (Fig 5-49b)
     - Convex profile
     - Deficient mandible
     - Deficient chin
2. Dental (Fig 5-49c)
   - Mixed dentition
   - Mandibular dental midline displaced to the left
   - Narrow maxillary arch
   - Tendency to an anterior open bite
   - Class II molar relation on the left
   - Slight cant of the occlusal plane
   - Tendency to bilateral crossbites
3. Skeletal (Fig 5-49d)
   - Mandibular asymmetry to the left
   - The mandible swings toward the left on mouth opening
   - Several unerupted permanent teeth
4. CT scan (Figs 5-49e and 5-49f)
   - Deformed left condyle
   - Condyle rotated
   - Medially displaced left mandibular ramus and condyle
   - Vertical deficient left mandibular ramus
   - Cant of the mandibular lower borders
   - Elongated left coronoid process
   - Anteroposterior deficient left mandibular corpus
   - Cant in the occlusal plane
   - Mandible rotated to the left

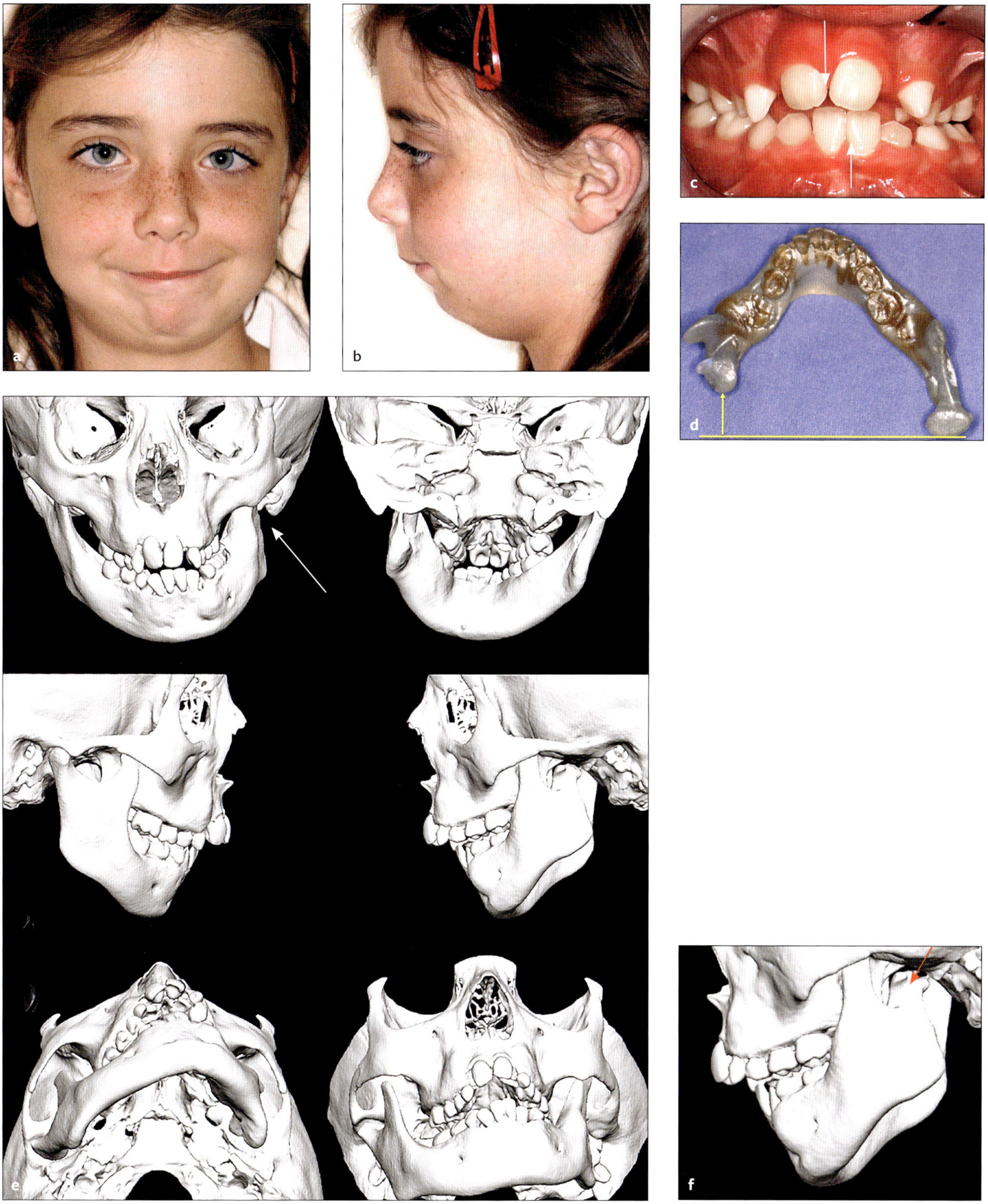

Fig 5-49 Case 11. An 8-year-old girl presented with Kaban Type IIB hemifacial microsomia. Frontal view (*a*), profile view (*b*), and occlusion (*c*). Note the severe facial asymmetry, deficient mandible, and the mandibular dental midline asymmetric to the affected side (*arrows*). (*d*) The 3D model of the mandible constructed from the CT scan. The severe anteroposterior deficiency of the left mandibular ramus and body as well as the medially displaced malformed condyle is well demonstrated (*arrow*). (*e*) The 3D CT scan illustrates the mandibular deformity and absence of the glenoid fossa. (*f*) Note the elongated coronoid process, deformed and medially displaced ramus (*arrows*), and condyle and absent glenoid fossa. →

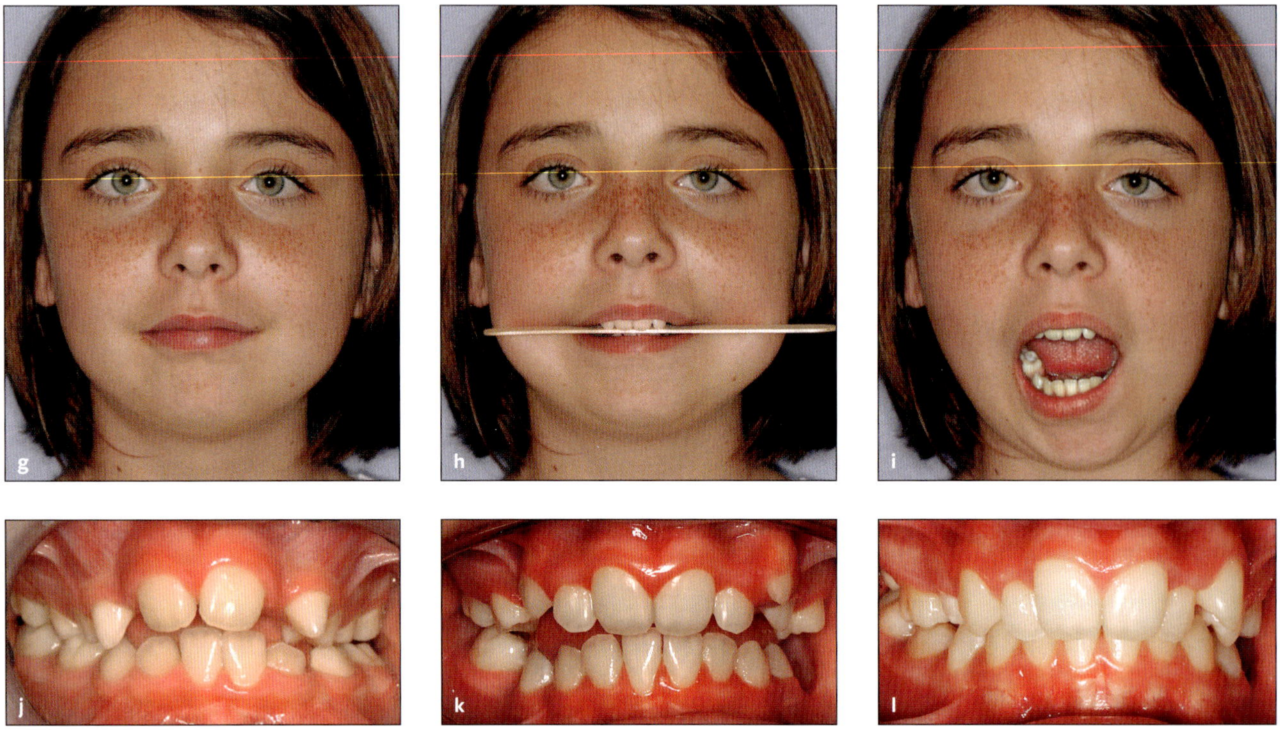

Fig 5-49 *(cont)* Improved facial symmetry (*g*), occlusal cant (*h*), and mouth opening (*i*) 3 years after surgery. Presurgical (*j*), immediate postsurgical (*k*), and 3-year postsurgical occlusion (*l*).

Problem list

- Severely deficient and deformed left condyle and ramus
- Mandibular anteroposterior deficiency (more on the left)
- Cant in the occlusal plane
- Mandibular dental midline is displaced to the left
- Mixed dentition with impacted right mandibular second molar
- The maxilla is vertically deficient on the left
- Microgenia

Presurgical orthodontics

No presurgical orthodontic treatment was contemplated before reconstruction of the TMJ.

Surgical treatment

Considering the patient's main complaint and age, the decision was made to perform the TMJ surgery rather than waiting for further growth. Three surgical options were considered:

1. Reconstruction of the TMJ using a costochondral graft
2. Reconstruction of the TMJ using an alloplastic patient-matched implant
3. Distraction of the malformed condyle

The literature and the author's experience have shown poor results with condyle distraction, and the inaccuracy of the vector of distraction of the condyle and the absence of a glenoid fossa are further disadvantages for this option. Considering the disadvantages of costochondral grafts (see page 214), it was decided to use a patient-matched alloplastic prosthesis. 3D CT scans of the facial bones were obtained and a prosthetic condyle and glenoid fossa designed (see Figs 5-49e and 5-49f). The existing condyle and muscle attachments to the condyle and coronoid process were maintained. This facilitated symmetric mouth opening. Vertical and anteroposterior overcorrection was planned with the lower dental midline to the right and a posterior open bite on the left.

Postsurgical orthodontics

The patient was referred to the orthodontist for orthodontic observation, and preliminary orthodontic correction started at age 11 years. The 3-year postsurgical results are demonstrated in Figs 5-49g to 5-49l.

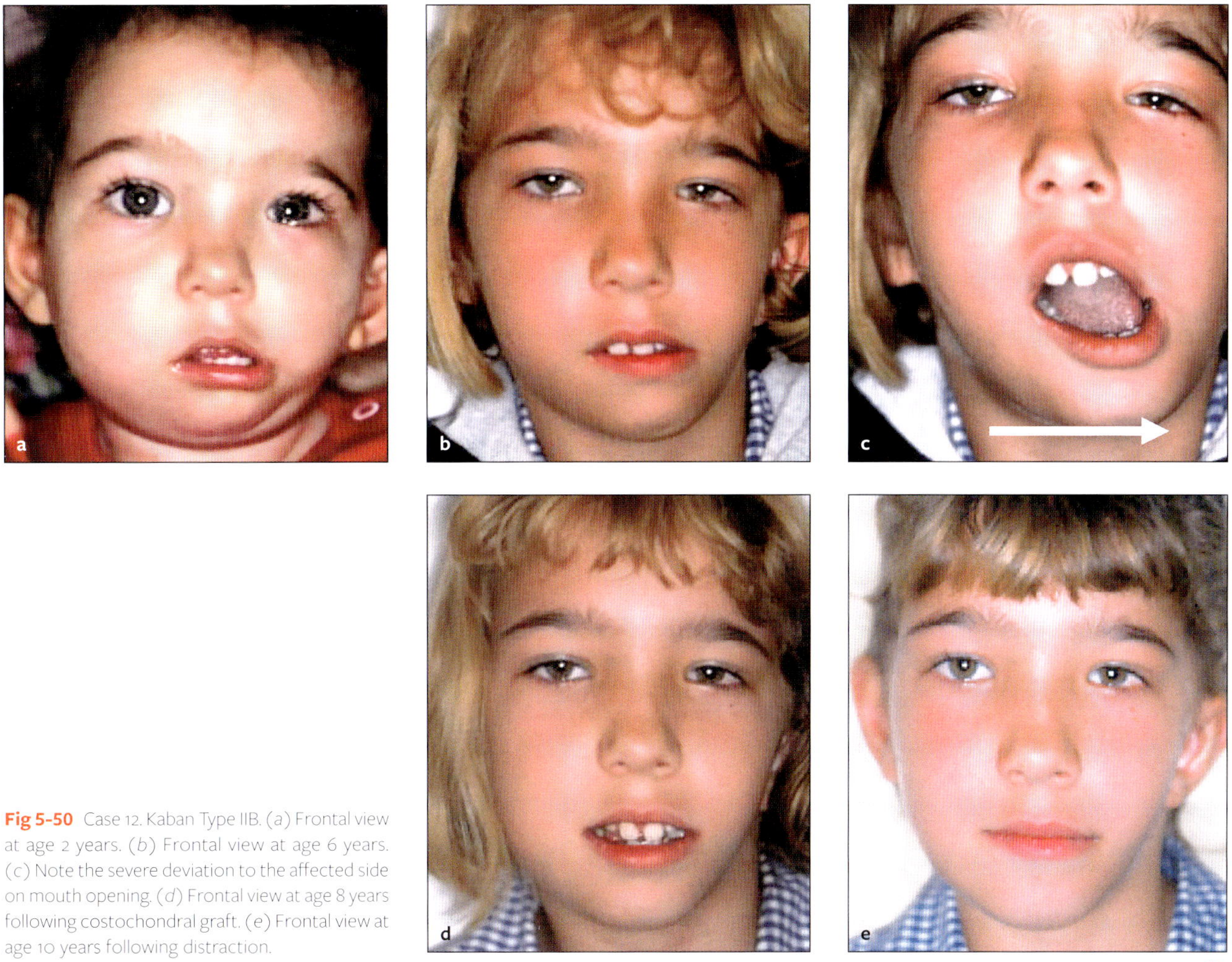

Fig 5-50 Case 12. Kaban Type IIB. (*a*) Frontal view at age 2 years. (*b*) Frontal view at age 6 years. (*c*) Note the severe deviation to the affected side on mouth opening. (*d*) Frontal view at age 8 years following costochondral graft. (*e*) Frontal view at age 10 years following distraction.

Case 12

This patient first presented with Kaban Type IIB hemifacial microsomia at age 2 years (Fig 5-50a). At the age of 8 years, her function and asymmetry deteriorated severely (Figs 5-50b to 5-50e; see Figs 5-50m and 5-50n). Note the severe mandibular deviation on mouth opening (see Fig 5-50c). The mandibular defect was augmented with a costochondral graft (Figs 5-50f to 5-50h), and the occlusion was slightly overcorrected. Unfortunately, the graft did not show any growth potential, and the left side of the mandible was distracted by means of an intraoral distraction device 2 years later, when the patient was 10 (Figs 5-50i to 5-50l). The patient was referred for orthodontic treatment at age 11 years (Figs 5-50m to 5-50o). Soft tissue augmentation will be performed once growth has been completed.

Type III

Clinical signs

- Absence of the glenoid fossa, condyle, and ramus.
- Masticatory muscles have a severe degree of hypoplasia.
- Retrognathia with chin displaced to the ipsilateral side.
- Anterior open bite and posterior crossbites.
- Transverse cant of the maxillary occlusal plane.
- No translation on the affected side.

Treatment options

- Reconstruction of the TMJ with a costochondral graft.
- Reconstruction of the TMJ with a patient-matched implant.
- Orthognathic surgery can be performed at the same time as the joint reconstruction. Patient-matched implants allow for more accurate orthognathic surgery.

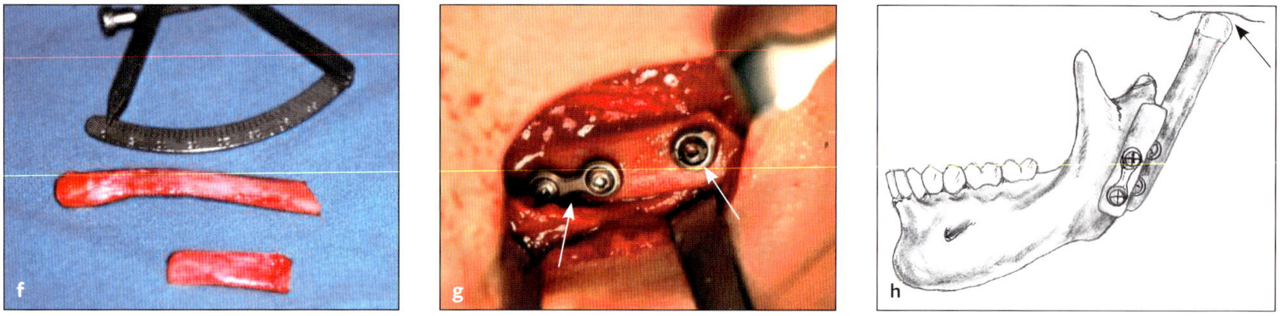

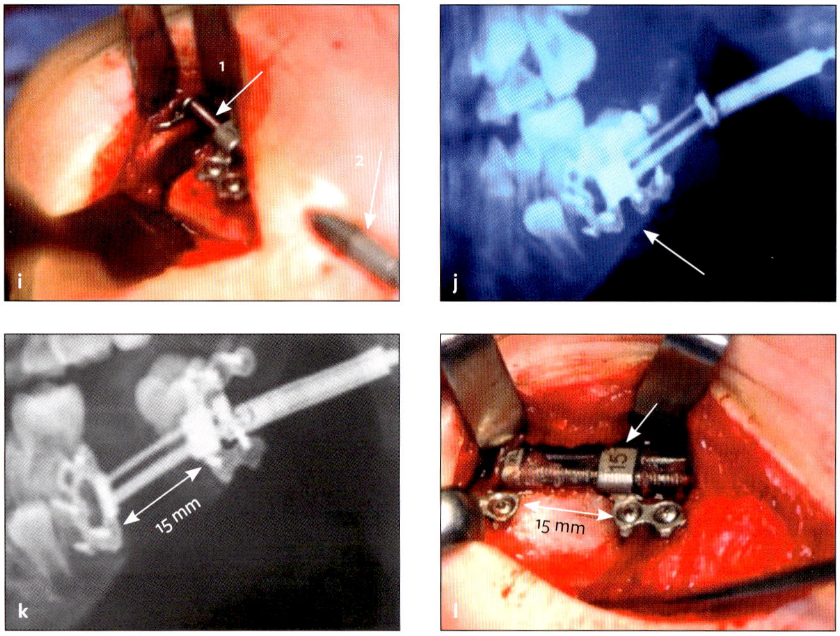

Fig 5-50 *(cont)* (*f*) The ramus and TMJ are reconstructed with a costochondral graft. At least 5 mm of cartilage is harvested with the bone, and a second bone graft is harvested to add stability and bulk. (*g*) The grafts are secured using rigid fixation plates and screws (*arrows*). (*h*) Although the glenoid fossa is usually poorly developed (*arrow*), the cartilaginous part of the graft is positioned onto the cranial base in the rudimentary fossa. (*i*) At the age of 10 years, the left side of the mandibular body was distracted with an intraoral distractor. The distractor is tested intraoperatively (*arrow 1*), and the driver exits infra-auricular posterior to the mandible (*arrow 2*). (*j*) Immediate postoperative radiograph before activation of distractor. (*k*) At termination of distraction and removal of the driver, a distraction of 15 mm was achieved. (*l*) The new bone (15 mm) is visualized and the distractor removed. (*m*) Occlusion before distraction. Note the severe dental midline discrepancy (*arrows*). (*n*) The mandibular deficiency on the left is overcorrected by distraction. Note the anterior crossbite and overcorrected dental midline (*arrows*). (*o*) The occlusion during lingual orthodontic finalization.

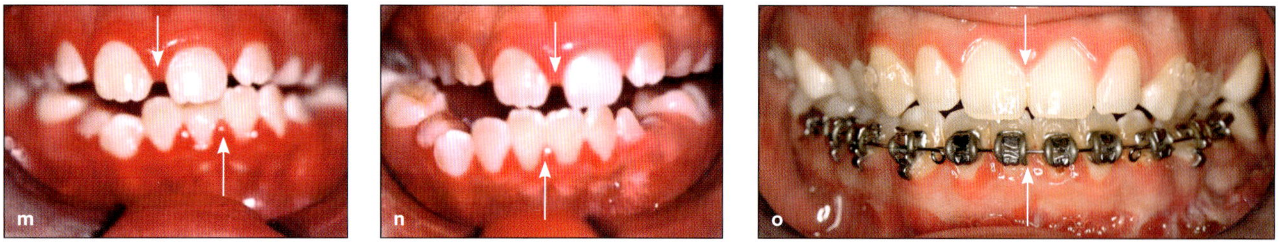

Case 13

A 21-year-old woman was referred for the correction of her facial asymmetry. She had been receiving orthodontic treatment for 10 months by an orthodontist in a different country before her orthognathic surgery consultation.

Main complaint

Her facial asymmetry was of major concern for her, and her malocclusion was of secondary concern.

Medical history

The diagnosis of hemifacial microsomia was only made in her late teens. Her medical history was noncontributory.

Clinical examination

1. Soft tissue
   - Frontal view (Figs 5-51a to 5-51c).
     - Mandibular asymmetry to the left
     - Chin is asymmetric to the left
     - Left masseter muscle deficiency
     - Tendency to macrostomia on the left
     - Left microtia
     - Coloboma on the left eye
   - Profile and three-quarter view (Figs 5-51d to 5-51f)
     - Acute nasolabial angle
     - Prominent upper and lower lips
     - Convex profile

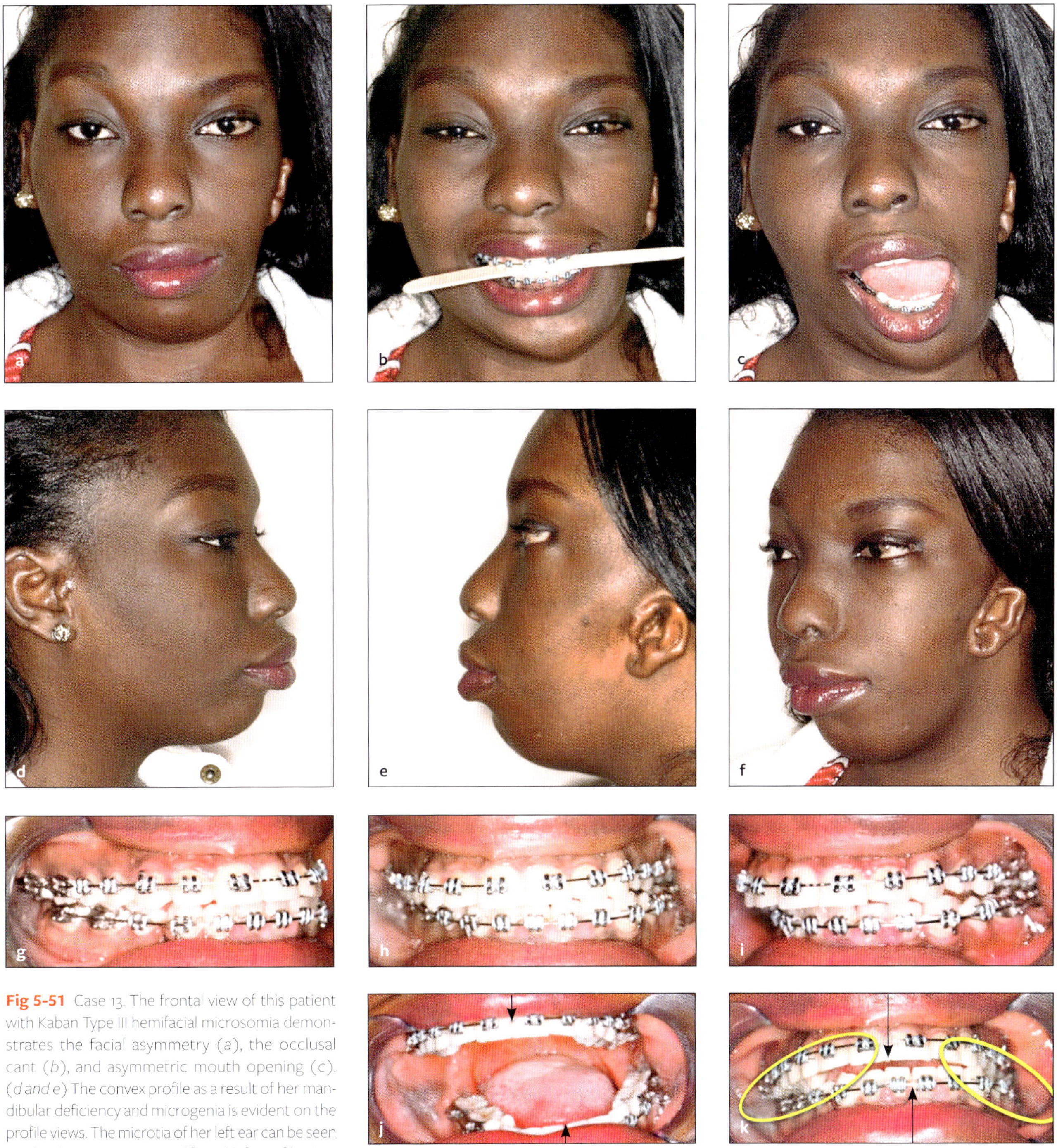

Fig 5-51 Case 13. The frontal view of this patient with Kaban Type III hemifacial microsomia demonstrates the facial asymmetry (*a*), the occlusal cant (*b*), and asymmetric mouth opening (*c*). (*d and e*) The convex profile as a result of her mandibular deficiency and microgenia is evident on the profile views. The microtia of her left ear can be seen on the three-quarter view (*f*) and left profile view. (*g to i*) Dental occlusal views. (*j and k*) Note the asymmetric mouth opening (*arrows*), dental midline discrepancy (*arrows*), and crossbites (*circles*).

- Everted lower lip
- Microtia of the left ear
- Increased lip-chin-throat angle
- Microgenia

2. Dental (Figs 5-51g to 5-51k)
   - Increased overjet
   - Bimaxillary protrusion
   - Class II molar and canine relationship on the left
   - Super Class II occlusion on the right
   - Bilateral crossbites
   - Lower dental midline 5 mm to the left
   - Transverse cant of the occlusal plane
3. Skeletal (Fig 5-51l)
   - Absent left mandibular ramus and condyle (Kaban IIB/III)
   - Absence of the left glenoid fossa

    - Mandibular anteroposterior deficiency
    - Microgenia
    - Mandibular asymmetry to the left
    - Chin asymmetry to the left

4. Radiographic
   - Panoramic (see Fig 4-51u)
     - Absent third molars
     - Absent left ramus, mandibular angle, and condyle
     - A separate bony segment is visible in the inferior temporal area
   - Cephalometric (see Fig 5-51w)
     - Convex profile
     - Increased lip-chin-throat angle
     - Mandibular anteroposterior deficiency
     - Bimaxillary protrusion
     - Prominent lips
     - Microgenia
   - 3D CT scan (see Fig 5-51l)
     - The skeletal observations as identified on the panoramic and cephalometric radiographs are observed in a 3D fashion.
     - A separate bony segment is identified in the infratemporal area.

Problem list

- Severe facial asymmetry
- Absent mandibular condyle and ramus
- Absent glenoid fossa on the left
- Deficient masseter and temporal muscles
- Microtia of the left ear
- Coloboma on the left eye
- Tendency to macrostomia of the left side of the mouth
- Microgenia of the left ear
- Convex profile
- Increased incisor overjet
- Bimaxillary protrusion
- Bilateral crossbites
- Transverse cant of the occlusal plane

Presurgical orthodontics

The initial orthodontic treatment consisted of leveling and coordination of both dental arches. No attempt was made to correct the dental midlines or the posterior crossbites. The mandibular incisor midline was placed in the middle of the mandible. No attempt was made to correct the bimaxillary protrusion.

Surgical treatment

First phase. A 3D virtual treatment plan was designed and consisted of the following:

- A unilateral sagittal split ramus osteotomy on the right side of the mandible advancing the mandible, assisting with the correction of the asymmetry and the correction of the occlusal cant (Fig 5-51m). A prefabricated intermediate surgical splint was used (see Figs 5-51o and 5-51q).
- Surgical removal of the "floating" bone in the infratemporal area (Figs 5-51n to 5-51p). The left mandibular TMJ and the mandibular angle were reconstructed with a patient-matched implant. The patient-matched implant corrected the mandibular asymmetry and the occlusal cant and advanced the left side of the mandible and reconstructed the left mandibular angle (Figs 5-51q to 5-51t).
- Superior repositioning of the left maxilla to correct the cant in the maxillary occlusal plane.
- The chin was advanced and mandibular symmetry refined by means of a sliding genioplasty.

The postoperative results are demonstrated in Figs 5-51u to 5-51gg.

Second phase

- Augmentation of the left masseter muscle and preauricular area using a free fat graft harvested from the buttock (Figs 5-51hh to 5-51ll).

Third phase

- Reconstruction of the left ear using rib cartilage.

Postsurgical orthodontics

- Finalizing the occlusion and retention.

There are several advantages to postponing definitive reconstruction until skeletal maturity:

- Avoid injury to dentition and inferior alveolar nerve.
- Avoid soft tissue scarring.
- Avoid reduction of mandibular marrow space that will complicate future surgery.
- Minimize negative psychosocial memories of earlier jaw surgery.
- Avoid iatrogenic 3D deformities that may result in multiple corrective procedures that will limit long-term results.

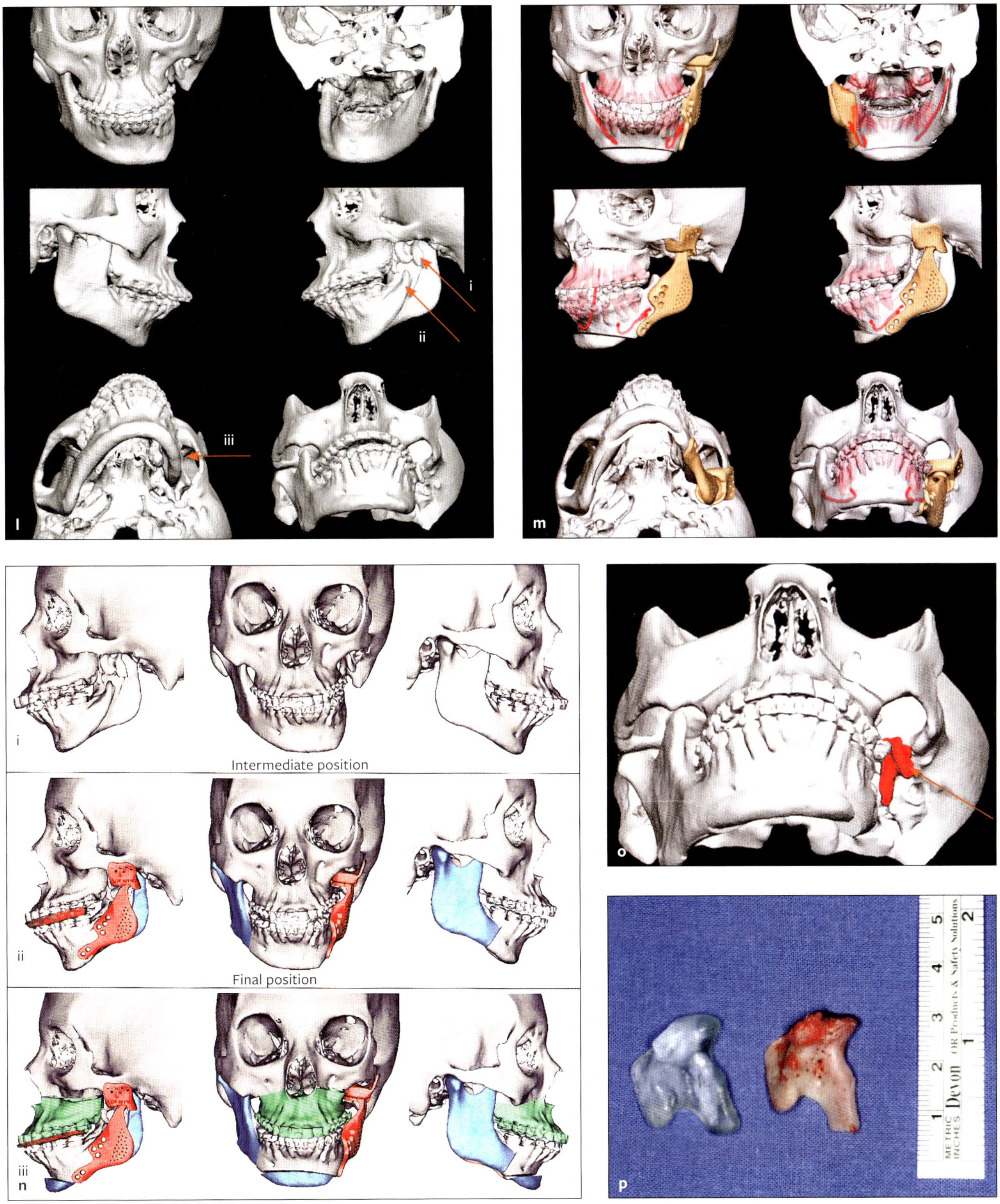

Fig 5-51 *(cont)* (*l*) The 3D CT scan. Note the "floating" bone in the left infratemporal area (*arrow i*), the deformed and deficient condyle and ramus (ii), and the medially displaced condyle and ramus (iii). (*m*) An overview of the 3D virtual treatment planning results following left TMJ, mandibular ramus, and angle reconstruction; Le Fort I osteotomy; right sagittal split ramus osteotomy; and sliding genioplasty. (*n*) The 3D skeletal deformities (i). The TMJ (*red*), mandibular advancement, and correction of the occlusal plane cant (*blue*) was first performed using an intermediate surgical splint (ii). The Le Fort I maxillary osteotomy was then performed using a final splint (*green*). The sliding genioplasty was performed last (*blue*) (iii). (*o*) The amorphous "floating" bone in the infratemporal area (*arrow*) is indicated in *red*. (*p*) The bone was removed during TMJ reconstruction and resembled an amorphous condyle and coronoid process. →

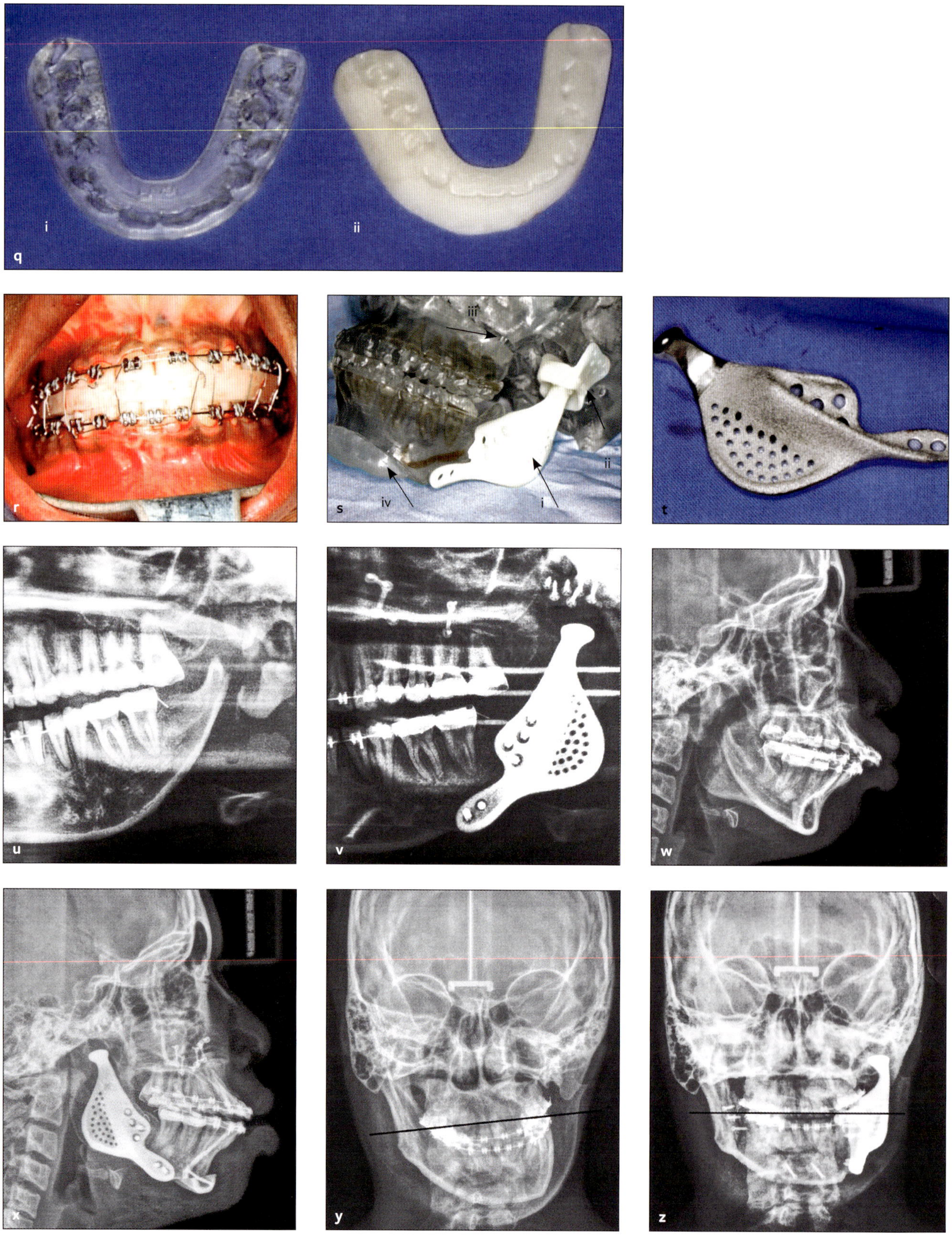

Fig 5-51 *(cont)* (*q*) The final (i) and intermediate (ii) surgical splints. (*r*) The intermediate splint and intermaxillary fixation in place during the first surgical phase. (*s*) The 3D virtual model of the patient. Note the Le Fort I maxillary osteotomy (i) and genioplasty (ii) on the model. TMJ (iii) and glenoid fossa (iv) templates are used to prepare the surgical site and an accurate fit of the implants before the final patient matched implants are placed. (*t*) The patient-matched TMJ, mandibular ramus, and angle before implantation. The radiographic left panoramic image before (*u*) and following surgery (*v*). The presurgical (*w*) and postsurgical (*x*) lateral cephalometric radiographs. The presurgical (*y*) and postsurgical (*z*) posteroanterior cephalometric radiographs.

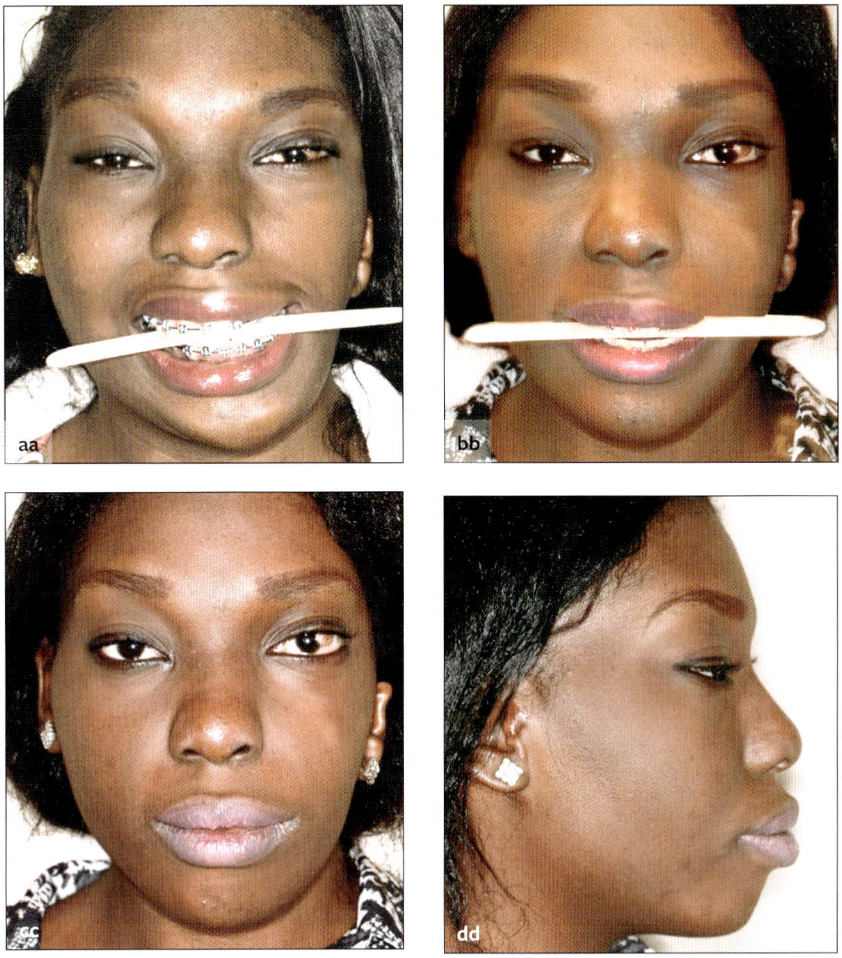

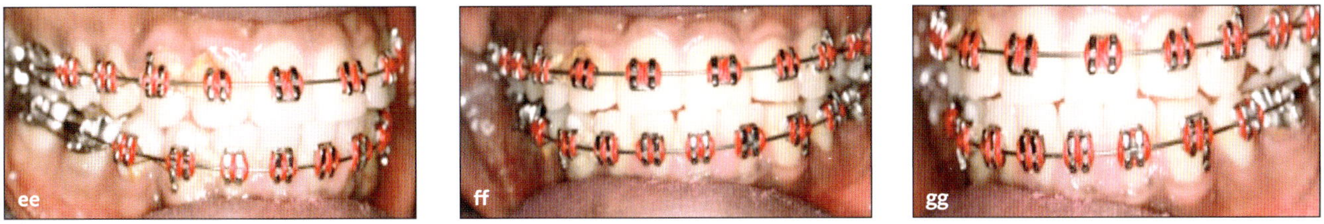

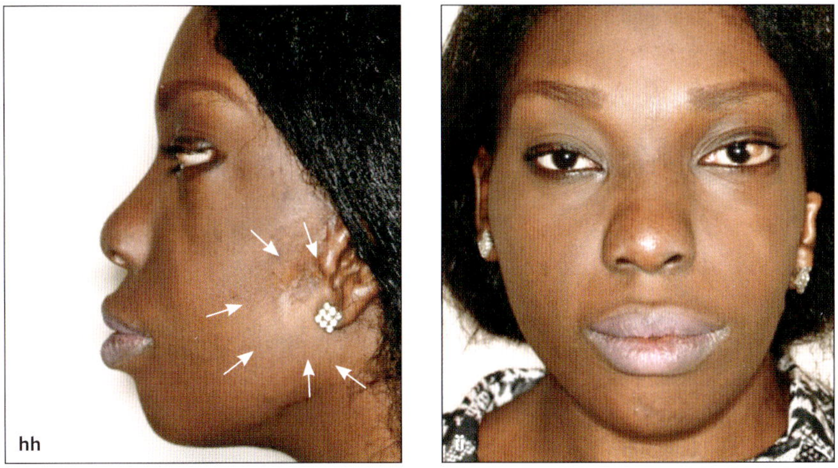

Fig 5-51 *(cont)* The pretreatment (*aa*) and postsurgical (*bb*) frontal views. Note the correction of the transverse occlusal cant. The postsurgical frontal view (*cc*), profile view (*dd*), and occlusion (*ee to gg*). (*hh*) Postoperative left profile view following skeletal reconstruction. The preauricular scar after removal of cartilaginous tags at age 7 years can be seen, as well as the soft tissue deficiency as a result of the masseter muscle deficiency and left ear microtia (*arrows*). (*ii*) Following skeletal reconstruction, there is still noticeable preauricular soft tissue deficiency present seen in the frontal view (*arrows*).

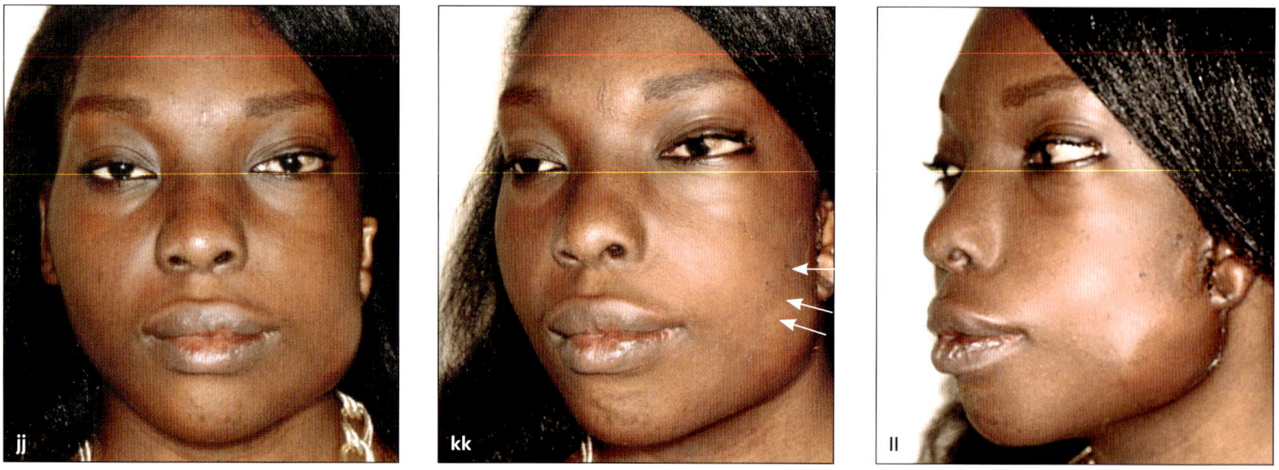

Fig 5-51 (*cont*) (*jj to ll*) Postoperative frontal, three-quarter, and profile views 7 days after soft tissue augmentation using a subdermal fat graft. Note that the augmentation was overcorrected (*arrows*), as a certain amount of postoperative resorption is to be expected.

TMJ ankylosis

True ankylosis is caused by either fibrous or bony fusion of the structures contained within the TMJ capsule. In its most severe state, it is characterized by a bony union of the condyle and the glenoid fossa. Mandibular movements are restricted and, depending on the patient's age, will limit normal growth on the affected side, causing significant facial asymmetry. Early surgery that releases the ankylosis followed by active functional therapy is indicated for these patients. Surgical release should include removal of all soft and hard tissue (including the coronoid process) as well as mandible release. This surgical procedure may be technically difficult, and it is futile to perform it without physical therapy to maintain the mouth opening obtained at surgery; either reankylosis of the joint will occur, or scarred soft tissue will limit mouth opening. In adult patients with ankylosis, the joint can be reconstructed by either placing a joint prosthesis or leaving an adequate gap between the mandible and the glenoid fossa, the so-called gap arthroplasty. The importance of postoperative physiotherapy cannot be overstated.

The surgical treatment for young patients with ankylosis can be performed in two stages.

First stage (5 to 7 years old)

The first stage is surgical release of the ankylosis, followed by long-term physical therapy. A costochondral graft may be indicated to reconstruct the TMJ and correct the vertical and anteroposterior dimensions of the mandible on the affected side. This will create an open bite, which will allow vertical maxillary growth under orthodontic control. The unpredictable tendency for either resorption of the graft, excessive growth potential of the costochondral graft, and the tendency to reankylose should be considered. Due to the low success rate of costochonral grafts, the graft often requires replacement by means of an alloplastic TMJ prosthesis (see case 15).

Second stage (14 to 16 years old)

The second surgical stage involves the final correction of facial asymmetry and occlusal cants with orthognathic surgery.

Case 14

This patient developed ankylosis of her TMJ after trauma to her chin at 3 years of age. When her orthodontist saw her at the age of 6 years, she had a severe malocclusion and a maximum mouth opening of 1 mm. Her parents recalled that she had fallen on her chin in a park when she was 3 years old. Although she experienced some pain at the time, she recovered uneventfully.

Main complaint

The patient's main concerns were limited mouth opening, an inability to eat properly, and a "crooked" face.

Medical history

Her medical history was noncontributory.

Clinical examination

1. Soft tissue
   - Frontal view (Fig 5-52a)
     - Severe asymmetry of the mandible toward the left side
     - Everted lower lip
     - Flat appearance of the right side of the chin and mandible

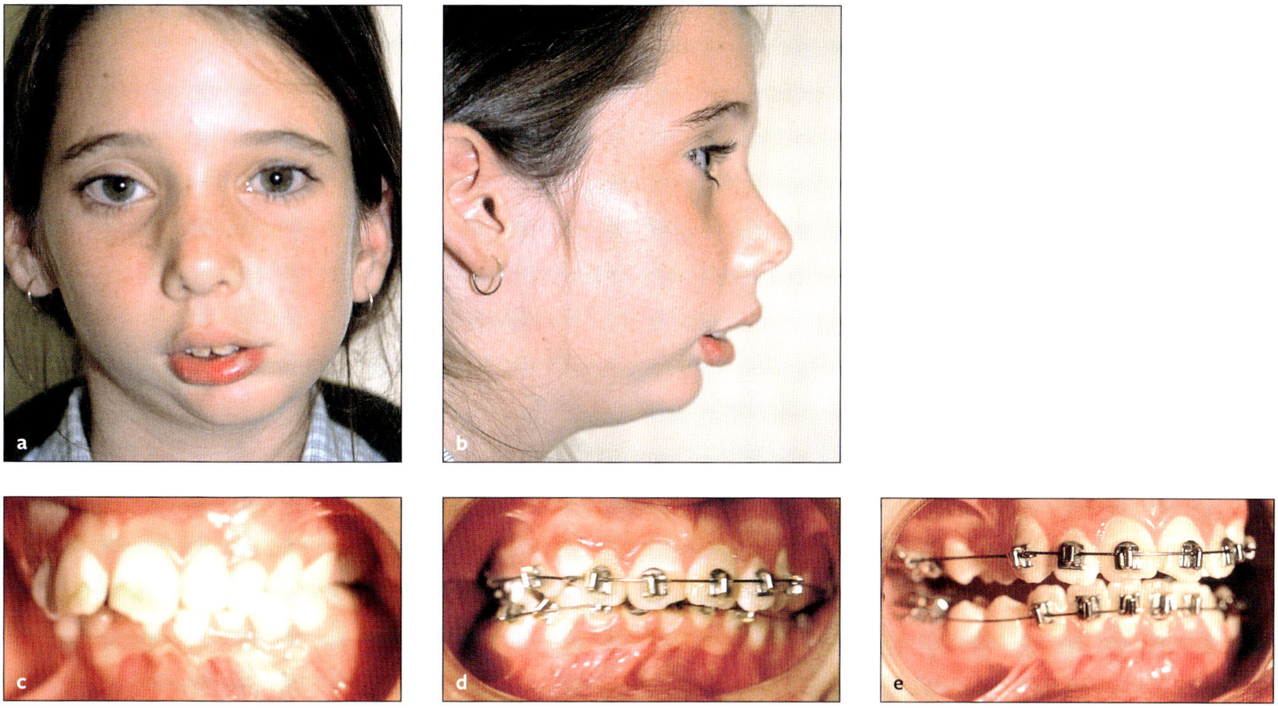

Fig 5-52 Case 14. Pretreatment frontal view (*a*), profile view (*b*), and right side of the occlusion (*c*). The presurgical occlusion (*d*) and maximal mouth opening before surgery (*e*) also are shown.

- Excessively rounded appearance of the left side of the mandible
- Profile view (Fig 5-52b)
  - Mandibular anteroposterior deficiency
  - Microgenia
  - Everted lower lip
  - Increased interlabial gap

2. Dental (Figs 5-52c and 5-52d)
   - Class II malocclusion, more on the left side
   - Increased overjet
   - Crowding in both arches
   - Mandibular dental midline toward the left
   - Maximal mouth opening of 1 mm (Fig 5-52e)
3. Skeletal
   - Mandibular anteroposterior deficiency
   - Microgenia
   - Mandibular asymmetry toward the left
   - Ankylosis of the left TMJ
4. Radiographic
   - Panoramic radiograph (Fig 5-52f)
     - Large bony mass in the left TMJ area
     - Elongated coronoid process
   - Lateral cephalometric radiograph (Fig 5-52g)
     - Severe mandibular anteroposterior deficiency
     - Anteroposterior cephalometric radiograph (Fig 5-52h)
     - Severe asymmetry of the mandible toward the left
     - Transverse cant of the occlusal plane

Problem list

- Ankylosis of the left TMJ
- Deficiency of the left side of the mandible
- Mouth opening of 1 mm
- Slight cant in the maxillary occlusal plane caused by deficient vertical growth of the maxilla on the left
- Class II malocclusion

Treatment plan

1. Surgical removal of bony ankylosis and creation of an articular fossa (Figs 5-52i and 5-52j)
2. Surgical removal of scar tissue that may inhibit normal mouth opening
3. Coronoidectomy of the left coronoid process (see Figs 5-52i and 5-52j)
4. Harvesting of a costochondral graft from the left eighth rib
5. Placement of a costochondral graft to reconstruct the left TMJ (Figs 5-55k and 5-52l)
6. Physical therapy to maintain the mouth opening achieved at surgery and to establish function to encourage growth of the deficient hard and soft tissues
7. Continuation of the orthodontic treatment to establish normal occlusion

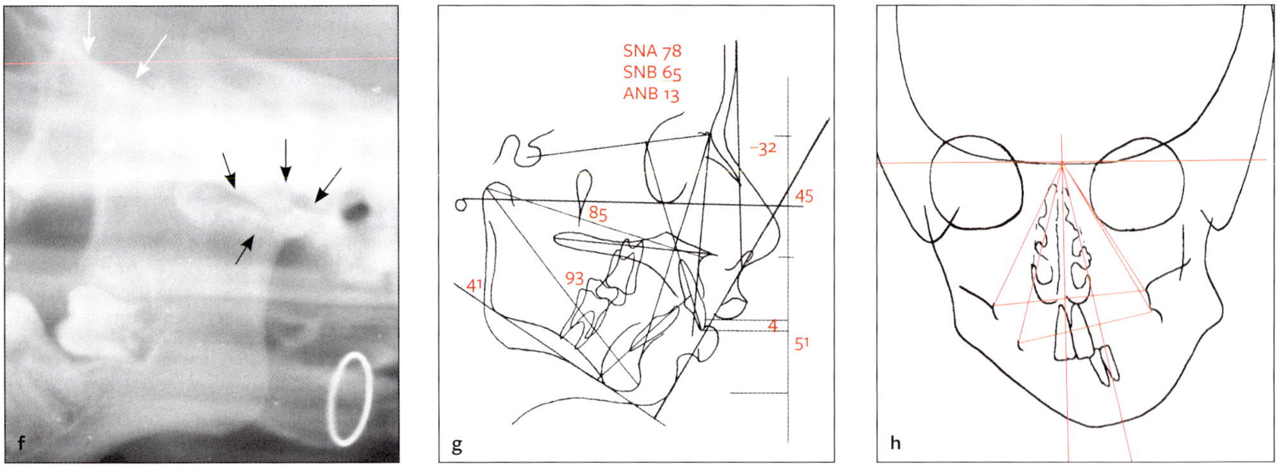

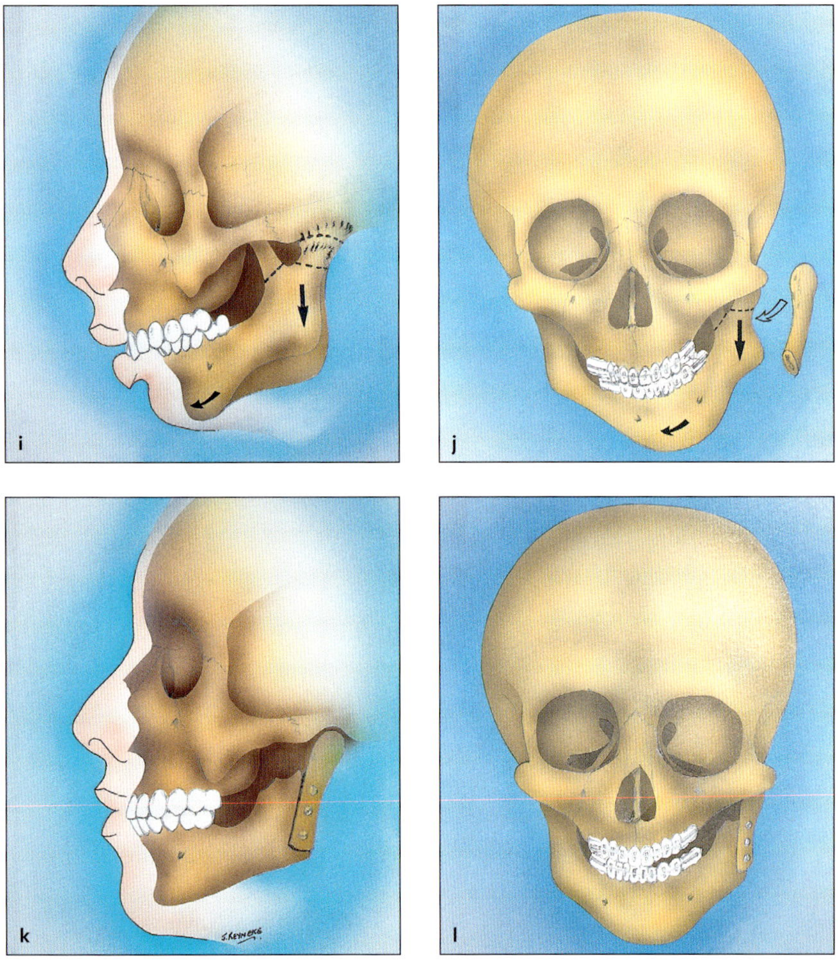

Fig 5-52 *(cont)* (*f*) Left side of the panoramic radiograph. The large bony mass obliterating the left TMJ (*black arrows*) and the elongated coronoid process (*white arrows*) are clearly visible. (*g*) The pretreatment lateral cephalometric tracing illustrates anteroposterior deficiency: SNB = 65 degrees, ANB = 13 degrees; convex profile: facial contour angle = −32 degrees; and the vertical difference of the left and right lower border of the mandible. (*h*) The presurgical anteroposterior cephalometric tracing clearly illustrates the severe asymmetry of the mandible. The transverse cant of the maxillary occlusion is only slightly affected at this stage and would probably respond favorably to functional correction of the mandible. The extent of the joint surgery and coronoidectomy as well as the surgical repositioning of the left side of the mandible is indicated from a lateral view (*i*) and a frontal view (*j*). Also depicted are the costochondral graft and mandibular position after surgery: lateral view (*k*) and frontal view (*l*).

Presurgical orthodontics

Because the patient could not open her mouth, the presurgical orthodontic treatment was limited.

Surgical treatment

The left TMJ was reconstructed with a costochondral graft, and a mouth opening of 35 mm was achieved at surgery. A gap was created between the maxillary and mandibular teeth on the left and was maintained with a splint (Figs 5-52m and 5-52n). A coronoidectomy was performed on the left side.

The patient followed an active physical therapy program, assisted by a mouth-opening appliance placed at the time of surgery. Excellent patient cooperation led to a mouth opening of 33 mm after 1 year.

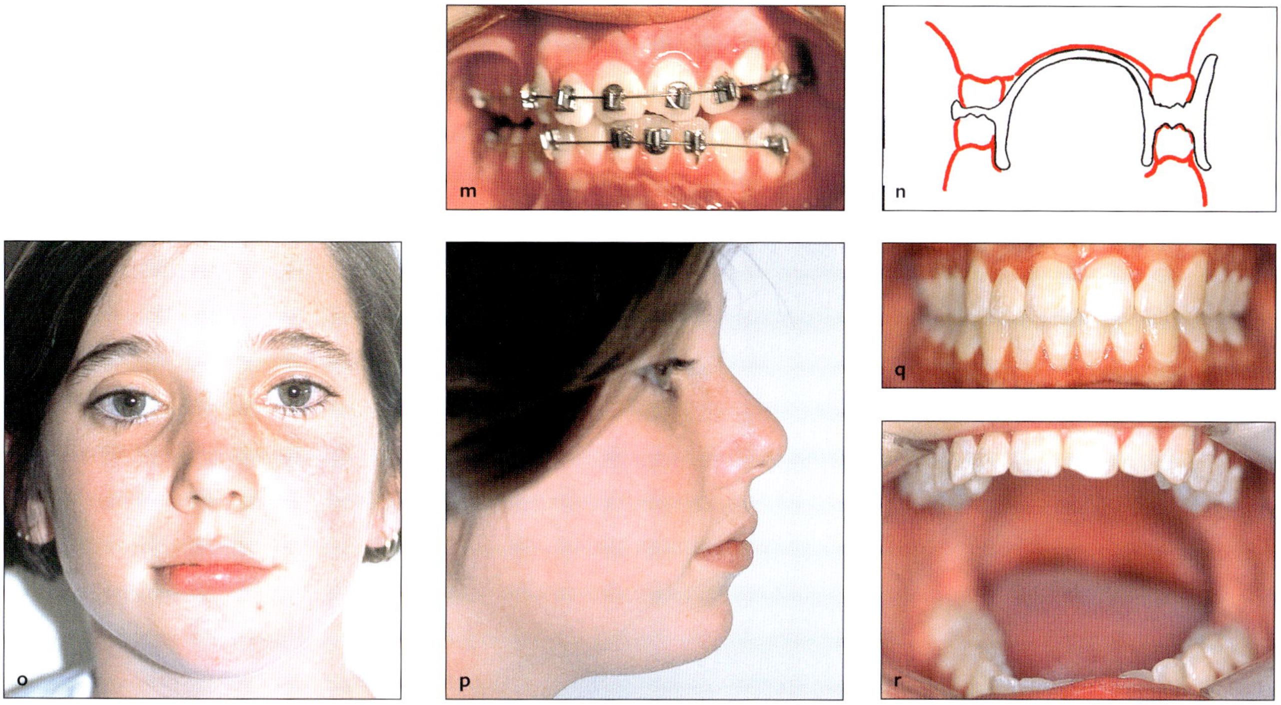

Fig 5-52 *(cont)* (*m*) The lateral open bite on the left was created by elongation of the left mandibular ramus by the rib graft. (*n*) The height of the left ramus is maintained by an acrylic splint placed at surgery. Postsurgical frontal view (*o*) and profile view (*p*) demonstrate the soft and hard tissue response to normal jaw function. The postsurgical occlusion (*q*) and mouth opening of 33 mm (*r*) are shown 2 years after surgery.

Postsurgical orthodontics

Postsurgical orthodontic treatment began only 6 months after surgery and was completed after 15 months. The postsurgical growth of the hard and soft tissue on the affected side and the final mouth opening are evident in Figs 5-52o to 5-52r. It is again important to stress that the success of surgical treatment of temporomandibular ankylosis is dependent on diligent postsurgical physical therapy.

Case 15

A 14-year-old boy was referred by his orthodontist for the treatment of left TMJ ankylosis. His mother gave the history that the patient developed septicemia at the age of 3 years. The infective process caused septic arthritis of both his right hip joint and right TMJ. He subsequently developed ankyloses of his right TMJ with a maximum mouth opening of 20 mm, facial asymmetry, and pain on mastication. At the age of 10 years, the ankylosis was treated with a costochondral graft, and his mouth opening improved to 35 mm. His orthodontist manufactured an appliance that would enhance vertical development of the maxilla on the affected side. Unfortunately, the costochondral graft reankylosed and overgrew, developing into facial asymmetry, lower dental midline to the left, bilateral crossbites, and a mouth opening of 4 mm (see Figs 5-53a and 5-53b).

Main complaint

The patient's main concern was the severe facial asymmetry caused by the overgrown graft and the decreased mouth opening.

Medical history

The patient's right hip was treated by an orthopedic surgeon at the age of 3 years; however, he walks with a slight limp and he is small in posture. No additional medical concerns were present.

Clinical examination

1. Soft tissue
   - Frontal view (Fig 5-53a)
     - The overgrowth of the graft is evident in the right temporomandibular area
     - The chin is displaced to the left
     - His right eye appears smaller than the left
     - Increased interlabial gap

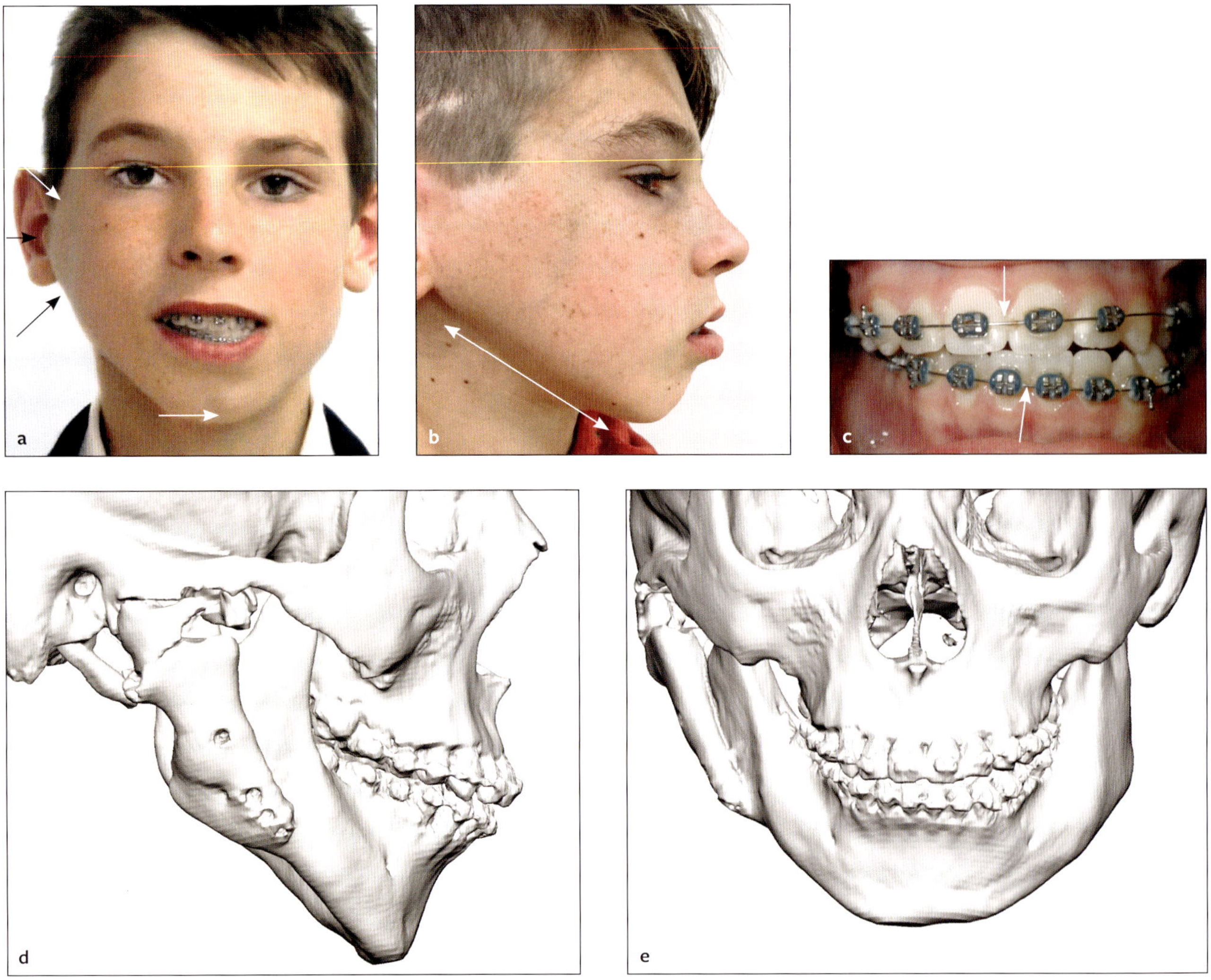

Fig 5-53 Case 15. (*a*) Frontal view: note the mandibular asymmetry to the left and the preauricular deformity (*arrows*). (*b*) Profile view: the mandibular elongation on the right side caused by the excessive costochondral graft growth is evident. (*c*) The limited mouth opening and dental midline displacement to the left is demonstrated. (*d and e*) The 3D frontal and lateral computer images. Note the excessive bone formation between the costochondral graft and the glenoid fossa. The skeletal asymmetry was caused by the overgrown graft with the chin displaced to the left.

- Profile view (Fig 5-53b)
  - Convex profile
  - Microgenia
  - Everted lower lip
  - Prominence of the temporomandibular area
  - Increased interlabial gap
2. Dental (Fig 5-53c)
   - Transverse cant in the occlusal plane
   - Mandibular dental midline displaced to the left
   - Bilateral crossbites
   - Root resorption of all first molars and absent mandibular left second premolar
   - Edge-to-edge incisor relationship
3. Skeletal
   - Mandibular asymmetry to the left.
   - The right side of the mandible is excessive.
   - The chin is deficient and asymmetric.
   - The overgrown bony mass of the graft appears prominent.
4. Radiographic
   - Panoramic root resorption of all four first molars
   - A large bone mass occupying the glenoid fossa is evident
   - Four screws placed during the reconstruction are present
- 3D CT scan (Figs 5-53d and 5-53e)
  - The large overgrown graft is evident
  - It seems as the graft has overgrown in all dimensions
  - The glenoid fossa is obliterated by bone
  - The mandibular body is asymmetrically shaped
  - The right coronoid process is elongated

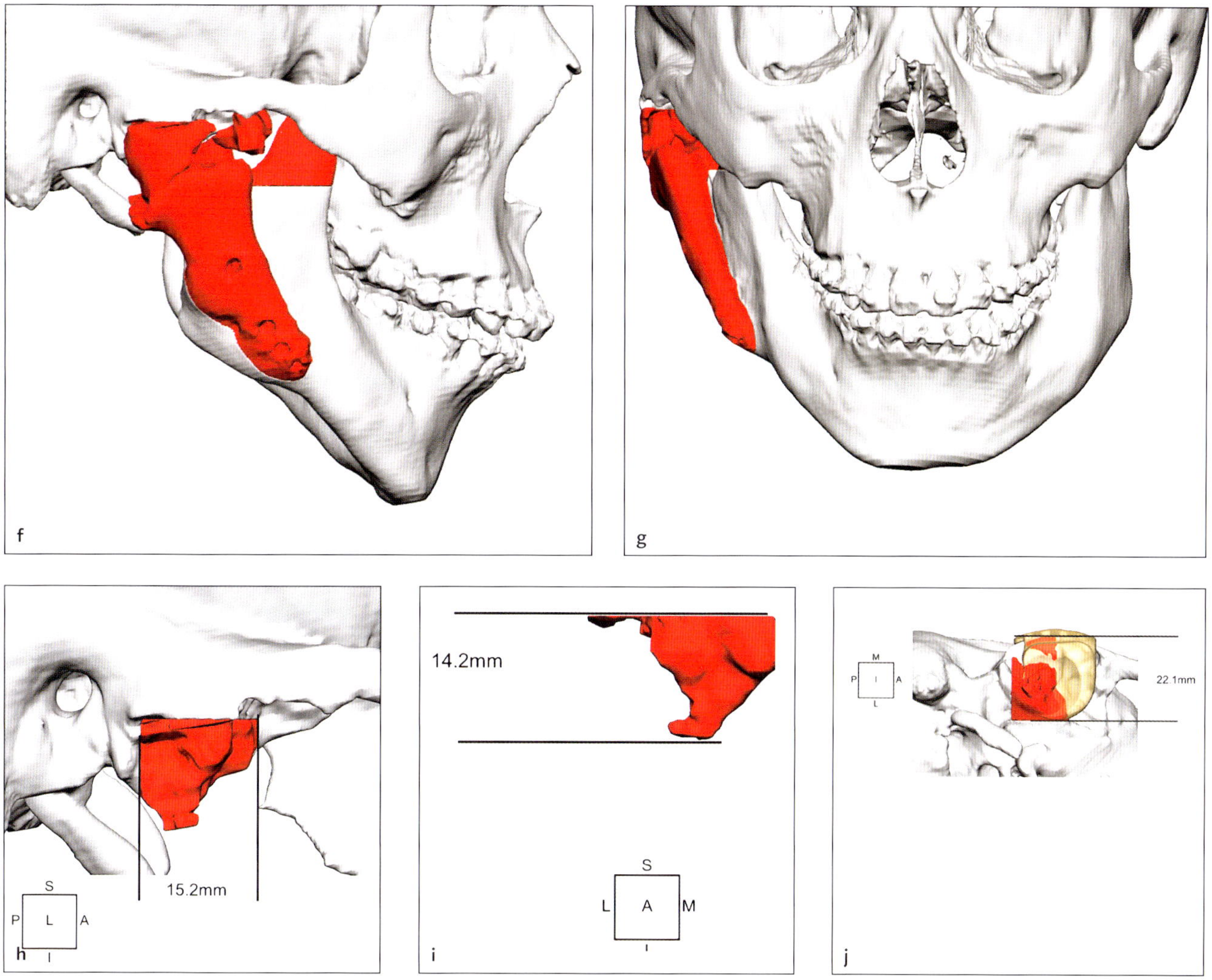

Fig 5-53 *(cont)* (*f and g*) Virtual surgical planning indicating the bone to be removed during surgery in *red*. (*h and i*) The 3D ventral computer images. The excessive bone medial to the glenoid fossa was to be removed. (*j*) Planned position of the custom-made fossa.

Problem list

- Mouth opening of 4 mm
- Malocclusion (crossbites, edge-to-edge incisor relationship, dental midline discrepancy)
- Large overgrown bone graft attached to the mandibular ramus (Figs 5-53f and 5-53g)
- Facial asymmetry
- Large mass of bone filling the glenoid fossa (Figs 5-53h and 5-53i)
- The bony mass in the glenoid fossa stretches 21 mm medially (Fig 5-53j)

Treatment

It was emphasized to the patient and his parents that postoperative exercise maintaining the mouth opening is mandatory for the treatment to be successful.

Presurgical orthodontics

The dental arches were aligned and arch compatibility was established.

Surgery

A 3D virtual treatment plan was developed (Figs 5-53k and 5-53l). A cutting guide was used to accurately remove the costochondral graft and the excessive bone occupying the glenoid fossa (see *red* on Figs 5-53f to 5-53j). A cutting guide was also used to remove the elongated coronoid process and to prepare the glenoid fossa for the patient-matched fossa. The mandible was manually stretched to an interincisal distance of 39 mm.

The teeth were placed into the planned occlusion and intermaxillary fixation. The condyle and fossa templates were used to ensure a perfect fit of the condyle and fossa.

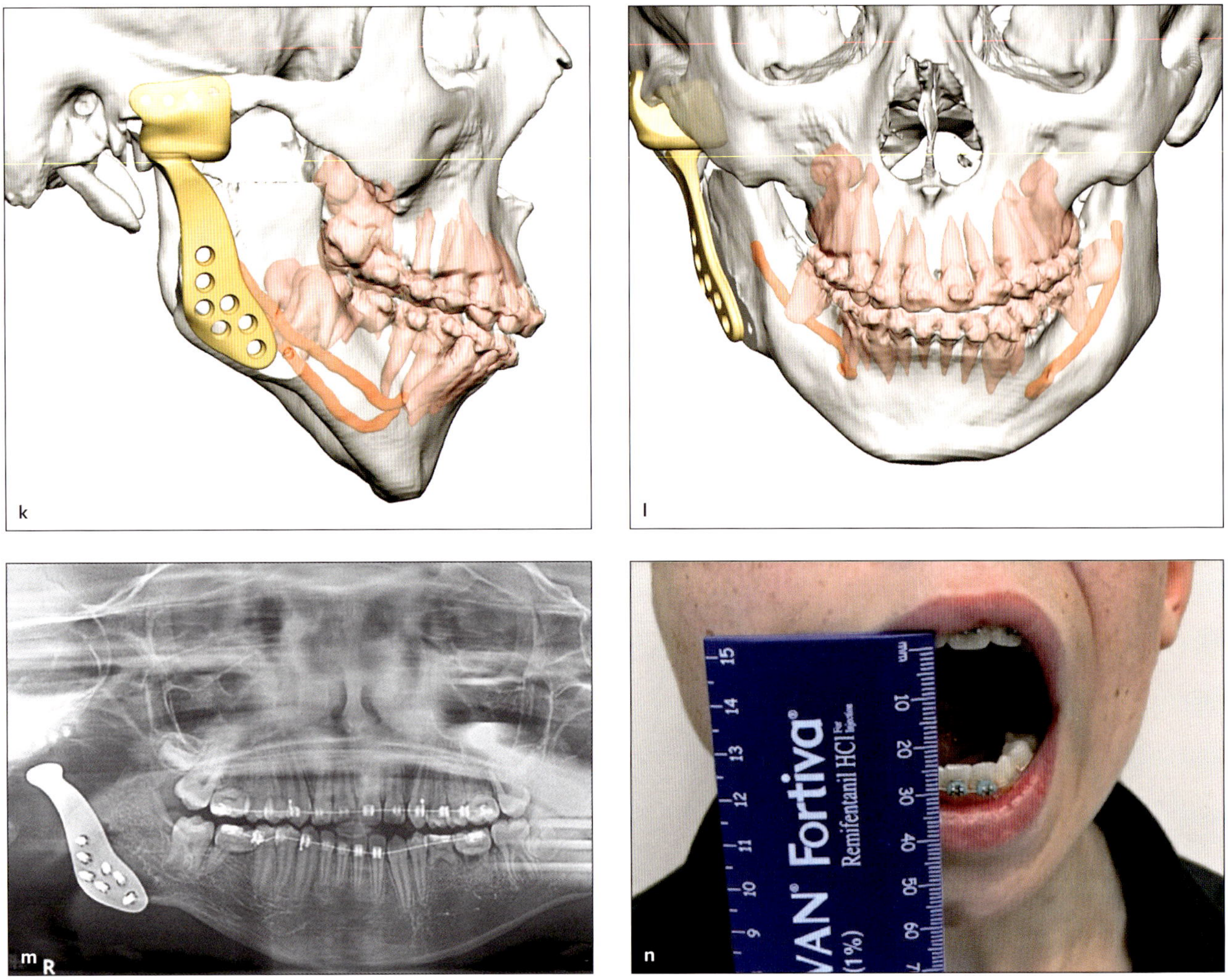

Fig 5-53 (cont) (*k and l*) The planned position of the patient-matched condyle and fossa. The dental roots and inferior alveolar nerve and planned correction of the occlusion are indicated in *red*. (*m*) A postoperative panoramic image following removal of the costochondral graft and placement of the patient-matched condyle and fossa. Note the dental root resorption as a result of the septicemia at age 3 years. (*n*) With active physiotherapy and excellent patient cooperation, a mouth opening of 44 mm was achieved 7 weeks after surgery.

The final components were then placed and rigidly fixated. After removal of the intermaxillary fixation and suturing of the incisions, two 3.5-oz 4-mm training elastics were placed (Fig 5-53m).

Postoperative treatment

Postoperative physiotherapy. Aggressive physiotherapy was started 1 day following surgery while the patient was instructed and motivated to maintain the mouth opening using tongue blades (Fig 5-53n).

Postoperative orthodontics. Finalization of the occlusion and retention.

Asymmetry in the adult

Facial asymmetry in adults will be discussed according to location.

Asymmetry of the chin

The fact that the chin is three-dimensional should always be considered during assessment and correction of chin asymmetry.

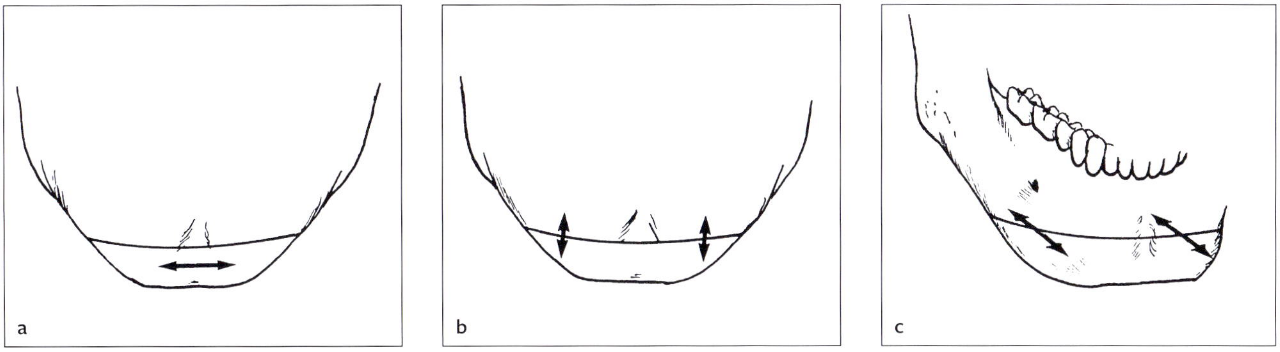

Fig 5-54 (*a*) Left or right sliding genioplasty for correction of transverse asymmetry of the chin. (*b*) Vertical reduction or downgraft of the chin to correct an asymmetric cant of the lower border. (*c*) Differential anterior or posterior repositioning of the chin to correct anteroposterior asymmetries.

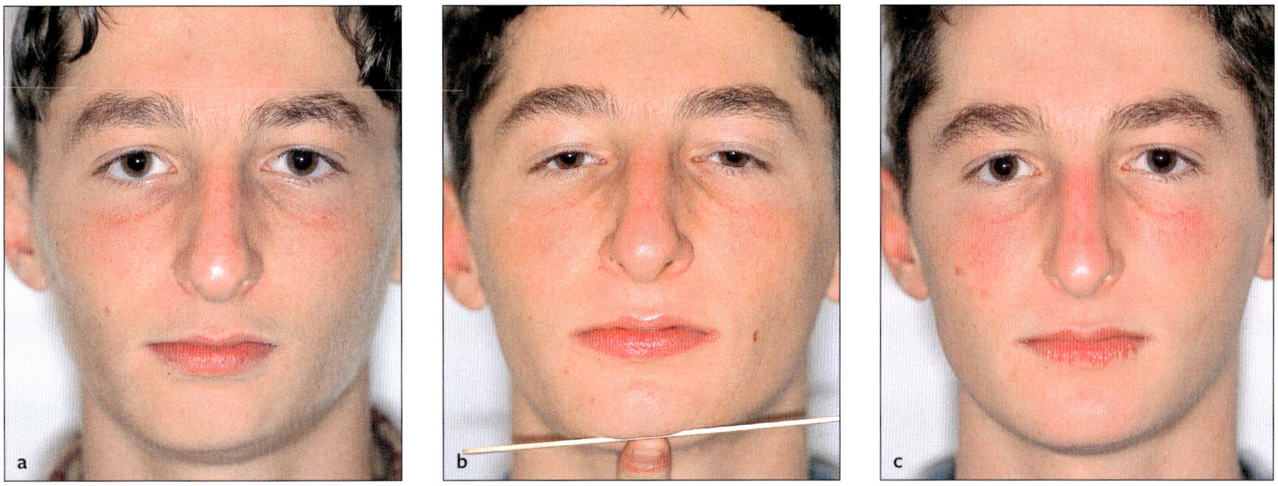

Fig 5-55 A patient with chin asymmetry. The transverse asymmetry of the chin toward the right (*a*) and the cant of the lower border of the chin (*b*) are evident. (*c*) A symmetric chin has been established by means of a genioplasty, sliding the chin toward the left side and downgrafting it on the left.

Transverse asymmetry

Transverse asymmetry of the chin is corrected by a sliding genioplasty that repositions the chin toward the left or right side (Fig 5-54a).

Cant of the lower border of the chin

A cant of the lower border of the chin is corrected by vertical change at the osteotomy site. The vertical height can be unilaterally reduced or increased by either downgrafting one side or performing an ostectomy on the other (Fig 5-54b). An alternative is a propeller osteotomy (see chapter 6).

Anteroposterior asymmetry

Anteroposterior asymmetry can be corrected by differential anterior or posterior repositioning of the chin (Fig 5-54c). Figure 5-55 demonstrates the correction of asymmetry of the chin in a transverse and vertical dimension.

Asymmetry of the mandible

Most patients with mandibular anteroposterior excess have some form of asymmetry. Facial asymmetry caused by mandibular asymmetry can be corrected by surgical repositioning of the mandible. It is important that the orthodontist position the mandibular incisors in the middle of the chin so that when the dental midlines are corrected,

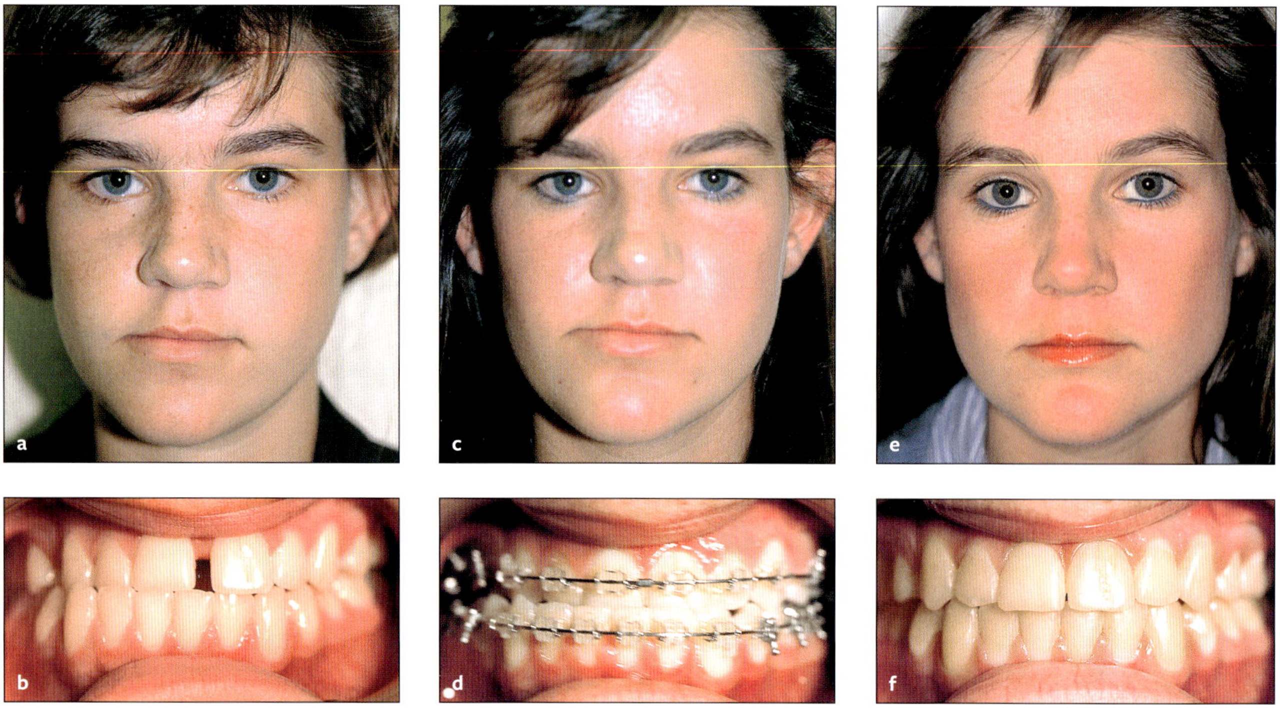

Fig 5-56 A patient with mandibular asymmetry. Facial asymmetry (*a*) and asymmetric Class III malocclusion (*b*). Slight worsening of the facial symmetry (*c*) and dental asymmetry after presurgical orthodontic treatment (*d*). Posttreatment results are demonstrated in frontal view (*e*) and occlusion (*f*) 2 years after debanding.

the middle of the chin is in the facial midline. The BSSO, also called *bilateral split ramus osteotomy or bilateral sagittal split ramus osteotomy*, is the procedure of choice for small corrections, whereas bilateral vertical osteotomies of the mandibular ramus are indicated for the correction of large asymmetries. When a BSSO is used to correct severe asymmetry, the proximal segments tend to flare, leading to poor bone contact, posterior mandibular asymmetry, and a greater tendency for peripheral condylar sag after placement of internal rigid fixation. Figure 5-56 illustrates the correction of mandibular asymmetry. The mandible was asymmetric toward the right, and there was mandibular anteroposterior excess. No attempt was made to correct the dental midlines during the preorthodontic preparation. The mandibular dental midline was positioned in the midline of the chin, and the maxillary incisor midline was positioned in the midline of the face (see Figs 5-56a to 5-56d). Facial and dental symmetry were established by a BSSO. The treatment results 2 years after debanding are seen in Figs 5-56e and 5-56f.

Unilateral sagittal split mandibular ramus osteotomy

A small asymmetric mandibular defect may be corrected by means of a unilateral sagittal split ramus osteotomy (USSO). However, several factors need to be considered when correcting mandibular asymmetry and operating only on one side of the mandible. The mandibular midline will be rotated around the condyle of the unoperated side until the mandibular dental midline coordinates with the maxillary dental midline and facial midline. This rotation will have certain geometrical limitations and possible functional implications (see Beukes et al, 2016, in Recommended Reading). Operating on only one side of the mandible will allow for rotation of the midline to either the left or the right by either advancing or setting the major segment back. The major segment will be rotated around the condyle and will have secondary anteroposterior implications (Fig 5-57).

When the USSO is performed on the left side, the midline can either be rotated to the right by advancing the major segment or to the left by setting the major segment back. Rotation to the right will result in a slight advance-

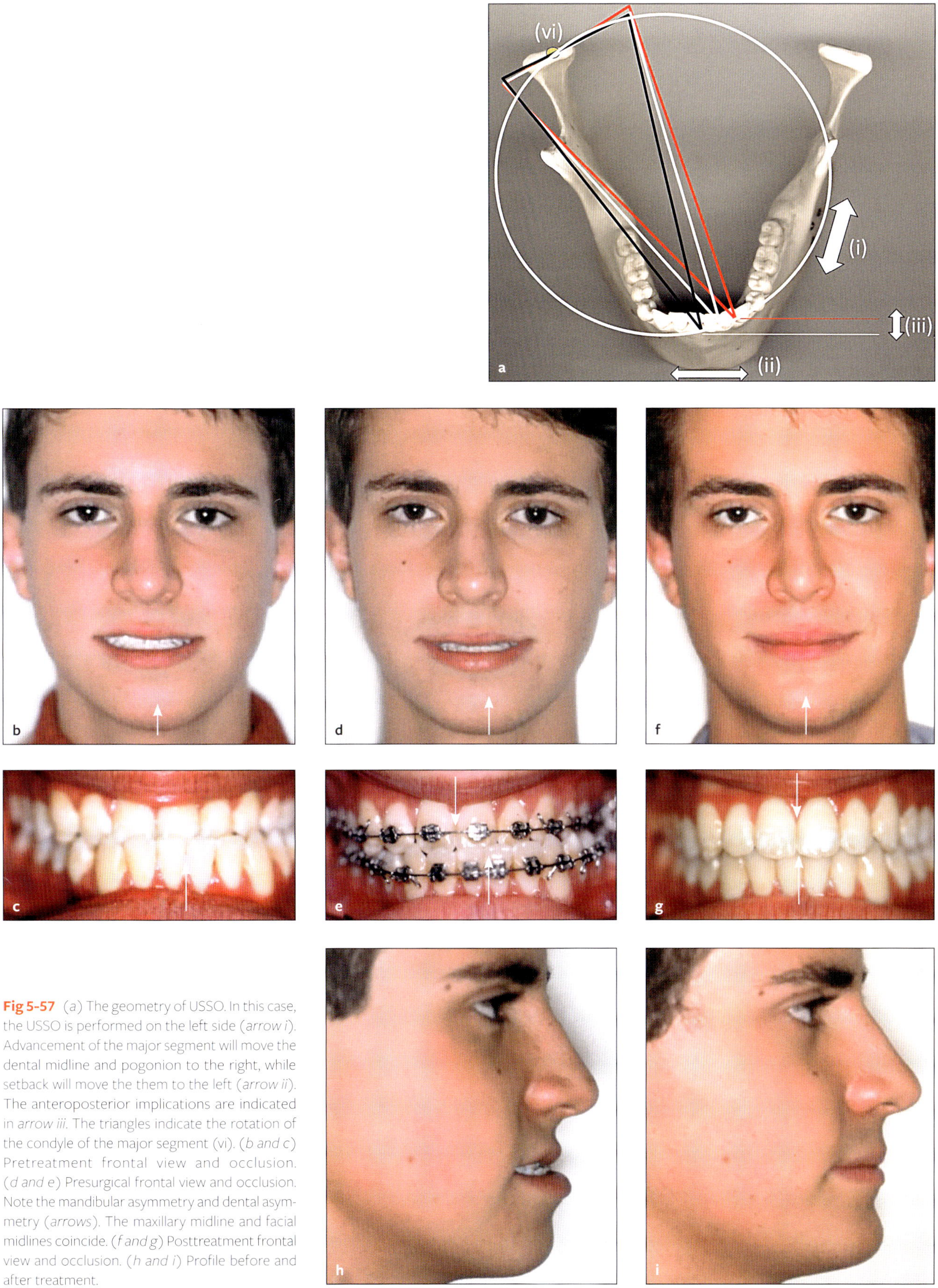

Fig 5-57 (*a*) The geometry of USSO. In this case, the USSO is performed on the left side (*arrow i*). Advancement of the major segment will move the dental midline and pogonion to the right, while setback will move the them to the left (*arrow ii*). The anteroposterior implications are indicated in *arrow iii*. The triangles indicate the rotation of the condyle of the major segment (vi). (*b and c*) Pretreatment frontal view and occlusion. (*d and e*) Presurgical frontal view and occlusion. Note the mandibular asymmetry and dental asymmetry (*arrows*). The maxillary midline and facial midlines coincide. (*f and g*) Posttreatment frontal view and occlusion. (*h and i*) Profile before and after treatment.

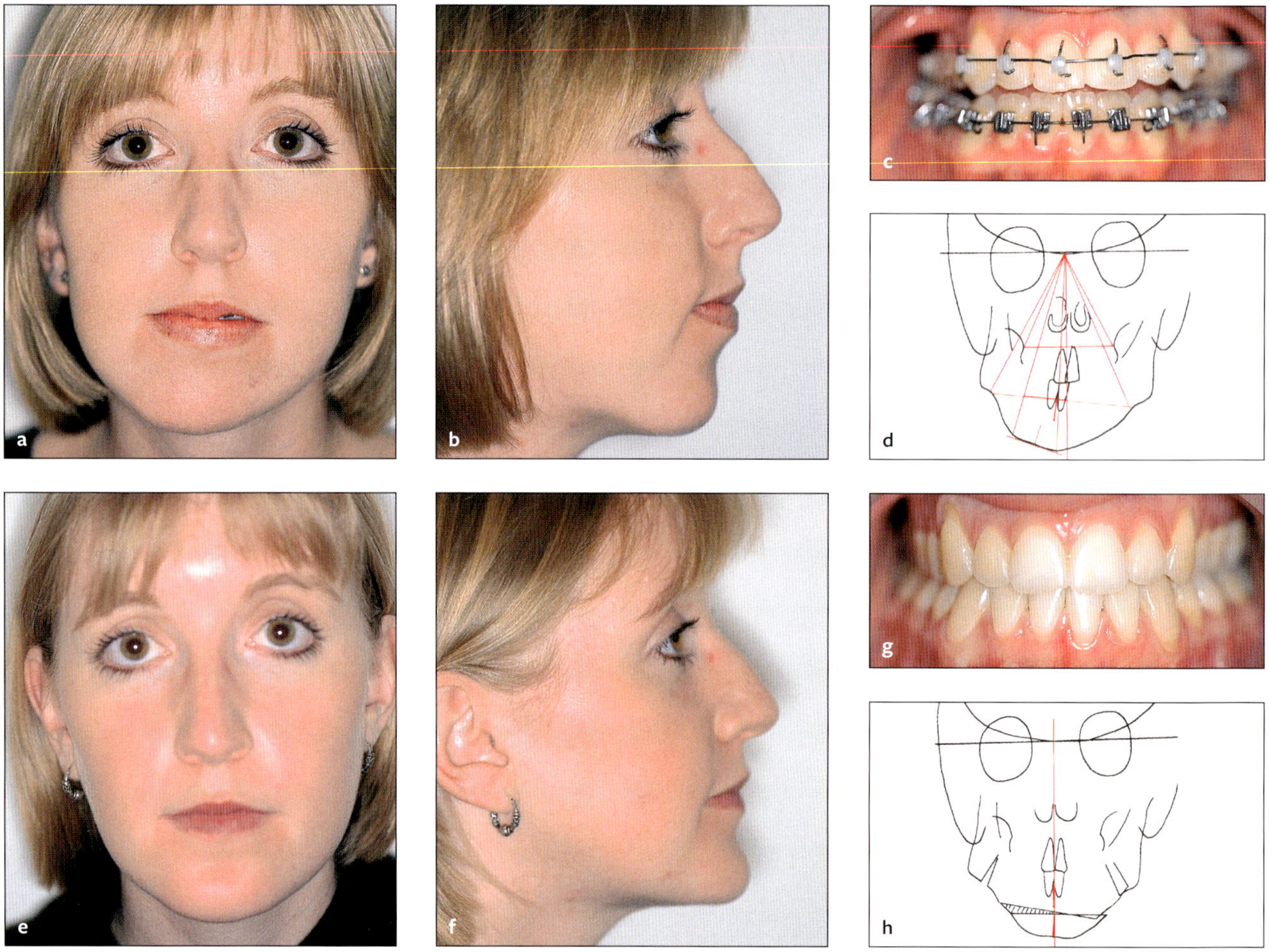

Fig 5-58 This patient presented with both chin and mandibular asymmetry. (*a*) In the frontal view, the asymmetry of the mandible and chin are clearly visible. (*b*) Mandibular anteroposterior deficiency and microgenia. (*c*) Presurgical occlusion. (*d*) Anteroposterior cephalometric tracing showing that the facial midline and maxillary dental midline coincide; however, the mandibular midline is displaced toward the right and the chin midline even further toward the right. Posttreatment frontal view (*e*), profile view (*f*), occlusion (*g*), and anteroposterior cephalometric tracing illustrating the surgical correction (*h*).

ment of pogonion, while rotation to the left will set pogonion back. These secondary anteroposterior changes will have esthetic implications that should be considered when planning treatment. The final anteroposterior position of the maxillary incisors and the maxilla will be dictated by the anteroposterior position of the mandibular incisors after correction of the midline and slight anteroposterior alteration. This will not be a consideration when a BSSO is performed, in which case the surgeon will not be "limited" by the unoperated side of the mandible.

The small rotational movement of the condyle on the major segment might have been a concern. Therefore, the author and colleagues investigated the indications for USSO, evaluated the geometry of the rotational movement of the mandible, and evaluated the long-term postoperative signs and symptoms in the TMJs of 23 patients who had undergone USSO for the correction of mandibular asymmetry. None of the patients experienced any long-term TMJ symptoms (Beukes et al, 2016).

Asymmetry of the mandible and chin

Mandibular asymmetry often occurs in combination with chin asymmetry. When both kinds of asymmetry are present, the dental midline does not coincide with the midline of the chin. After surgical correction of the mandibular asymmetry with correction of the dental midline, additional correction of the chin midline will be necessary. Accurate presurgical assessment of dental and chin midlines in relation to the facial midline is essential. When facial asymmetry will be corrected by mandibular surgery, the orthodontist must ensure that the maxillary dental midline is corrected orthodontically before surgery.

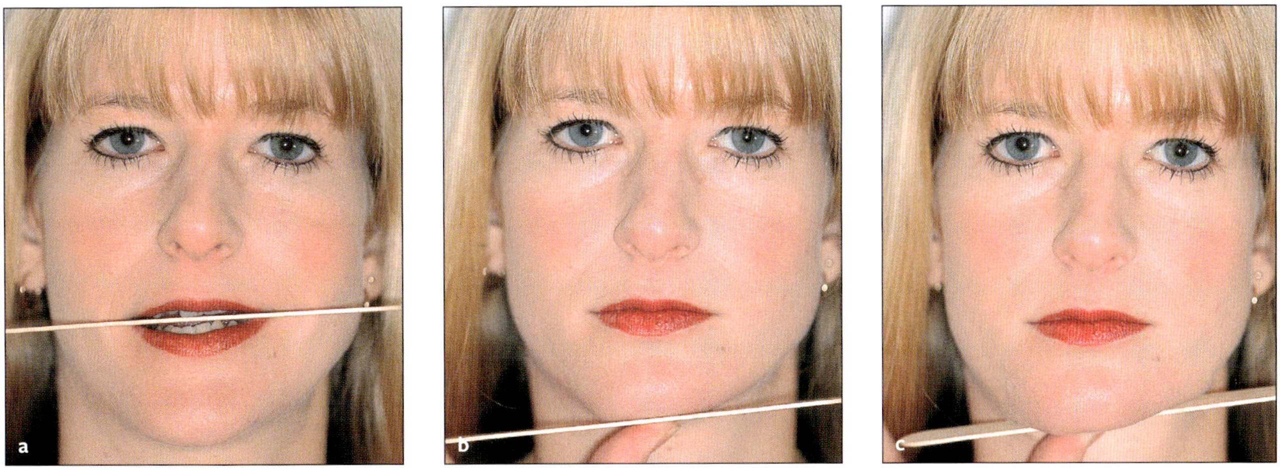

Fig 5-59 Transverse cant of the anterior maxillary occlusal plane (*a*), the lower border of the chin (*b*), and the lower borders of the posterior mandible (*c*) are illustrated using a tongue spatula.

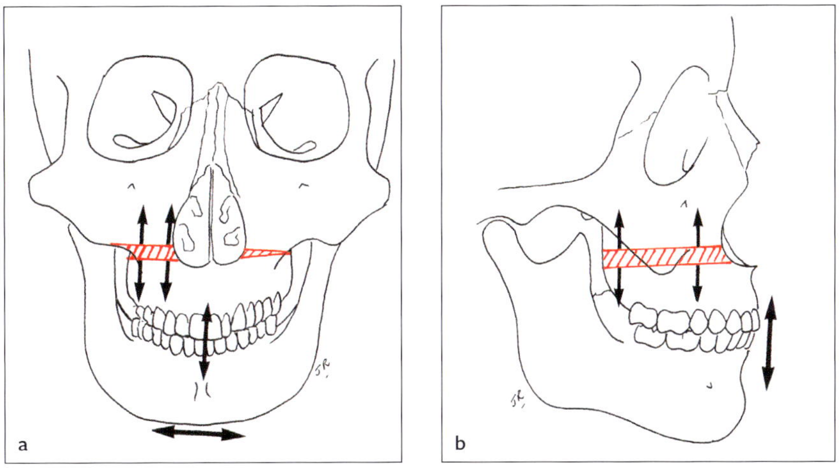

Fig 5-60 Correction of the cant of the occlusal plane in cases where the anterior and posterior cants are the same will involve two dimensions of change: vertical and transverse (*arrows*) as indicated by the arrows on the frontal view (*a*) and lateral view (*b*).

Correction of a combination of mandibular and chin asymmetry is demonstrated in Fig 5-58. The patient's mandible was asymmetric toward the right and anteroposteriorly deficient with a Class II malocclusion (more on the right side than the left side). The mandibular dental midline was 4 mm to the right of the maxillary incisor midline (facial midline); however, the midline of the chin was 11 mm to the right of the facial midline. There was a slight transverse cant in the maxillary occlusal plane, but it was not clinically significant (see Figs 5-58a to 5-58d). The mandibular asymmetry was corrected by a BSSO, advancing the mandible and rotating it toward the left to correct the dental midlines. Final facial symmetry was established by a genioplasty, which slid the chin to the left, downgrafted it on the right, and reduced the chin height on the left (see Figs 5-58e to 5-58h).

Asymmetry of the maxilla and mandible

Facial asymmetry involving both the maxilla and mandible often includes a cant in the occlusal plane. The cant can be assessed clinically using a dental fox plane plate or tongue spatula. Both the anterior and posterior cants of the occlusal plane as well as the lower border of the mandible should always be evaluated and noted (Fig 5-59). The cant in the occlusal plane of the maxilla is most easily and accurately evaluated on casts articulated on an adjustable articulator from a facebow recording. When the anterior and posterior cants are equal, the correction involves two dimensions: transverse and vertical (Fig 5-60). The maxillary incisor–lip relationship is very important in the correction of the occlusal cant of the maxilla (see chapter 3).

When surgery will involve both jaws, the orthodontist should not waste treatment time by correcting the dental midlines, which can be corrected surgically. Arch form,

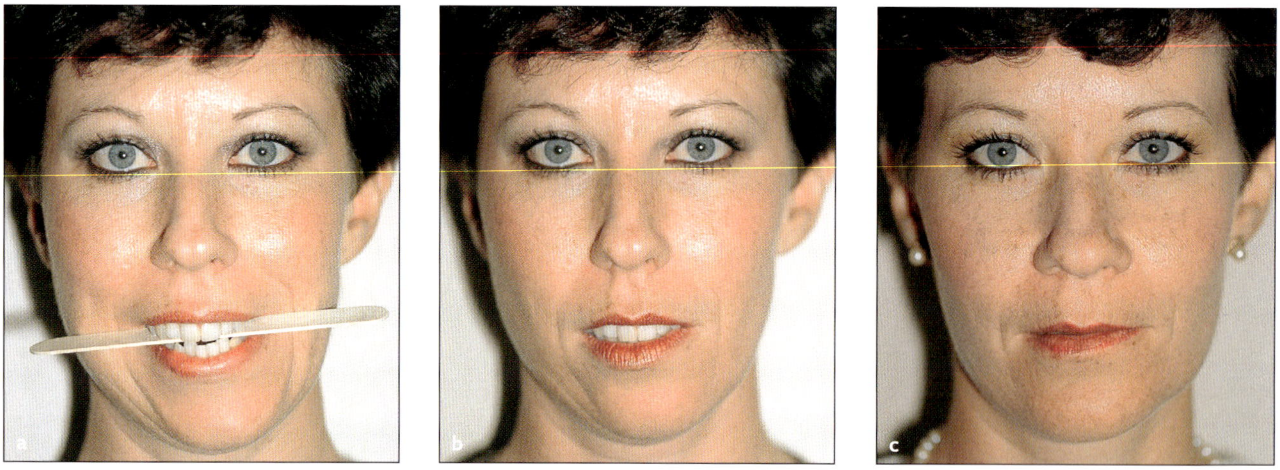

Fig 5-61 The tongue spatula demonstrates the cant of the occlusal plane (*a*), and the facial asymmetry involves the maxilla and mandible (*b*). (*c*) The postsurgical result after correction of the occlusal cant by means of a Le Fort I maxillary osteotomy and BSSO.

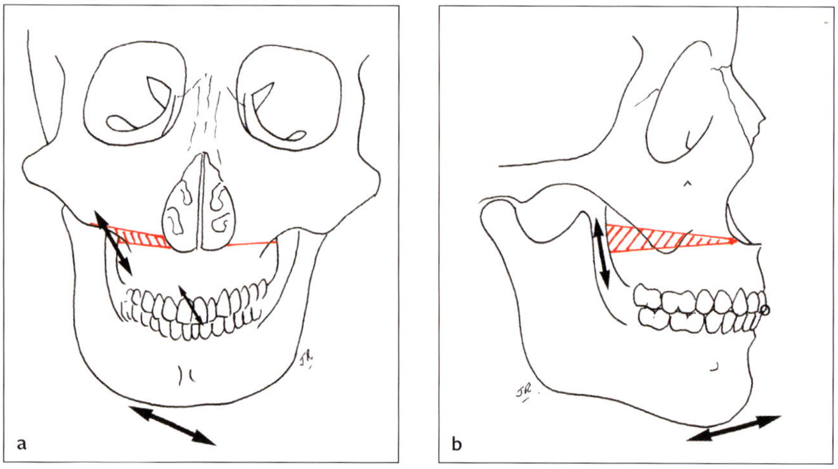

Fig 5-62 The 3D changes are indicated by the *arrows* following correction of the different cants in the anterior and posterior maxilla. (*a*) Frontal view. (*b*) Lateral view.

however, should be maintained to accommodate the rotational movement during the correction of dental midlines.

An example of facial asymmetry involving the maxilla and mandible is illustrated in Fig 5-61. There is a transverse cant of the occlusal plane, and the mandible is asymmetric toward the left. The patient has a Class I malocclusion, and the dental midlines coincide. The mandibular dental midline is in the middle of the chin. By correcting the occlusal cant (and, at the same time, the maxillary incisor-lip relationship), facial symmetry is restored (Fig 5-62).

Difference in anterior and posterior occlusal cants

A dual cant of the occlusal plane almost always results from unilateral excessive or deficient growth of the mandibular ramus—eg, patients with unilateral condylar hyperplasia or unilateral hypoplasia (hemifacial microsomia or temporomandibular ankylosis). The unilateral increase in or lack of vertical growth of the mandibular ramus secondarily influences the vertical growth of the maxilla and leads to a cant in the occlusal plane. The cant is more severe in the posterior than in the anterior maxilla, necessitating 3D correction.

Asymmetry of the maxilla, mandible, and chin

When the maxilla, mandible, and chin are all involved in the facial asymmetry, 3D correction is usually needed. Correction of the transverse cant of the maxillary occlusal plane will be more challenging than in patients whose anterior and posterior cants are equal. The posterior vertical change will differ on the right and left sides as well as in the anterior maxilla. This correction will eventually have a profound effect on the chin in the anteroposterior, vertical, and transverse dimensions (see Fig 5-52). Thus, these patients benefit from the propeller genioplasty (see chapter 6), a procedure that allows the surgeon to control

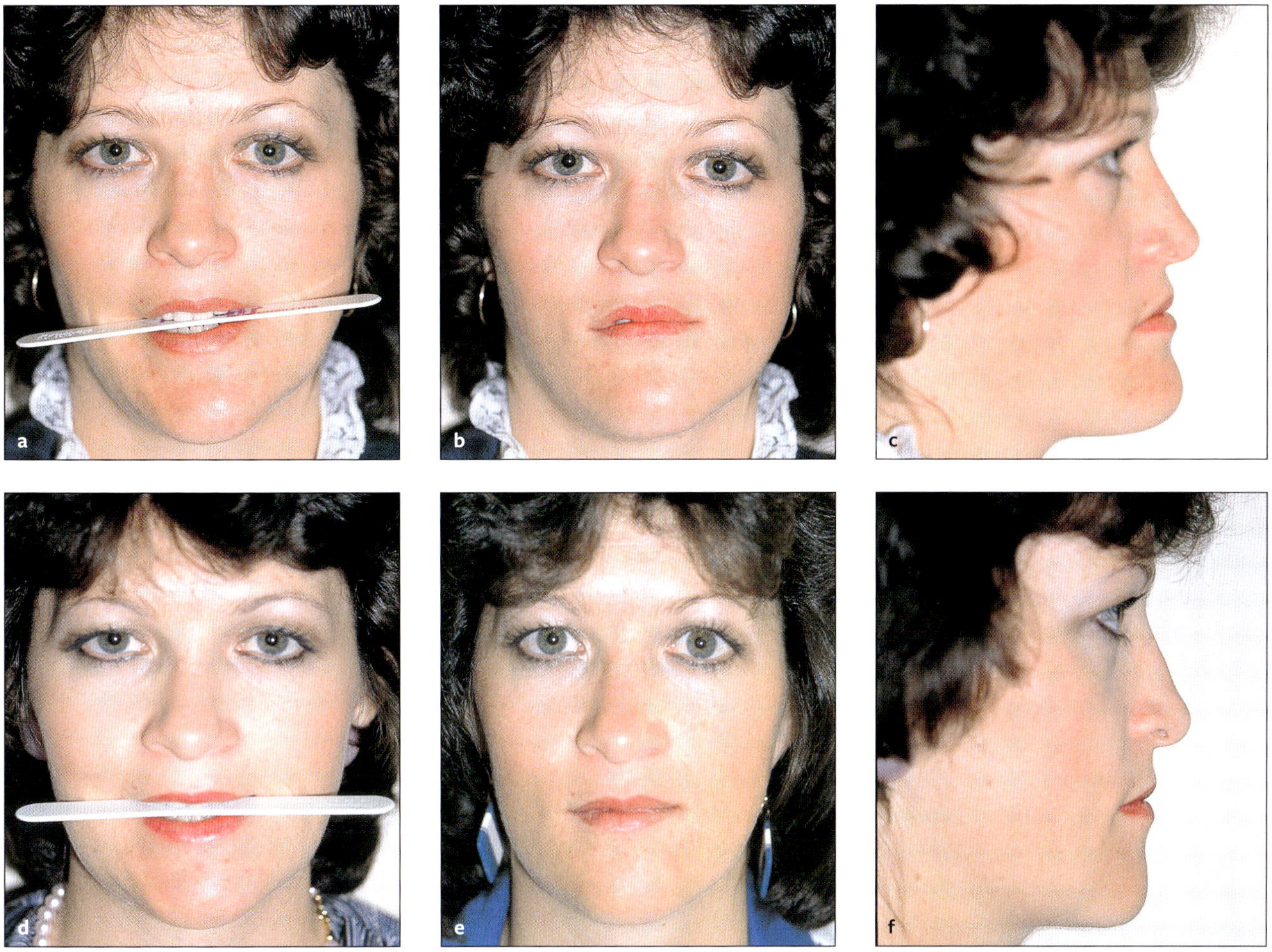

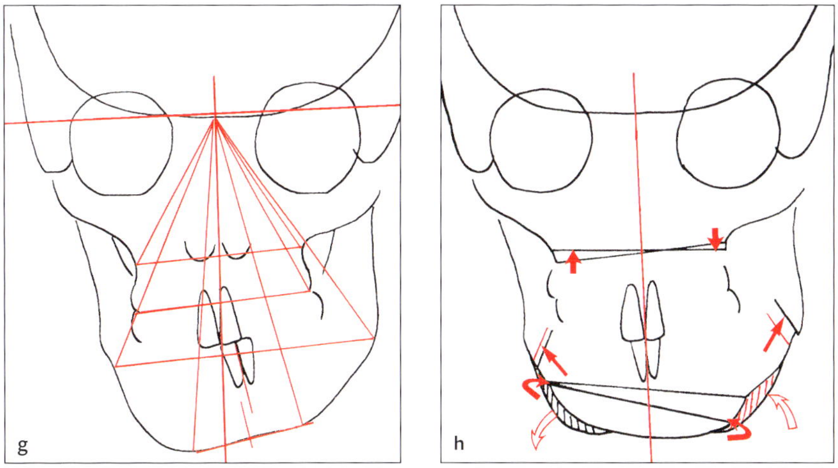

Fig 5-63 The presurgical cant of the occlusal plane is illustrated by the tongue spatula (*a*), while the presurgical transverse, vertical, and anteroposterior dimensions are demonstrated in frontal (*b*) and profile (*c*) views. The correction of facial asymmetry in all three dimensions is illustrated in frontal (*d and e*) and profile (*f*) views. (*g*) Presurgical anteroposterior cephalometric tracing. (*h*) Surgical correction.

the chin in the vertical, transverse, and anteroposterior dimensions. The patient shown in Fig 5-63 had unilateral condylar hyperplasia on the right side, and the asymmetry involved the maxilla, mandible, and chin. Surgical correction included the correction of the occlusal cant with a Le Fort I maxillary osteotomy. This change in the cant was followed by a BSSO in the mandible. A propeller genioplasty was performed to establish final chin symmetry. Better symmetry of the lower border of the posterior mandible was achieved with an ostectomy of the lower border of the right side of the mandible (after repositioning the inferior alveolar nerve) and the use of part of the ostectomized bone as a graft on the lateral side of the left mandibular body.

Asymmetry of the zygoma, nose, and frontal areas

The zygoma, nose, and frontal areas play an important role in the overall symmetry of the face and should be assessed carefully during the clinical examination. Correction of asymmetry in these areas should be an integral part of the correction of the total treatment of facial asymmetry; however, discussion of the treatment is beyond the scope of this text.

Distraction Osteogenesis and Orthognathic Surgery

During the International Congress of Cranial and Facial Distraction Osteogenesis held in Paris, France, in 1997, Dr Paul Tessier referred to distraction osteogenesis as the "end of facial osteotomies as we know them." New innovations to improve patient care are highly attractive and important; however, the use of distraction osteogenesis frequently exceeds and precedes its scientific evaluation. More than two decades have passed, and traditional osteotomies are still used; orthognathic surgical procedures are performed much more frequently. As with many new treatment concepts and surgical techniques, the learning curve regarding distraction of the facial bones was steep, and in many aspects, it is still continuing.

Following the first successful distraction of the mandible, the application of the treatment concept has developed rapidly. Numerous ingenious applications have been developed, ranging from the increase of alveolar bone height for dental implant placement and increase in maxillary and mandibular dental arch width to the transfer of bone in reconstruction following jaw resection. A multitude of distraction devices have been designed and developed, ranging from large extraoral appliances, minute intraoral devices, multivector devices, and even resorbable devices for neonates. A major advantage of distraction osteogenesis is that it provides solutions for the correction of severe and previously untreatable deficiencies of the craniofacial region. Distraction is advantageous because the surgeon can achieve large skeletal movements; in addition, distraction of soft tissue makes it an impressive and dynamic treatment modality that has become an essential part of the orthognathic surgeon's armamentarium.

There are several basic treatment principles for successful distraction of bone as initially described by Ilizarov (1997), including osteotomy of the bony cortex with minimal periosteal stripping. Depending on the surgical site, a latency period ranging from 3 to 7 days is necessary before activation of the distraction device. (The latency period should be shorter in young children.) The rate of distraction should be 0.5 to 2.0 mm per day; this rate is influenced by the surgical site and the age of the patient. In neonates, the distraction rate should be faster to prevent early ossification. Application of a continuous force is ideal; however, activation of the distraction device twice or three times per day is practical. Following distraction, a period of stabilization is essential for consolidation of the bone regenerate. The consolidation period depends on the magnitude of the distraction, the type of deformity, and the age of the patient. In adults, the consolidation period should be at least 3 months; in children, a shorter period may be indicated. Once consolidation has been confirmed radiographically, the distraction device can be removed.

Although orthopedic surgeons can correct angular and rotational long bone deformities with distraction, the basic shape of a long bone is cylindric. The 3D curvature of the facial skeleton, variation in bone thickness, the extreme accuracy demanded by the occlusion, the sensitivity of the TMJs, and the importance of facial esthetics are all factors adding to the difficulty of the technique. Another challenging aspect of placing a distractor in the facial region is to make the appliance as unobtrusive as possible. The treatment technique and protocol as described by Ilizarov had to be adjusted and refined for the application to facial bones. Since the first reports by Guerrero et al in 1990 and McCarthy et al in 1992 on gradual lengthening of the mandible by distraction, the initial enthusiasm and hype has settled, experience has been gained, and treatment protocols have been established for the treatment of the facial skeleton.

Successful distraction demands accurate presurgical planning that often requires 3D models. It is critical to determine the correct vector for lengthening, accurate positioning of the device on the bone, the size and design of the device, and the positioning of the driver for easy activation. Stereolithic models are often used to determine the best site of placement while allowing the surgeon to prebend the device. The presurgical adjustment of the device to conform to the anatomy of the bone saves considerable operating time. Following proper treatment planning, distraction osteogenesis can be divided into five treatment phases.

Treatment phases

Surgical phase

A minimum amount of periosteum should be dissected from the bone for placement of the distraction device. The device is first positioned and fixed to the bone according to the treatment plan. The osteotomy line is then accurately marked and the device removed. The osteotomy is performed through the cortex of the bone, taking care not to damage any underlying structures such as tooth roots, nerves, or blood vessels. The clinician will complete the osteotomy through the cancellous bone and carefully test the mobility of the bone segments. The distraction device is replaced and fixed. It is critical that the functionality of the device is then tested by activating the driver, ensuring movement of the segments while taking care not to injure underlying structures.

Latency period

Once the cortical osteotomies have been completed and the distraction device placed, a latent period is required to allow for resolution of the initial inflammatory response. The initial healing phase involves organization of the hematoma while mesenchymal, endosteal, and periosteal cells are induced into osteoblasts and fibroblasts. Osteoid is produced following deposition of type I collagen.

Distraction phase

The initial process of bone formation involves a regenerate chamber filled with a fibrous matrix that will ossify starting at the periphery and moving centrally over time. The fibrous matrix is lengthened by distraction and can occur at a rate of 1 mm per day. In children younger than 6 years, the rate may be increased. If the distraction is performed too fast, nonunion will result. On the other hand, distraction performed too slowly may result in early bone healing and failure of bone lengthening.

Consolidation phase

Once the required bone length has been obtained, the bone segments need to be stabilized to allow for the regenerate to consolidate into mature bone. The consolidation time in adults should be at least 12 weeks depending on the magnitude of distraction, anatomy of the bone, type of deformity, and age of the patient. An adequate length of consolidation time and stabilization of the bone segments are essential during this phase and will influence the stability of the results.

Removal of the distraction device

Confirmation of ossification of the bone is done by basic radiography or other imaging modalities such as computed tomography. In most patients, removal of the distraction device is tedious and cumbersome, necessitating a second surgical procedure. A major advantage of resorbable devices is that in most instances, the device does not require removal. Currently, the use of resorbable devices is indicated only in neonates.

Distraction osteogenesis offers several advantages over conventional orthognathic surgical techniques: large advances can be achieved; the surrounding soft tissue matrices are also expanded; the need for bone grafting is limited or eliminated; and it is thought that the potential for relapse is less than with traditional treatment methods. Despite these advantages over conventional orthognathic surgery, the following disadvantages should be kept in mind when choosing a treatment technique during treatment planning:

- Risk of premature bone formation, resulting in failure of bone lengthening
- Risk of distracting too fast, resulting in nonunion
- Higher rate of postoperative infection at the surgical site
- Risk of distraction device failure
- Difficulty of vector control, resulting in inaccurate segment positioning
- Removal of the distraction device requiring a second surgical procedure
- Patient discomfort during distraction
- Lack of patient compliance regarding activation of the distraction device
- Severe scars caused by mandibular extraoral devices
- Additional expense related to the cost of distractors and the need for a second procedure for removal of the device

Mandibular lengthening by distraction osteogenesis

The complex 3D anatomy of the mandible and bilateral involvement of the TMJs render distraction of the mandible challenging. Precise presurgical planning and accurate device orientation are paramount for predictable widening and lengthening of the mandible. The device should be placed parallel to the axis of distraction; in patients requiring bilateral distraction, the vectors of the devices should be parallel to each other. Because the mandible is narrower in the front and wider at the back, adjustments should be made by creating a step to compensate for the discrepancy in width of the anterior and posterior mandible. Failure to compensate for the variation in mandibular body width may result in loosening of the screws, bending of the device, development of a torque force on the condyles, and failure of distraction.

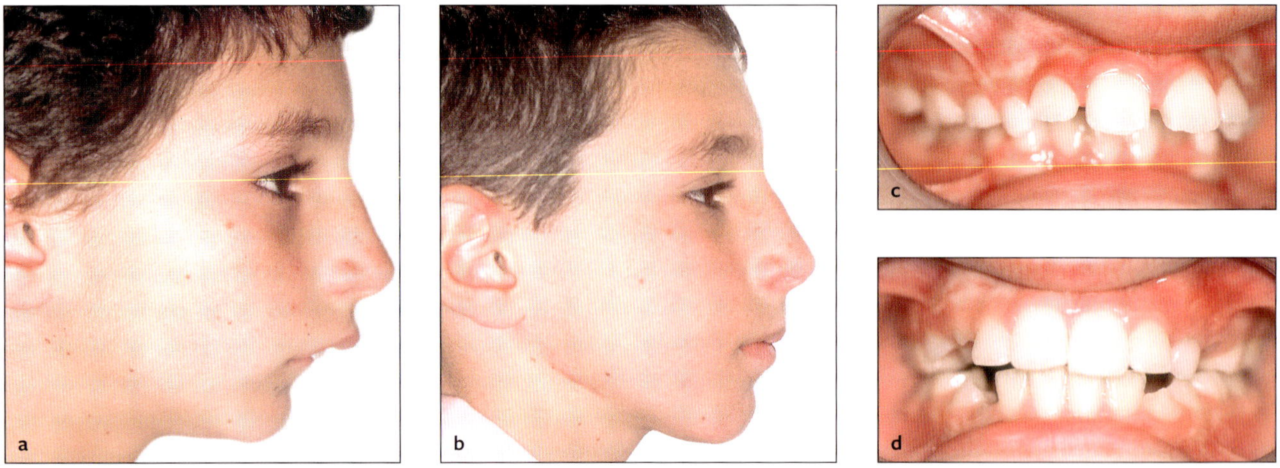

Fig 5-64 Profile views of a 5-year-old patient with severe mandibular anteroposterior deficiency before (*a*) and after 15-mm distraction of the mandible (*b*). (*c*) Pretreatment view shows severe Class II malocclusion, maxillary dental protrusion, and increased overjet. (*d*) Occlusion is improved following mandibular distraction and orthodontic retraction of maxillary incisors using a removable appliance.

TMJ considerations

Once the distractor is activated, reciprocal forces are placed on the glenoid fossa by the condyle. Flattening of the condyle, thinning and even perforation of the cartilaginous disc, subcondylar bone formation, and loss of the superior and inferior joint space have been reported. Some clinicians think that it is fundamental to unload the joints before distraction. It is recommended that during the presurgical orthodontic phase, the joints should be unloaded by Class II elastics, 6 oz per side. The unloading forces are continued during the distraction and consolidation phases and later discontinued by the orthodontist.

An open bite may develop during the distraction phase as a result of lack of parallelism or poor vector control of the devices. Open bite may be overcome by releasing the anteroposterior arm of the device following full activation. The bite is then closed by placement of strong maxillomandibular elastics that are maintained during the consolidation phase.

Postsurgical orthodontics

Once the distraction devices are removed, the patient is again referred to the orthodontist to finalize the occlusion. Some clinicians recommend the use of Class II elastics during the distraction and consolidation phases. The long-term effects of this action on the TMJs have not yet been established.

There are two main indications for distraction of the mandible: (1) in young children with severe mandibular deficiency where conventional orthognathic surgery cannot be performed (see Fig 5-65); and (2) in adult patients with abnormally shaped mandibles requiring large advancements (see Fig 4-70).

The patient in Fig 5-64 was referred at the age of 5 years with Pierre Robin sequence and had severe difficulty with chewing, speech, and nocturnal breathing. Bilateral distraction devices were placed with the distraction drivers exiting extraorally in the postauricular area. Following a latency period of 4 days, the distractor was turned twice daily (0.5 mm of distraction per turn), and the mandible was lengthened by 15 mm on each side during a 15-day period. The distraction devices were removed following a consolidation period of 4 months. The protrusion of the maxillary incisors was controlled by a removable orthodontic appliance.

The adult patient in Fig 5-65 was referred by his orthodontist for the correction of a severe Class II malocclusion by surgical advancement of the mandible. The patient required superior repositioning of the maxilla and a large advancement of his mandible to establish a normal occlusion. However, the shape of the patient's mandible was not favorable to sagittal split osteotomy (see Fig 5-65e). His maxilla was superiorly repositioned by performing a Le Fort I osteotomy and the occlusal plane manipulated, reducing the occlusal plane angle. Bilateral intraoral mandibular distractors were placed at the same time maxillary surgery was performed. His mandible was lengthened by 17 mm with bilateral intraoral distractors, with the drivers exiting intraorally. A genioplasty was performed at the time of distractor removal, 5 months after completion of the distraction.

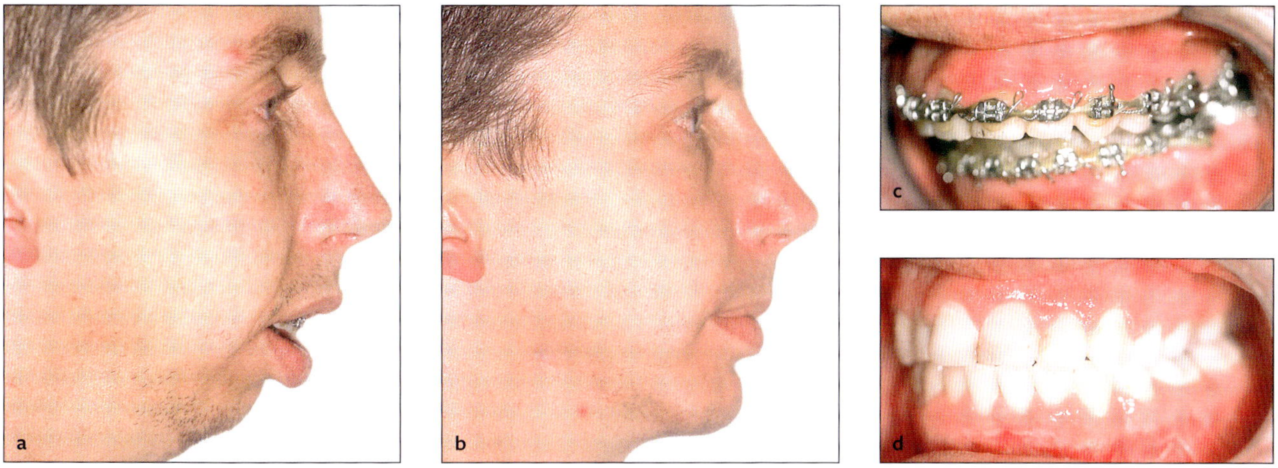

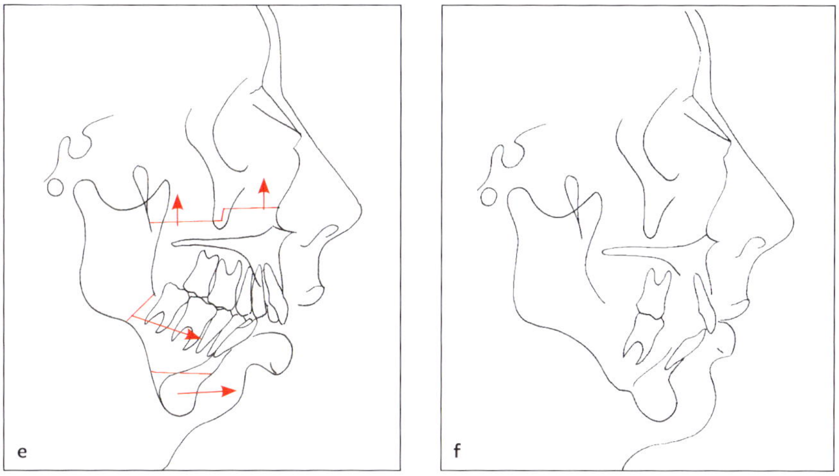

Fig 5-65 (*a*) A patient with vertical maxillary excess, severe mandibular deficiency, and microgenia. The surgical correction required superior repositioning of the maxilla with a Le Fort I osteotomy. The unfavorable mandibular anatomy as well as the amount of advancement planned required use of an intraoral distraction device on the mandible. The chin was advanced with a genioplasty performed when the distractor was removed. (*b*) The improved profile is evident posttreatment. Preoperative occlusion (*c*) and posttreatment occlusion (*d*) are shown. (*e*) Severe anteroposterior deficiency and unfavorable anatomy of the mandible are evident in the pretreatment cephalometric tracing. (*f*) Posttreatment cephalometric tracing demonstrates improved soft tissue, skeletal, and dental relationships.

Maxillary advancement by distraction osteogenesis

Midface deficiencies are traditionally treated by surgical advancement of the maxilla in the Le Fort I, II, or III level. Severe hypoplasia of the maxilla often occurs in syndromic patients and/or patients with cleft lip and palate. The maxillary skeletal hypoplasia in patients with cleft lip and palate is usually a manifestation of impaired growth as a result of multiple previous surgeries and related scar tissue formation. These patients often require large advancements of the maxilla with bone grafting and extensive rigid fixation, but postoperative stability proves to be questionable.

Anterior distraction of the maxilla should be considered as the preferred method of treatment in patients with obstructive sleep apnea. The distraction technique has the added advantage of monitoring the improvement of the posterior pharyngeal airflow and allowing titration of the advancement during the distraction phase. Intraoral devices can be used for distraction of the maxilla on the modified Le Fort I and modified Le Fort III levels; it is recommended that extraoral distractors be used to advance the midface on the classic Le Fort III level (see Fig 5-66).

The use of stereolithic models is an essential aspect of the treatment planning process. The model allows for accurate calculation of the vectors of distraction, assessment of the bone stock in the area of placement of the device, and prebending of the device by the surgeon.

Extraoral distraction for the craniofacial skeleton

For distraction of the midface at the Le Fort I level, an extraoral device should be considered. However, it is very difficult to control the occlusion and simultaneously achieve optimal esthetics in these patients. Patients

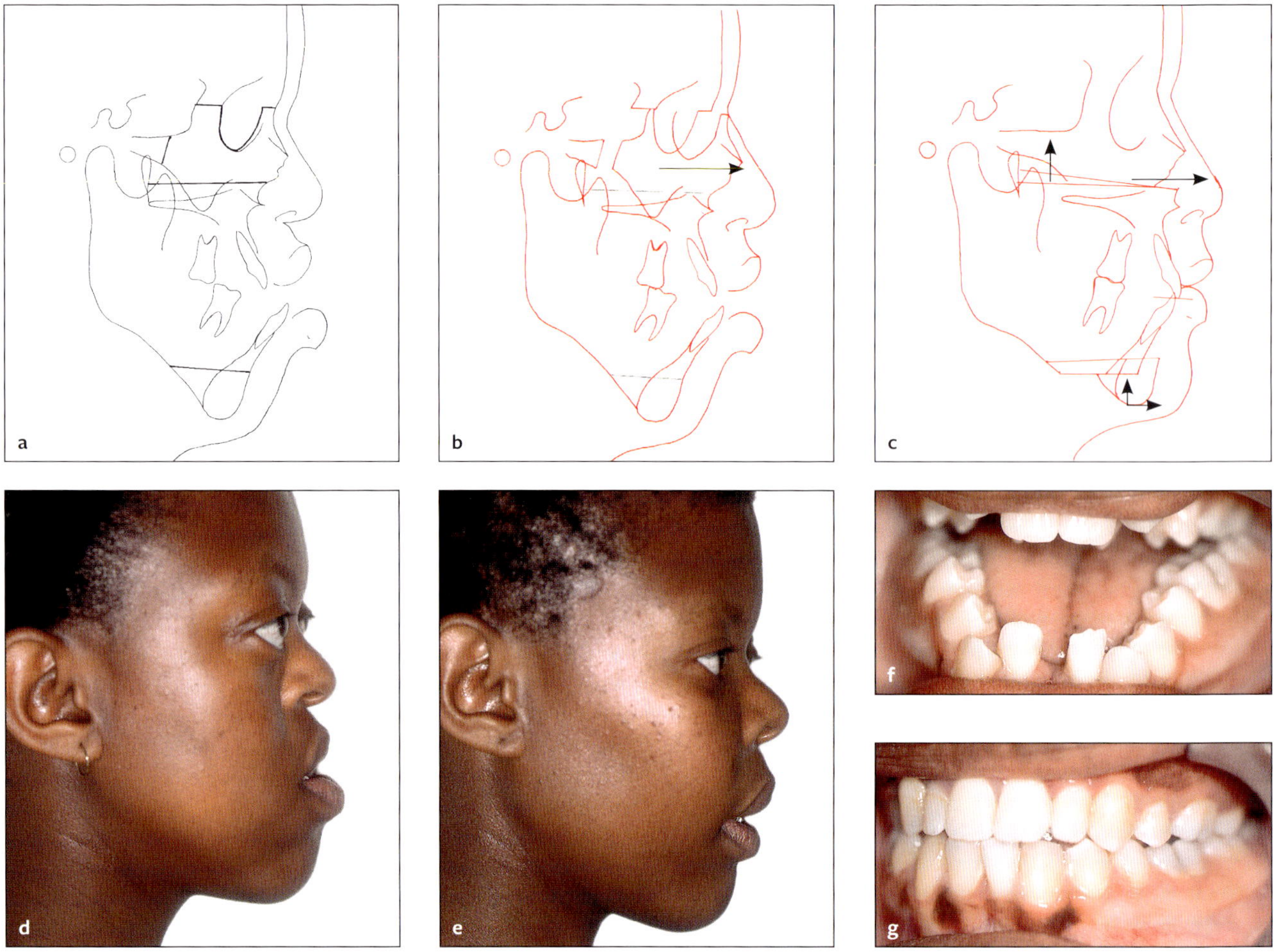

Fig 5-66 (*a*) The cephalometric tracing of a patient with a severe Class III open bite malocclusion and midface deficiency. (*b*) The prediction tracing for the first treatment stage consisting of distraction of the midface (*arrow*). (*c*) The prediction tracing of the second surgical stage consisting of superior repositioning of the maxilla to close the open bite and advancement of the chin with a sliding genioplasty (*arrows*). Presurgical profile (*d*), postsurgical profile (*e*), pretreatment malocclusion (*f*), and posttreatment occlusion (*g*).

with Crouzon, Apert, and Pfeiffer syndromes often have severe Class III open bite occlusions that require not only midface advancement but also a rotational movement of the segment to close the open bite. In addition, these patients usually require a Le Fort I osteotomy in combination with the Le Fort III distraction to manage both the occlusion and esthetic expectations. The author prefers to perform the midface advancement by distraction as a first procedure, followed by conventional maxillary advancement for final correction of the occlusion.

Figure 5-66 demonstrates the treatment of a patient with Crouzon syndrome who presented with a severe Class III anterior open bite malocclusion and midface deformity.

Following the orthodontic alignment of her dental arches, the patient's midface was advanced with an extraoral distractor. The midface was advanced by 12 mm; however, the occlusion was not corrected. Extraoral devices proved to be extremely uncomfortable for the patient, and the consolidation period had to be adjusted. The occlusion was finally corrected 6 months after removal of the distraction device by means of a Le Fort I maxillary osteotomy, and the facial contour was improved with an advancement genioplasty.

Widening the maxilla by distraction osteogenesis

It is relatively easy to widen the maxilla by opening the midpalatal suture before or during adolescence, but this procedure becomes increasingly difficult as the patient becomes older. Orthodontic expansion of the maxillary dental arch in adults is limited to dental movement and often involves tipping of the teeth. Orthodontic expansion of the teeth beyond the alveolar bony base will likely lead to transverse relapse.

Skeletal constriction of the maxilla rarely occurs without coexisting vertical and/or sagittal problems. Surgical expansion of the maxilla in patients with this condition can be easily accomplished with segmental surgery in the course of a Le Fort I downfracture to correct other problems. When skeletal expansion of the maxilla is the only objective, distraction should be considered. Increase of the skeletal width of the maxilla by distraction is also called *surgically assisted rapid palatal expansion* (SARPE), a form of rapid palatal expansion in adult patients whose midline palatal suture has ossified and been surgically recreated by a palatal osteotomy (see Fig 4-4 in chapter 4).

Surgically assisted expansion of the maxilla is indicated in the following cases:

- When there are no other indications for the maxilla to be downfractured on the Le Fort I level, such as advancement or superior repositioning
- When only unilateral expansion is required
- When an increase in arch length is required to accommodate all the teeth (ie, the first premolar has been removed and orthodontic anchorage loss resulted in loss of extraction spaces and severe crowding)
- When space needs to be created for unerupted teeth in preparation for orthodontic treatment
- When a transverse increase of more than 7 mm is required
- For patients whose previous orthodontic palatal expansion failed

The art of repositioning and lengthening the facial bones by distraction has eventually found its place in the field of surgical reconstruction of the face and has proved to be a powerful treatment modality. Continued research, critical evaluation of outcomes, and technical refinements will certainly improve both the decision-making process of surgeons and patient treatment outcomes.

Recommended Reading

Acebal-Bianco F, Vuylsteke PL, Mommaerts MY, De Clercq CA. Perioperative complications in corrective facial orthopedic surgery: A 5-year retrospective study. J Oral Maxillofac Surg 2000; 58:754–760.

Adlam DM, Yau CK, Banks PA. A retrospective study of the stability of midface osteotomies in cleft lip and palate patients. Br J Maxillofac Surg 1989;27:265–276.

Booth RP. Reflections on distraction osteogenesis. A surgical distraction or the "future"? Br J Oral Maxillofac Surg 2001;39:179–180.

Beukes J, Reyneke JP, Damstra J. Unilateral sagittal split mandibular ramus osteotomy: Indications and geometry. Brit J Oral Maxillofac Surg 2016;54:219–223.

Blæhr TL, Mommaerts MY, Kjellerup AD, Starch-Jensen T. Surgically assisted rapid maxillary expansion with bone-borne versus tooth-borne distraction appliances—A systematic review. Int J Oral Maxillofac Surg 2019;48:492–501.

Bütow KW, van der Walt PJ. The "Stellenbosch"—Triangle analysis of posteroanterior and basilar cephalograms. J Dent Assoc S Afr 1981;36:461–467.

Bütow KW, van der Walt PJ. The use of triangle analysis for cephalometric analysis in three dimensions. J Maxillofac Surg 1984;12:62–70.

Cupar I. Die chirurgische Behandlung der Form und Stellungs Veränderungen des Oberkiefers. Öst Z Stomatol 1954;51:565–577.

Diner PA, Vasquez MP (eds). Transactions of the International Congress of Cranial and Facial Bone Distraction Osteogenesis. Bologna, Italy: Mondozzi, 1997.

Ellis E 3rd, McNamara JA Jr. Components of adult Class III open-bite malocclusion. Am J Orthod 1984;86:277–290.

Ellis E 3rd, McNamara JA Jr, Lawrence TM. Components of adult Class II open-bite malocclusion. J Oral Maxillofac Surg 1985;43:92–103.

Enlow DH. Facial Growth, ed 3. Philadelphia: Saunders, 1990.

Epker BN. Modifications in the sagittal osteotomy of the mandible. J Oral Surg 1977;35:157–159.

Ferrario VF, Sforza C, Ciusa V, Dellavia C, Tartaglia GM. The effect of sex and age on facial asymmetry in healthy subjects: A cross-section study from adolescence to mid-adulthood. J Oral Maxillofac Surg 2001;59:382–388.

Gonzales M, Bell WH, Guerrero CA, Buschang PH, Samchukov ML. Positional changes and stability of bone segments during simultaneous bilateral mandibular lengthening and widening by distraction osteogenesis. Br J Oral Maxillofac Surg 2001;39:169–178.

Gonzalez-Perez LM, Fakih-Gomez N, Gonzalez-Perez-Somarriba B, Centeno G, Montes-Carmona JF. Two-year prospective study of outcomes following total temporomandibular joint replacement. Int J Oral Maxillofac Surg 2016;45:78–84.

Grenlich WW, Pyler SI. Radiographic Atlas of Skeletal Development of the Hand and Wrist, ed 2. Stanford: Stanford UP, 1959.

Guerrero CA, Figueroe F, Bell WH, Olmos-Malave Y, Rojas A, Gonzalez M. Surgical orthodontics in mandibular lengthening. In: Guerrero CA (ed). Distraction Osteogenesis of the Facial Skeleton. Hamilton, ON: BC Decker, 2007.

Hamamci N, Basaran G, Sahin S. Nonsurgical correction of an adult skeletal class III and open-bite malocclusion. Angle Orthod 2006;76:527–532.

Houston WJ, James DR, Jones E, Kavvadia S. Le Fort I maxillary osteotomies in cleft palate cases. Surgical changes and stability. J Craniomaxillofac Surg 1989;17:9–15.

Hugo A, Reyneke JP, Weber ZJ. Lingual orthodontics and orthognathic surgery. Int J Orthodon Orthognath Surg 2000;15:153–162.

Hunsuck EE. A modified intraoral sagittal splitting technic for correction of mandibular prognathism. J Oral Surg 1968;26:250–253.

Ilizarov GA. The principles of the Ilizarov method. 1988. Bull Hosp Jt Dis 1997;56:49–53.

Jacobs JD, Bell WH, Williams CE, Kennedy JW 3rd. Control of the transverse dimension with surgery and orthodontics. Am J Orthod 1980;77(3):284–306.

Johnson NR, Roberts MJ, Doi SA, Batstone MD. Total temporomandibular joint replacement prostheses; A systematic review and bias-adjusted meta-analysis. Int J Oral Maxillofac Surg 2017;46:86–92.

Kaban LB, Mulliken JB, Murray JE. Three-dimensional approach to analysis and treatment of hemifacial microsomia. Cleft Palate J 1981;18:90–99.

Kaban LB, Troulis MJ. Hemifacial microsomia. In: Pediatric Oral and Maxillofacial Surgery. Philadelphia: Elsevier, 2004.

Kleinheinz J, Jung S. Alloplastic total temporomandibular joint replacement—Indications prognosis, and benefit. J Craniomand Func 2015;7:117–134.

Koudstaal MJ, Poort LJ, van der Wal KG, Wolvius EB, Prahl-Andersen B, Schulten AJ. Surgically assisted rapid maxillary expansion (SASME): A review of the literature. Int J Oral Maxillofac Surg 2005;34:709–714.

Letzer GM, Kronman JH. A posteroanterior cephalometric evaluation of craniofacial asymmetry. Angle Orthod 1967;37:205–211.

Liu F, Steinkeler A. Epidemiology, diagnosis, and treatment of temporomandibular disorders. Dent Clin North Am 2013; 57:465–497.

McCarthy JG, Grayson BH, Williams J. Distraction of the mandible: The New York University experience. In: McCarthy J (ed). Distraction of the Craniofacial Skeleton. New York: Springer-Verlag, 1999.

McCarthy JG, Schreiber JS, Karp N, Thorne CH, Grayson BH. Lengthening of the human mandible by gradual distraction. Plast Reconstr Surg 1992;89:1–8.

McNamara JA Jr. Components of Class II malocclusion in children 8–10 years of age. Angle Orthod 1981;51:177–202.

Mercuri LG. Alloplastic temporomandibular joint replacement: Rationale for the use of custom devices. Int J Oral Maxillofac Surg 2012;41:1033–1040.

Mommaerts MY. Transpalatal distraction as a method of maxillary expansion. Br J Oral Maxillofac Surg 1999;37:268–272.

Mommaerts MY, Lipperns F, Abeloos JV, Neyt LF. Nasal profile changes after maxillary impaction and advancement surgery. J Oral Maxillofac Surg 2000;58:470–474.

Obwegeser H, Trauner R. Zur Operationstechnik bei der Progenie und anderen Unterkieferanomalien. Dtsch Zahn Mund Kieferheilkd 1955;23:1–26.

O'Ryan F, Schendel S. Nasal anatomy and maxillary surgery. I. Esthetic and anatomic principles. Int J Adult Orthodon Orthognath Surg 1989;4:27–37.

Posnick JC. Hemifacial microsomia: Evaluation and treatment. In: Posnick JC (ed). Orthognathic Surgery, Principles and Practice. St Louis: Elsevier, 2014:1059-1094.

Proffit WR, White RP. Surgical-Orthodontic Treatment. St Louis: Mosby, 1992.

Reyneke JP. Basic guidelines for the surgical correction of mandibular anteroposterior deficiencies and excess. In: Patel PK (ed). Clinics in Plastic Surgery, Orthognathic Surgery, vol 34. Philadelphia: Elsevier, 2007:501–518.

Reyneke JP. Reflections on: Distraction osteogenesis—The future? Br J Oral Maxillofac Surg 2001;39:180–181.

Reyneke JP. Rotation of the maxillomandibular complex: An alternative in orthognathic treatment planning [thesis]. Acta Univ Tamparensis 2006;35:142.

Reyneke JP. Rotation of the occlusal plane. In: Fonseca E (ed). Oral and Maxillofacial Surgery, ed 2, vol 3. Philadelphia: Saunders, 2009:249–271.

Reyneke JP, Ferretti C. Anterior open bite correction by Le Fort I or bilateral sagittal split osteotomy. In: Van Sickels JE (ed). Oral and Maxillofacial Surgery Clinics of North America, Orthognathics, vol 19. Philadelphia: Saunders, 2007:21–338.

Reyneke JP, Masureik CJ. Treatment of maxillary deficiency by a Le Fort I downsliding technique. J Oral Maxillofac Surg 1985;43:914–916.

Saito I, Yamaki M, Hanada K. Nonsurgical treatment of adult open bite using edgewise appliance combined with high-pull headgear and class III elastics. Angle Orthod 2005;75:277–283.

Sandor GKB, McGuire TP, Ylokontiola LP, Serlo WS, Pirttiniemi PM. Management of facial asymmetry. In: Van Sickels JE (ed). Oral and Maxillofacial Surgery Clinics of North America, Orthognathics, vol 19. Philadelphia: Saunders, 2007:395–422.

Vandersea BA, Ruvo AT, Frost DE. Maxillary transverse deficiency—Surgical alternatives and management. In: Van Sickels JE (ed). Oral and Maxillofacial Surgery of North America, Orthognathics, vol 19. Philadelphia: Saunders, 2007:351–368.

Wagner S, Reyneke JP. The Le Fort I downsliding osteotomy: A study of long-term hard tissue stability. Int J Adult Orthodon Orthognath Surg 2000;15:37–49.

Wolford LM, Mercuri LG, Schneiderman ED, Movahed R, Allen W. Twenty-year follow-up study on a patient-fitted temporomandibular joint prosthesis: The Techmedica/TMJ Concepts device. J Oral Maxillofac Surg 2015;73:952–60.

Wassmund M. Lehrbuch der Probleschen Chirurgie des Mundes und der Kiefer, vol 1. Leipzig: Meuser, 1935.

Wunderer S. Erfahrungen mit der operativen Behandlung hochgradiger Prognathien. Dtsch Zahn Mund Kieferheilkd 1963;39:451.

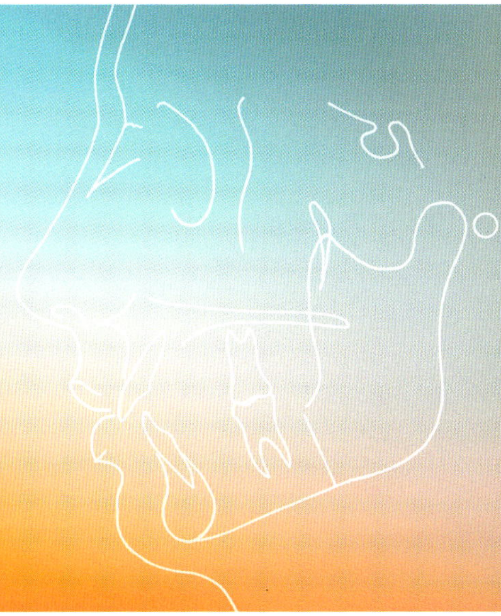

6 Surgical Technique

Knowledge and understanding of all aspects of orthognathic surgery have grown considerably during the past few decades. Diagnostic skills and treatment planning have become more sophisticated, and surgical techniques have been developed that enable clinicians to treat even the most complex jaw deformities with confidence. This chapter presents surgical techniques for the four procedures most often used in the correction of dentofacial deformities in a concise, step-by-step format. Complications and their possible solutions are also included.

Orthognathic surgery requires not only sophisticated and accurate technique but also the utmost respect for the hard and soft tissues involved. The formulation of a treatment plan involving accurate tooth movement by the orthodontist does no good if what follows is inaccurate surgery, sloppy technique, and disregard for soft tissue, all of which lead to unsatisfactory results.

Good surgical technique involves the following:

- *Treatment planning.* Before surgery, accurate and comprehensive surgical treatment planning should be carried out, including cephalometric treatment objectives, 3D computer visual treatment planning (when required), and model surgery.
- *Surgical routine.* As much as possible, the surgeon should develop a routine for each procedure that will enable assistants and the rest of the surgical team to anticipate each step, thus increasing efficiency and decreasing operating time. The surgeon should clearly understand the surgical steps of each procedure and be aware of complications that may arise with each step. It is essential to have a basic routine, from the selection of scalpel blades to suture material. An established step-by-step operating technique also prevents intraoperative uncertainty and often eliminates postoperative complications. The details and sequence of a surgical procedure may vary from surgeon to surgeon, but the ultimate objective is the same. The surgeon must be able to clearly visualize every step as well as the sequence of the surgical procedure to operate with confidence and achieve the surgical goal and optimal results.
- *Instrumentation.* A large number of instruments are available to help the surgeon achieve the same goals. However, it is much less confusing to both the surgeon and the surgical team when a small, select group rather than an entire range of instruments is used.

Bilateral Split Mandibular Ramus Osteotomy

The first report of surgical repositioning of the mandible was written by Blair and published in July 1907 in the medical journal *Surgery, Gynecology and Obstetrics*. Since then, the surgical correction of dentofacial deformities has developed into not only a well-defined science but also a fascinating art form.

The development of surgical repositioning of the mandible includes ingenious work by surgeons such as New and Erich; Dingman; and Burch, Bowden, and Woodward, who described body osteotomy procedures. Procedures to reposition the mandible using various ramus osteotomies were described by Caldwell and Letterman,

Hinds and Girotti, and Robinson. In 1955, Obwegeser and Trauner described a surgical procedure involving a sagittal split osteotomy through the ramus of the mandible. This technique was later modified by Dal Pont and further refined by Hunsuck in 1968 and Epker in 1977.

The surgical repositioning of the mandible has developed from a life-threatening procedure to outpatient surgery (in some parts of the world). The ingenuity of the procedures, development of special instruments, and improvement of surgical skills have made it possible to achieve surgical goals relatively quickly and atraumatically. The advent of rigid fixation has also made postoperative recovery safer and more comfortable and with improved stability of the results. The technique described in the following pages has evolved over many years and, because of its simplicity, has been found beneficial in the training of postgraduate students at the University of the Witwatersrand in Johannesburg, South Africa.

Standard surgery

Step 1: Infiltration of soft tissue with a vasoconstrictor

Infiltrate the area of dissection with a local anesthetic containing a vasoconstrictor (epinephrine in a concentration of 1:100,000) 10 minutes before surgery. Place the needle deep in the soft tissue, aspirate, and infiltrate the area as the needle is slowly retracted. The patient's lips should be kept lubricated with steroid ointment throughout the surgical procedure.

Step 2: Soft tissue incision

Make an incision through mucosa, muscle, and periosteum from just lingual of the external oblique ridge halfway up the mandibular ramus superiorly to mesial of the second molar inferiorly (Fig 6-1a). Leave at least 5 mm of nonkeratinized mucosa buccally at the lower end of the incision for later ease of suturing.

Ideally, third molars should be removed 9 months before surgery, and their removal should be part of the treatment plan. If these teeth are still present at the completion of the preoperative orthodontic phase, one option is for the surgeon to remove the impacted teeth at this stage and delay definitive surgery for at least 9 months to allow for bone healing. However, this is often not possible, in which case the third molars can be removed during surgery. A partially erupted or erupted third molar present at the time of surgery should be included in the soft tissue incision. However, an impacted third molar increases the difficulty of the sagittal split osteotomy procedure in several ways. (1) It weakens the retromolar part of the distal segment and may lead to a Type 4 bad split (see page 264). (2) The tooth increases involvement of the inferior alveolar nerve and will increase morbidity of sensation. (3) It increases the prevalence of postoperative infection. (4) If the tooth is not removed during surgery, it may interfere with optimal bone contact. (5) The presence of a third molar or tooth socket will limit the positioning of rigid fixation screws (Figs 6-1b and 6-1c).

Step 3: Buccal subperiosteal dissection

The dissection must remain subperiosteal, decisive, clean, and neat. The masseter muscle attachment should be maintained as far as possible without sacrificing adequate exposure. Strip enough of the masseter muscle to allow easy visualization of the osteotomy area. However, it is not necessary to strip the entire masseter muscle attachment off the mandible. The proximal segments of the mandible will not be repositioned. In fact, apart from autorotation, it is important for this segment to be maintained in its original position and not totally detached from the masseter muscle. Total stripping of the muscle increases dead space, which encourages swelling and hematoma formation and may cause devascularization of part of the bone, leading to necrosis.

Step 4: Superior subperiosteal dissection

Once the buccal and lingual sides of the anterior ramus have been exposed, place a notched ramus retractor over the anterior border of the mandibular ramus, and strip the lower fibers of the temporalis muscle attachment from the anterior border and coronoid process. Alternatively, a coronoid clamp may be used to retract the soft tissue superiorly. Dissect the periosteum from the internal oblique ridge down to the medial aspect of the retromolar area.

Step 5: Medial subperiosteal dissection and exposure of the lingula

The dissection must remain subperiosteal by keeping the periosteal dissector against the bone at all times. Start the dissection from the internal oblique ridge above, and then dissect inferiorly to the region of the lingula (Fig 6-2). The lingula must be carefully identified and well visualized (see step 6).

Step 6: Identification of the lingula

The medial osteotomy should never be performed without positive identification of the lingula. The panoramic radiograph may be a helpful guide. However, the lingula is often difficult to see because of the convexity of the internal oblique ridge. If visualization is difficult, the ridge should

Fig 6-1 (*a*) The soft tissue incision is made from just lingual of the external oblique ridge above to mesial of the second molar below. At least 5 mm of nonkeratinized mucosa is left buccally for ease of suturing. (*b*) A lateral view of the mandible. The pattern area (i) indicates the areas where bicortical screw fixation can be safely placed avoiding the inferior alveolar neurovascular bundle and the roots of the second molar. Unicortical screws can be safely placed in areas (ii). (*c*) Safe placement of rigid fixation screws are limited by the presence of an impacted third molar (or tooth socket following removal) (iii) and roots of the second molar (iv).

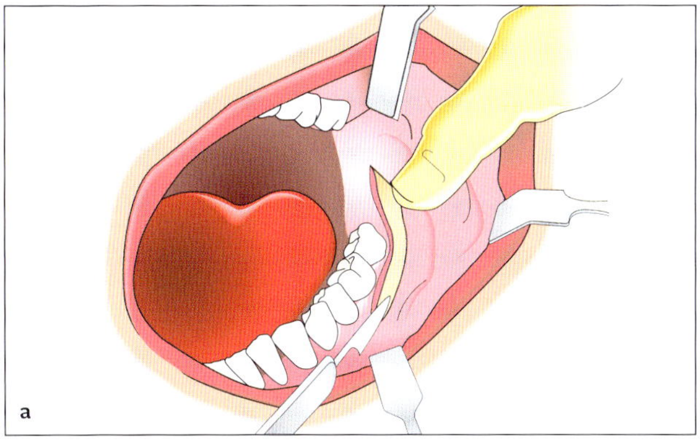

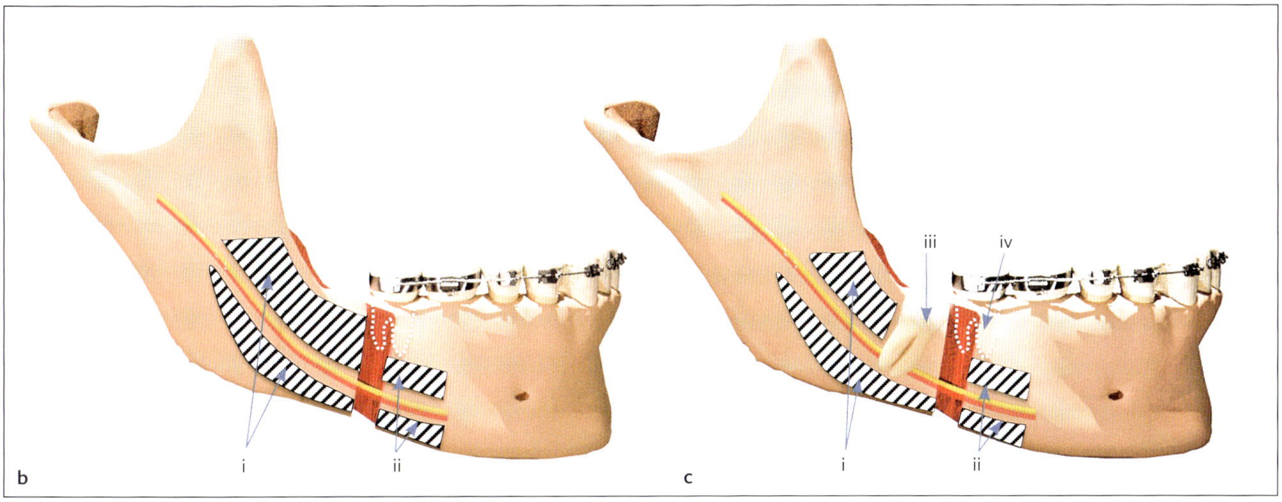

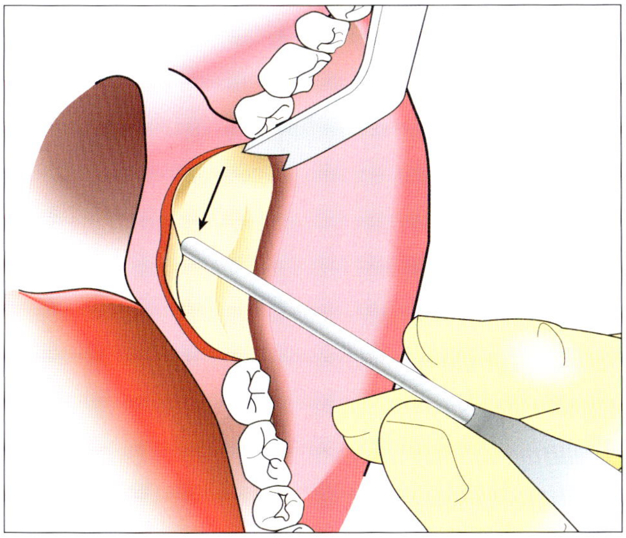

Fig 6-2 Subperiosteal dissection is carried out posteriorly to identify the lingula. Start from above and dissect downward. The panoramic radiograph may be helpful in determining the relative position of the lingula.

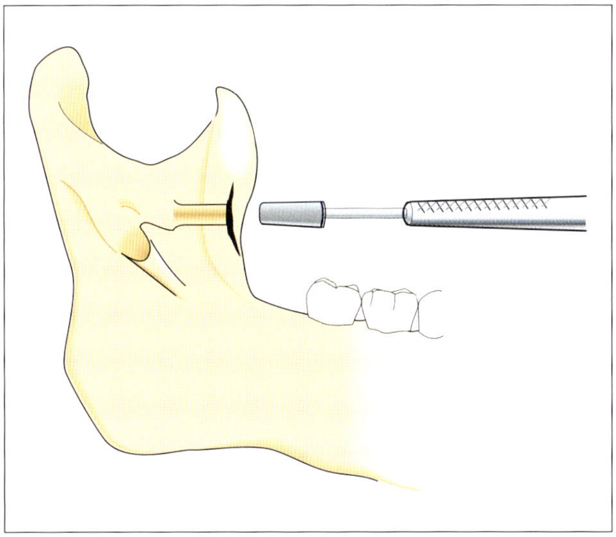

Fig 6-3 Visualization of the lingula can be improved by reduction of a convex internal oblique ridge using a large trimming bur.

be reduced with a large trimming bur (Fig 6-3). If the periosteum is perforated, a brisk hemorrhage may result (probably originating from the vessels of the medial pterygoid muscle); however, it often subsides spontaneously. Do not stretch the inferior alveolar nerve at its entrance to the foramen because this may result in prolonged anesthesia of the lower lip.

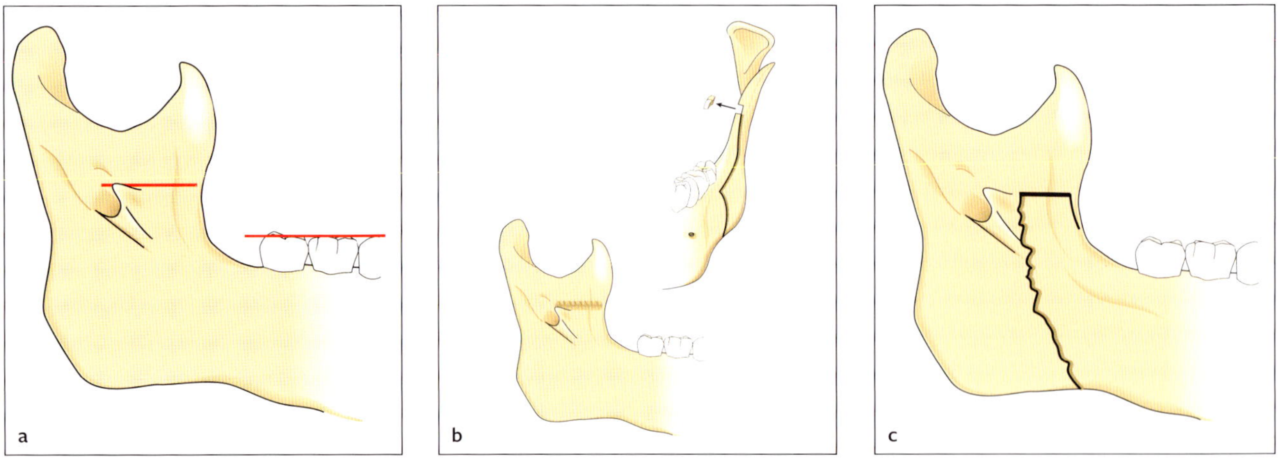

Fig 6-4 (*a*) The horizontal ramus osteotomy should be made parallel to the occlusal plane. The osteotomy should end posterior to the lingula in the fossa. (*b*) The distal segment will be positioned posteriorly and also tend to move superiorly in patients with mandibular setback and high occlusal plane angles. In these patients, a small segment of bone should be removed superior to the horizontal osteotomy line to prevent interference between the segments. (*c*) The horizontal osteotomy should be carried past the lingula; otherwise, there will be a strong tendency for the mandible to split anterior to the lingula.

Step 7: Medial ramus osteotomy

While aiming at the notch of the lingula, angle the medial ramus osteotomy parallel to the occlusal plane using a 701 fissure bur or a Lindeman bur (Fig 6-4a). Terminate the osteotomy just posterior to the lingula (see Fig 6-4a), and ensure that the osteotomy is carried through the lingual cortex into the medullary bone of the mandibular ramus. When mandibular setback procedures will be performed, a small segment of bone should be removed superior to the horizontal osteotomy line (Fig 6-4b). When the medial ramus osteotomy is terminated anterior to the lingula, the bone tends to split anterior to the lingula. The lingula and superior part of the alveolar canal (including the nerve) thus remain attached to the proximal segment during the splitting procedure (Fig 6-4c). This is one of the most common reasons surgeons have difficulty splitting bone at the superior aspect of the sagittal split osteotomy.

Step 8: Vertical section of the osteotomy

Start the vertical section of the osteotomy from the medial osteotomy superiorly, staying just inside the buccal cortex of the mandibular ramus. End inferiorly just mesial to the second molar. Ensure that the osteotomy is made through the cortex well into medullary bone (approximately 5 mm). The presence of an impacted third molar may make the osteotomy difficult (ideally, third molars should be removed at least 9 months prior to surgery). However, it should be treated as bone and the osteotomy made through the tooth.

Step 9: Removing the notched ramus retractor and placing a channel retractor

Place the channel retractor around the inferior border of the mandible. Remain subperiosteal at all times. Visibility may be increased by removing the mouth prop and closing the mandible slightly.

Step 10: Buccal osteotomy of the mandibular body

Start the buccal osteotomy of the mandibular body at the lower border, and join it superiorly with the vertical part of the ramus osteotomy (Fig 6-5a). Cut toward the mandible, "feel" the bur perforate the buccal cortex, and angle the osteotomy slightly obliquely and posteriorly (Fig 6-5b). Ensure that the cortex of the lower border of the body of the mandible is included in the osteotomy. The actual start of the sagittal split osteotomy should be at the lower border and must include part of the lingual cortex (Fig 6-5c). When placing the sagittal separator instrument, make sure it engages the lower border so that this part of the mandible stays attached to the proximal segment (see the discussion of the "bad" split on page 264). The surgeon should be careful in patients with mandibular anteroposterior excess, mandibular asymmetry (the excessive side), and unilateral condylar hyperplasia, in whom the inferior alveolar neurovascular bundle tends to be situated very close to the buccal cortex and lower border.

Step 11: Drilling holes for a holding wire

The holes for a holding wire should be positioned in such a way that the proximal segment is directed distally. The direction of the anterior hole (ie, proximal segment) should be posterior, and the direction of the posterior hole (ie, distal segment) should be anterior. The placement of holding wires is optional. However, the author believes that condylar positioning (the most important step of the procedure) is more accurate if performed as a separate step prior to the placement of the screws. Once the condyle has been

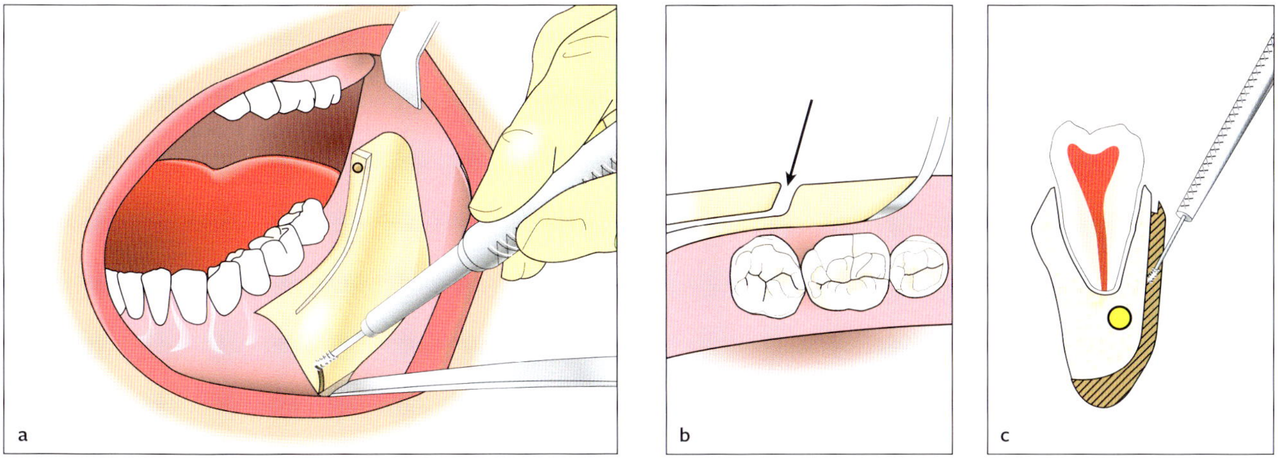

Fig 6-5 (*a*) The buccal osteotomy is started at the lower border of the mandible and joined superiorly with the vertical ramus osteotomy. (*b*) The buccal osteotomy is angled slightly obliquely and posteriorly to enhance the start of the split. (*c*) It is mandatory to include the lingual cortex in the buccal osteotomy to ensure that it forms part of the proximal segment at the start of the split.

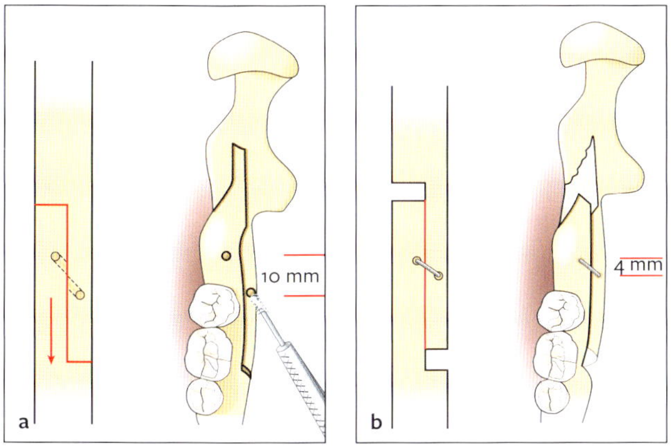

Fig 6-6 Positioning of the holes for mandibular advancement. (*a*) For a 4-mm advancement, the holes are placed 10 mm apart (the hole in the distal segment should be posterior to that in the proximal segment). (*b*) After a 6-mm mandibular advancement, the holes will be 4 mm apart, ensuring a vector that will support the advancement of the tooth-bearing segment and seat the condyle.

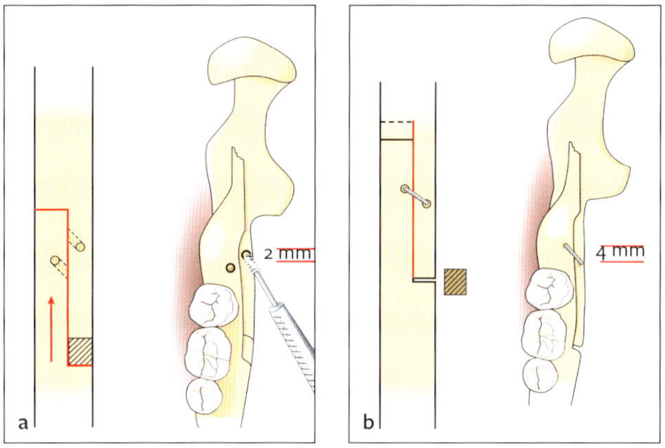

Fig 6-7 Positioning of holes for mandibular setback. (*a*) For a mandibular setback of 6 mm, the holes are placed 2 mm apart, with the hole in the proximal segment posterior to that in the distal segment. (*b*) After a 6-mm setback, the holes will be 4 mm apart with the vector of the holding wire supporting the tooth-bearing segment and the condyle.

positioned (see step 27), it is held in place using a condylar-positioning instrument and digital pressure while the assistant tightens the holding wire. This process will be facilitated if the interrelationship of the segments and the condylar position was established and maintained by the holding wire at the time of rigid fixation. This is particularly helpful in the placement of resorbable fixation when the drilled holes have to be tapped before placement of the screws.

The ideal distance between the holes after repositioning the segments is 4 mm, with the hole in the proximal segment positioned anteriorly. The vectors of pull should always be in the proximal segment posteriorly and in the distal segment anteriorly (the direction of the wire must always be Class II). Two examples follow:

1. In a patient for whom a mandibular advancement of 6 mm is planned, the holes should be drilled 10 mm apart (Fig 6-6a). After advancement of the distal segment by 6 mm, the holes will be 4 mm apart (Fig 6-6b).
2. In a patient for whom a mandibular setback procedure of 6 mm is planned, the holes should be drilled 2 mm apart, with the hole in the distal segment positioned anteriorly (Fig 6-7a). If the holes are more than 4 mm apart after jaw repositioning, bone approximation between distal and proximal segments will be less accurate because of the long span of the wire and may lead to inaccurate placement of rigid fixation (Fig 6-7b).

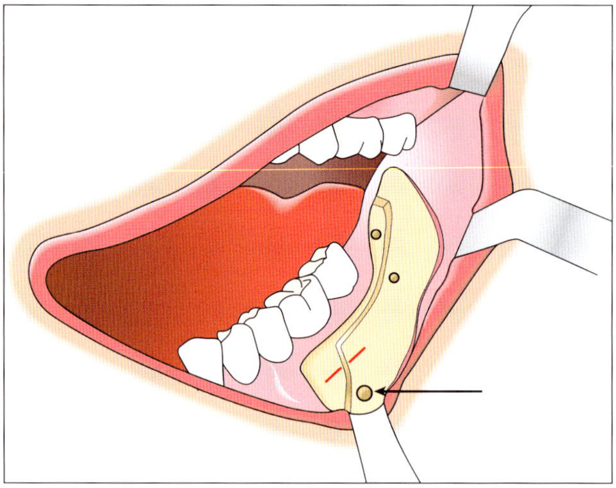

Fig 6-8 The hole for the engagement of the condylar positioner is placed in a low, anterior position on the proximal segment (see step 28).

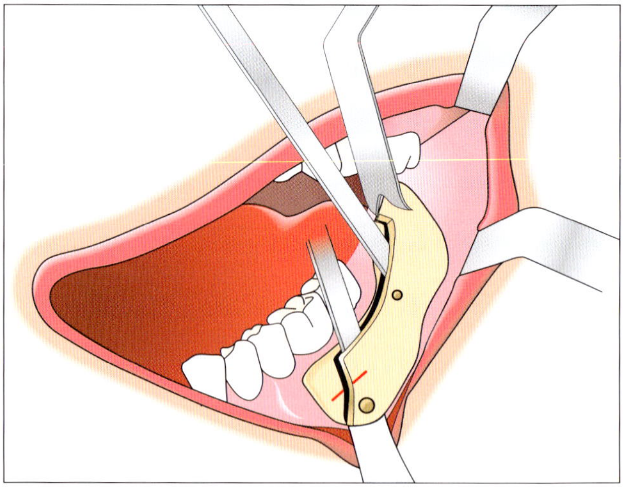

Fig 6-9 The split is started by tapping a 10-mm-wide osteotome along the vertical osteotomy, from the medial to the buccal osteotomy.

Alternative techniques

A bone clamp may be used as an alternative to a holding wire. Some surgeons prefer simply to hold the proximal segment in position with a condylar positioner (ramus pusher or wire director) while placing the bicortical screws. Whatever method is used, the proximal segment and condyle must be secured in the ideal relationship to the glenoid fossa when the bicortical screws are placed (see step 27).

Step 12: Drilling a hole for the condylar positioner

A hole is drilled in the buccal cortex of the proximal segment and angled posteriorly (Fig 6-8). This hole will serve as a purchase point for the condylar positioner during condylar positioning before the tightening of the holding wire.

Step 13: Placing reference marks

Reference marks are now placed on opposite sides of the vertical body osteotomy (see Fig 6-8). The alignment of these marks during condylar positioning (positioning the proximal segment) will prevent any rotation of the proximal segment. Clockwise or counterclockwise rotation of this segment will influence the stability of the result.

Step 14: Lavage

Wash the surgical area thoroughly with saline solution, and gently place a small, wet sponge in it. Once the osteotomy cuts have been performed on one side, it is recommended that the surgeon complete them on the other side before splitting the mandible.

Step 15: Defining the osteotomy cut with an osteotome

It is important not to manipulate the jaw unnecessarily when splitting the contralateral side because this may cause hard and soft tissue damage on the side that has already been split. A thin but rigid 10-mm-wide osteotome is used to tap along the vertical osteotomy from the medial osteotomy downward to the buccal osteotomy (Fig 6-9). Keep the osteotome just inside the buccal cortex, and support the mandible at the inferior border with the channel retractor. The osteotomy cuts are only defined during this step; make no attempt to completely separate the segments. Vigorous indiscriminate tapping may fracture the buccal cortical plate from the distal segment, and failure to support the mandible during this step may cause trauma to the temporomandibular joint (TMJ), such as hemarthrosis or disc displacement.

Step 16: Splitting the mandible

The actual splitting of the mandible can be divided into two stages. The first stage involves the initiation of the split. At the start of the split, the surgeon must be able to see that (*1*) the lower border of the mandible splits toward the proximal segment and (*2*) the neurovascular bundle

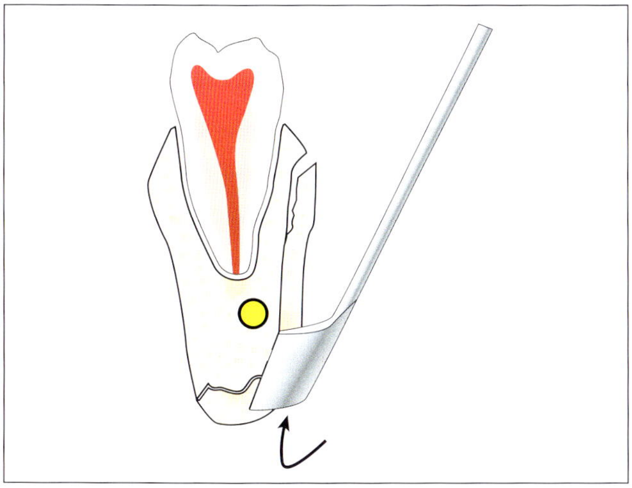

Fig 6-10 A small Reyneke Sagittal Split Separator (Zimmer Biomet) is placed deep into the buccal osteotomy, and the lower border is engaged.

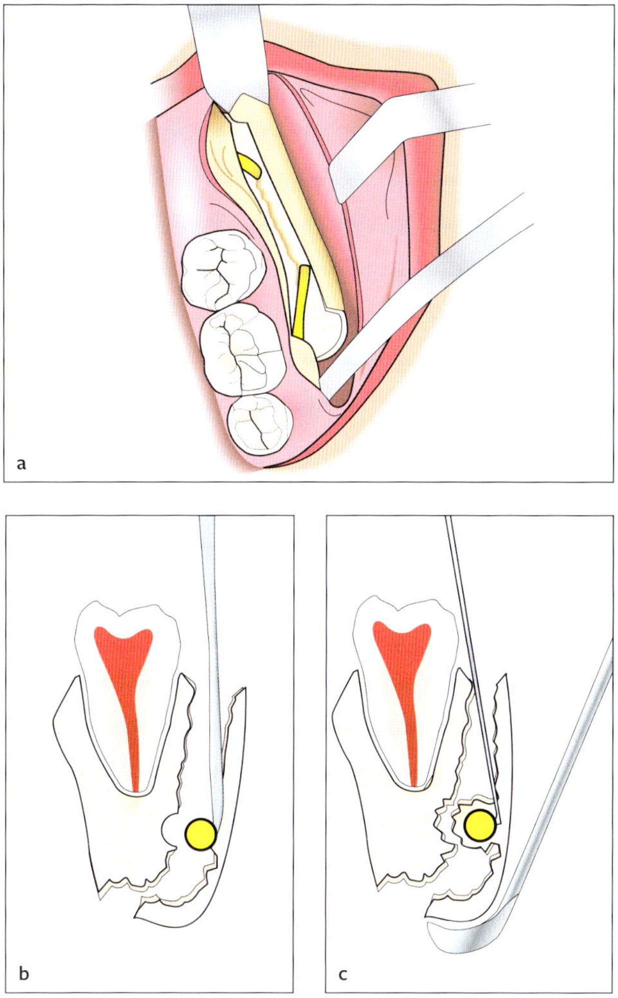

Fig 6-11 (*a*) The neurovascular bundle is attached to the proximal segment. (*b*) Before continuing with the split, carefully dissect the neurovascular bundle from the bone using a blunt instrument. (*c*) The neurovascular bundle may still be encased in the bony canal. An osteotome should be used to very carefully dissect the canal from the proximal segment and the bundle from the canal.

is intact and separates from the proximal segment. In the second stage, the split is completed. Here the surgeon must be able to see that (1) the lower border continues to split with the proximal segment, (2) the neurovascular bundle detaches from the proximal segment as the split continues, and (3) the inferior alveolar foramen and proximal part of the canal detach from the proximal segment. The surgeon places a large osteotome superiorly into the vertical osteotomy of the ramus and a small sagittal split separator into the buccal osteotomy of the lower body of the mandible to engage the lower border (Fig 6-10). It is very important that the mandible be supported at all times by a channel retractor and digital pressure to protect the TMJ. If the split does not begin spontaneously, stop and redefine all the osteotomies.

Step 17: Completion of the split

To continue the separation between the distal and proximal segments, the osteotome is now replaced by a larger osteotome and the small sagittal split separator by a larger separator, and the instruments are rotated. Always ensure that the lower border continues to split with the proximal segment and that the neurovascular bundle is protected and intact. The neurovascular canal is often attached to the proximal segment, especially when the mandible is anteroposteriorly excessive or asymmetric (excessive side), when there is unilateral condylar hyperplasia (excessive side), and when there is an unerupted third molar (Fig 6-11a). As soon as the surgeon realizes that the neurovascular bundle is still attached to the proximal segment, the split should be stopped and the bundle very carefully dissected from the proximal segment using a blunt (Howarth) dissector (Fig 6-11b). When the inferior alveolar canal splits toward the proximal segment, the surgeon should stop the split and very carefully dissect the medial wall of the canal from the proximal segment using a small osteotome (Fig 6-11c). Carefully remove the bone from the neurovascular bundle with a small, nontoothed forceps. During the splitting, it is important not to use the retromolar bone (on the distal segment) as a fulcrum, especially if an impacted third molar is still present, because this will fracture the thin retromolar segment and make fixation difficult. Again, it is important to handle the proximal segment with care to maintain the integrity of the TMJ.

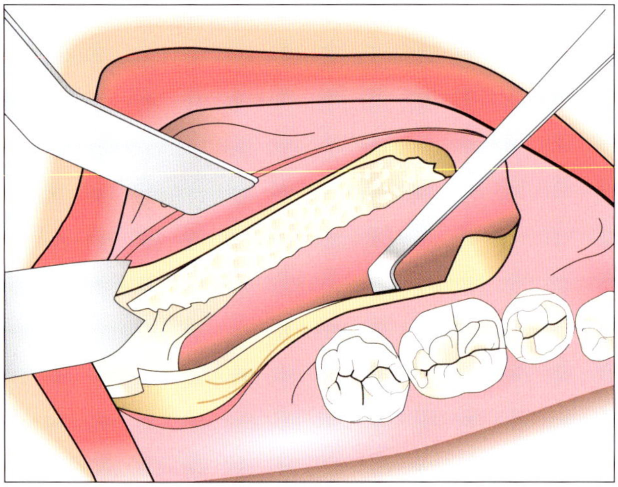

Fig 6-12 A curved periosteal elevator is used to strip the pterygomasseteric sling from the distal bone segment and also to ensure that the split is complete at the lower and posterior borders.

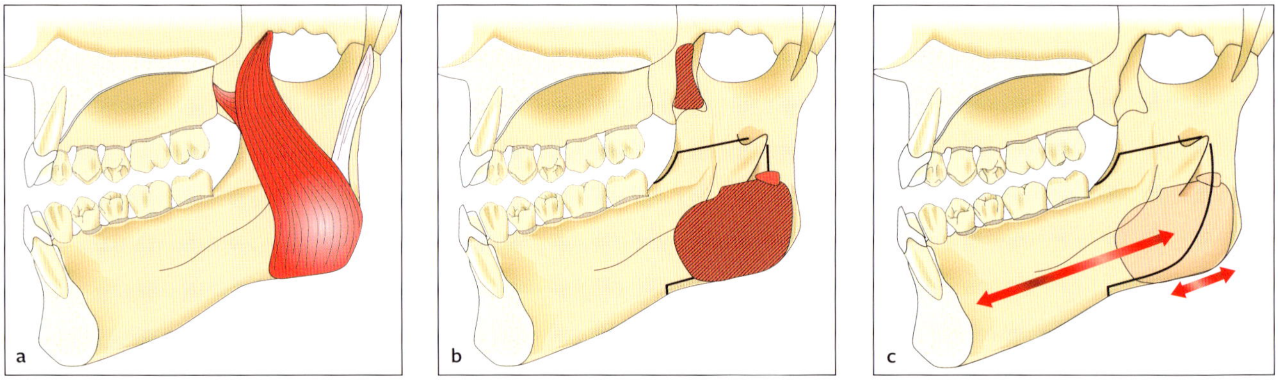

Fig 6-13 (*a*) The positions of the medial pterygoid muscle (anterior and inferior) and the stylomandibular ligament (posterior and superior) on the medial aspect of the mandibular angle. (*b*) The attachments of the muscle and ligament on the bone and their relation to the sagittal osteotomy are demonstrated. (*c*) These attachments will interfere when the proximal segment is repositioned anteriorly or posteriorly and may lead to rotation of the proximal segment.

The following fractures may cause resistance to the split:

- A greenstick fracture of the bone in which the lower border starts fracturing superiorly toward the distal part of the medial ramus osteotomy, posterior to the lingula. The solution is to use a large osteotome to carefully separate the bone attachment between the segments under good visualization.
- A fracture of the vertical osteotomy of the ramus anterior to the inferior alveolar foramen (caused by the medial osteotomy of the ramus stopping short of the lingula). The solution is to revise the horizontal osteotomy and carefully separate the canal and foramen from the distal segment using a small osteotome. Support both segments during detachment to prevent nerve damage.

Step 18: Stripping the pterygomasseteric sling

Place a curved periosteal elevator between the bone segments and at the inferior border of the distal segment, and proceed to strip the pterygomasseteric sling from the distal segment (Fig 6-12). This step will ensure that no greenstick bony attachments have remained between the distal and proximal segments. The neurovascular bundle should be protected at all times. Insufficient stripping of the pterygomasseteric sling or inadequate removal of bony attachments between the proximal and distal segments will lead to difficulty in repositioning the distal segment and inaccurate positioning of the condyle.

Step 19: Stripping the medial pterygoid muscle and stylomandibular ligament

The medial pterygoid muscle and the stylomandibular ligament are attached to the medial side of the angle of the mandible. Failure to strip them from the bone may interfere with the repositioning of the distal segment and may lead to unfavorable rotation of the proximal segment (Fig 6-13). This may distract the condyle from the glenoid fossa or rotate the proximal segment posteriorly, thereby increasing the potential for relapse.

Step 20: Removal of impacted third molars

It is the author's policy to remove impacted third molars at least 9 months before performing a bilateral sagittal split osteotomy (BSSO). Because this is not always possible, it is often necessary to remove third molars during the sagittal split procedure if they prevent optimal bone contact between the proximal and distal segments. The clinician should be careful not to fracture the retromolar bone (lingual cortex) or damage the neurovascular bundle during tooth removal. The presence of an impacted third molar or an empty tooth socket (after removal of the tooth) will limit the availability of bone and thus the placement of bicortical screws.

Step 21: Smoothing contact areas of bone segments

A large pear-shaped vulcanite bur is used to smooth the medial aspect of the proximal segment to ensure good bone contact between the segments and prevent nerve damage by sharp bony edges. Bone should not be removed from the lateral aspect of the distal segment because of potential damage to the alveolar neurovascular bundle.

Step 22: Placement of a holding wire

Place a 0.018-inch wire through the holes (see step 11) in the distal (medial) segment. Support the distal segment when the wires are pulled through to prevent any damage to the TMJ.

Step 23: Noting the position of the inferior alveolar neurovascular bundle

The inferior alveolar neurovascular bundle is often seen (and dissected) during the splitting procedure. The surgeon should take advantage of this visualization and make a mental note of the position of the neurovascular bundle to ensure safe placement of bicortical screws.

Step 24: Noting the position of the third molar (or its socket)

The third molar (or its socket after removal of the tooth) will influence the placement of the bicortical screws. Thus, the position and size of the tooth or socket should be noted to ensure safe, efficient placement of bicortical screws later in the procedure.

Step 25: Mobilization of the distal segment

Remove the sponge placed during lavage (see step 13). Mobilize the distal segment on each side by pulling it anteriorly while supporting the proximal segment with the index finger (Fig 6-14).

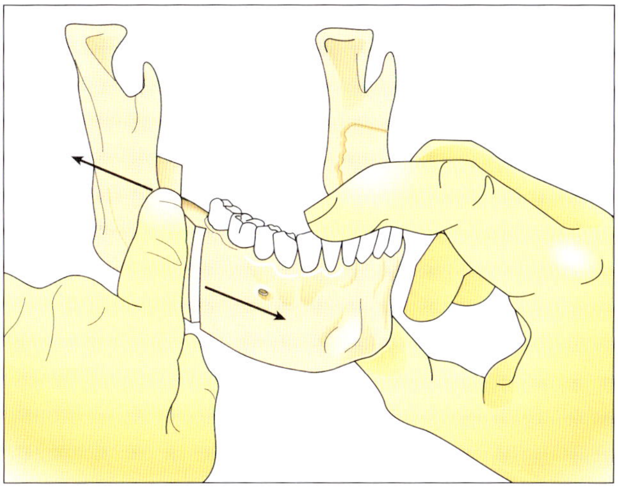

Fig 6-14 The proximal segment is mobilized by pulling the mandible forward while supporting the distal segment with digital pressure.

Step 26: Selective odontoplasty and maxillomandibular fixation

The selective odontoplasty should now be performed as indicated by the model surgery using a diamond bur and copious water cooling. Maxillomandibular fixation is then applied with the teeth in the planned occlusion. A prefabricated splint may be used when necessary. The use of an acrylic splint is not always indicated, and it is superfluous when it is possible to achieve a stable occlusion and no segmental surgery is contemplated. The intercuspation of the teeth can be observed better without the use of a splint. Fixation of the central incisors is done first to establish the planned incisor relationship; the maxillomandibular fixation is then applied to the posterior teeth. It is important to place the wires with a vector assisting the surgical repositioning.

Ensure that the teeth are placed into the planned occlusion without any bony or soft tissue interference. At this stage, interference may be caused by (1) an incomplete split, (2) a pterygomasseteric sling that has not been completely stripped, or (3) sharp, bony interference between the proximal and distal segments that prevents free movement between segments. Forcing the teeth into occlusion against muscular, bony, or dental interference will result in inaccurate positioning and poor stability. Poor immediate preoperative orthodontic preparation (loose orthodontic brackets, lack of or too few K-hooks, or incorrect positioning of the K-hooks) may make it impossible to maintain the occlusion because of inadequate wire fixation. A surgical acrylic splint may be helpful in these cases.

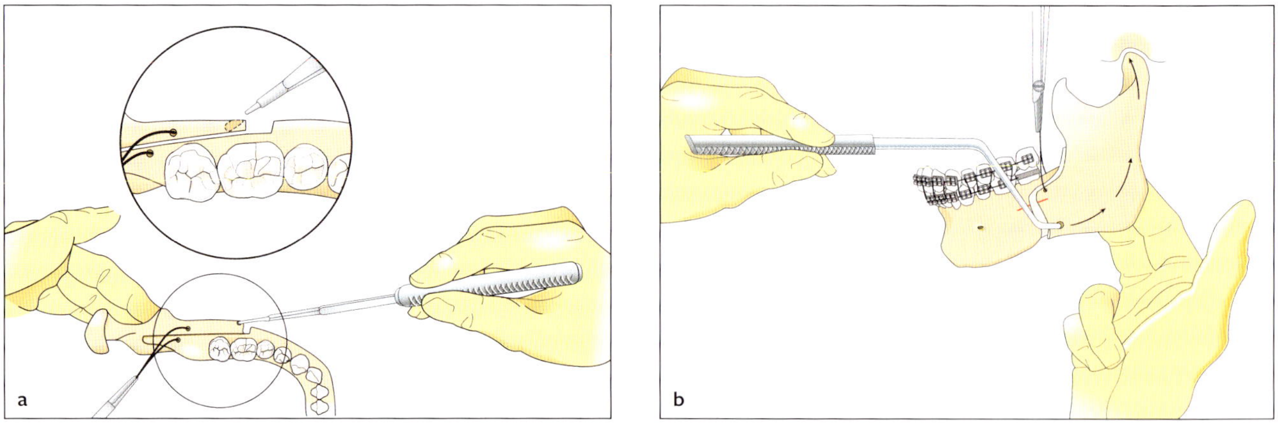

Fig 6-15 (*a*) The condylar positioner is placed in a hole drilled into the buccal cortex (see step 12). (*b*) The condyle is carefully pushed superiorly and slightly anteriorly in the fossa by the condylar positioner and digital force on the mandibular angle. The assistant can now tighten the positioning wire.

Step 27: Removal of bone from the proximal segment

When the teeth have been wired into occlusion and the proximal segment has been gently pushed back, the bony overlap (which should coincide with the planned setback amount) will be evident. The overlapping bone should now be removed, with the surgeon taking care not to damage the neurovascular bundle or facial artery during bone removal. There is no advantage to an accurate fit of bone at the buccal osteotomy. In contrast, if the proximal segment is forced to fit tightly against the distal segment at the buccal osteotomy site, the condyle may be forced too far posteriorly or eccentrically in the fossa, leading to condylar sag (see page 268). The result will also be less stable if the segments are forced together at the vertical osteotomy because the proximal segment may also rotate backward and downward. The small piece of bone removed may be used as a bone graft in other areas (eg, where there are intersegmental bone defects in BSSOs or Le Fort I osteotomies).

Step 28: Condylar positioning

A condylar positioner is placed into the hole drilled into the buccal cortex (see step 12). While the angle of the mandible is supported by extraoral digital pressure (Fig 6-15a), the condyle should be positioned in its preoperative relationship to the fossa. Posterior digital pressure on the positioning instrument and superior and slightly anterior extraoral digital pressure at the angle of the mandible will give the surgeon control of the proximal segment (Fig 6-15b). This control combined with both an awareness of the anatomical relationship between the condyle and glenoid fossa and an alignment of the reference marks should enable the surgeon to achieve the correct condylar position. Excessive force on the proximal segment during this maneuver may displace the articular disc in the fossa or lead to hemarthrosis or joint effusion.

The positioning of the proximal segment (condyle) in its preoperative relationship to the glenoid fossa is the most challenging and important aspect of the BSSO procedure. Numerous techniques and devices to position the condyle have been described and used with varying degrees of success. The technique described here has been developed during the performance of more than 5,100 BSSOs in 35 years.

Step 29: Tightening the holding wire

Hold the proximal segment in its desired position (described in step 27) while the assistant gently tightens the holding wire. View the segments while carefully tightening the holding wire, and ensure that the wire is twisted until it passively holds the segments in position. Do not force the segments together. Incorrect positioning of the holes may place unfavorable vectors of force on the bony segments and thus prevent correct condylar positioning. Excessive tightening of the holding wire may cause undesirable force on the condyle and lead to condylar sag. The use of a bone clamp is not recommended because it has a tendency to displace the condyle.

Step 30: Placement of the trocar

An extraoral stab incision is made on the lower border of the mandible, just behind the gonial notch. The surgeon places the trocar through the skin incision, ensuring that the tip of the trocar perforates the periosteum intraorally. The initial placement should be superior to the bone, avoiding damage to the neurovascular bundle or bony

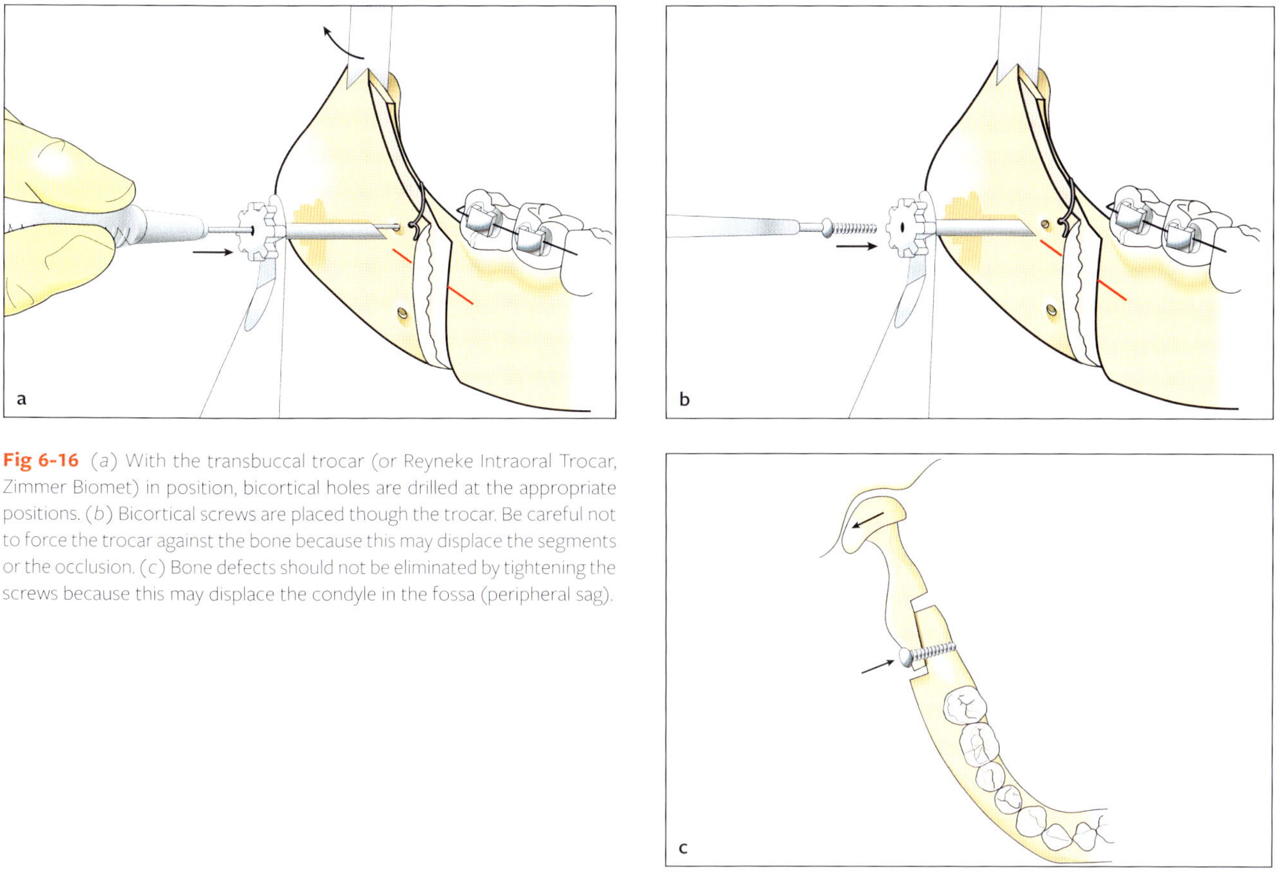

Fig 6-16 (*a*) With the transbuccal trocar (or Reyneke Intraoral Trocar, Zimmer Biomet) in position, bicortical holes are drilled at the appropriate positions. (*b*) Bicortical screws are placed though the trocar. Be careful not to force the trocar against the bone because this may displace the segments or the occlusion. (*c*) Bone defects should not be eliminated by tightening the screws because this may displace the condyle in the fossa (peripheral sag).

segments. Incorrect placement of the skin incision may damage the mandibular branch of the facial nerve, resulting in palsy of the lower lip.

Step 31: Drilling bicortical holes and placing screws

When drilling bicortical holes and placing screws, keep in mind the following factors:

- The position of the inferior alveolar neurovascular bundle (noted in step 23)
- The bone thickness (a depth gauge may be used) to assist in estimating the screw length
- The position of an impacted third molar (or socket, if the tooth has been removed)
- The distal root of the second molar
- Both cortices must be engaged

Drill the holes with a sharp drill while applying light pressure (Fig 6-16a). Keep in mind that if the shaft of the bur is forced against the trocar while drilling, it will generate heat and, without sufficient water cooling, may burn the skin and subcutaneous tissue in contact with the tube of the trocar. Position three holes in either a triangle or a straight line along the superior border. Angle the holes slightly backward to support the repositioning of the condyle. In the absence of an impacted or partially erupted third molar, a Reyneke intraoral trocar may be used for the placement of the screws.

Once a hole has been drilled, keep the trocar absolutely still to avoid "losing" the hole or its direction. While keeping the trocar in position, measure the depth of the hole. (With increased experience, the surgeon may estimate the length of the screw.) The screw is now "fed" into the trocar and gently tightened (a motorized screwdriver is a handy instrument at this stage; Fig 6-16b). View the cortex of the distal segment while tightening the screw to ensure that the screw engages the lingual cortex. If the two segments are pushed apart, the screw should be removed and a new hole drilled. The screwdriver should be pushed gently; keep in mind that positioning screws are self-tapping and need only be turned to engage.

After placing the first screw, place two more screws in appropriate positions. Make sure the screws do not compress the bone segments or close any intersegmental gaps because this may result in displacement of the condyle and peripheral condylar sag (Fig 6-16c; see discussion of peripheral condylar sag). Small bone grafts may be placed into bone defects.

Step 32: Removing maxillomandibular fixation and checking the occlusion

The occlusion should not be checked immediately after removal of fixation wires. Before assessing the final occlusion, open and close the mandible, and gently translate it to the left and right. Then wait 1 minute, and with light digital pressure under the chin, close the mandible and assess the occlusion. The occlusion should be exactly as planned. Do not accept an incorrect occlusion; there is no better time to correct a problem than at this stage.

Step 33: Intraoperative diagnosis of a malocclusion

A malocclusion caused by incorrect positioning of the condyle in the glenoid fossa should be apparent immediately after removal of maxillomandibular fixation (see step 31). However, if the proximal segment is not handled with care during the surgery, intracapsular edema, hemarthrosis, condylar disc displacement, or condylar disc damage may result. These problems will become apparent only postoperatively and may require further surgery. The causes of incorrect occlusion at this stage of the procedure include incorrect condylar position (condylar sag), mobility at the osteotomy site, and movement of the occlusion during placement of rigid fixation. The differential diagnosis of an incorrect occlusion and correction of the cause are discussed later in this chapter (see page 268).

Step 34: Placement of intraoral and extraoral sutures

Resorbable sutures are used intraorally, and 5-0 nylon sutures are used extraorally. Extraoral sutures are removed 2 days after surgery.

Step 35: Placement of elastics

A 4-oz, 0.25-inch elastic is placed on each side to assist in directing the surgical positioning of the jaw. The direction of the elastics should reinforce the movement (ie, use Class II elastics for patients with mandibular advancement and Class III elastics for patients with mandibular setback). Immediate postoperative placement of a strong vertical component is advocated.

Step 36: Placement of a pressure bandage

A pressure bandage should remain on the face for 2 days.

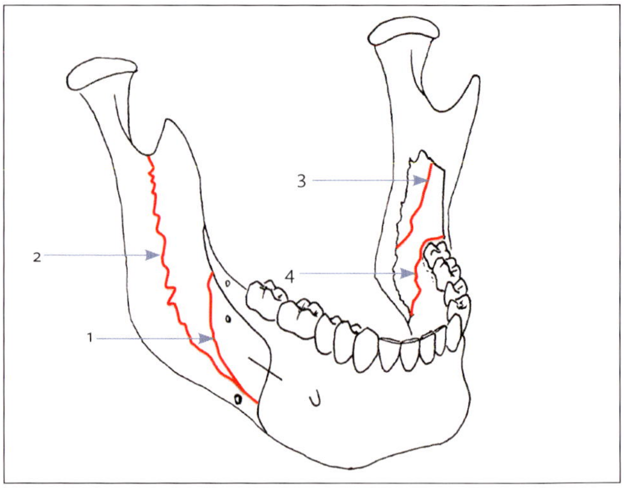

Fig 6-17 The 4 typical fracture lines of bad splits: (1) buccal plate fracture, (2) buccal plate fracture including the coronoid process, (3) a fracture short of the lingula, and (4) a retromolar fracture.

Complications

The "bad" split

An unfavorable split can by prevented by following the surgical steps meticulously. However, if the split does not seem to be proceeding favorably, stop and identify the problem area under good visualization. It is much easier to salvage the split if a potential problem is recognized early. The clinical features of an unfavorable split may occur either alone or in combination. Figure 6-17 demonstrates the four typical fracture lines of bad splits.

Fracture of the buccal cortex of the body of the mandible

Early diagnosis. If a fracture of the buccal cortex of the body of the mandible is diagnosed early, the beginning of a fracture that does not include the lower border is seen (Fig 6-18a). If this is detected, redefine the buccal osteotomy, especially around the lower border. Place the sagittal split separator down low into the osteotomy, and recapture the lower border to fracture it with the buccal cortex. When applying rigid fixation, place bicortical screws in the nonfractured part of the proximal segment while also securing the buccal cortex (Fig 6-18b).

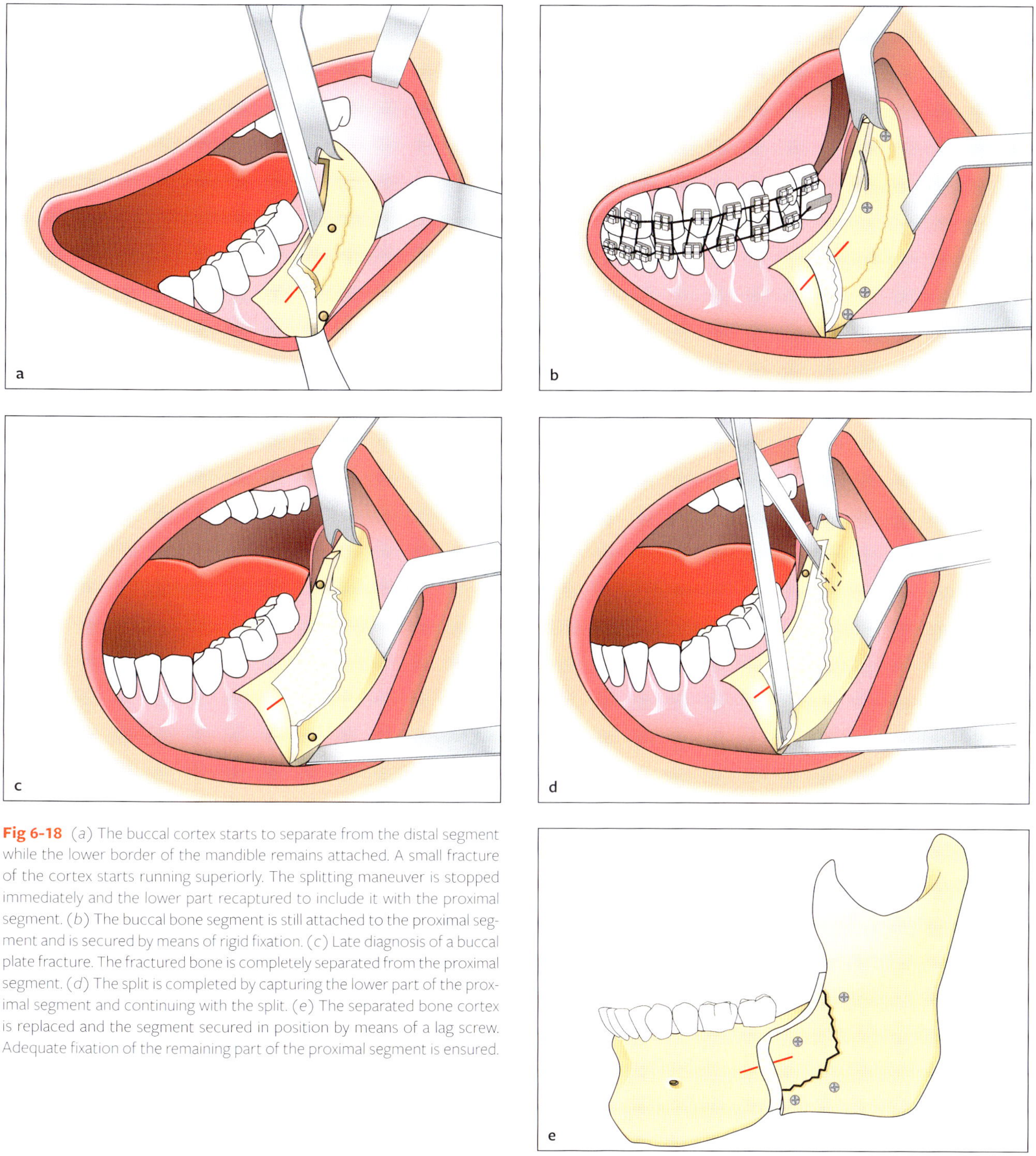

Fig 6-18 (*a*) The buccal cortex starts to separate from the distal segment while the lower border of the mandible remains attached. A small fracture of the cortex starts running superiorly. The splitting maneuver is stopped immediately and the lower part recaptured to include it with the proximal segment. (*b*) The buccal bone segment is still attached to the proximal segment and is secured by means of rigid fixation. (*c*) Late diagnosis of a buccal plate fracture. The fractured bone is completely separated from the proximal segment. (*d*) The split is completed by capturing the lower part of the proximal segment and continuing with the split. (*e*) The separated bone cortex is replaced and the segment secured in position by means of a lag screw. Adequate fixation of the remaining part of the proximal segment is ensured.

Late diagnosis. If a fracture of the buccal cortex of the body of the mandible is diagnosed late, the buccal cortex will have fractured unfavorably and be totally separated from the mandible (Fig 6-18c). In this case, remove the buccal plate and save the bone in a wet saline sponge. Redefine the remaining part of the buccal osteotomy, especially around the lower border. The osteotomy at the buccal cortex fracture line may also be redefined; pay particular attention not to damage the inferior alveolar neurovascular bundle. Proceed with the split, using a straight osteotome positioned at the superior aspect of the vertical ramus osteotomy and placing the sagittal split separator down low in the buccal osteotomy (Fig 6-18d). The separated buccal cortex can be replaced when rigid fixation is completed (Fig 6-18e). Use a lag screw to secure this bone segment back into position.

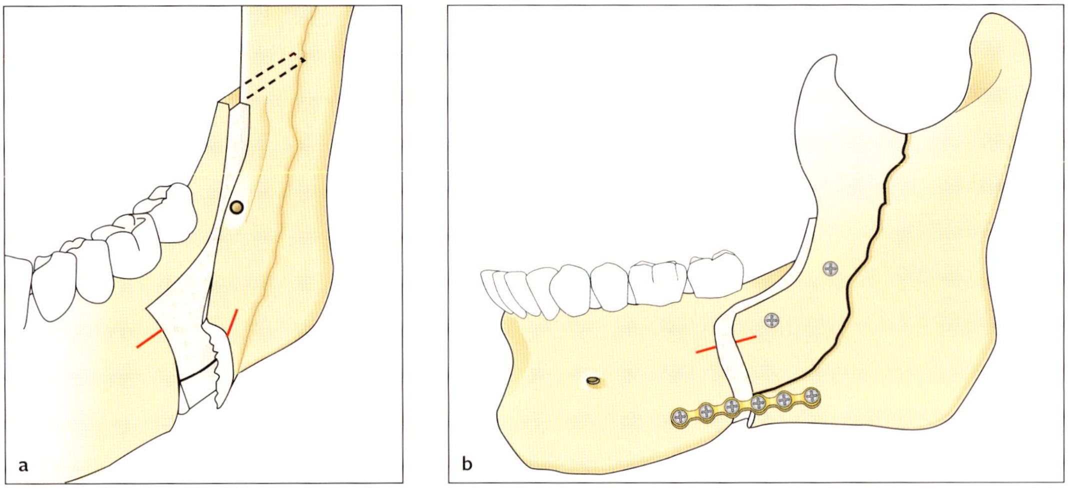

Fig 6-19 (*a*) The buccal cortex fractures separately from the lower border, while the fracture runs superiorly toward the coronoid notch. The splitting maneuver is stopped and the lower border captured to form part of the proximal segment. (*b*) The buccal cortex fracture continues superiorly and includes the coronoid process. The buccal osteotomy is redefined and the lower border captured. Rigid fixation is achieved by using a bone plate and by securing the fractured cortex by means of bicortical screws.

Fracture of the buccal cortex involving the body and ramus of the mandible

Early diagnosis. If fracture of the buccal cortex involving the body and ramus of the mandible is detected early, the cortex is seen as starting to fracture separately from the lower border (Fig 6-19a). The buccal osteotomy should be redefined, especially around the lower border. The sagittal split separator should be placed down low into the osteotomy and the lower border captured to facilitate fracture with the rest of the buccal cortex.

Late diagnosis. The buccal cortex, including the coronoid process, will have fractured and become separate from the rest of the mandible. Because the bone is still attached to the temporalis muscle, it should not be removed. Redefine the buccal osteotomy of the body with what remains of the attachment at the lower border. Carefully attempt to start the split along the fracture line of the cortex. Using an osteotome in the fracture line and the sagittal split separator down low in the buccal osteotomy, recapture the split. Very little bone will overlap after repositioning of the distal segment, which makes the placement of rigid fixation difficult. A bone plate should be used to fixate the fragments. Monocortical screws can be placed on the distal fragment, and the fractured segment can be secured with bicortical screws (Fig 6-19b).

Fracture of the vertical osteotomy on the medial aspect of the mandibular ramus anterior to the inferior alveolar foramen

Early diagnosis. If diagnosed early, fracture of the vertical osteotomy on the medial aspect of the mandibular ramus anterior to the inferior alveolar foramen may be detected by the surgeon as resistance to the splitting maneuver at the superior aspect of the osteotomy. If this occurs, redefine the medial osteotomy of the ramus. Make sure that the osteotomy extends past the lingula. Take care not to damage the inferior alveolar neurovascular bundle, and define the osteotomy with a small osteotome. Proceed with the osteotomy.

Late diagnosis. If the condition is diagnosed late, the split will have been completed. However, the proximal part of the inferior alveolar canal and lingula will be attached to the proximal segment because the vertical ramus osteotomy fractured anterior to the lingula (Fig 6-20a). Support both segments to protect the inferior alveolar neurovascular bundle, and redefine the medial ramus osteotomy. Carefully split the lingula and inferior canal off the proximal segment of the mandible using a small osteotome (Fig 6-20b).

Fig 6-20 (*a*) The lingula and proximal part of the nerve canal are still attached to the proximal bone segment. This usually occurs when the horizontal osteotomy is terminated short of the lingula. (*b*) The canal containing the inferior alveolar neurovascular bundle is carefully dissected from the proximal bone segment.

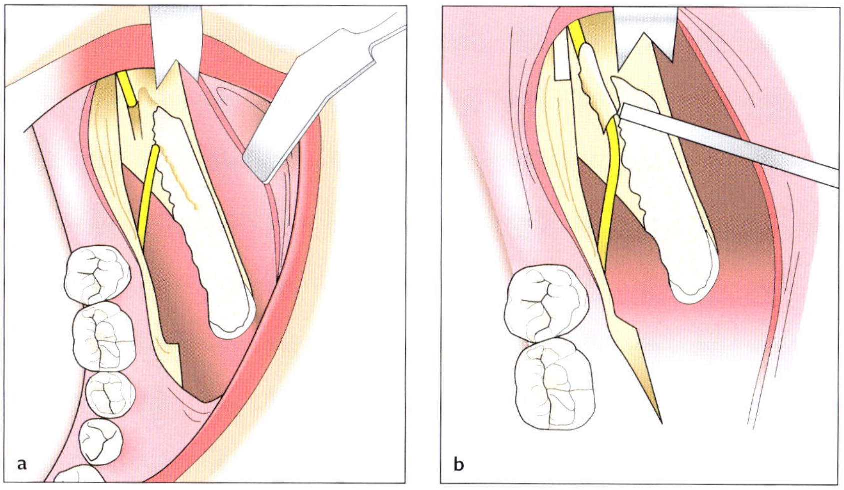

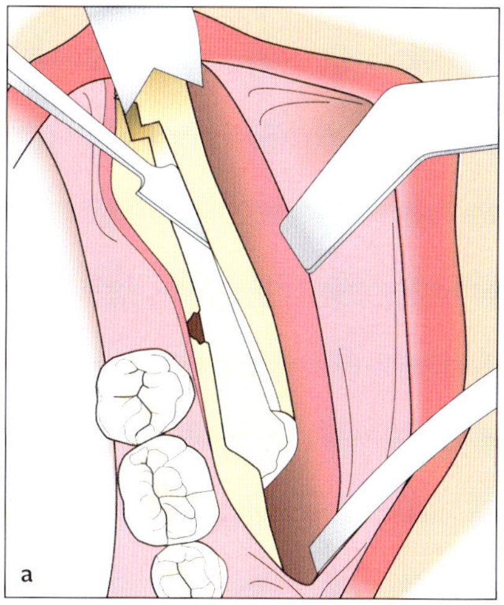

Fig 6-21 (*a*) Indiscriminate force applied to the fragile retromolar bone may cause this part to fracture. (*b*) The posterior lingual aspect of the proximal segment. An impacted third molar often weakens this part of the bone, rendering it more fragile. A fracture of this part of the proximal segment is demonstrated. (*c*) A bone plate is used to fixate the bone segments, while the fractured lingual part is secured by means of the bicortical screws.

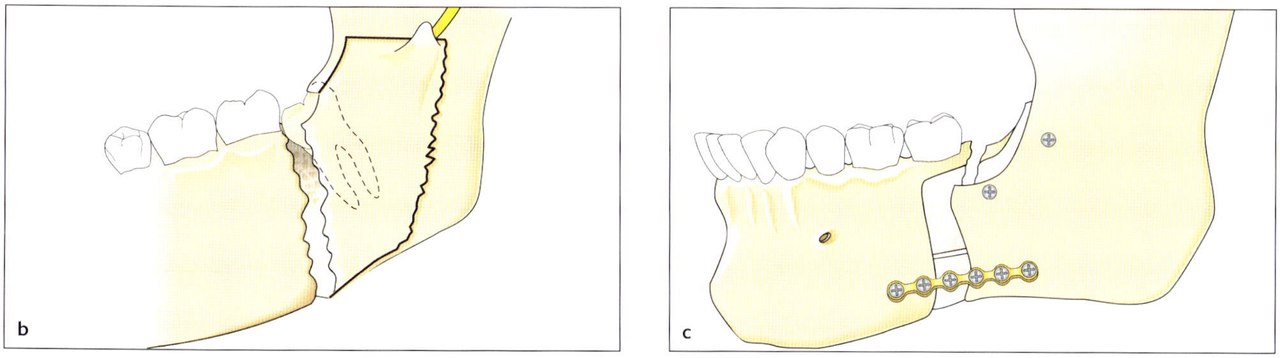

Fracture of the retromolar segment of the mandible distal to the second molar

Early diagnosis. The retromolar segment of the mandible distal to the second molar is particularly fragile, especially when an impacted third molar is present. When the surgeon finds that this segment is fragile, extreme care should be taken not to lever against this part of the jaw during the splitting procedure (Fig 6-21a).

Late diagnosis. If this aspect of the bone is fractured (Fig 6-21b), rigid fixation with bicortical screws will be impossible. The surgeon will be forced to use bone plates, as previously described (Fig 6-21c).

Intraoperative diagnosis of condylar sag

The need to accurately position the condyle in the glenoid fossa has been underlined by the increasingly common application of rigid fixation in bilateral sagittal split ramus osteotomies. However, there is no consensus as to what constitutes an ideal functional and stable relationship between the condyle, meniscus, and glenoid fossa. The literature not only contains contradictions about the functional relationship of the components of the TMJ, but more importantly, it is vague about how a functional and stable relationship can be achieved during surgical repositioning of the jaws.

Condylar sag can be defined as an immediate or late caudal movement of the condyle in the glenoid fossa after surgical establishment of a preplanned occlusion and rigid fixation of the bone fragments, leading to a change in the occlusion. Relapse of the occlusion due to a change in the condylar position may occur immediately after removal of the maxillomandibular fixation or later during the postoperative course.

Avoiding an unfavorable condylar position intraoperatively is obviously highly desirable and therefore the subject of ongoing research that has focused primarily on two management philosophies:

1. The condyle is maintained in its preoperative position prior to bilateral sagittal split ramus osteotomies. This is achieved by means of a device recording the relationship of the proximal segments to a skeletal structure that will remain constant and not be repositioned during surgery.
2. Sophisticated imaging modalities or computer-assisted navigation are used to replace the condyle in its preoperative position.

These techniques, although relatively successful, are either cumbersome or rely on expensive hardware that is not universally available. A simple technique that can reliably identify a malpositioned condyle intraoperatively has obvious advantages. It is highly desirable to be able to diagnose an incorrect occlusion at the time of surgery, and it is just as important to be able to recognize the cause of the problem. This section discusses possible etiologies of malocclusion after intraoperative removal of intermaxillary fixation and patterns of malocclusion that should assist the clinician in differentiating the various etiologic factors.

Intraoperative diagnosis of an incorrect occlusion

A disclusion is often apparent shortly after intraoperative removal of maxillomandibular fixation. Figure 6-22 shows

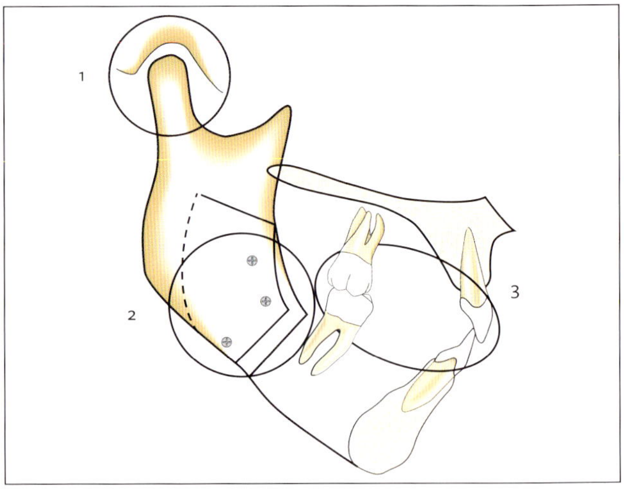

Fig 6-22 An incorrect occlusion immediately following intraoperative removal of maxillomandibular fixation may be caused by condylar sag (1), mobility at the osteotomy site (2), or a shift in the occlusion during placement of rigid fixation (3).

possible causes of an incorrect occlusion at this stage of the procedure: (1) condylar sag, (2) mobility at the osteotomy site, or (3) a shift of the occlusion during placement of rigid fixation.

Condylar sag

Two types of condylar sag may occur: central and peripheral. In central condylar sag type I, the condyle is positioned inferiorly in the glenoid fossa and makes no contact with any part of the fossa (Fig 6-23a). In the absence of intracapsular edema or hemarthrosis (causing hydraulic pressure), the condyle will move superiorly after removal of maxillomandibular fixation, leading to a malocclusion (Fig 6-23b).

In central condylar sag type II, the condyle is pushed posterioroly in the fossa, sliding down on the posterior surface of the fossa (Fig 6-23c). Once the intermaxillary fixation is removed, the condyle will slide superiorly into the fossa, leading to a Class II anterior open bite malocclusion (Fig 6-23d).

Peripheral condylar sag may also be split into two types. In type I, the condyle is positioned inferiorly, with some fossa contact (lateral, medial, posterior, or anterior) with the maxillomandibular fixation in position (teeth in occlusion) and rigid fixation placed. This type of condylar malpositioning provides physical support to the occlusion (Fig 6-24a). Postoperative resorption or a change in condylar shape will lead to late relapse (Fig 6-24b). In type II, the condyle is positioned correctly in the fossa with the maxillomandibular fixation in position (teeth in occlusion); however, with the placement of rigid fixation, a torquing force is applied to the condyle and ramus of the mandible (Figs 6-25a and 6-25b). The tension on

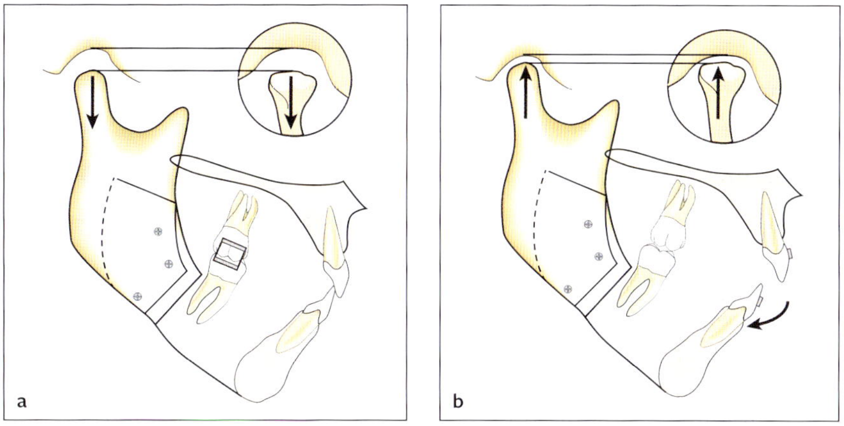

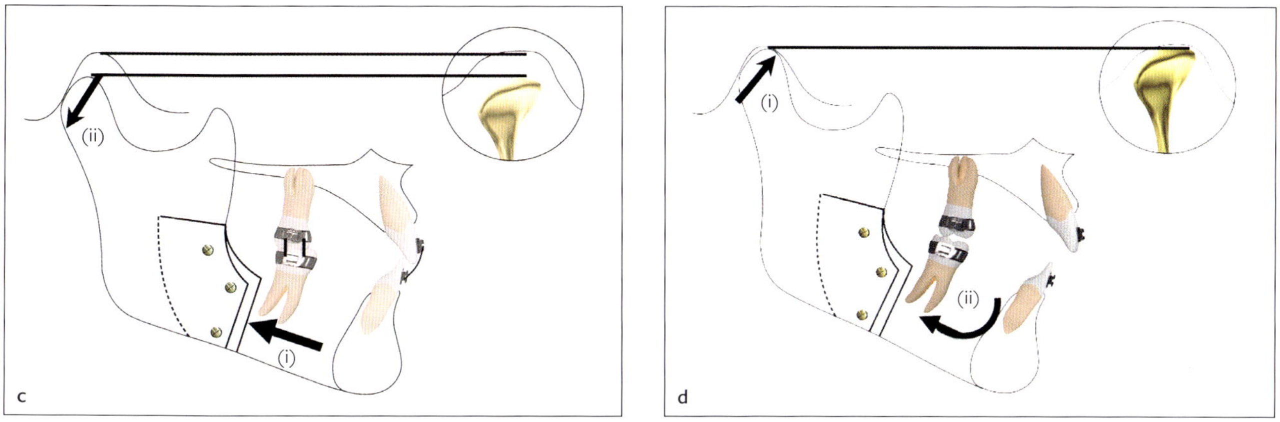

Fig 6-23 (*a*) Central condylar sag type I. The condyle is positioned inferiorly in the glenoid fossa with no bone contact while the teeth are in occlusion (maxillomandibular fixation) and rigid fixation is placed. (*b*) After removal of maxillomandibular fixation, the condyle will move superiorly, causing immediate relapse. (*c*) Central sag type I. Excessive posterior force during condylar positioning (*arrow i*) has pushed the condyle posteriorly, and it slides downward and inferiorly on the posterior wall of the glenoid fossa (*arrow ii*). (*d*) Following removal of the intermaxilary fixation, the condyle will slide superiorly into the fossa (*arrow i*), leading to a Class II anterior open bite (*arrow ii*).

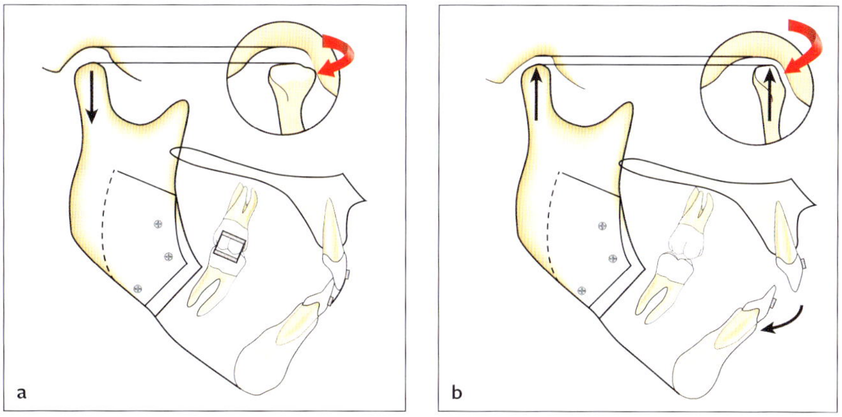

Fig 6-24 (*a*) Type I peripheral condylar sag. The condyle is displaced inferiorly with (in this case) medial fossa contact. After removal of the maxillomandibular fixation, the condyle-fossa contact provides physical support to the occlusion. (*b*) Postoperative condylar resorption will lead to superior positioning of the condyle, which will later cause relapse.

the ramus is released when the maxillomandibular fixation is removed, and the condyle will move either laterally or medially and slide inferiorly in the fossa (Fig 6-25c).

Peripheral sag occurs more often in bilateral sagittal split ramus osteotomy procedures where a defect develops between the two bone segments because of the repositioning of the distal segment. When these intersegmental defects are closed by forcing the segments together during the application of rigid fixation, the condyle is often displaced in the glenoid fossa. In procedures for the correction of mandibular asymmetry (Fig 6-26a)—large setback or advancement procedures (especially in V-shaped mandibles) with the use of lag screws for rigid fixation—special care should be taken not to displace the condyle in the fossa during the placement of fixation (Figs 6-26b and 6-26c). The step at the horizontal osteotomy on the medial side of the mandibular ramus may also interfere with bone contact (Fig 6-26d) and act as a fulcrum during the placement of rigid fixation.

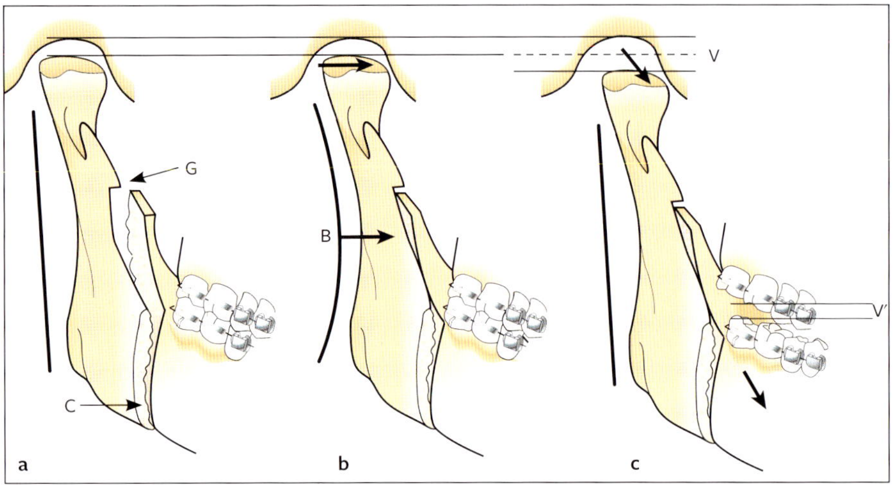

Fig 6-25 Frontolateral view of the glenoid fossa, condyle, and proximal and distal bone segments. (*a*) The condyle is in the correct relationship to the glenoid fossa. Note, however, the gap (G) and the contact area (C) between the bone segments. (*b*) The placement of rigid fixation forces the bone segments together, which applies tension on the condyle and ramus, causing a bowing effect (B). (*c*) Once the maxillomandibular fixation is removed, the tension on the ramus is released, causing the condyle to move medially and slide inferiorly on the medial wall of the fossa; this creates a posterior open bite. The vertical change in condylar position (V) is equal to the posterior open bite (V′).

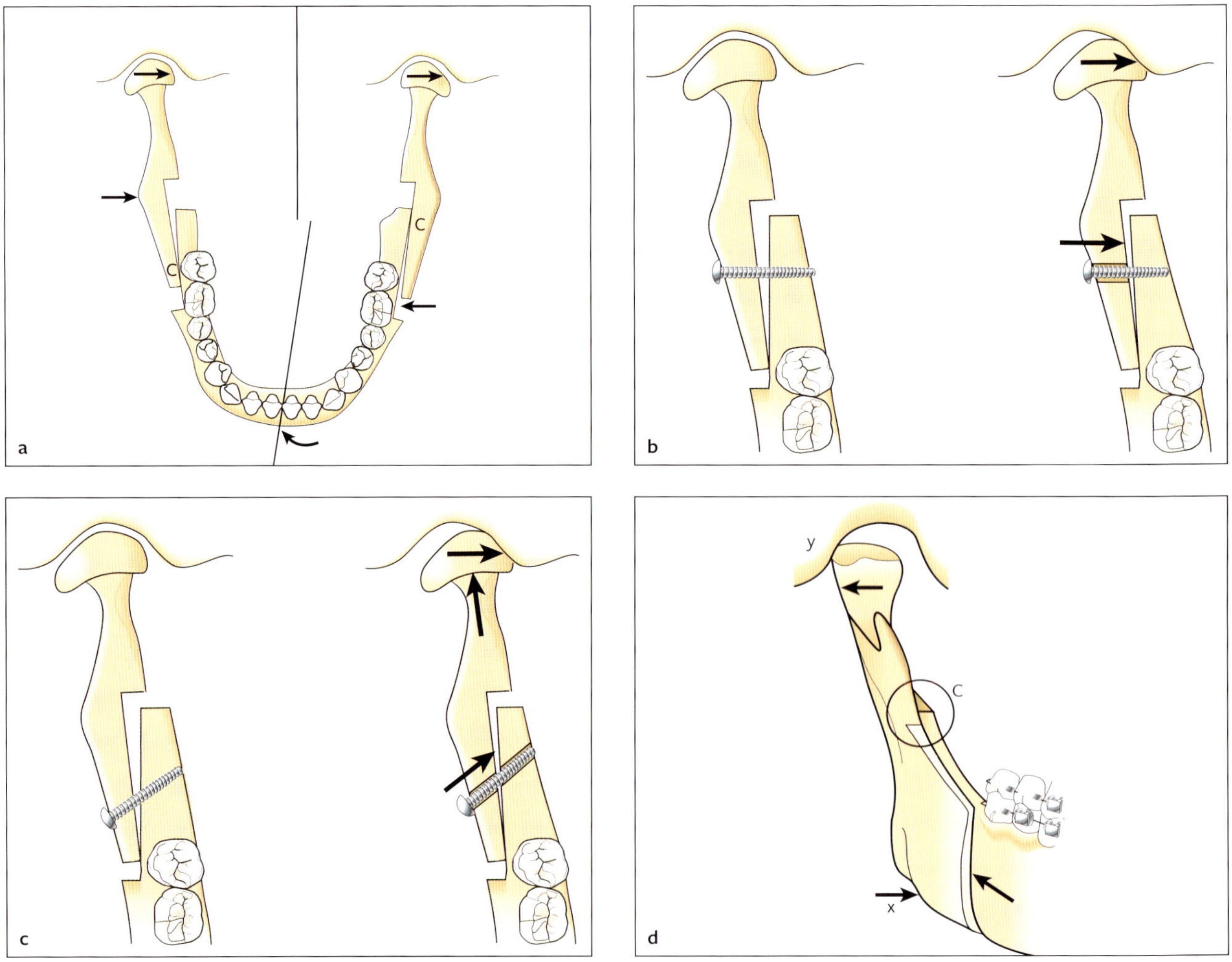

Fig 6-26 (*a*) The intersegmental defects are demonstrated after correction of mandibular asymmetry. The only bone contact is at C, which acts as a fulcrum if the segments are forced together by rigid fixation. Both condyles will be forced to the left side in the glenoid fossa. (*b*) The positioning screw (*left*) will tend to maintain the intersegmental gap. A lag screw (*right*) readily allows the bone segments to be forced together, secondarily displacing the condyle medially in the fossa. (*c*) Bicortical screws must be placed at an angle when the procedure is done intraorally. The lag screw (*right*) will tend to force the condyle medially and distally in the fossa, whereas the positional screw (*left*) will maintain the intersegmental position. (*d*) During large setback procedures with shortening of the mandibular ramus, the horizontal step (of the medial osteotomy) may act as a fulcrum (C). Medial force to achieve bone contact (x) will displace the condyle laterally in the fossa (y).

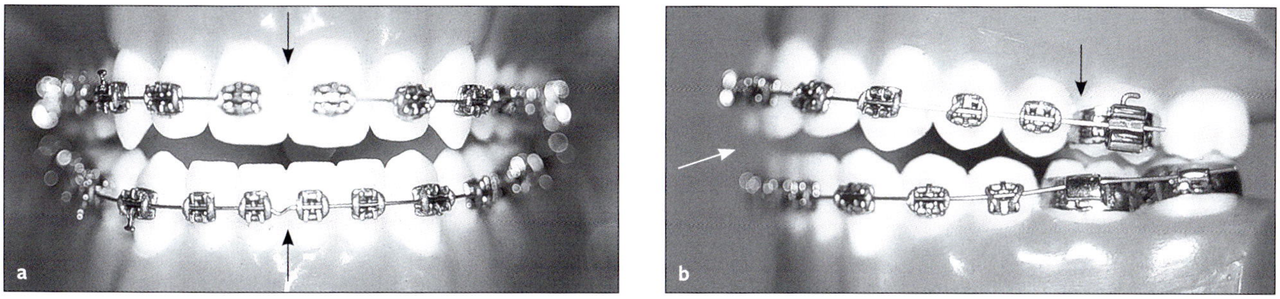

Fig 6-27 Bilateral central condylar sag. (*a*) Frontal view of occlusion. The dental midlines are correct (*arrows*), and there is a tendency for anterior open bite. (*b*) Left view of occlusion. Note the increased overjet, tendency for anterior open bite (*white arrow*), and Class II dental relationship (*black arrow*). The right side of the occlusion is similar.

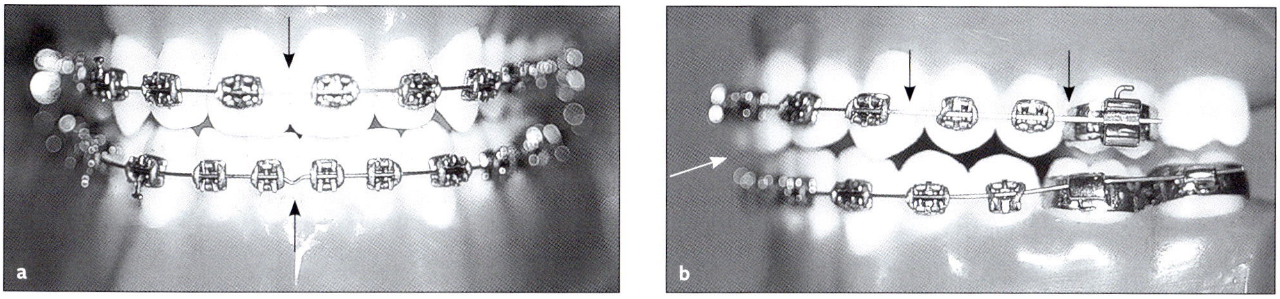

Fig 6-28 Unilateral central condylar sag, left condyle. (*a*) Frontal view of occlusion. The mandibular dental midline is displaced toward the left (*arrows*). (*b*) Left side of occlusion. Note the increased overjet (*white arrow*) and Class II dental relationship (*black arrows*). The right side of the occlusion has a Class I dental relationship.

An occlusal shift may be identified by careful clinical examination following the removal of maxillomandibular fixation. Condylar sag produces repeatable patterns of occlusal shift that will help the surgeon identify the offending condyle. Following are the clinical signs of condylar sag:

1. Central condylar sag (see Fig 6-23)
   - Bilateral central condylar sag (Fig 6-27)
     - Dental midlines correct
     - Overjet increased
     - Anterior open bite
     - Class II malocclusion (bilaterally)
   - Unilateral central condylar sag (Fig 6-28)
     - Mandibular dental midline toward the offending side
     - Overjet increased (more on the offending side)
     - Class II dental relationship on the offending side
     - Overjet corrected and the correct occlusion reestablished if the mandible is moved until the midlines coincide
2. Peripheral condylar sag
   - Type I (see Fig 6-24)
     - Difficult to diagnose intraoperatively because the contact between the condyle and glenoid fossa supports the occlusion, which may lead to late relapse due to condylar resorption
   - Type II
     - Bilateral peripheral condylar sag (Fig 6-29)
       - Dental midlines correct
       - Anterior crossbite or edge-to-edge incisal relationship
       - Tendency for Class III dental relationship
       - Tendency for bilateral posterior open bites
     - Unilateral peripheral condylar sag (Fig 6-30)
       - Dental midline of the mandible toward the contralateral side
       - Edge-to-edge incisal relationship with tendency for crossbite on the offending side
       - Posterior open bite on the offending side with teeth in occlusion
       - Incisal relationship edge to edge or in crossbite, with tendency for a Class III dental relationship between canines and molars when the mandible is moved toward the left to correct dental midlines

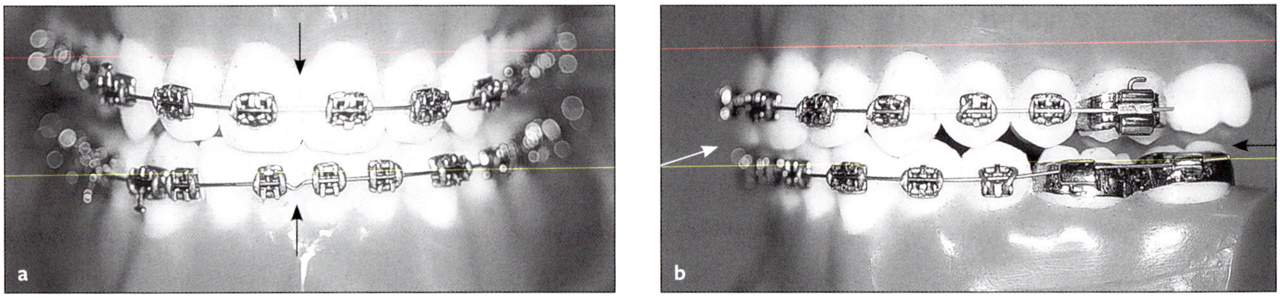

Fig 6-29 Bilateral Type II peripheral condylar sag. (*a*) Frontal view of occlusion. The dental midlines are correct (*arrows*), and there is a tendency toward an edge-to-edge incisal relationship. (*b*) Left side of occlusion. There is a tendency toward a Class III dental relationship, posterior open bite (*black arrow*), and edge-to-edge incisal relationship (*white arrow*). The right side of the occlusion is similar.

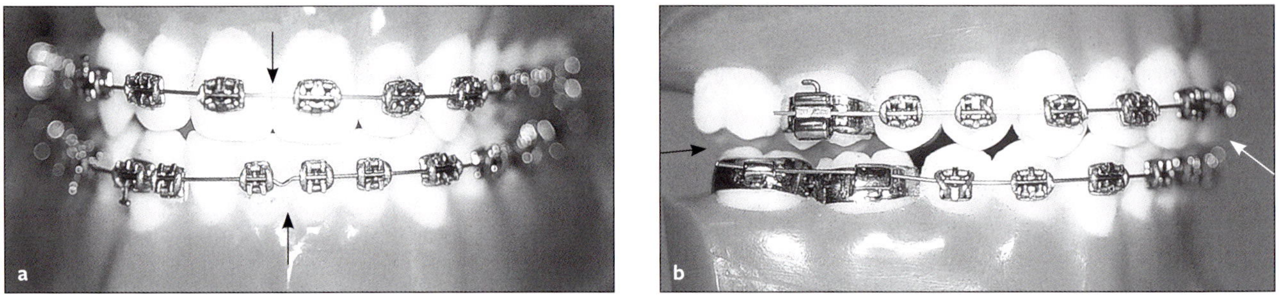

Fig 6-30 Unilateral Type II peripheral condylar sag of the right condyle. (*a*) Frontal view of occlusion. The dental midline of the mandible is displaced toward the left (*black arrows*). (*b*) Right side of occlusion. Note the edge-to-edge incisal relationship (*white arrow*), Class III dental relationship, and posterior open bite (*black arrow*). The left side of the occlusion has a Class I dental relationship.

It is possible to diagnose central condylar sag and type II peripheral condylar sag intraoperatively immediately after removal of the maxillomandibular fixation. With type I, however, where condyle–glenoid fossa contact supports the occlusion, the condylar sag will become apparent only when resorption of the condyle has taken place.

Mobility at the osteotomy site

Inadequate rigid fixation at the osteotomy site will lead to mobility between the distal and proximal segments of the mandible. The occlusal signs will mimic those of central condylar sag on the same side. The surgeon should consider this complication when a malocclusion occurs after the removal of maxillomandibular fixation. By applying light, controlled force on either side of the osteotomy site, the surgeon should be able to detect mobility between the two bone segments.

Shift of the occlusion during placement of rigid fixation

Inadequate occlusal fixation combined with excessive lateral force during placement of bicortical screws may displace the occlusion. This displacement may go undetected until after maxillomandibular fixation has been removed and the occlusion checked. Thus, the occlusion should be checked before the removal of maxillomandibular fixation.

Intra-articular hemorrhage or edema. The step-by-step description of the surgical technique stressed careful handling of and respect for hard and soft tissue during surgery. This is especially important during the actual splitting procedure and in handling the proximal segment after splitting. Rough, indiscriminate manipulation of this segment (and the condyle) may lead to intracapsular hemorrhage and/or edema or may displace the articulating disc.

Hemorrhage or edema in the TMJ capsule may cause increased intracapsular pressure, which makes subsequent condylar positioning difficult. Also, when the hemorrhage or edema resolves postoperatively, the condyle will move superiorly in the fossa (condylar sag) (Figs 6-31a and 6-31b). If increased pressure develops postoperatively, the condyle will be pushed inferiorly in the fossa—a situation that is usually accompanied by pain. The clinical signs mimic those of peripheral condylar sag. There is a posterior open bite on the affected side, and the bite will improve as the intracapsular hemorrhage or edema resolves (Fig 6-31c).

Disc displacement. A preoperative history of TMJ clicking or locking indicates that the proximal segment should be handled with even more care than usual during surgery. The integrity of the joint structures must be carefully

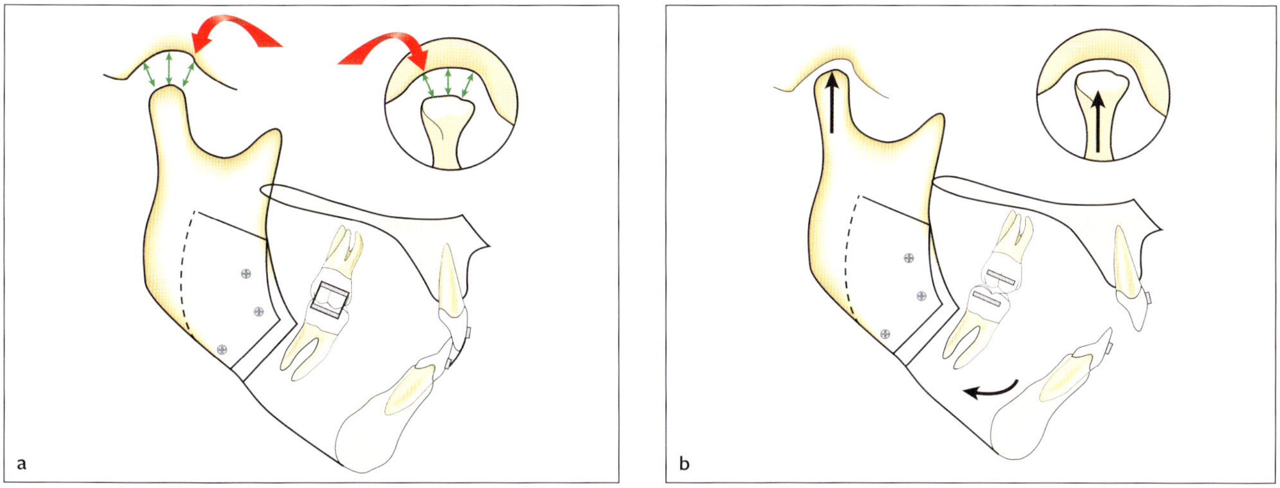

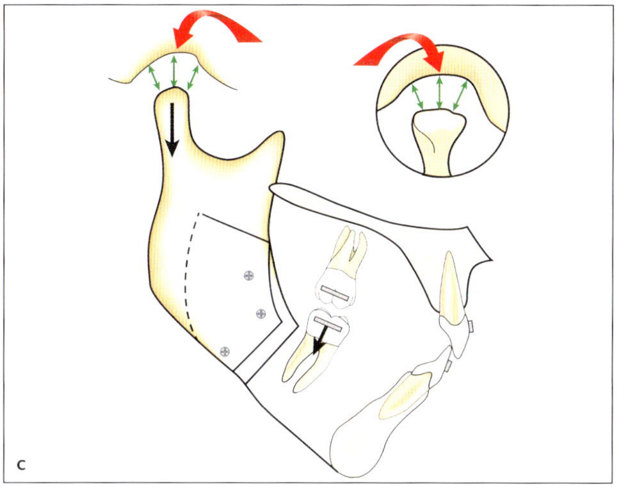

Fig 6-31 (*a*) Intracapsular hemarthrosis and/or edema before condylar positioning. The increase in intracapsular hydraulic pressure tends to displace the condyle inferiorly and make condylar positioning difficult. This may lead to postoperative central sag. (*b*) As the hemarthrosis and/or edema resolves postoperatively, the condyle moves superiorly, leading to malocclusion. (*c*) Intracapsular hemarthrosis and/or edema after condylar positioning. The increased intracapsular hydraulic pressure tends to push the condyle inferiorly, leading to postoperative posterior open bite (mimicking peripheral sag). With resolution of the intracapsular hemarthrosis and/or edema, the condyle will move superiorly, reestablishing the occlusion.

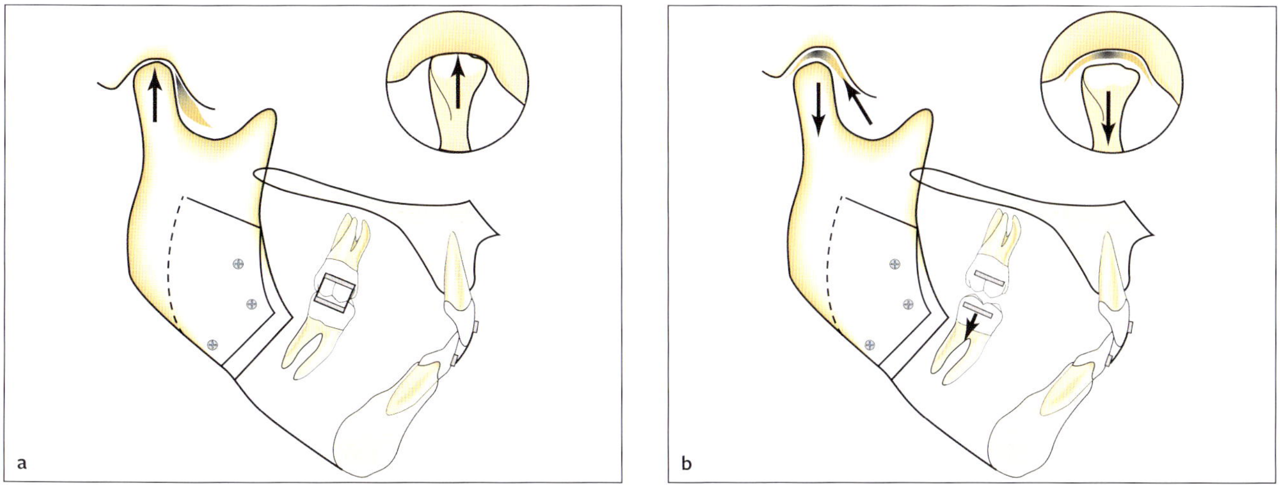

Fig 6-32 (*a*) The articulator disc is displaced anteriorly in the fossa during condylar positioning. (*b*) Once the disc returns to its normal position in the fossa, the condyle will be pushed downward, leading to a posterior open bite on the affected side.

maintained, and displacement of the articulator disc must be avoided as much as possible. If the disc is not in its normal relation to the condyle and fossa during condylar positioning, the bite will open posteriorly once the disc returns to its normal position in the fossa (Fig 6-32).

Condylar orientation in the glenoid fossa is critical and probably the most demanding step of the bilateral sagittal split ramus osteotomy procedure. During the condylar-positioning maneuver, the surgeon cannot see the condyle or glenoid fossa; however, its position is influenced by numerous intracapsular and extracapsular factors, including the following:

- Incorrect vector during condylar positioning
- Incorrect direction of the holding wire or bone clamp
- An incomplete or greenstick split that prevents condylar seating
- Muscular, ligamentous, or periosteal interference
- Intra-articular hemorrhage or edema
- Flexing the proximal segment while placing rigid fixation (with stress in the segment being released once the maxillomandibular fixation is removed)
- Displacement of the articulator disc
- Resistance to movement between the distal and proximal segments during condylar positioning

The technique for condylar positioning is discussed in the surgical technique section. As previously emphasized, the surgeon who develops the ability to diagnose an incorrect occlusion and understands what leads to malocclusion during surgery has immense advantages. Intraoperative correction will prevent a disappointing occlusal result and many hours of hard work and irritation for the orthodontist, not to mention further surgery. The surgeon should not depend on extensive, prolonged postoperative orthodontics to correct a poor surgical outcome.

Intraoral Vertical Mandibular Ramus Osteotomy

The bilateral sagittal split ramus osteotomy is currently the procedure of choice for the correction of most mandibular dentoskeletal deformities. The intraoral vertical ramus osteotomy is traditionally used when large setback of the mandible is required as well as for the correction of severe mandibular asymmetry. This procedure has several advantages over the BSSO:

1. It has less inferior alveolar nerve morbidity.
2. It can be performed on an outpatient basis.
3. It causes less flaring of the proximal segments.
4. There is no need for rigid fixation.
5. Existing TMJ dysfunction can be treated concurrently as the condylar heads freely move into a physiologically equilibrated position.

However, the intraoral vertical ramus osteotomy also has certain disadvantages, such as the need for postoperative maxillomandibular fixation and the need for a strict protocol of active physiotherapy for at least 2 weeks after release of the fixation. A limiting factor with large setback procedures is the anatomical interference between the coronoid process and the skull base or with the TMJ capsule. If this interference occurs, coronoidectomy should be considered, but it may impose difficulties in physiotherapy.

Standard surgery

Step 1: Infiltration of the soft tissue with a vasoconstrictor

Ten minutes before surgery begins, the retromolar area and deep layer of the masseter muscle are infiltrated with local anesthetic containing vasoconstrictor (epinephrine in a concentration of 1:100,000).

Step 2: Mucosal incision

A mucosal incision is made over the external oblique ridge close to the mucogingival junction. Start the incision just above the level of the occlusal plane, and end 30 mm anterior and inferior. Take care to leave sufficient nonkeratinized epithelium superiorly on the body of the mandible to facilitate ease of suturing later.

Step 3: Periosteal incision

Place the scalpel firmly on the bone, and incise the periosteum along the anterior border of the ramus of the mandible.

Step 4: Subperiosteal dissection

The overlying periosteum and muscle attachments (lower parts of the temporalis muscle, masseter muscle, and posterior part of the buccinator muscle) are dissected. The periosteum is reflected broadly from the sigmoid notch superiorly to the antigonial notch inferiorly. Carry the dissection posteriorly to include the angle of the mandible to facilitate adjustment to the proximal segment after the osteotomy has been completed. Clean and complete stripping is essential for ease of placement of the Bauer retractors as well as for proper visualization during surgery.

Step 5: Placement of the retractors

Two Bauer retractors are now placed. One retractor is placed in the sigmoid notch and the other in the antigonial notch (Fig 6-33). The lateral surface of the mandibular ramus is now copiously washed by lavage with saline solution and suction so that important landmarks can be identified.

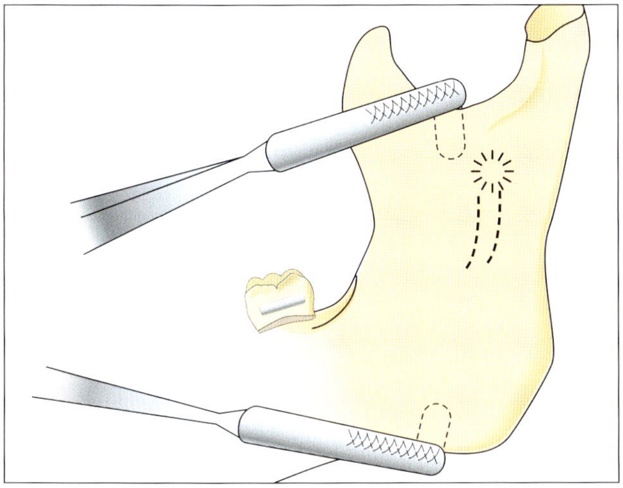

Fig 6-33 The Bauer retractors are placed to retract the soft tissue and expose the lateral surface of the ramus. One retractor is hooked into the sigmoid notch, while the other is hooked around the lower border of the mandible into the antigonial notch.

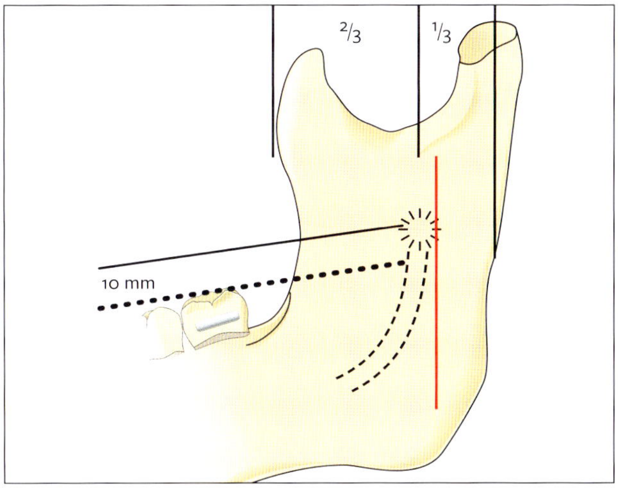

Fig 6-34 The antilingular eminence corresponds to the alveolar foramen on the medial side of the ramus and gives the clinician an indication of the position of the inferior alveolar foramen. The eminence is usually situated about 10 mm above the occlusal plane, and it can be found about two-thirds posterior of the width of the mandibular ramus. A reference line (*red line*) is marked 2 mm posterior to the eminence from the sigmoid notch superior to the antigonial notch inferior.

Step 6: Identification of landmarks

Various methods to establish the position of the mandibular foramen on the lingual side of the ramus can be implemented: (1) The antilingular eminence on the lateral surface of the ramus can be identified and marked with a pen. This small protuberance is usually situated about 10 mm above the level of the occlusal plane and two-thirds posterior to the width of the ramus. The protuberance corresponds to the mandibular foramen on the lingual side of the ramus. (2) Hall (2002) recommends that it is safe to perform the vertical osteotomy 6 mm to 7 mm anterior to the posterior border of the ramus. (3) Da Fontura et al (2002) described that the mandibular foramen is most often located horizontally in the middle third of the ramus and vertically in the superior third. (4) Park (2009) relies on location of the antilingular eminence and the radiographic location of the foramen to accurately identify the mandibular foramen. A guideline can now be drawn from the antilingular notch toward the antigonial notch parallel to the posterior border of the ramus (Fig 6-34).

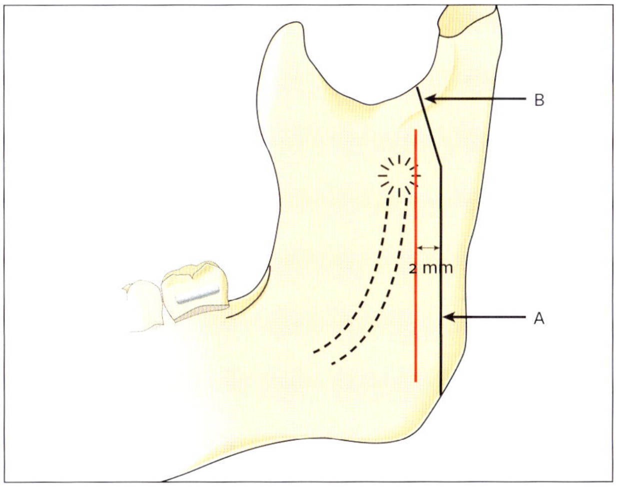

Fig 6-35 A round oscillating saw is used to perform the first osteotomy 2 mm posterior to the reference line (shown at A). A second osteotomy, shown at B, is angulated slightly anteriorly and performed from the superior end of the reference line into the sigmoid notch.

Step 7: First vertical osteotomy

The osteotomy is first performed only through the outer cortex of the bone. The cut is started just above the marked protuberance, 2 mm posterior and parallel to the guideline, with an oscillating saw and a rounded blade. Before the osteotomy is completed, the position and direction should be checked with a dental mirror. The completion of the osteotomy is started superiorly, and once the surgeon feels the saw perforate the medial cortex, the blade is moved downward to the antigonial notch. The osteotomy should be performed under copious irrigation with cooling saline solution. The inferior alveolar neurovascular bundle is situated anterior to the osteotomy, and there are no major vessels located in the depth of the saw blade along the osteotomy line (Fig 6-35).

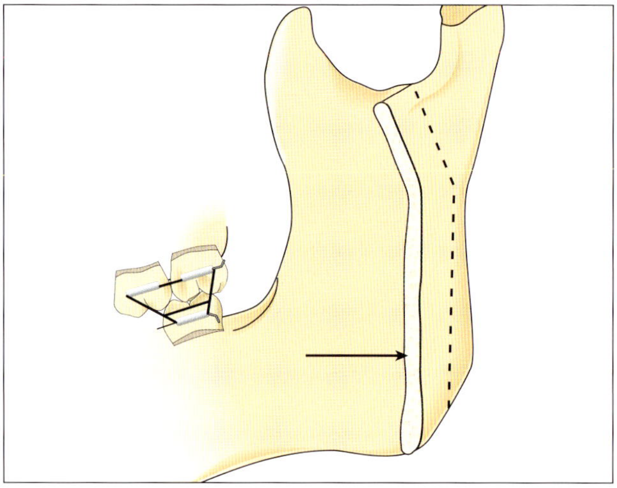

Fig 6-36 The distal segment can now be easily mobilized and the osteotomized surface of the distal segment seen (*arrow*).

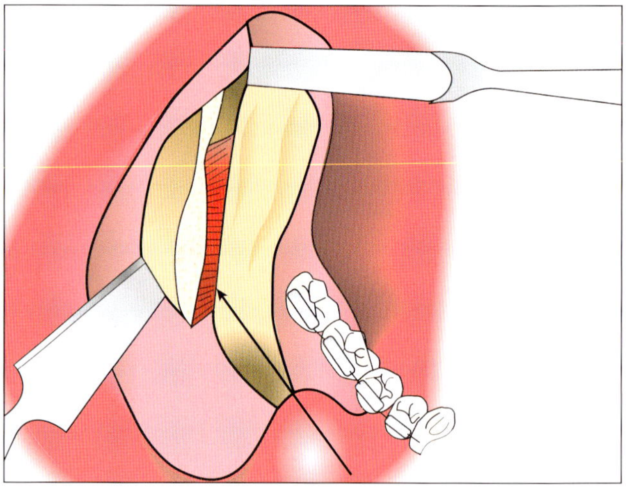

Fig 6-37 The medial pterygoid muscle and stylomandibular ligament attachments on the medial surface of the distal segment should be carefully dissected off the bone (*arrow*).

Step 8: Second vertical osteotomy

The second osteotomy is started at the superior end of the first and carried upward and obliquely to the midpoint of the sigmoid notch (see Fig 6-35). Because of the increased risk of damage to the branches of the maxillary artery, which are located medially near the mandibular foramen, the oscillating saw blade should not be inserted deeply when performing this part of the procedure. It is recommended that the blade be held slightly obliquely at this stage. The Bauer retractor in the sigmoid notch serves as protection to the masseteric branches of the maxillary artery. Following the completion of the second osteotomy, the distal segment will be mobile, and its lateromedial cut surface will be partially visible (Fig 6-36).

Step 9: Subperiosteal stripping on the medial aspect of the distal segment

All the periosteal attachments (medial pterygoid muscle and stylomandibular ligament) on the medial aspect of the distal segment are now carefully stripped to facilitate easy setback of the proximal segment without soft tissue interference. Careful stripping is advised to avoid displacement of the condyle from the fossa or damage to joint structures (Fig 6-37).

Step 10: Repeating the procedure on the opposite side

Repeat steps 1 through 9 of the intraoral vertical mandibular ramus osteotomy on the opposite side.

Step 11: Throat pack removal

The throat pack is removed, and the oral cavity is washed by copious irrigation with saline solution. A nasogastric tube is inserted to remove gastric fluids that may have accumulated during the operation and ensure that the throat is clear.

Step 12: Maxillomandibular fixation

The teeth are now placed into the planned occlusion, and maxillomandibular fixation is applied. A surgical splint may be used to guide the teeth into the final occlusion.

Step 13: Checking the bone contacts

The overlapping of the bone segments should be checked. The lateral side of the distal segment and the medial side of the proximal segment can be contoured to improve the bone contact and prevent flaring. Finally, the level of the inferior border of the proximal segment should be evaluated. If the lower border of this segment extends lower than the mandibular lower border, it should be trimmed to prevent soft tissue irritation and a prominent mandibular angle.

Step 14: Suturing

The wounds are closed via routine suturing procedures with 4-0 resorbable sutures.

Postoperative physiotherapy

Postoperative physiotherapy is mandatory following the intraoral vertical ramus osteotomy and should commence immediately following removal of maxillomandibular

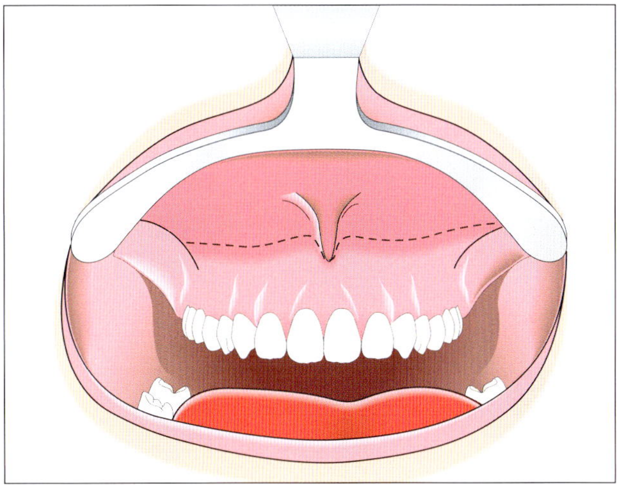

Fig 6-38 Mucosal incision (*dotted line*). Leave at least 5 mm of nonkeratinized epithelium inferior to the incision.

fixation. The exercises should include mouth opening, lateral excursions, and protrusive movements. There is a tendency for anterior open bite to develop, and it should be controlled by elastic therapy when the patient is not exercising. Open bites of more than 2 mm should be controlled by a longer period of maxillomandibular fixation.

Complications

Although not strictly a complication, the main disadvantage of the procedure is the fact that intermaxillary fixation is required for 8 to 10 days postoperatively. No rigid fixation between the bone segments is required, and the incidence of inferior alveolar nerve damage is significantly lower than with BSSO.

Complications are rare and include fibrous union, infection, and hemorrhage originating from the masseteric artery.

Le Fort I Maxillary Osteotomy

After Le Fort described the natural planes of fracture of the midface in 1901, maxillary surgery developed through the work of Wassmund, Axhauser, Schuchardt, Obwegeser, Willmar, and others. However, it was not until the excellent research by Bell et al in the mid 1970s on the biologic basis of the hemodynamics and vascular supply of the maxilla during and after maxillary downfracture surgery that the Le Fort I maxillary osteotomy developed into the refined science and art that it is today.

Maxillary abnormalities contribute to many facial deformities that should be recognized and treated successfully by adhering to basic biologic and technical treatment principles. Numerous techniques for Le Fort I maxillary osteotomy have been described and reflect a strong tendency to operator preference. The technique described here has been developed during the performance of almost 5,000 Le Fort I maxillary osteotomies over the course of the past 35 years. It has been found to be beneficial in the training of many residents participating in the oral and maxillofacial program at the University of the Witwatersrand in Johannesburg, South Africa.

Standard surgery

Step 1: Infiltration of the soft tissue with a vasoconstrictor

Infiltrate the area of dissection with local anesthetic containing a vasoconstrictor (epinephrine in a concentration of 1:100,000) 10 minutes before surgery. Inject the soft tissue areas at the intended osteotomies by placing the needle deep into the maxillary buccal sulcus, aspirating, and then injecting the anesthetic as the needle is withdrawn.

Step 2: Mucosal incision

Make an incision in the maxillary buccal sulcus, through the mucosa only, with a no. 15 blade or diathermy knife. The incision is started at the buttress area and then carried forward to the centerline, leaving approximately 5 mm of nonkeratinized mucosa on the alveolar side for later ease of suturing. This incision should be increased posteriorly to approximately 10 mm at the buttress area. A V-shaped incision at the labial frenum helps with alignment in later suturing (Fig 6-38).

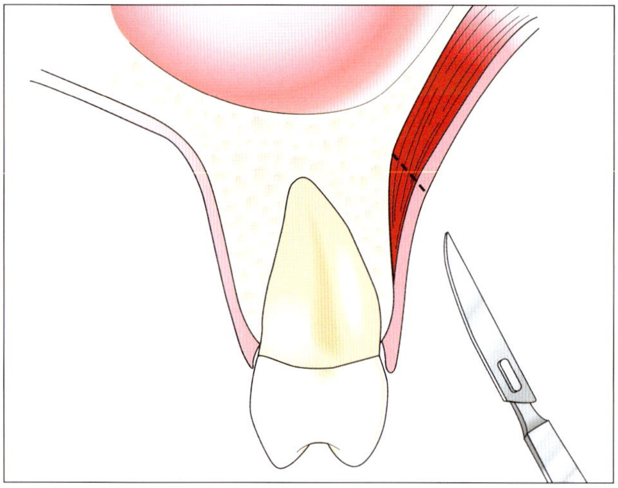

Fig 6-39 The incision is angled superiorly so more soft tissue is left inferiorly for later ease of suturing and for sufficient blood supply support to the downfractued maxilla.

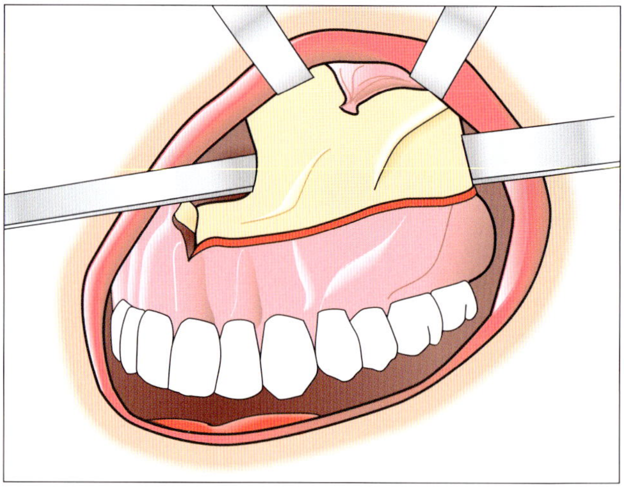

Fig 6-40 The subperiosteal dissection is carried superiorly and posteriorly to identify the piriform rim, infraorbital nerve, zygomatic buttress, and posterior maxilla.

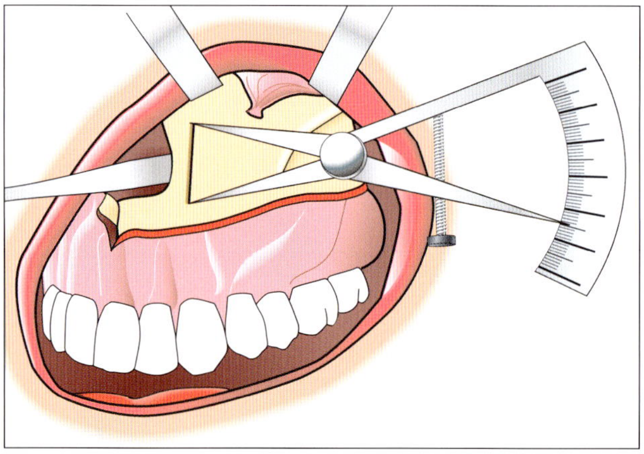

Fig 6-41 Vertical and horizontal reference marks are scored on the bone and the distances between them measured.

Step 3: Completing the soft tissue incision through the periosteum

The blade is angled superiorly to leave more submucosal tissue on the alveolar side for later submucosal suturing (Fig 6-39). The incision onto bone should be clean and decisive to facilitate neat subperiosteal dissection. If the incision is carried too far posteriorly or too high, it may cause herniation of the buccal fat pad and make surgery cumbersome.

Step 4: Subperiosteal dissection

1. Dissect the buccal periosteum from anterior to posterior around the tuberosity, and place the pterygoid retractor subperiosteally.
2. Identify the piriform rim, and carefully elevate the nasal periosteum from the rim, nasal floor, and lateral nasal wall.
3. Place a Howarth dissector laterally in the nasal cavity to protect the nasal mucosa.
4. Dissect neatly. Do not perforate the periosteum, especially not posteriorly, to prevent herniation of the buccal fat pad through the periosteum.
5. Push the nasal mucosa inward with the back of the periosteal dissector to tent the mucosa for the beginning of the nasal dissection.
6. Continue the nasal dissection laterally from the floor of the nose to the lateral wall of the nose and medially to the nasal septum.
7. Identify the position of the infraorbital foramen and nerve both to protect the nerve and to influence the height of the osteotomy cut (especially with superior repositioning of the maxilla; Fig 6-40).
8. If the buccal fat pad is exposed, it should be covered with a small, wet sponge and retracted with the pterygoid retractor.

Step 5: Placement of reference marks

Vertical and horizontal reference marks are scored (approximately 10 mm apart) on either side at the canine and buttress area using a 701 bur. The distance between the marks is recorded (Fig 6-41). The height of the osteotomy is significant in more than one way, and the reference marks should be made accordingly:

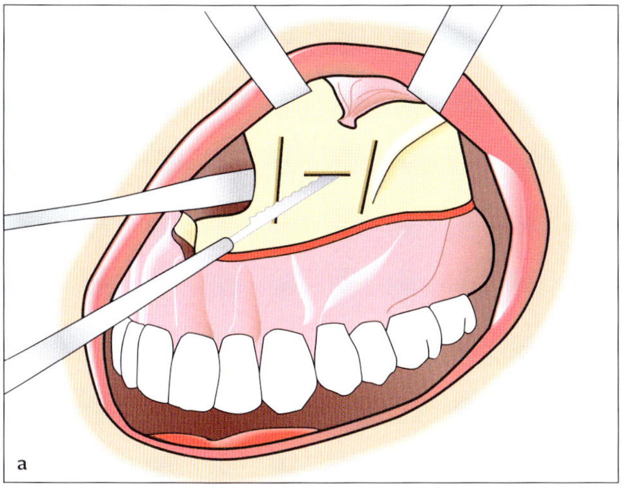

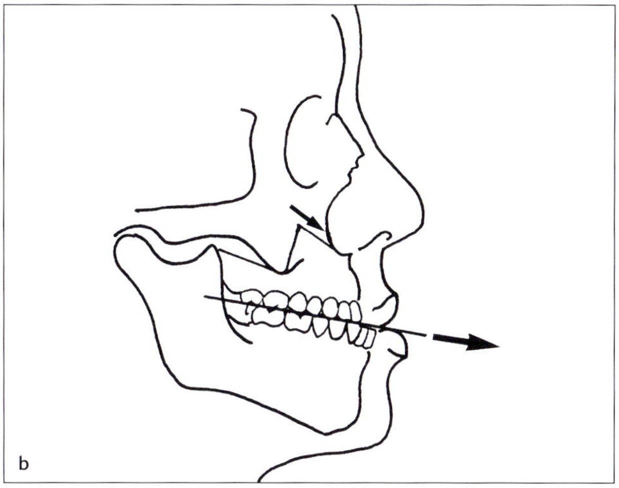

Fig 6-42 (*a*) A reciprocating saw is used to perform the osteotomy. In most patients, the osteotomy should be kept parallel to the occlusal plane. (*b*) The osteotomy is angled to allow the maxilla to slide downward along this plane as it is advanced. Bone contact is therefore maintained as the height of the maxilla is increased. (*c*) The osteotomy is angled superiorly. This will result in an open bite, and the height of the maxilla will be reduced as it is advanced to correct the Class III malocclusion.

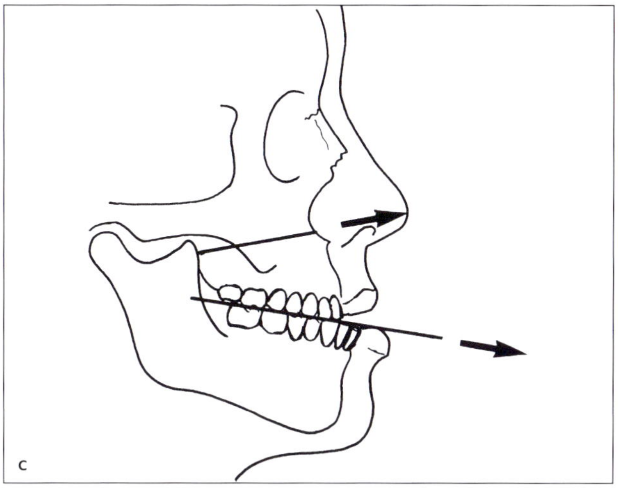

- With maxillary advancement procedures, osteotomy height depends on the esthetic requirements of the patient. The osteotomy can be made high (just inferior to the infraorbital nerve in the "high Le Fort I" osteotomy) or low (not less than 5 mm above the tooth apices).
- When superiorly repositioning the maxilla, the amount of bone removed dictates the positioning of the osteotomies. Other determining factors include structures such as the infraorbital nerve and tooth apices as well as the positioning of rigid fixation.

Step 6: Anterior buccal osteotomy

Use a reciprocating saw to perform the osteotomy from the buttress to the piriform rim at least 5 mm superior to the apex of the canine (Fig 6-42a). In principle, horizontal Le Fort I osteotomies should be parallel to the occlusal plane to allow repositioning to take place along it. Therefore, during the planning phase, the osteotomy must be performed on the same plane, both in model surgery and cephalometric visual treatment objective tracing; measurements on these records are then more accurate when applied during surgery. Although the osteotomy may be angled intentionally in the downsliding Le Fort I technique (Fig 6-42b), incorrect angulation of the osteotomy will make it difficult to achieve the surgical treatment objective because the maxilla will be moved along this plane and may vertically shorten as it is advanced (Fig 6-42c).

Step 7: Posterior buccal osteotomy

Perform the posterior buccal osteotomy with a reciprocating saw on a plane approximately 3 mm lower than the anterior osteotomy, extending from the buttress to the tuberosity. This will create a step between the anterior and posterior osteotomies. This osteotomy design has certain advantages:

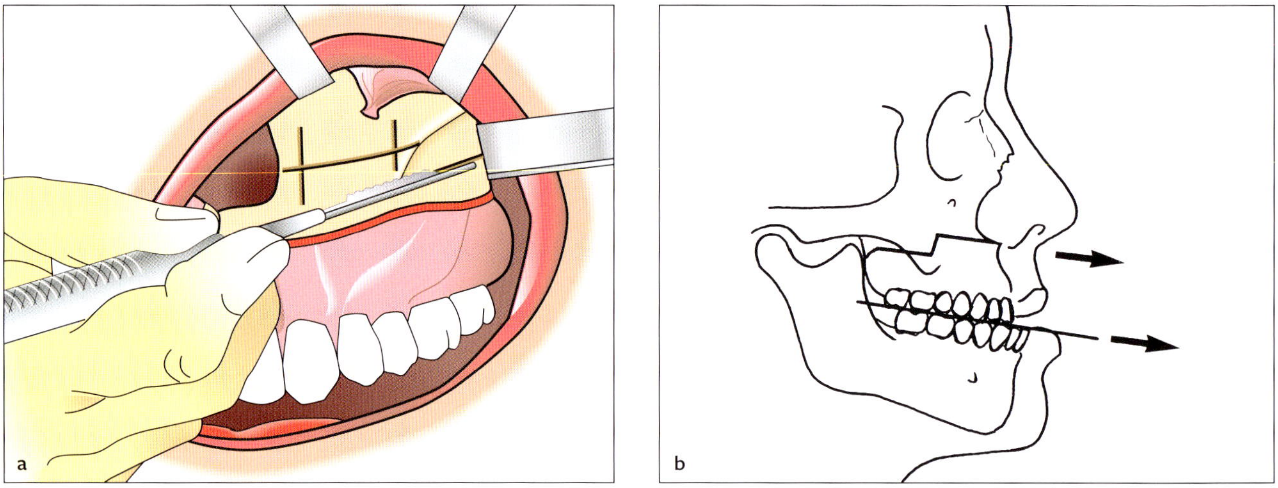

Fig 6-43 (a) The osteotomies can be kept parallel to the occlusal plane by placing a vertical step at the buttress area. (b) The maxilla can now be advanced parallel to the occlusal plane without any vertical changes.

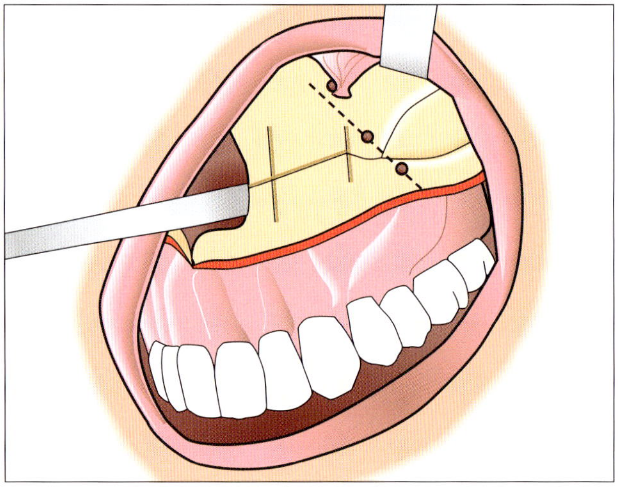

Fig 6-44 For maxillary advancement procedures, the holes for interosseous wires are positioned to support the movement. The lower hole is placed posterior to the top hole.

- It enables the surgeon to keep the osteotomies parallel to the occlusal plane (Fig 6-43a).
- It enables the surgeon to make the posterior osteotomy lower at the tuberosity, thus facilitating easier and safer downfracture.
- The steps act as a guide in repositioning the maxilla, and the extent of the advancement or any rotations of the maxilla can be measured and monitored at these steps (Fig 6-43b).
- After advancement of the maxilla, the defect created at the step area facilitates placement of a bone graft. The osteotomy should be limited to the lateral wall of the maxilla and not carried too far medially. Rotating the pterygoid retractor upward when performing the osteotomy not only protects the periosteum and thus prevents buccal fat pad herniation but also improves visualization.

Step 8: Connecting the anterior and posterior osteotomies

Connect the two horizontal osteotomies with a vertical osteotomy at the buttress using a 701 bur.

Step 9: Placement of holes for interosseous wires

The holes should be placed in thick bone at the buttress areas and positioned in such a way that the vector of the positioning wire will support the repositioning of the maxilla (Fig 6-44).

Step 10: Separation of the tuberosity from the pterygoid plates

The pterygoid osteotome is placed between the tuberosity and pterygoid plates while the hamulus is palpated pala-

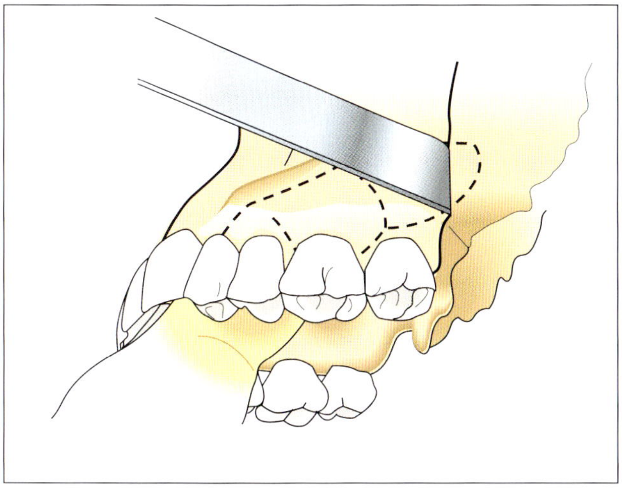

Fig 6-45 The contents of the pterygoid maxillary fissure and soft palate are protected by placing the index finger at the hamulus palatally to feel the osteotome as it separates the tuberosity and the pterygoid plates. Note that the osteotome is directed medially and downward.

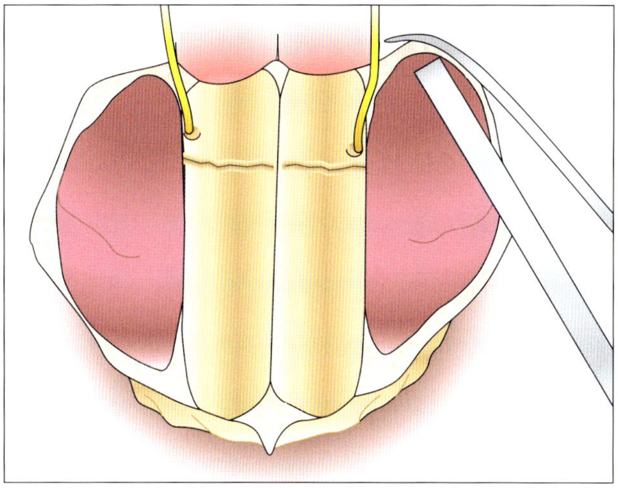

Fig 6-46 The osteotomy is completed using a small osteotome while the pterygoid osteotome is still in position, protecting the soft tissue behind the maxilla.

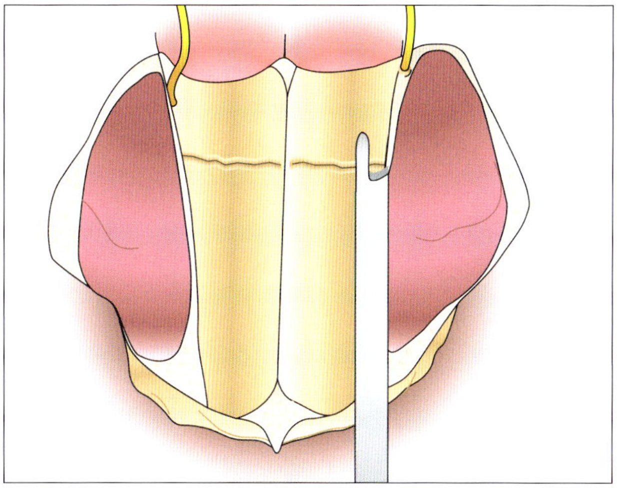

Fig 6-47 The lateral nasal wall is separated. Note that the wall deviates posteriorly; therefore, care should be taken not to damage the descending palatine neurovascular bundle at the posterior end of the wall.

tally with the index finger. The assistant then carefully taps the osteotome, which is directed medially and downward (Fig 6-45). Avoid overstretching the buccal mucosa and periosteum. Take extreme care not to damage the palatal soft tissue; perforation of the palatal mucosa with the osteotome may compromise the blood supply and lead to catastrophic consequences. Failure to separate the tuberosity from the pterygoid plates will lead to failure or difficulty in downfracturing the maxilla or to an unfavorable fracture (through the palatine bone or through the pterygoid plates).

Step 11: Completion of the posterior osteotomy

With the pterygoid osteotome still in position, use a thin osteotome to complete the osteotomy of the posterior wall of the maxilla. The osteotome should protect the contents of the pterygopalatine fossa during completion of the osteotomy (Fig 6-46). Do not stray too far medially because the osteotome may damage the descending palatine artery or tear the soft palate.

Step 12: Osteotomy of the lateral nasal wall

A lateral nasal osteotome is placed on the piriform rim and directed slightly laterally (keep in mind that the nasal fossa widens posteriorly; Fig 6-47). The nasal mucosa should be protected to prevent tearing during the osteotomy.

Step 13: Repeating the procedure on the opposite side

A small, wet sponge is placed on the completed side. The osteotomies should be placed at the same level and angle on both sides according to the surgical treatment plan.

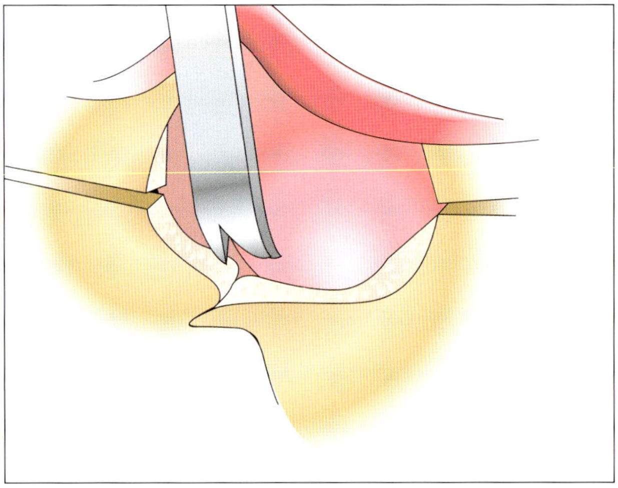

Fig 6-48 The nasal mucosa is dissected from the ANS, nasal septum, and piriform rim.

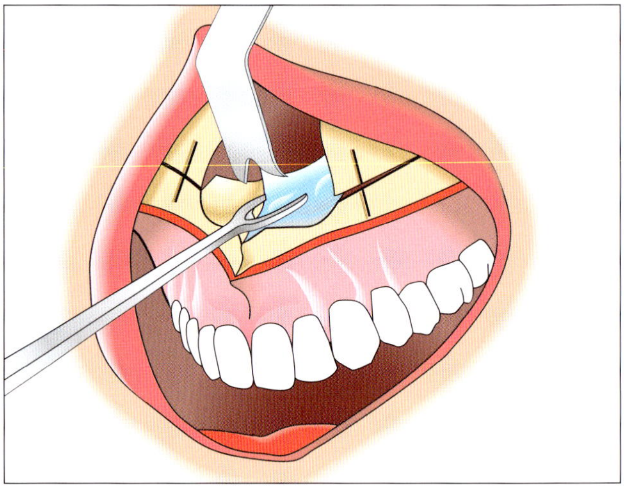

Fig 6-49 The nasal cartilage and bony septum are separated from the maxillary bone using a nasal septal osteotome.

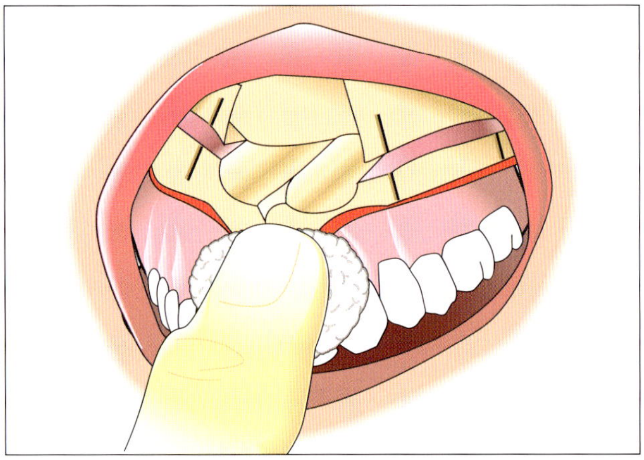

Fig 6-50 The maxilla is downfractured with downward pressure on the anterior maxilla.

Step 14: Completing the nasal spine subperiosteal dissection

Place a ramus retractor subperiosteally in the midline over the anterior nasal spine (ANS). Dissect the rest of the periosteum from the ANS.

Step 15: Completing the nasal mucosa dissection

Separate the septal cartilage from the ANS. Complete the dissection of the nasal mucosa from the nasal septum and floor (Fig 6-48):

- Protect the nasal mucosa; do not perforate or tear it.
- A light tug on the ramus retractor (swallowtail retractor) will separate the septal cartilage from the ANS and facilitate further dissection.
- Dissection of the nasal mucosa from the septum and floor will be facilitated by removal of the ANS.
- Remove the ANS with a bone nibbler but leave enough bone at the base of the spine to accommodate a hole, which will later be used for a cinch and septal suture.
- Keep in mind that removal of the nasal spine will have soft tissue implications.

Step 16: Osteotomy of the septal cartilage and vomer

Complete the separation of the septal cartilage and vomer from the maxillary bone using a nasal septal osteotome (Fig 6-49). Angle the osteotome toward the nasal floor to prevent tearing of the nasal mucosa.

Step 17: Maxillary downfracture

Downfracture the maxilla by pushing downward on the anterior maxilla. Place a small, wet sponge between the thumb and the maxilla (Fig 6-50). The assistant should stabilize the patient's superior midface. The maxilla should downfracture

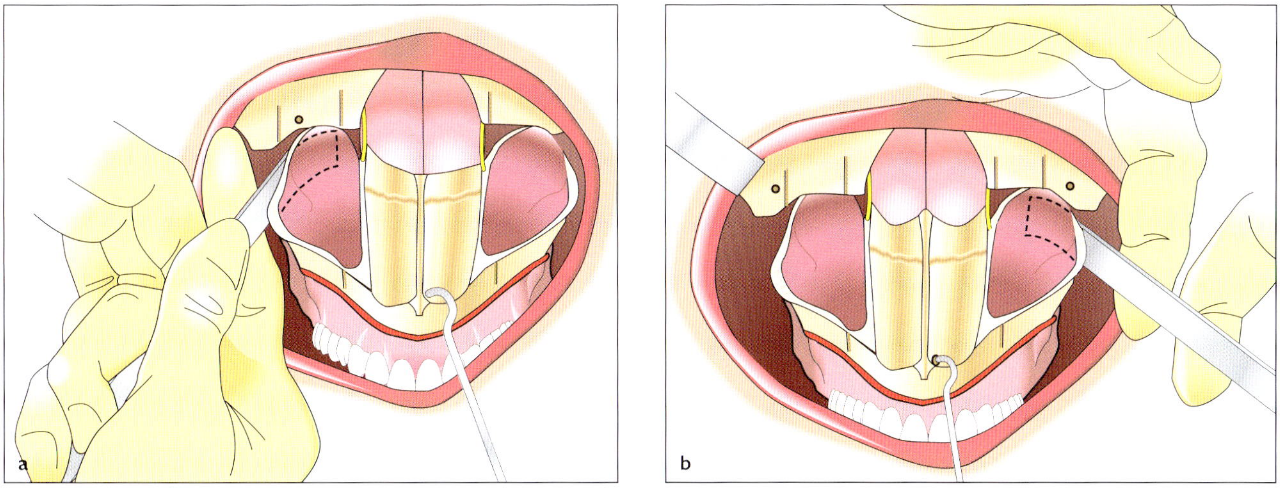

Fig 6-51 (*a*) The right side of the maxilla is mobilized by pushing the maxilla anteriorly using a mobilizer (or pterygoid osteotome). (*b*) The left side of the maxilla is mobilized; use a finger as a fulcrum, and protect the soft tissue at all times.

easily; if it does not, revise all the osteotomies, especially at the junction between the tuberosity and the pterygoid plates (see step 18). If necessary, complete the elevation of the nasal mucosa from the nasal floor under direct visualization, once the maxilla has been downfractured. Do not use excessive force for the following reasons:

- Excessive pressure may mobilize the maxillary teeth. (Remember that the teeth may be slightly mobile because of the orthodontic tooth movement.)
- Prolonged and excessive pressure on the maxillary gingiva may compromise the blood supply.
- Excessive force may loosen the orthodontic brackets on the anterior teeth.
- Excessive force may cause the maxilla to fracture unfavorably (eg, fracture through the palatine bone or the pterygoid plates, resulting in excessive hemorrhage and/or difficult repositioning of the maxilla).

Step 18: Redefining osteotomies when maxillary downfracture fails

The maxilla should downfracture with ease. If it does not, following are the most probable reasons for the failure:

- The pterygoid plates and tuberosity are not sufficiently separated.
- The lateral nasal wall osteotomy is incomplete (too short).
- Occasionally, the bone of the maxilla is very thick, making downfracture difficult. In such cases, tap the lateral nasal wall osteotomes into position (bilaterally), and carefully push down on the osteotomes to assist in the downfracture.

Step 19: Mobilization of the maxilla

Place the maxillary mobilizer securely behind the tuberosity while the assistant pulls the maxilla downward using a cricoid hook placed in the incisive canal. Push the maxilla carefully anteriorly, finally separating the maxilla from the pterygoid plates (Fig 6-51). Mobilization can also be completed by placing a sponge on each side at the posterior osteotomies and then pushing the anterior maxilla superiorly so that the posterior maxilla is distracted, thus separating it from the pterygoid plates.

The following are a few helpful hints at this stage:

- Protect the soft tissue; take care not to tear the buccal mucosa with the mobilizing instrument.
- Ensure that the maxilla is completely mobile and separated from the pterygoid plates.
- Ensure that the cricoid hook is positioned securely in the incisive canal.
- Use controlled force.
- Keep the osteotome securely down behind the tuberosity to prevent fracture of the posterior maxillary wall and keep the instrument from slipping.
- Support the instrument with one finger, using it as a fulcrum, while pushing forward with the other hand (see Fig 6-51).

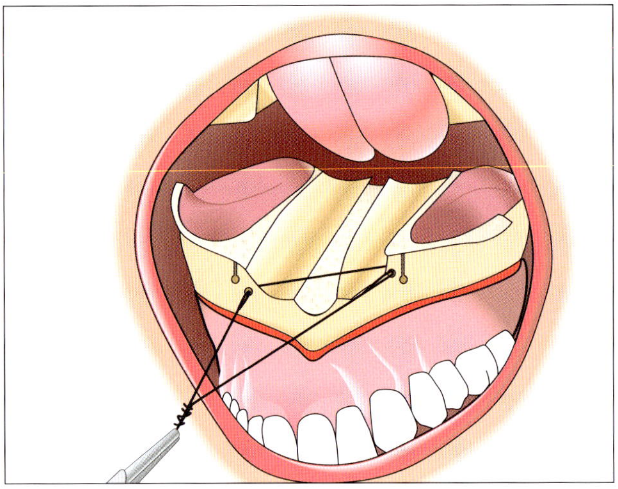

Fig 6-52 Attach a 0.018-inch wire through holes lateral to the piriform rims bilaterally. This wire is helpful in mobilizing the maxilla, improving the visualization of the posterior maxilla, and final positioning of the maxilla.

Step 20: Placement of a maxillary positioning wire

Drill a hole through the lateral part of the piriform rim on each side of the downfractured maxilla. Feed a 0.018-inch wire through the holes, and attach a wire twister to the wire (Fig 6-52). The wire is removed when rigid fixation has been completed. The positioning wire is helpful to assist with the final mobilization of the maxilla, pull the maxilla anteriorly for better visualization of and access to the posterior area of the maxilla, and assist in the final positioning of the maxilla.

Step 21: Exposure of the posterior maxilla

Place one pterygoid retractor on the medial side of the lateral nasal wall to completely visualize the posteromedial area of the maxillary sinus. Place another pterygoid retractor subperiosteally on the buccal aspect of the maxilla around the tuberosity (Fig 6-53a). This retraction will expose one side of the posterior maxilla sufficiently to allow the surgeon to do the following:

1. Identify the descending palatine neurovascular bundle.
2. Examine the osteotomies for refinement.
3. Recheck all the osteotomies, especially the level of the fracture in the area of the perpendicular plate of the palatine bone and posterior wall of the maxilla.
4. Examine the maxillary sinus mucosal lining and, when necessary, remove pathologic mucosa.

It is extremely important to be able to visualize the posterior wall of the maxilla, the descending palatine neurovascular bundle, the posterior part of the lateral nasal wall (containing the neurovascular bundle), and the anterior aspect of the pterygoid plates. Bony interference in these areas is often the cause of incorrect maxillary repositioning and condylar sag. Sharp bony edges may perforate blood vessels (ie, descending palatine vessels) and lead to intraoperative or postoperative hemorrhage. Removal of irregular bony edges in this area without adequate visualization may damage the contents of the pterygopalatine fossa (ie, the maxillary artery; Fig 6-53b).

Step 22: Checking fracture level in the perpendicular plate of the palatine bone

Ideally, the fracture should be at the junction between the tuberosity and pterygoid plates. If the fracture is high and not visible, an osteotomy should be performed lower, at a visible level. The fracture may also be too short, occurring through the tuberosity (involving an unerupted third molar) and continuing between the horizontal plate of the palatine bone and the maxilla, making accurate repositioning of the maxilla impossible. Using the pterygoid chisel placed between the tuberosity and pterygoid plate, carefully establish the separation at the correct site.

Step 23: Trimming the lateral nasal wall

The lateral nasal wall should be trimmed according to the treatment plan using a bone nibbler and a vulcanite bur. Take care not to damage the descending palatine neurovascular bundle (Fig 6-54).

Step 24: Refining the osteotomy at the posterior maxillary wall

Refining the osteotomy at the posterior maxillary wall is an important step. Take special care in removing bony interference in the following areas (Fig 6-55): the posterior part of the lateral wall, the palatine bones, the maxillary tuberosities, the posterior wall of the maxilla, the pterygoid plates, and the nasal septum.

It is important to remove all bony interferences to facilitate unhindered and accurate repositioning of the maxilla. Bone should be removed from the posterior maxilla at the inferior aspect rather than from the superior aspect of the maxilla or pterygoid plates. The descending palatine neurovascular bundle should be protected at all times, especially when removing the bony interferences posterior to this structure.

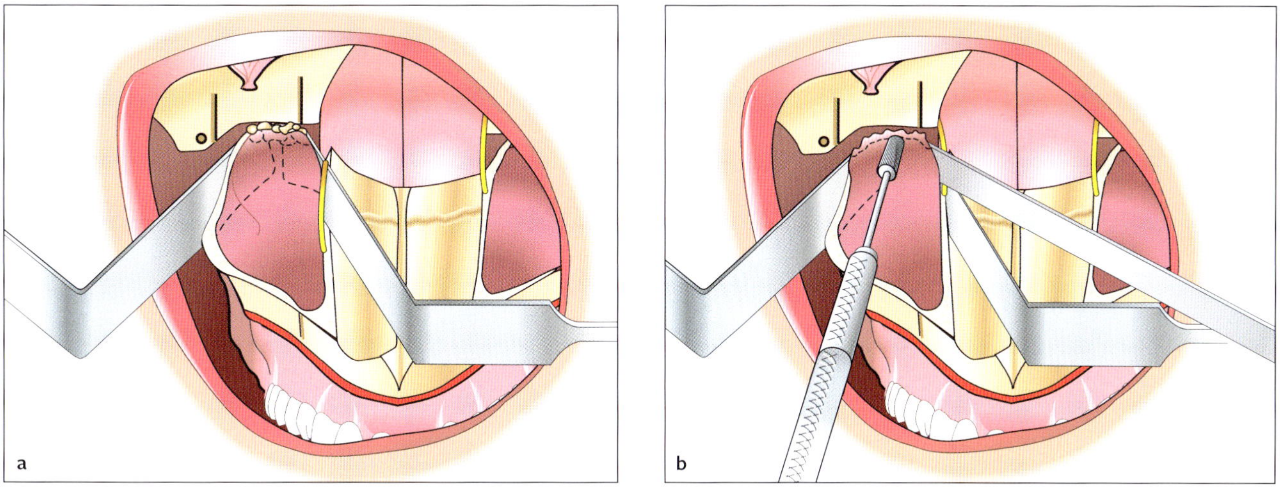

Fig 6-53 (*a*) Visualization of the posterior maxilla is improved by placing pterygoid retractors around the tuberosity. (*b*) Bone irregularities at the posterior wall of the maxillary sinus should be removed under good vision while the soft tissue is protected adequately.

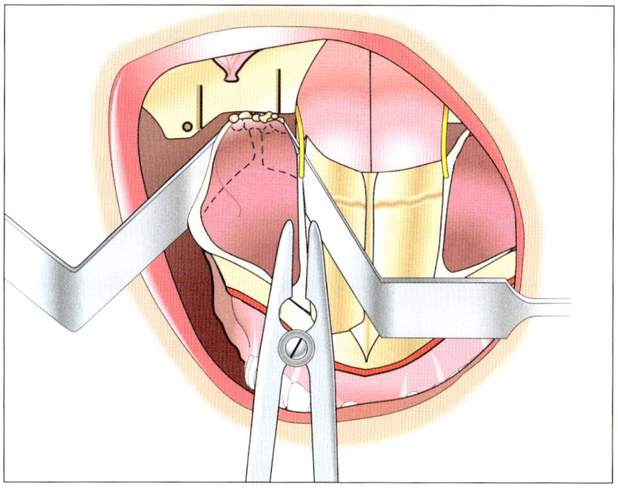

Fig 6-54 The lateral nasal wall is trimmed with a bone nibbler; care is taken to carefully remove bone around the descending palatine neurovascular bundle.

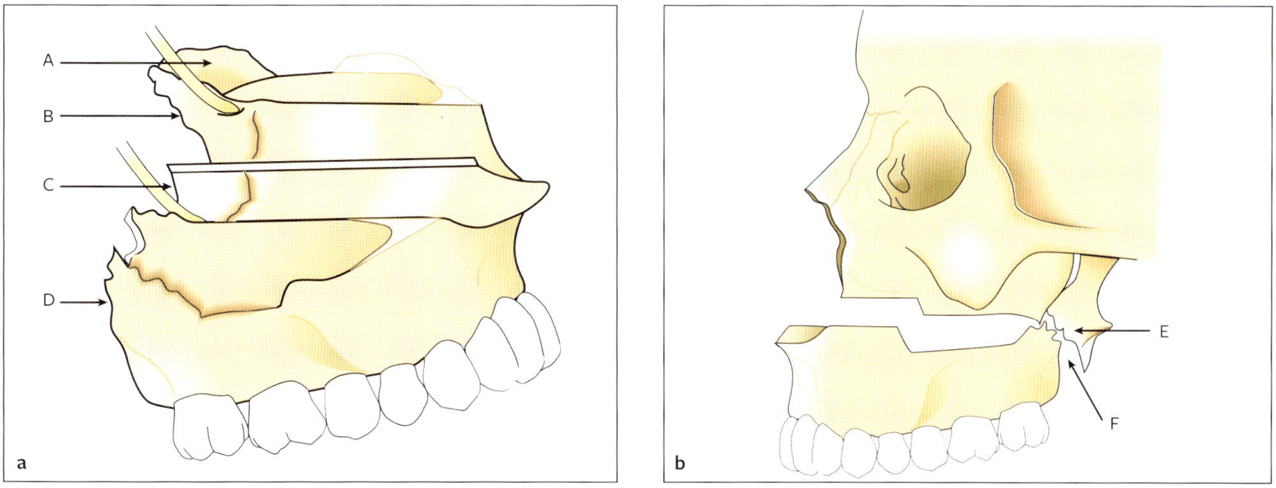

Fig 6-55 (*a*) Refinement of the osteotomy at the posterior maxillary wall and adequate removal of bone is mandatory. Pay special attention to the posterior part of the lateral wall (A), the palatine bone (B), the nasal septum (C), and the maxillary tuberosity (D). (*b*) It is important to remove adequate bone from the pterygoid plates (E) and the tuberosities (F), especially when the maxilla will be superiorly repositioned. It is preferable to remove bone from the tuberosities rather than from the pterygoid plates.

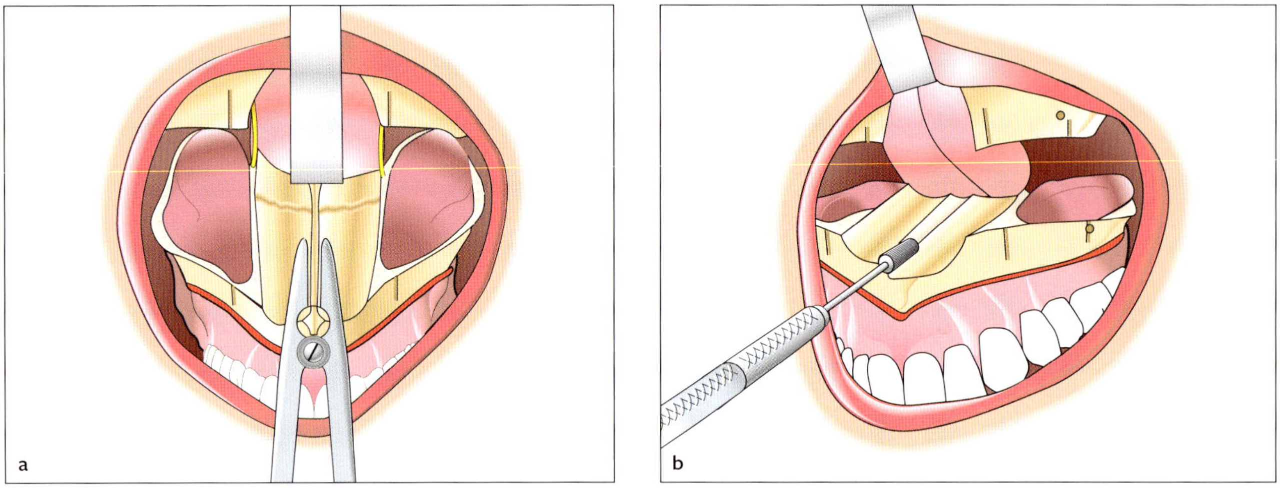

Fig 6-56 (*a*) The nasal septum and remaining part of the vomer is trimmed from the nasal floor with a bone nibbler. (*b*) Adequate trimming of the vomer and even creation of a trough in the nasal floor is essential to accommodate the nasal septum after maxillary repositioning. This is especially important when the maxilla will be superiorly repositioned.

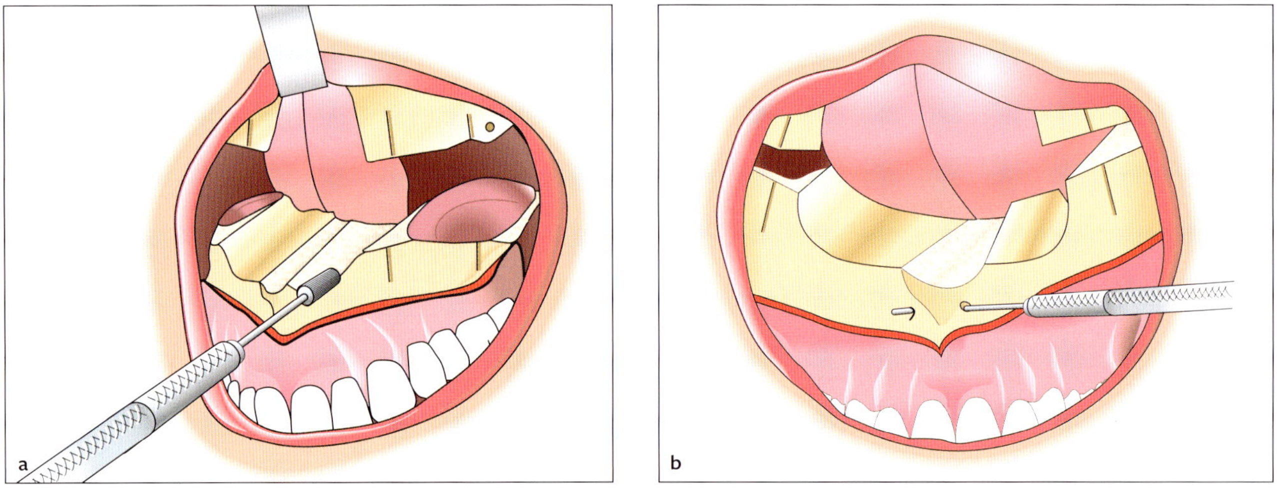

Fig 6-57 (*a*) The piriform rim should be contoured with a vulcanite bur to accommodate the soft tissue of the base of the nose after maxillary repositioning. (*b*) A hole is drilled horizontally through the ANS. This hole will be used later for the placement of a cinch suture and for securing the nasal septum.

Step 25: Reduction of the palatal aspect of the nasal septum

The remaining part of the nasal septum is removed from the nasal floor with a bone nibbler (Fig 6-56a). Then, with a large trimming bur, a trough is created on the nasal floor to accommodate the nasal septum after maxillary repositioning (Fig 6-56b). This is especially important when the maxilla is superiorly repositioned. Failure to remove enough bone will result in a deviated septum, an asymmetric columella, and an unpredictable soft tissue result.

Step 26: Contouring the piriform rim

The piriform rim should be contoured to accommodate the nasal tissue after maxillary repositioning (Fig 6-57a). At the same time, a hole is drilled horizontally through the base of the ANS (Fig 6-57b). This hole will later be used to position and secure the nasal septum as well as to assist in the placement of a cinch suture. Insufficient removal of the bone at the piriform rim areas, especially when the maxilla will be superiorly repositioned, may lead to flaring of the alae, lifting of the nasal tip, and/or asymmetry of the nose.

Step 27: Reversing the hypotensive anesthesia and checking for hemorrhage

Before final repositioning and fixation of the maxilla, it may be wise to reverse the hypotensive anesthesia. While the patient is normotensive, undetected arterial hemorrhage can be discovered and addressed, which will help prevent postoperative hemorrhage.

Step 28: Feeding a wire through the holes at the buttress

In most patients, semirigid fixation of the maxilla is achieved with two bone plates (1.5 mm) placed anteriorly in the thick bone of the piriform rim and 0.018-inch interosseous wires placed at the buttress area bilaterally. After a Le Fort I maxillary osteotomy, semirigid fixation provides the necessary fixation as well as the flexibility for optimal results. When more rigidity is required (eg, maxillary expansion, maxillary downgrafting, multi-piece Le Fort I procedures, and large movements [greater than 6 mm]), more plates are recommended.

Step 29: Maxillomandibular wire fixation

The vector of pull of the fixation wires should support the direction of jaw positioning. Place the first maxillomandibular wire around the four central incisors to achieve the planned interincisal relationship. Place the wires around the orthodontic brackets, guided by Kobayashi hooks (or Lewis brackets with integral hooks). However, be careful not to detach the orthodontic brackets.

Orthodontic movement causes more tooth mobility than normal. The teeth could easily be "pulled into occlusion" or into the acrylic splint by the maxillomandibular fixation wires. Once the wires are removed, the teeth will return to their original position. For example, the bone next to the midpalate is often very thin, and once alveolar bone support is removed by segmental surgery (eg, an anterior maxillary segment), the palate may be bent easily by the force of the maxillomandibular fixation. However, when maxillomandibular fixation is removed, relapse will occur immediately because the maxilla will return to its original shape.

Step 30: Maxillary repositioning

Rotate the maxillomandibular complex closed, and check the reference marks for accurate maxillary positioning. Positioning the condyles in their ideal relationship to the fossa while the maxilla is repositioned is the most challenging and difficult part of the procedure. With experience, the surgeon will develop a feel for positioning the condyles and will usually be able to detect bony interferences that might distract the condyles out of the glenoid fossa. Numerous devices have been designed to achieve condylar positioning by recording the preoperative mandibular position in relation to a fixed part of the facial skeleton. This position is then reproduced after repositioning the maxilla. However, the use of these devices is time consuming and leads to varying degrees of success.

The following are a few hints for the maxillary repositioning stage:

- Take great care during this step to ensure that the maxilla is in its planned position while both mandibular condyles are in an ideal relationship with the glenoid fossa.
- Place one hand on either side of the mandible, and rotate the maxillomandibular complex closed with light, controlled digital pressure on the chin and the angles of the mandible until bone contact is achieved (Fig 6-58a).
- The vectors of force in positioning the condyles are a slight backward pressure on the chin and an upward and slightly anterior pressure on the angles.
- Make sure there are no bony interferences during the rotation (Fig 6-58b).
- Do not force the mandible closed to achieve the planned maxillary position. When any bony interferences are detected, rotate the mandible open, inspect the area where interferences are suspected, and remove them under good visualization (see the discussion of condylar sag, page 268).

Step 31: Turbinectomy

If an enlarged inferior turbinate interferes with superior repositioning of the maxilla, it should be reduced. Enlargement of the turbinate could be caused by soft tissue hypertrophy alone or both soft tissue and bone hypertrophy. A turbinectomy can be performed via a ventral approach through an incision or tear in the nasal mucosa by grasping the hypertrophied soft tissue with an artery clamp and resecting the tissue above the clamp using a diathermy knife (Fig 6-59). Hypertrophied bone may be removed by elevating the mucoperiosteum above the bone and then removing the desired portion of bone with a small bone nibbler. The overlying hypertrophied mucoperiosteum may be removed with a diathermy knife and need not be sutured. The nasal mucosa incision (tear) is sutured with a 4-0 chromic suture.

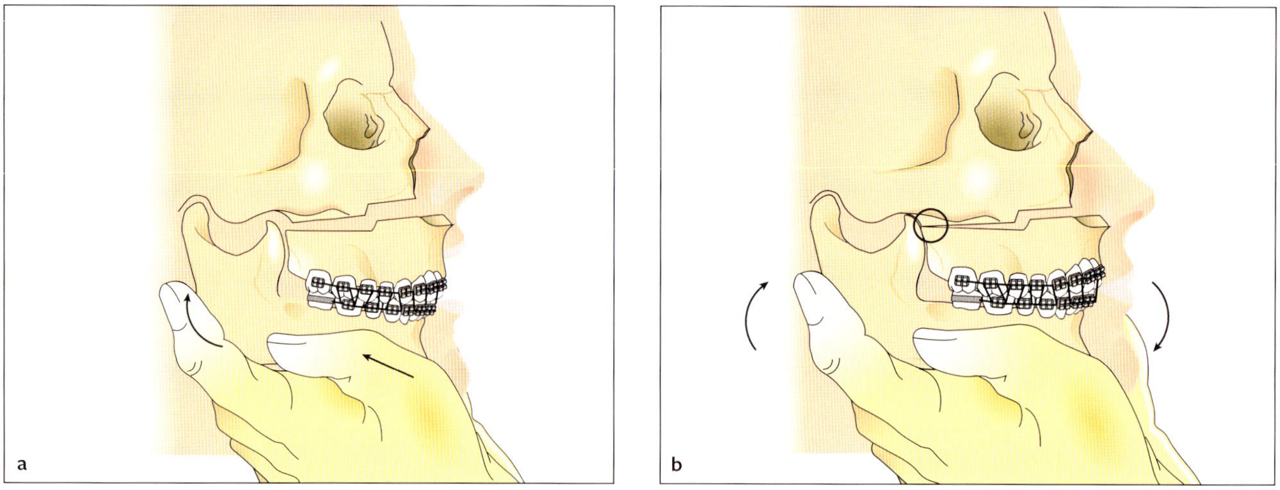

Fig 6-58 (*a*) With maxillomandibular fixation in position, the maxillomandibular complex is rotated to achieve bone contact. The vector of force on the condyle should be superior and slightly anterior. There should be no bony interferences during the rotation. (*b*) Bony interferences usually occur at the posterior maxilla (*circle*). As the maxilla is rotated, the interference will cause the condyle to be distracted downward. Once the maxillomandibular fixation is removed, the condyle will move superiorly, creating an anterior open bite (see the section on intraoperative diagnosis of condylar sag during Le Fort I osteotomy, pages 268 to 271).

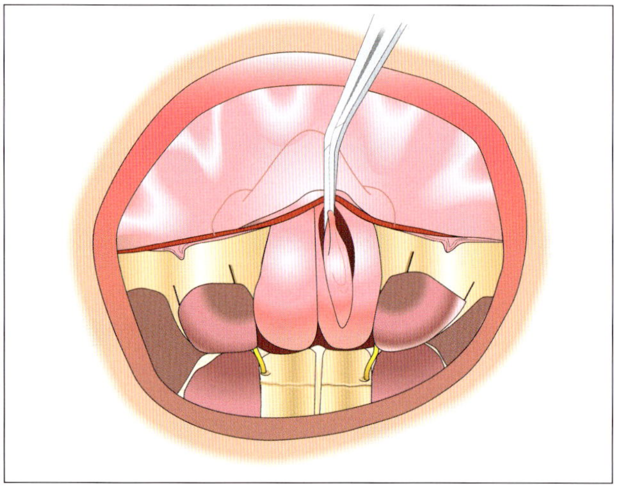

Fig 6-59 The hypertrophied turbinate is grasped with a tissue clamp and then removed using a diathermy knife.

Step 32: Suturing the nasal mucosa

Identify any tears in the nasal mucosa, and repair them with a 4-0 chromic suture. Failure to repair a tear in the nasal mucosa may cause excessive intraoperative and/or postoperative hemorrhage and may also jeopardize the success of any bone grafts in the palate.

Step 33: Checking the position of the nasal septum

Rotate the maxillomandibular complex closed to achieve the predetermined maxillary position. Ensure that the condyles are seated in the glenoid fossa, and then check the position of the nasal septum. The septum should lie freely, without any interference in the trough created in the nasal floor (see step 25). The nasal septum cartilage and vomer may be trimmed to ensure that the septum lies passively. The nasal septum may be secured in position by placing a suture through it and through the horizontal hole in the base of the nasal spine after maxillary fixation (see step 39). If nasal reconstruction with cartilage graft is contemplated, the cartilage can be harvested from the septum at this stage. If nasal reconstruction will be deferred for a second operation, the harvested cartilage can be "stored" subperiosteally on the lateral wall of the maxilla for later use. See the section on simultaneous management of functional and esthetic nasal problems with Le Fort I osteotomy (pages 292 and 293).

Step 34: Tightening the buttress wires

Copious lavage of the maxillary sinuses and nasal floor with saline solution should be carried out before tightening the buttress wires; small bone fragments remaining in the sinus or nasal cavities will lead to postoperative infection. Retract the soft tissue bilaterally away from the osteotomy line using pterygoid retractors to allow the necessary bone contact and avoid soft tissue entrapment. Carefully rotate the maxillomandibular complex superiorly to achieve bone apposition, and tighten the interosseous buttress holding wires. Avoid overtightening the wires in an attempt to achieve better bone apposition because the tension it would place on the bone would result in displacement and occlusal discrepancy once maxillomandibular fixation is removed.

Step 35: Checking maxillary position using a caliper

If there is any doubt about the condylar position at this stage, the maxillomandibular fixation should be removed and the occlusion checked by referring to intraoral bony reference marks or to an extraoral reference point (eg, a Kirschner wire in the frontal bone). The interosseous wires are usually sufficient (in single-piece maxillary or segmental surgery with the teeth wired into an acrylic splint) to maintain the maxilla in position while the occlusion is checked. If necessary, small adjustments in the maxillary position can now be made to achieve the planned occlusion. An unacceptable occlusion should be corrected by removing the interosseous wires, finding the reason for the discrepancy, and correcting the problem.

Step 36: Replacing the maxillomandibular fixation

Recheck the position of the maxilla using a caliper and the reference marks made in step 5. If the maxillary position and occlusion are satisfactory, replace the maxillomandibular fixation.

Step 37: Placement of bone plates

Selection and adaptation of plates

Use 1.5-mm titanium bone plates or resorbable bone plates. The decisions about the method of stabilization and type of plate (titanium or resorbable) are influenced by several factors, including bone thickness, bone quality and contact, amount of surgical movement, and direction of movement. The methods of fixation are interosseous wires, suspension wires, bone plating (titanium or resorbable), and a combination of these methods.

For most patients, the author uses semirigid fixation, which consists of bilateral titanium (1.5-mm) bone plates or resorbable (2.0-mm) plates placed anteriorly in the thick bone at the piriform areas and two interosseous (0.018-inch) wires placed at the zygomatic buttresses. However, some patients may require additional fixation—for example, in those with large movements (more than 6 mm) and poor bone contact, downgrafting procedures, or segmental osteotomies of the maxilla. Suspension wires are seldom used.

The plates should be adapted to fit passively. Two screws should be placed on either side of the osteotomy, and care should be taken not to place screws into the roots of teeth, too close to the edge of the bone, or in thin bone. If thin bone must be used, self-drilling screws are recommended.

Segmental maxillary surgery

Segmental surgery should be used to facilitate narrowing or widening of the maxillary dental arch, to close interdental spaces, or to surgically level the occlusal plane.

Interdental osteotomy

The surgeon should ensure that there is sufficient space between the roots of the teeth adjacent to the proposed interdental osteotomy site. For vertical movements of the segments, the roots should be at least parallel; when closure of an interdental space is contemplated, the roots should be divergent. The interdental osteotomy should be initiated before the maxilla is downfractured. This technique has two distinct advantages: (1) When the maxilla is stable, the initial bur cut and tapping with the interdental osteotome are easier; (2) because the osteotome is tapped while the maxilla is stable, the technique prevents stretching of the vital soft tissue pedicle of the maxilla. The interdental osteotomy may also be performed by using piezoelectric surgery. The author prefers to make the initial cut with a bur only through the buccal cortex and then to complete the interdental osteotomy using piezoelectric surgery (Fig 6-60).

The interdental bone should be exposed by careful reflection of the mucoperiosteum inferiorly. Using a small fissure bur (no. 701), penetrate only the cortical bone between the roots of the adjacent teeth (Fig 6-61a). Place a finger on the palate to palpate the osteotome as the interdental osteotomy is completed with a thin spatula osteotome. Hold the osteotome in one hand while placing a finger of the other hand in the palate. The assistant should then carefully tap the osteotome. As the osteotome passes through the alveolar bone and thick palatal bone, the resistance to the tapping helps in determining the position of the osteotome tip. To avoid damaging the periodontal tissue, do not tap the osteotome right down to the alveolar crest (Fig 6-61b). The segment should be mobilized only

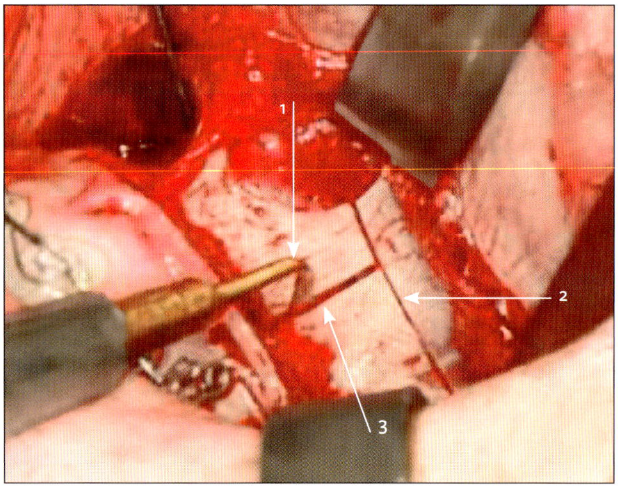

Fig 6-60 Piezoelectric surgery may be used to perform the interdental osteotomy (1), the Le Fort I osteotomy line (2), and the interdental osteotomy line (3).

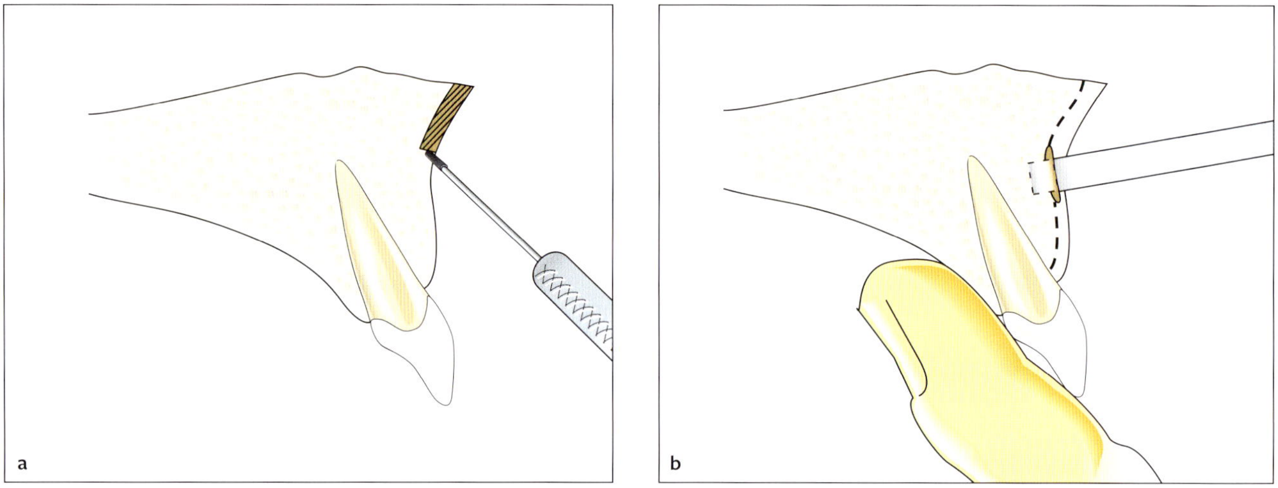

Fig 6-61 (*a*) Interdental osteotomy. First, only the cortical bone between the roots of the adjacent teeth is penetrated by the drill. (*b*) The interdental osteotomy is completed by tapping a thin, sharp osteotome between the roots. The position of the osteotome is monitored by placing a finger on the palate behind the teeth.

once the maxilla is downfractured; mobilization should be achieved by completion of the palatal osteotomy through the nasal floor. Mobilize the segment using finger pressure or rotation of a flat instrument placed into the line of the interdental osteotomy.

Nasal floor or palatal osteotomy

The palatal osteotomy in the nasal floor is performed once the maxilla is downfractured. Protect the mucoperiosteal pedicles by supporting the maxilla while the osteotomies are performed. Perimidline sagittal osteotomies are performed lateral to the nasal septum, where the bone is thin and the palatal mucosa is slightly thicker than in the midline of the palate. Use a fissure bur to drill through the bone lateral to the nasal septum, taking care not to perforate the palatal periosteum (Fig 6-62). The palatal osteotomy is connected to the interdental osteotomy and completed with a thin osteotome. Be extremely careful not to tear the palatal mucosa, especially in a transverse direction, because this will limit blood supply. Mobilize the segments with finger pressure or by placing a small, flat instrument in the interdental osteotomy areas and rotating it. Bilateral osteotomies should be contemplated for palatal expansion of more than 5 mm.

For large expansions, it may be desirable to graft the defect. When doing so, ensure that the nasal and palatal mucosa are intact. Large palatal expansions may result in tension in the palatal soft tissue, which may be released by

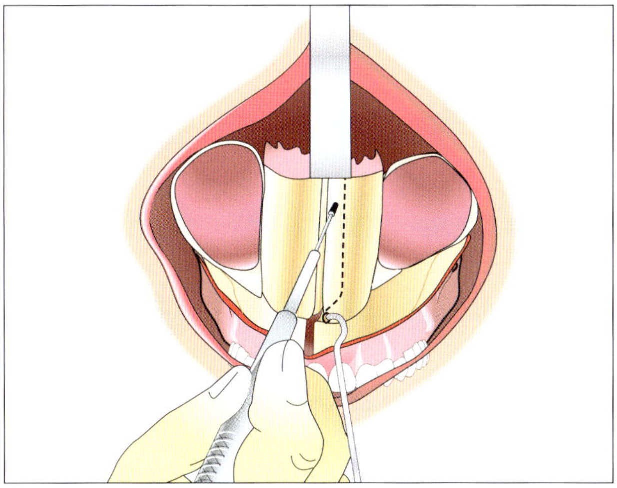

Fig 6-62 The palatal osteotomy is placed just lateral to the nasal septum. The bone is thin here and the mucosa thick. Placement of the osteotomy too far laterally may damage the greater palatine neurovascular bundle. For large palatal expansions, a second osteotomy may be placed on the contralateral side.

further lateral mucoperiosteal dissection or by incising the periosteum (anteroposteriorly) in an area that is not overlying the osteotomy. Ensure that the nasal mucosa is intact, and never incise or tear the palatal mucosa transversely.

Fixation and stabilization after segmental osteotomies

To establish the planned occlusion, use an acrylic splint prefabricated according to the model surgery. Place a two-hole bone plate across the interdental osteotomy, one screw on either side, to secure the segment. Using the orthodontic brackets, place an interdental wire around the teeth adjacent to the osteotomy. The bone plates should be bent accurately to conform passively to the bony contour and must be secured with two screws on either side of the Le Fort I osteotomy. Each segment should be secured with a bone plate.

Bone defects may be grafted to promote more rapid healing of bone at the osteotomy sites without forcing bone into the defects and thus displacing the segments. It is recommended that palatal bone defects larger than 3 mm be grafted to enhance the stability of the result. Bone grafts at the piriform rim and zygomatic buttress areas should be stabilized with wire or screw fixation because unsupported bone grafts may be dislodged in the maxillary sinus and thus lead to infection.

Step 38: Removing the maxillomandibular fixation and checking the occlusion

Before the occlusion is checked, the mandible should be gently opened and closed as well as translated forward and from side to side to ensure that the articulating disc was not displaced while teeth were in maxillomandibular fixation. Any displacement of the articulating disc will produce a malocclusion and may cause TMJ dysfunction later. Wait a few minutes after removing the maxillomandibular fixation before checking the occlusion. Then, with slight pressure on the chin, close the mandible until the teeth occlude. If the planned occlusion has not been achieved, remove the rigid fixation and identify and correct the reason for failure. Keep in mind that the occlusal splint may be at fault. Accepting an incorrect occlusion may necessitate another operation. There is no better time to correct a problem than now.

Step 39: Placement of nasal septum and cinch sutures

Secure the septum in the trough created in the nasal floor by a suture through the septum and the hole in the base of the ANS. Depending on the esthetic requirements, the width of the alar base may need to be controlled by a cinch suture. Roll the upper lip outward with the thumb while placing the index finger extraorally at the alar rim. With the lip everted, grasp the lateral alar soft tissues opposite the index finger using a toothed forceps (Fig 6-63a). Release the lip while lightly pulling the toothed forceps medially. Observe the alar base moving medially with the forceps. Insufficient movement of the alar base indicates that the correct tissue (fibroareolar extension of the lower lateral cartilage) has not been grasped, and another attempt should be made to grasp it.

Place a 3-0 Vicryl suture (Johnson & Johnson) through the tissue held by the forceps, feed the suture through the hole at the base of the ANS, and repeat the procedure on the contralateral side in a figure-eight configuration (Fig 6-63b). Tighten the suture to narrow the base to approximately 3 mm less than the desired width to allow for postoperative widening.

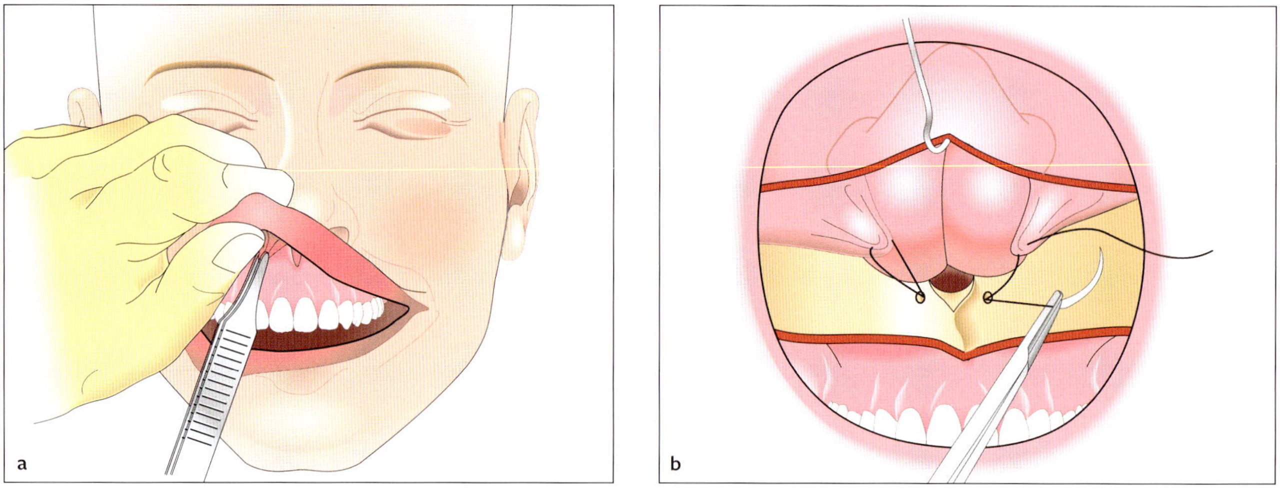

Fig 6-63 (*a*) The lateral alar soft tissue is grasped with a toothed forceps. (*b*) The cinch suture is placed in a figure-eight fashion through the hole in the ANS.

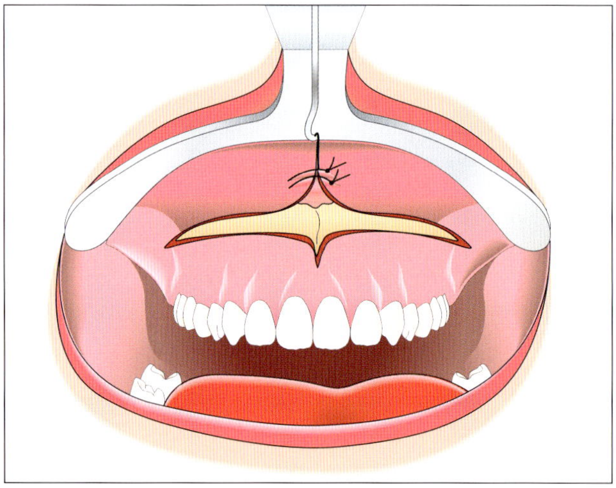

Fig 6-64 V-Y closure of the upper lip.

Step 40: Submucosal suturing

The soft tissue incision is closed in layers—first the submucosal tissue and then the mucosa. Suturing is one of the most important steps of the procedure and should be performed meticulously. It is the last step of the surgical procedure, and the surgeon may be tired at this stage and not give this important step enough attention. It is essential to realize that incorrect suturing may result in poor esthetic results. Start posteriorly, and end at the piriform rim on both sides by pulling the superior tissues slightly forward.

Step 41: Mucosal suturing

Perform a V-Y closure (Fig 6-64), and reapproximate the mucosal midline using 4-0 chromic sutures. Place two interrupted sutures on both sides of the midline to reapproximate it. Complete the mucosal suturing using a continuous suture, starting posteriorly and pulling the superior tissue slightly forward. When lip lengthening is indicated, more horizontal sutures (or even bilateral V-Y suturing) may be used.

Step 42: Placement of elastics or maxillomandibular fixation

Maxillomandibular fixation is seldom used and may be reserved for patients requiring immobilization because of multiple segmental surgery or large movements that require an occlusal splint. The period of maxillomandibular fixation may vary from a few days to 3 weeks. Alternatively, for most patients, two to four interocclusally placed elastics (0.25 inch, 3.5 oz) are sufficient to guide the teeth into the new occlusion. The direction of the elastics should support the repositioning. Long elastics should be avoided.

Step 43: Applying a pressure dressing

A pressure dressing is applied to help control swelling and/or prevent hematoma formation.

Alternatives and complications

Simultaneous management of functional and esthetic nasal problems

Much attention has been given to the effects that Le Fort I osteotomies have on nasal morphology (esthetics), and adjunctive soft tissue techniques (eg, cinch sutures) have been recommended to limit suboptimal esthetic outcomes caused by maxillary repositioning. However, little atten-

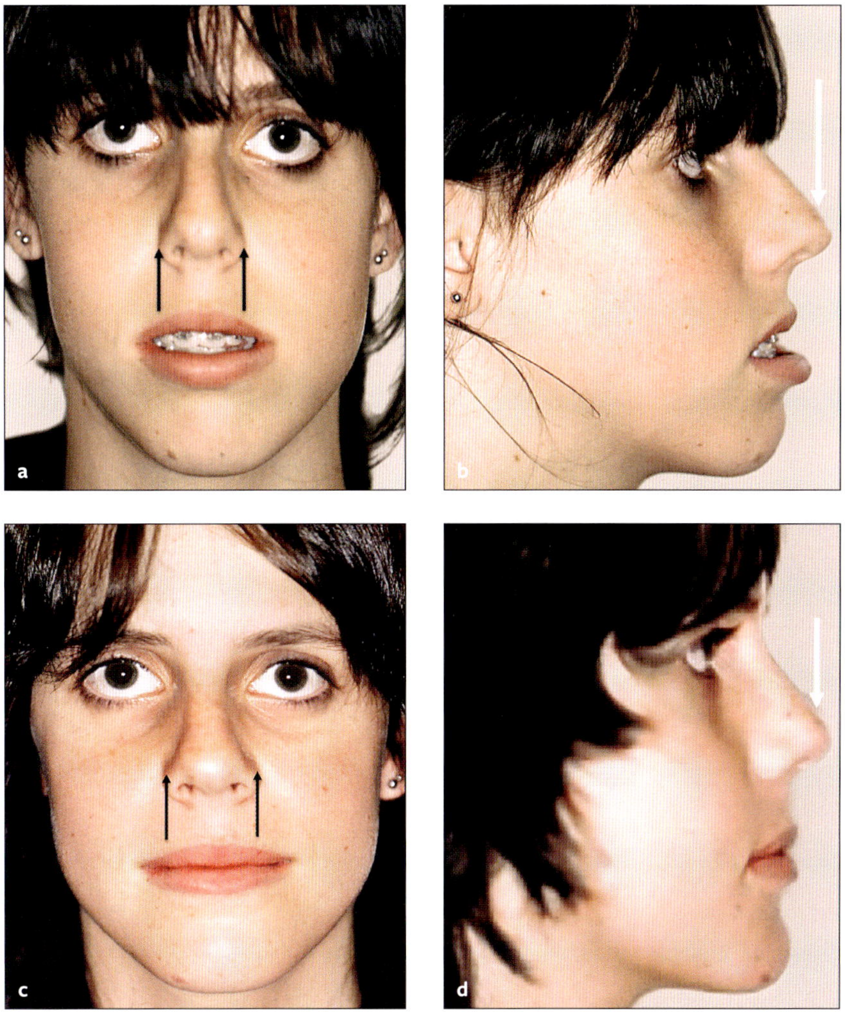

Fig 6-65 (*a*) The frontal view of a patient with vertical maxillary excess and maxillary anteroposterior deficiency. Note the relatively narrow alar base (*arrows*). (*b*) The ill-defined supratip brake and somewhat downturned nasal tip is demonstrated in the profile view (*arrow*). (*c*) Following maxillary superior repositioning and advancement, the slightly widened alar base has improved the nasal esthetics (*arrows*). (*d*) In profile view, the nasal dorsum has improved by the slight tipping up of the nasal tip (*arrow*).

tion has been given to the preoperative assessment of the upper airway and how maxillary surgery may affect long-term nasal breathing.

Excessive vertical growth of the anterior maxilla above the roots of the teeth results in a high nasal floor with constricted nasal aperture and increased nasal airway resistance. Obstruction of nasal airflow can be caused by narrow nasal apertures, an elevated nasal floor, enlarged turbinates, and a deviated nasal septum. A thorough presurgical functional and esthetic assessment of the airway and nose should be done before maxillary orthognathic surgery (see the section on the nose in chapter 2). Problems should be noted, and if any unfavorable nasal esthetic features or airway obstruction are present, a baseline problem list should be established. Individuals with vertical maxillary excess and/or maxillary anteroposterior deficiency often display narrow noses and slightly tipped down nasal tips (Figs 6-65a and 6-65b). Soft tissue nasal changes as discussed would actually improve the nasal esthetics (Figs 6-65c and 6-65d). Keep in mind that existing airflow problems and/or unfavorable nasal esthetics may be worsened by Le Fort I maxillary surgery. Most existing upper airflow problems can be addressed simultaneously once the maxilla is downfractured, while care should be taken not to cause restriction of normal airflow due to poor surgical technique.

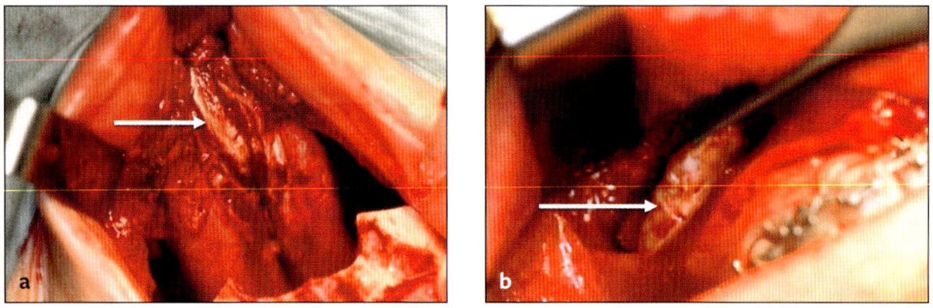

Fig 6-66 (*a*) The nasal septum is trimmed to allow for maxillary superior repositioning. (*b*) In cases where rhinoplasty is considered as a second procedure, the cartilage is "saved" in the buccal sulcus.

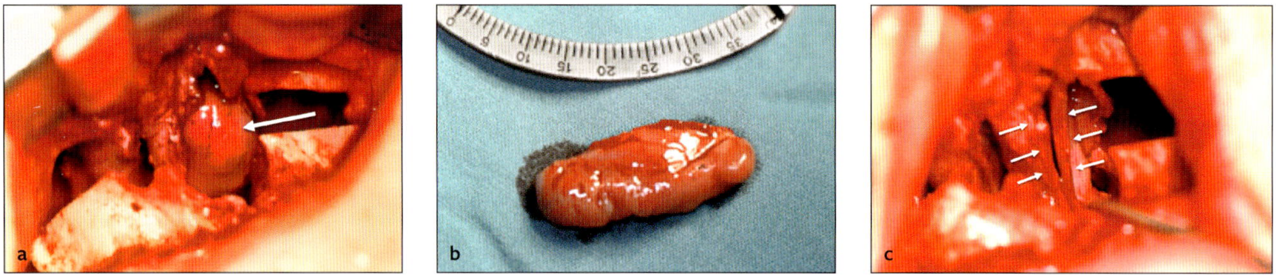

Fig 6-67 (*a*) The hyperplastic turbinate is exposed through a nasal mucosa incision (or tear). (*b*) A resected turbinate. (*c*) The nasal mucosa is sutured (*arrows*).

Simultaneous management of chronic obstructive nasal breathing

A downfractured maxilla provides excellent access to the nasal septum, the piriform rims, the nasal floor, the inferior turbinates, the anterior nasal spine, the maxillary sinuses, and the ostium. Downfracturing the maxilla to access these structures allows for correction of preexisting functional problems as well as control of unfavorable functional and esthetic problems that may be caused by surgery.

Septoplasty following downfracture and disimpaction of the maxilla

Care is always taken to maintain the integrity of the nasal mucosa when downfracturing the maxilla; however, tears in the mucosa may occur. With the maxilla in the downfractured position, the nasal mucosa is gently elevated from the bony and cartilaginous septum using a periosteal elevator. The buckled and deviated portions of the deviated septum are exposed and removed by using a rongeur bone nibbler. Make sure to preserve adequate dorsal and caudal components of the cartilaginous septum for structural nasal support. If cosmetic rhinoplasty is a consideration in the future, the useful cartilage removed can be saved as a tip graft for the second procedure. The cartilage is placed in the buccal sulcus mucosa and sutured in the submucosa when completing the procedure (Fig 6-66). Make sure this is noted, including which side the cartilage is kept on.

Turbinectomy

An incision is made through the nasal mucosa, parallel and just inferior to each turbinate. If the mucosa was torn during dissection, the access is used and can be extended for additional visualization of each turbinate (Fig 6-67a). Partial resection of the turbinate can now be performed using large dissection scissors (Fig 6-67b). The endotracheal tube is usually cephalically positioned and allows the surgeon sufficient room and visualization to adequately perform the procedure. Ensure that there are no oxygen leaks in the ventilation system before cauterizing the exposed raw surface of each turbinate, and ensure that adequate hemostasis has been achieved. The nasal mucosa is then sutured with resorbable sutures (Fig 6-67c).

There are six unfavorable esthetic and functional complications that may occur following Le Fort I maxillary osteotomy (Fig 6-68):

1. Tipping up of the nasal tip
2. Buckling of the nasal septum
3. Increased nostril visibility
4. Widening of the nasal alae
5. Increased nasolabial angle
6. Compression of the inferior turbinates

By completing a thorough presurgical assessment, existing unfavorable nasal features (both functional and

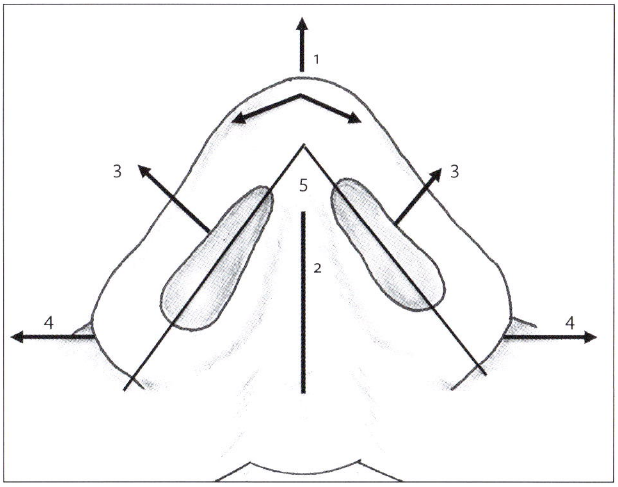

Fig 6-68 Worm's-eye view of the nose. Unfavorable nasal effects following Le Fort I maxillary osteotomy include (1) tipping up of the nasal tip, (2) displacement of the nasal septum, (3) increased nostril show, (4) widening of the alar base, and (5) increasing the nostril angle. Compression of the turbinates (which cannot be seen in the figure) is an additional unfavorable effect.

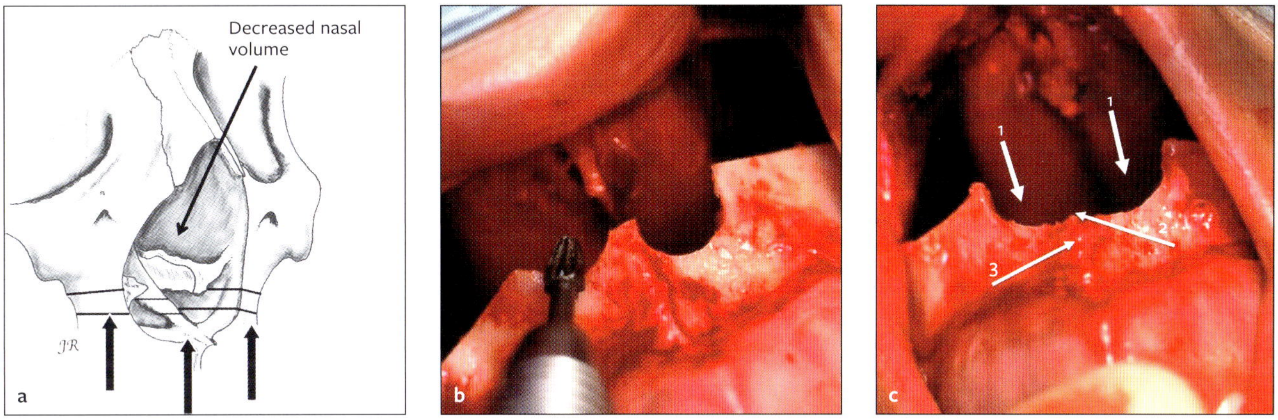

Fig 6-69 (*a*) Superior repositioning of the maxilla will reduce the volume of the bony cavity and encroach on the nasal tissues (*arrows*). (*b*) The piriform rims and nasal floor should be reduced to accommodate the nasal tissues after superior repositioning of the maxilla. To ensure symmetry, complete one side first and then the other. (*c*) The increased volume will allow the nasal tissues to fill the space (*arrows 1*). Also trim the nasal septum (*arrow 2*) and anterior nasal spine (*arrow 3*) when indicated.

esthetic) should be identified, and complications can be avoided by taking certain precautions. Before surgery, identify unfavorable nasal features such as a wide alar base, an accentuated supratip break, a deviated nasal septum, poorly defined nasal tip, hypertrophied turbinates (usually in cleft palate patients), and a hanging columella.

Ala width

The width of the ala should coincide with the width of the inner cantus of the eyes, delineated as the middle fifth of the face (see the section on transverse dimensions in chapter 2). For patients in whom maxillary advancement and/or superior repositioning is considered and the ala falls on or outside the middle fifth lines, control of ala width is indicated during surgery. The nasal tissues are contained in a specific volume created by the maxillary and nasal bones. Maxillary advancement and/or superior repositioning of the maxilla will reduce this volume and encroach on the nasal tissues (Fig 6-69a). In patients with vertical maxillary excess, the nasal floor is high with excessive bone between the incisor apices and nasal floor. Surgical lowering of the anterior nasal floor is therefore indicated and carried out in the downfractured maxilla (Fig 6-69b). The amount of bone removal is determent by the amount of superior repositioning of the maxilla and should be equal. To ensure symmetric bone removal, the piriform aperture is first completed on one side and then performed on the contralateral side. This will allow the nasal tissues to fill the increased space (Fig 6-69c). Control of the ala width is further enhanced by the placement of a cinch suture (see step 39).

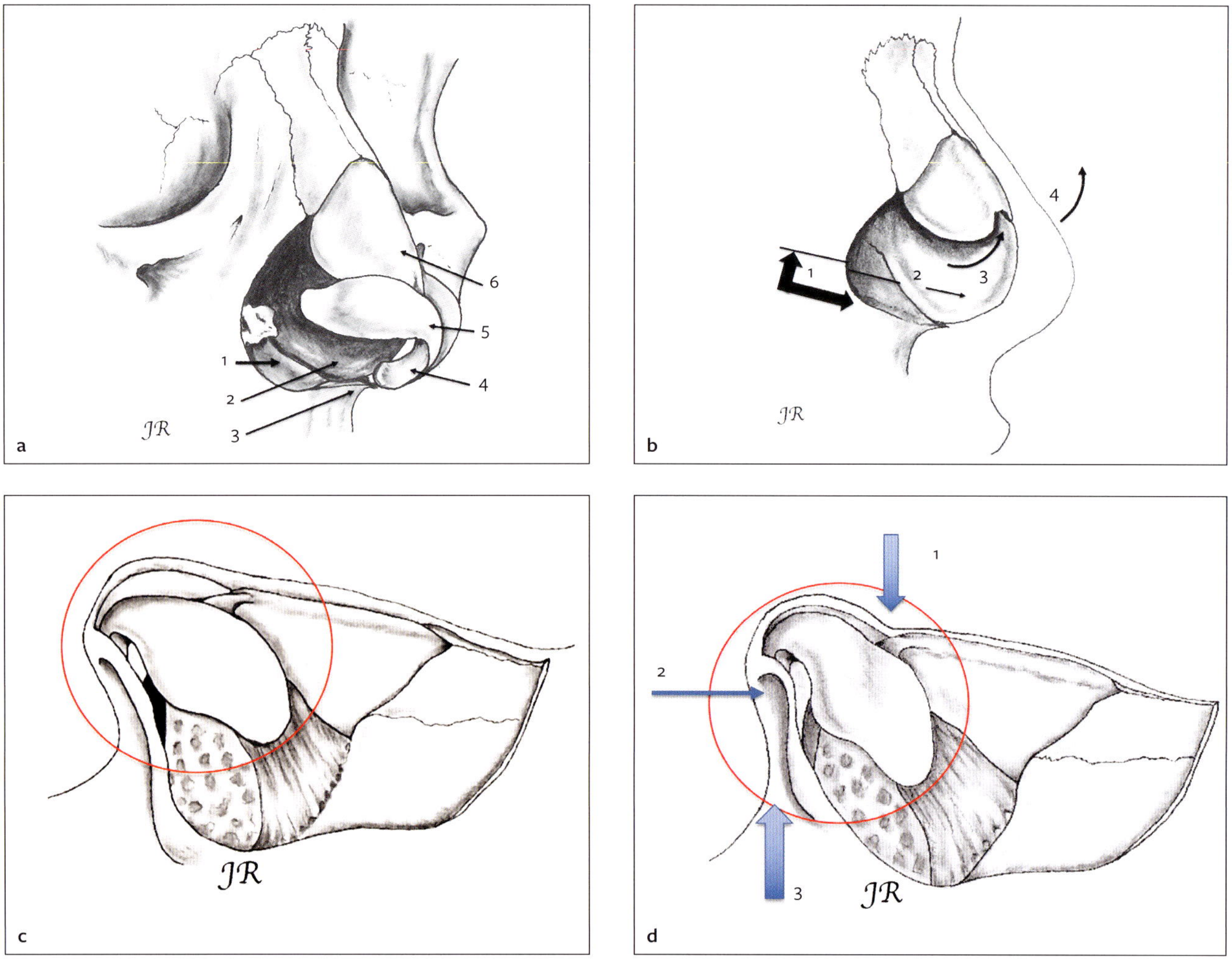

Fig 6-70 (*a*) The relationship between the bony septum (1), the quadrangular cartilage (2), the anterior nasal spine (3), the medial crus of the lower lateral cartilage (4), the lateral crus of the lower lateral cartilage (5), and the upper lateral cartilages (6) is demonstrated. (*b*) The lower lateral nasal cartilages are removed. *Arrows 3* and *4* show the results of advancement and/or superior repositioning of the maxilla without trimming the septum, reducing the anterior nasal spine, and contouring the piriform rims. (*c*) A lateral view of the nasal structures with the skin removed. (*d*) Without nasal control, the nasal tip will turn up (1) and the nostril show will increase (2), following a Le Fort I osteotomy (3).

Management of the nasal septum

Vertical reduction of the maxilla will inevitably impact the nasal septum and result in a deviated septum. Preventing this complication will require either reduction of the nasal septum height and/or creation of a trough in the nasal floor. This can be performed by trimming the cartilaginous septum and bony septum using a rongeur bone nibbler and/or creating a trough in the floor of the nose (the palatal aspect of the septum; see step 25). To stabilize and to centralize the septum in the trough, a septal suture is placed through the septum and then through a hole in the anterior nasal spine. It is wise to also reduce part of the ventral part of the septum when the maxilla is advanced to prevent any septal interferences.

Control of the nasal tip

Maxillary superior repositioning and/or advancement of the maxilla will increase the soft tissue and septal support of the medial crus of the lower lateral cartilages and the anterior nasal cartilaginous septum (Figs 6-70a and 6-70b). The above in combination with poor nasal volume control will tend to cause tipping up of the nasal tip and increase the nostril show (Figs 6-70c and 6-70d). Contouring the nasal floor and trimming the anterior nasal spine will prevent this unfavorable effect (see Figs 6-71a to 6-71d).

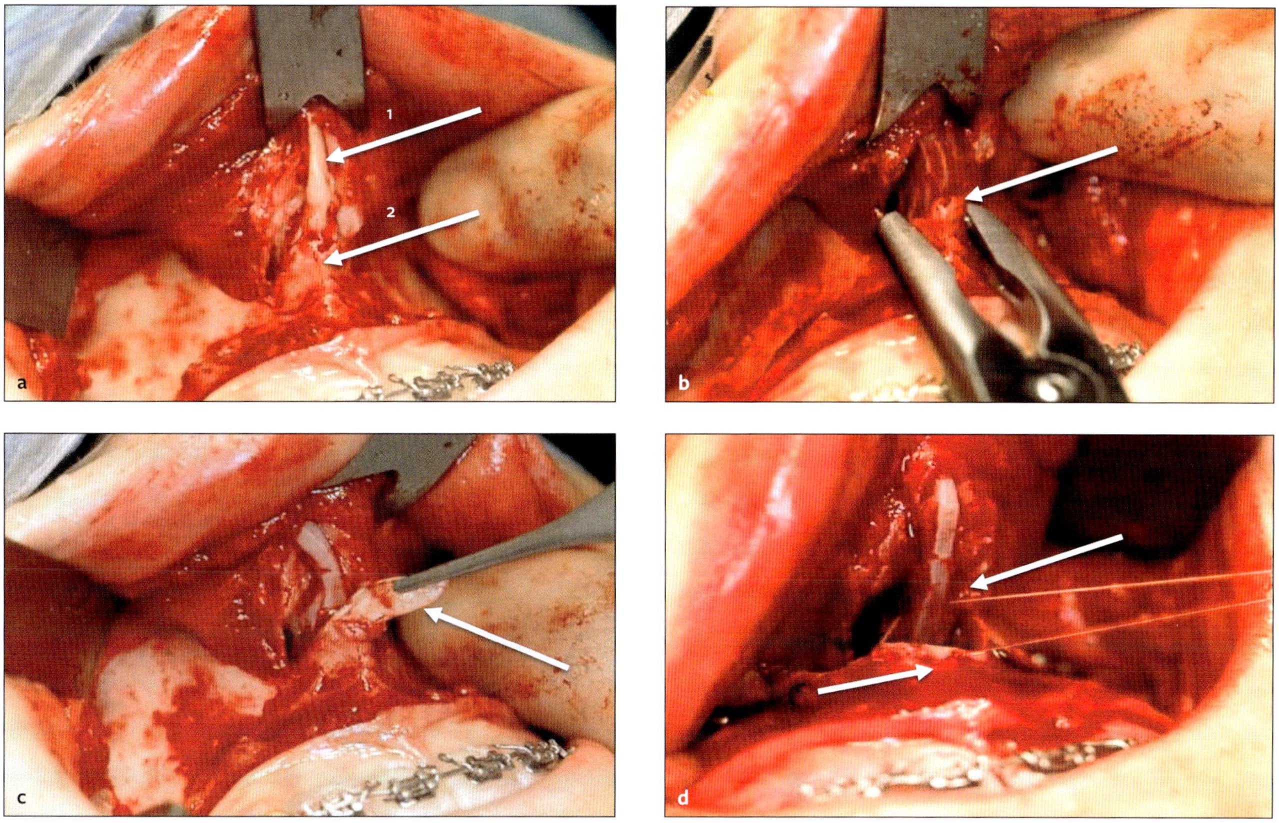

Fig 6-71 (*a*) The anterior nasal cartilage (1) and anterior nasal spine (2) are exposed. (*b*) A section of the inferior aspect is trimmed (*arrow*). (*c*) The anterior nasal spine is trimmed using a rongeur bone nibbler (*arrow*). (*d*) A nonresorbable suture is placed through the septum and through a hole in the remaining bone of the anterior nasal spine (*arrows*).

Control of the nasolabial angle

Increased support will tip the nasal tip up. Soft tissue subnasale (Sn′) will advance and the nasolabial angle will increase (see the section on nasolabial angle in chapter 2). The anterior nasal spine should be contoured. An existing increased nasolabial angle may also be caused by a hanging columella. The excessive cartilage should be trimmed and a septal suture placed through a hole in the anterior nasal spine (Fig 6-71) The septal discrepancy is addressed on the nasal floor area as well as reducing the cartilaginous septum (see Fig 6-71l).

Rhinoplasty and orthognathic surgery

The author prefers to perform formal rhinoplasty as a secondary procedure and not at the same time as jaw surgery. However, the reduction of a prominent nasal dorsum can be performed in combination with mandibular surgery.

Intraoperative diagnosis of condylar sag

During condylar positioning, the maxillomandibular complex (the mobilized maxilla fixed to the mandible by maxillomandibular fixation with the teeth in the planned occlusion) must rotate around a point at the condyle. If too little bone is removed at the posterior maxilla, the bone will act as a fulcrum, which will interfere with the rotation (Fig 6-72a). To achieve bone contact at the osteotomy site, the maxillomandibular complex is forced superiorly, which pulls the condyles inferiorly in the fossa (Fig 6-72b). Once the maxillomandibular fixation is released, the condyles will move superiorly into their normal position in the fossa, causing the mandible to rotate clockwise and the bite to open anteriorly, with a tendency for Class II malocclusion (Fig 6-72c). Slight upward force on the chin will allow the mandible to rotate counterclockwise, with the fulcrum now at the second molars.

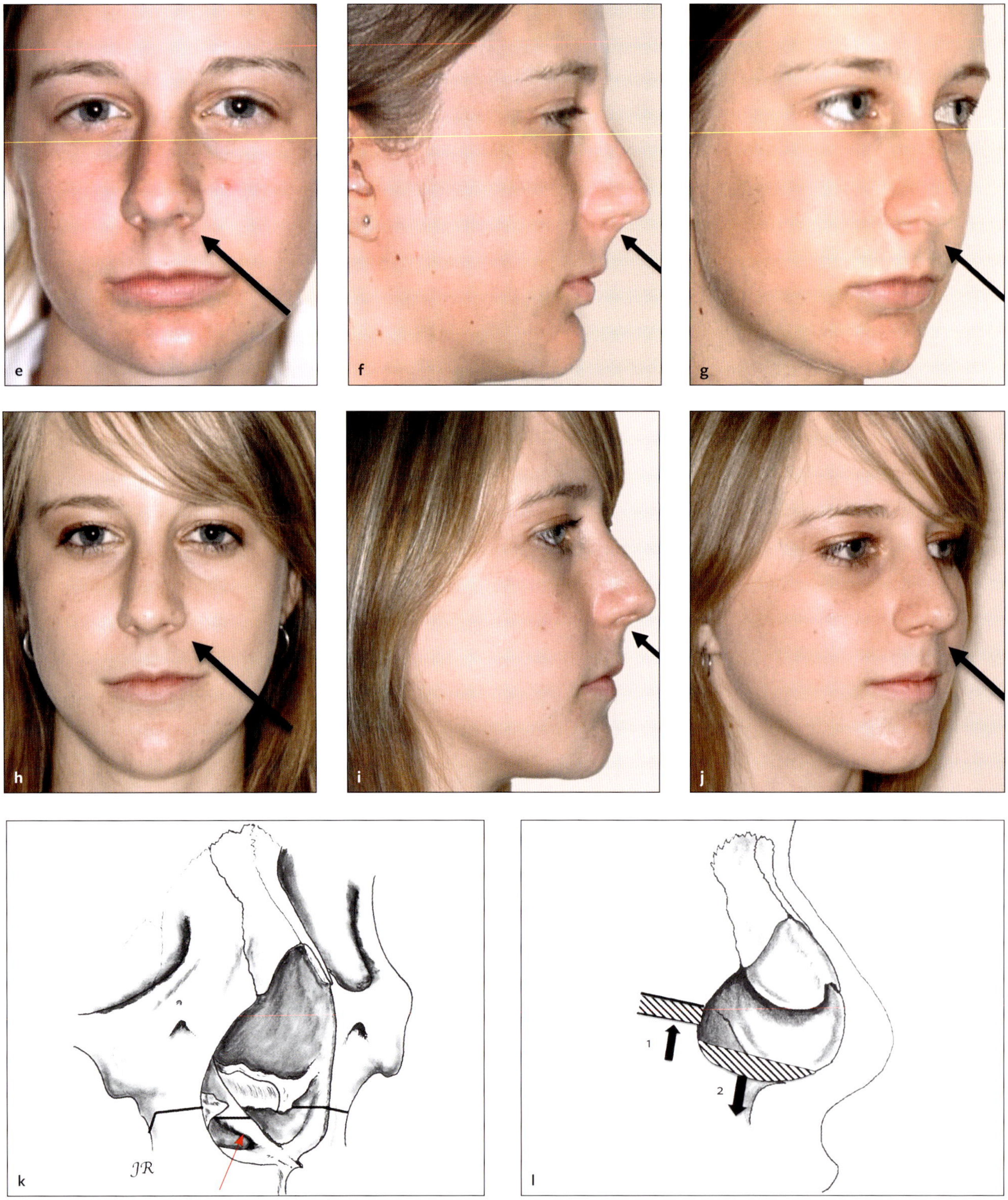

Fig 6-71 (*cont*) (*e to g*) The hanging columella and obtuse nasolabial is indicated by the *arrows* in the frontal, profile, and three-quarter views. (*h to j*) The esthetics improved after mandibular advancement and chin reduction combined with columella reshaping. Note the improved nasolabial angle and increased columella length (*arrows*). (k) Following the Le Fort I osteotomy, the septum needs to be reduced on the nasal floor to prevent any interference as a result of maxillary repositioning (*arrow*). (*l*) When the maxilla is superiorly repositioned (1), adequate septum reduction is necessary. Reduction of the anterior septum on the columella is required to control the nasolabial angulation (2).

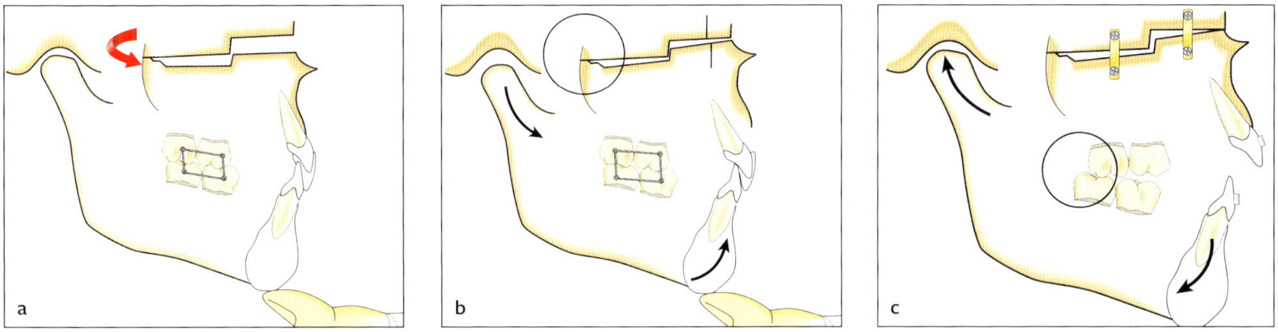

Fig 6-72 (*a*) The bony interference (*arrow*) at the posterior maxilla prevents rotation of the maxillomandibular complex around a point at the condyle to achieve ideal bone contact. (*b*) To achieve bone contact at the anterior maxilla, the maxillomandibular complex is rotated around the bony interference (*circle*), while the condyle moves inferiorly in the fossa. (*c*) Once the maxillomandibular fixation is released, the mandible rotates back in a clockwise direction, this time with the posterior molars (*circle*) as the fulcrum. This results in an anterior open bite and Class II dental relationship.

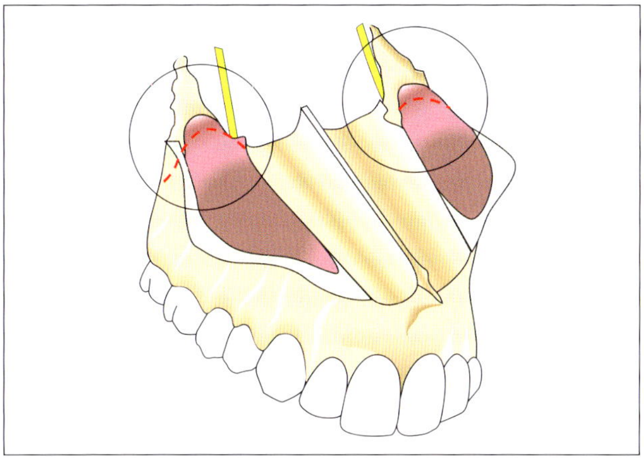

Fig 6-73 Bone interferences occur most often at the posterior maxilla (*circles*). The areas where bone should be removed are indicated by *dotted lines*.

The surgeon should be extremely critical when evaluating the occlusion at this stage. In the evaluation, the following issues should be kept in mind. First, the mandibular condyles should be treated with great care during the entire procedure to prevent intracapsular edema, hemarthrosis, or disc displacement—problems that would make condylar positioning difficult.

Second, during the placement of rigid fixation after Le Fort I maxillary osteotomies, the condyle may not be in its correct position. Sometimes the placement of rigid fixation takes a substantial amount of time, during which the condyle is held in an "abnormal" position. After the release of maxillomandibular fixation, the condyle may tend to remain in this position and make it appear that the occlusion and condyle are well positioned. Therefore, the mandible should be translated gently laterally and anteroposteriorly after removal of maxillomandibular fixation. Then, by light digital pressure on the chin, the mandible is rotated closed and the occlusion assessed. Any tendency to an anterior open bite due to interference of the molars indicates possible incorrect condylar positioning. This effect will only get worse postoperatively. Thus, a surgeon who suspects that the condyle may be displaced by posterior bone interferences should carefully investigate after the removal of rigid fixation.

Third, posterior bone interference usually occurs in the posteromedial area of the maxillary tuberosities (Fig 6-73). It is better to remove bone inferiorly at the posterior area of the downfractured maxilla than at the superior aspect.

Genioplasty

To correct a chin deformity, a sliding genioplasty may be performed as an isolated procedure or in conjunction with other surgical procedures. Over the past 40 years or so, the versatility of an osteotomy of the anterior part of the inferior border of the mandible has enabled the surgeon to modify the genial area in all three dimensions. The chin is one of the most noticeable facial structures; therefore, the surgeon must develop both artistry and surgical technique.

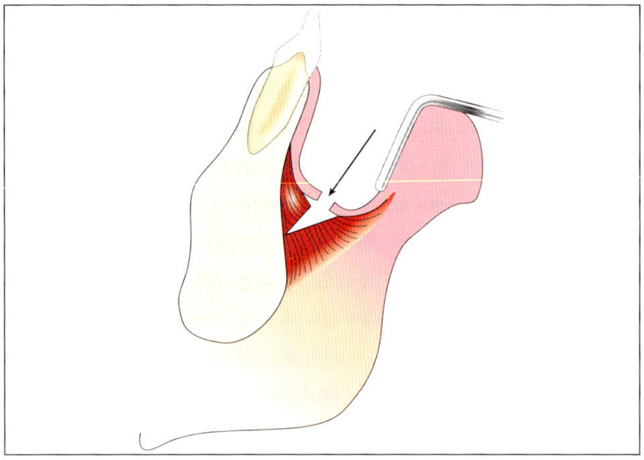

Fig 6-74 The soft tissue incision is angled to maintain more submucosal tissue for later ease of suturing.

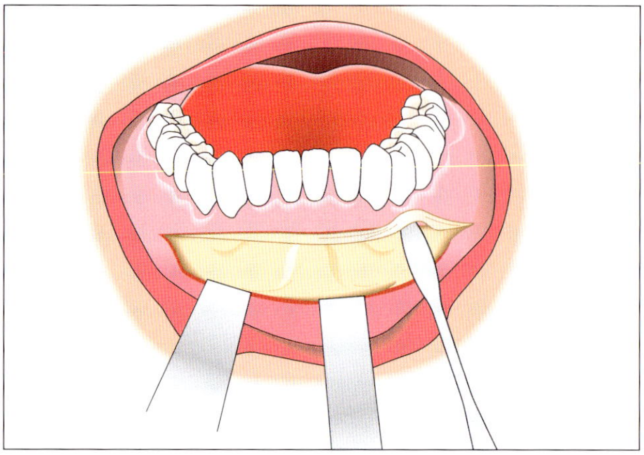

Fig 6-75 Subperiosteal dissection is carried downward and laterally to identify the mental nerve. The mucoperiosteum at the superior aspect is also elevated to make reapproximation of the mentalis muscle and mucosa easier.

Standard surgery

Step 1: Infiltration of soft tissue with a vasoconstrictor

Infiltrate the area of dissection with 2 mL of local anesthetic containing a vasoconstrictor (epinephrine in a concentration of 1:100,000) 10 minutes before surgery. Do not inject more than 2 mL of local anesthetic into this tissue because a large volume will distort the shape of the chin and make it difficult to clinically judge the esthetics at the time of surgery. Avoid injecting anesthetic into the mental neurovascular bundle.

Step 2: Mucosal incision

Make the first soft tissue incision through the labial mucosa of the mandible from just distal to the canine to a similar point on the contralateral side. Branches of the mental nerve can often be identified in the submucosal tissue laterally. Leave at least 5 mm of nonkeratinized mucosa superiorly to make later suturing easier.

Step 3: Submucosal incision

Make the second incision through the submucosal tissue and periosteum onto the bone, avoiding damage to the mental nerve at the lateral aspects of the incision. This incision is angled at 45 degrees to the bone so that more submucosal tissue and periosteum remain at the superior aspect, which will make later suturing easier (Fig 6-74).

Step 4: Mucoperiosteal dissection

Start the mucoperiosteal dissection from the center, and dissect laterally and inferiorly. Identify the mental nerves bilaterally. Also elevate the mucoperiosteum at the superior aspect (Fig 6-75) to make later suturing easier.

Step 5: Establishing reference points

Use a 701 bur to mark the dental midline on the bone superiorly and inferiorly to the intended osteotomy. Make small, shallow holes, keeping the roots of the incisors in mind, and score a line into the cortex to connect the holes (Fig 6-76a). Deepen the inferior hole by angling the bur superiorly and extending the hole well through the cortex. This hole is intended for the placement of a positioning wire later in the procedure. Place the hole in thick bone to ensure that the wire will not pull through (Fig 6-76b). For accurate repositioning of the chin, place reference marks approximately 15 mm lateral to the midline to assist with symmetric repositioning.

Step 6: Osteotomy design

The osteotomy should be created at least 5 mm below the roots of the incisors and 5 mm below the mental foramen. View and mark the angle of the osteotomy as planned on the surgical visual treatment objective (Fig 6-77a).

The following text will discuss the basic technique for the advancement of the chin using tricortical screw and bone plate fixation. The techniques for anteroposterior

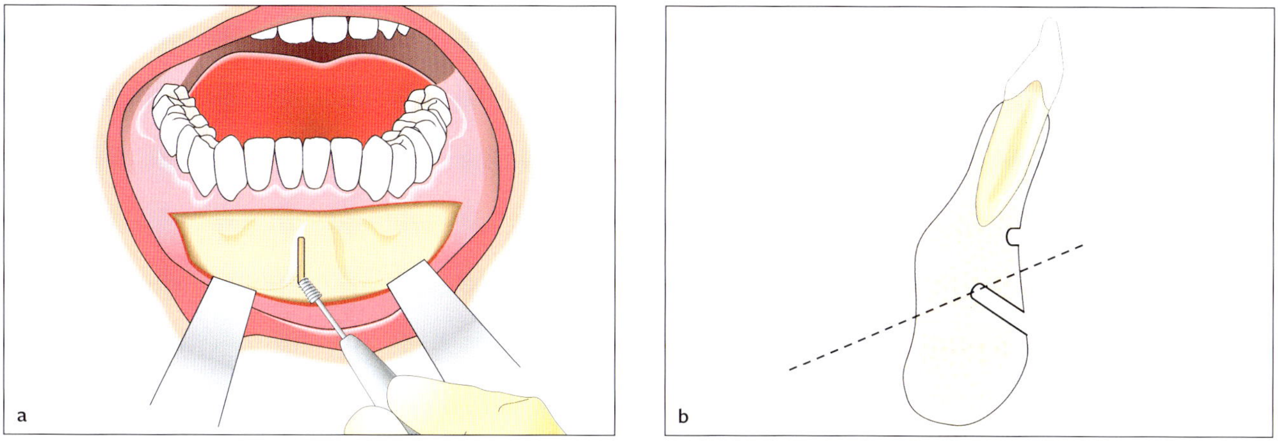

Fig 6-76 (*a*) The dental midline is marked on the bone. Two vertical reference lines are placed lateral to this line. (*b*) A superiorly angled hole is drilled in the midline below the intended osteotomy line. A positioning wire will be placed through this hole once the chin has been mobilized.

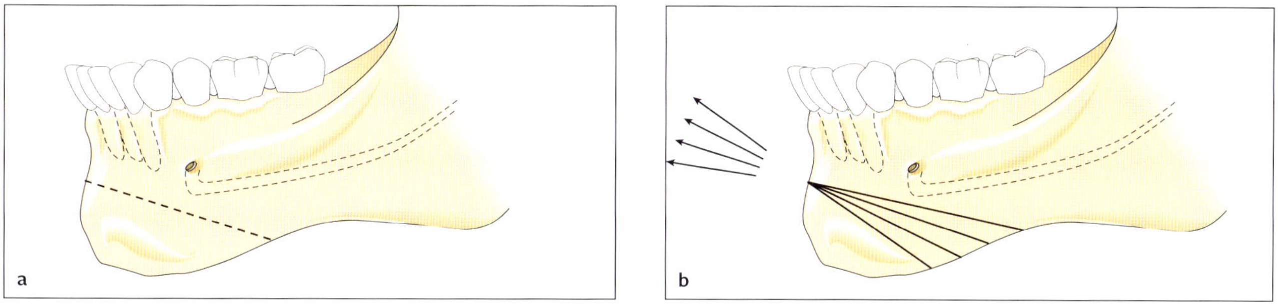

Fig 6-77 (*a*) The angle and position of the osteotomy is seen. The position of the mental nerve and the roots of the incisors and canines should be kept in mind. (*b*) The change of the angulation of the osteotomy and its effects on the vertical dimension after repositioning are demonstrated.

reduction, vertical change, correction of asymmetry, and change in width are discussed in steps 16 through 20.

Most genioplasty procedures are performed to improve the anteroposterior position of the chin. However, consideration must be given to the angulation of the osteotomy because variations in the angle will lead to changes in the vertical dimension of the chin, with obvious esthetic consequences. The angle of the osteotomy creates a plane along which the bony segment will slide (Fig 6-77b). The steepness of the angle of the osteotomy will be influenced by the esthetic requirements, the roots of the incisors and canines, and the position of the mental foramen. Keep in mind that the course of the mental nerve prior to its exit through the mental foramen is approximately 5 mm inferior and anterior to the foramen.

Step 7: Osteotomy of the chin

Perform the osteotomy with an oscillating saw by starting in the center and cutting laterally. Ensure that both cortices are osteotomized. Failure to include the lower border in the osteotomy will lead to an unfavorable fracture at the inferior border of the bone segment and thus inaccurate repositioning of the chin (unless contoured).

Step 8: Mobilization of the chin

After completion of the osteotomy, the chin segment should be mobile. However, it may be necessary to finally mobilize it with a light tap and then rotate a small osteotome in the osteotomy line. The need for excessive force to mobilize the chin indicates that the osteotomy is not completely through both cortices or the inferior border of the mandible, which may lead to an unpredicted fracture of the lower border.

When the genioplasty is combined with a bilateral sagittal split osteotomy of the mandible, it is preferable to perform the genioplasty after completing the sagittal split osteotomy. At this stage, the mandible is still held in position by maxillomandibular fixation. Performing

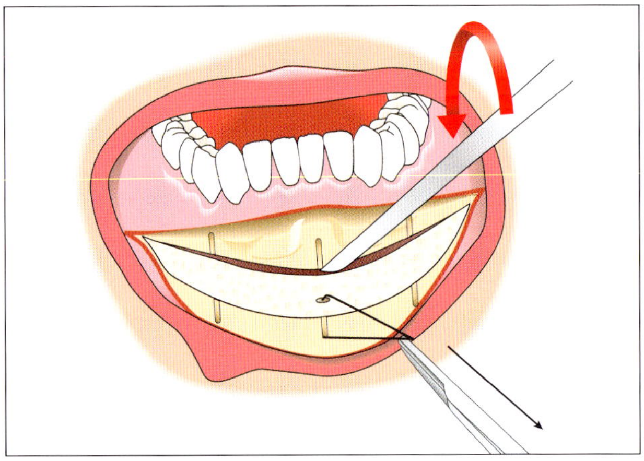

Fig 6-78 Mobilizing the chin. A Howarth elevator is placed behind the chin segment while the chin is pulled forward by the positioning wire.

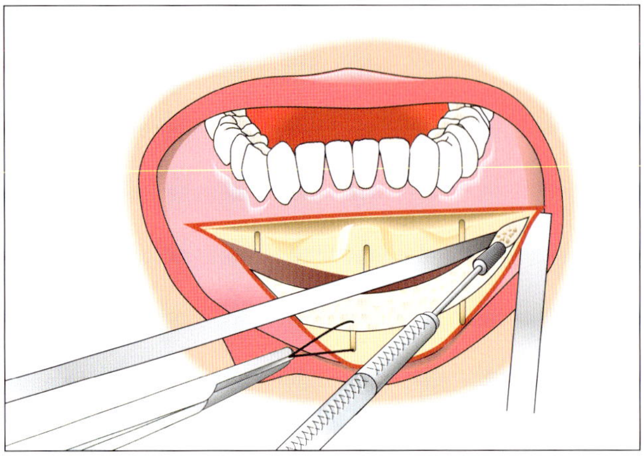

Fig 6-79 All bony interferences should be removed and irregularities smoothed prior to repositioning. Special attention should be given to the posterior area of the chin segment.

the genioplasty at this point allows the surgeon to evaluate the esthetics and, if necessary, make small positional changes to the chin to improve the appearance. Keeping the teeth in occlusion while performing the genioplasty provides the added advantage of supporting the mandible and reducing the forces on the rigid fixation screws that were recently placed. Avoid applying too much force to the mandible, however, because this may dislodge the orthodontic brackets.

Step 9: Engaging the positioning wire

Place a 0.018-inch wire through the hole drilled in the osteotomized segment during marking (see step 5), and attach a wire twister to it. This wire will be helpful both during the mobilization phase (see step 10) and in accurate repositioning of the chin.

Step 10: Final mobilization of the chin segment

Place a Howarth elevator behind the lingual cortex, and pull the chin forward by stretching the soft tissue (the suprahyoid muscles and periosteum; Fig 6-78). Adequate mobilization of the segment will facilitate easy and accurate repositioning of the chin.

Step 11: Refinement of the osteotomy

Check the posterior aspect of the osteotomized segment for any sharp or irregular edges, and remove the interferences using a large round vulcanite bur (Fig 6-79). Failure to smooth any irregularities will prevent accurate repositioning of the chin. Interferences are often found at the posterolingual area of the mobilized segment and the soft tissue. The sublingual salivary gland, facial artery, mentalis nerve, and geniohyoid muscles should also be protected during removal of these bony interferences.

Step 12: Repositioning the chin

Use the positioning wire and extraoral digital pressure to accurately reposition the chin according to the treatment plan (Fig 6-80). Although a golden rule in orthognathic surgery is "Never change your treatment plan on the operating table," genioplasty may be the exception. The surgeon may use clinical judgment at the time of surgery to slightly alter the repositioning of the chin for a better esthetic result.

Step 13: Countersinking holes for tricortical screw fixation

When tricortical bone screw fixation is contemplated, countersink two holes in the buccal cortex approximately 8 mm on either side of the marked midline of the osteotomized segment. Position the countersunk holes at least 5 mm from the superior edge of the segment to accommodate the head of the screw (Fig 6-81).

Step 14: Placement of tricortical screws

Drill the holes, and place the bone screws while the assistant holds the chin in its planned position using the holding wire and digital pressure. Drill the holes into the center of the countersunk holes using a trocar to protect the soft tissue, and simultaneously guide the drill at an appropriate angle to engage all three cortices (Fig 6-82a). Ensure that the screw is long enough to engage all three cortices (Fig 6-82b).

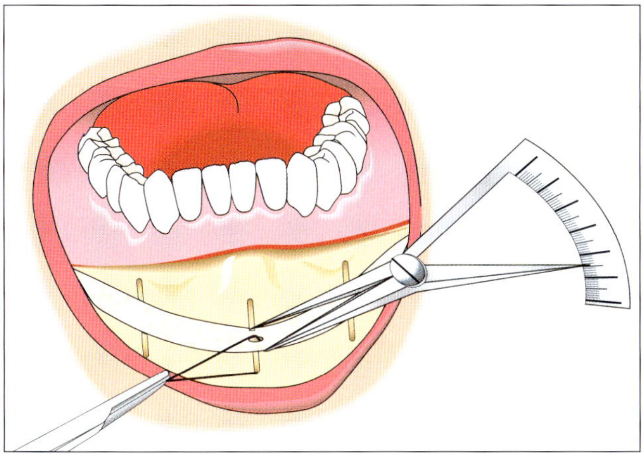

Fig 6-80 The chin segment is placed in its planned position via the positioning wire.

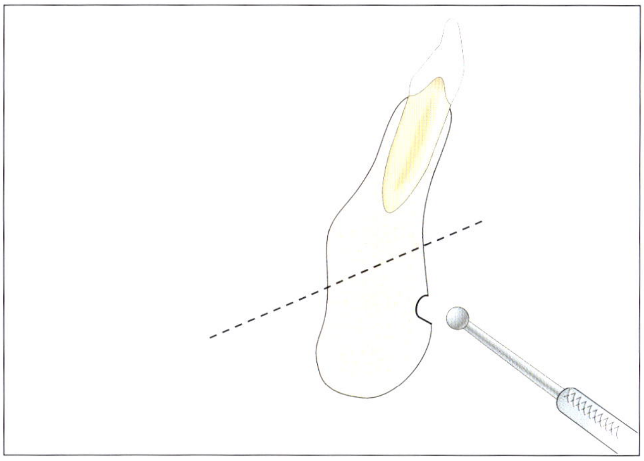

Fig 6-81 A countersink hole is placed to accommodate the head of the screw.

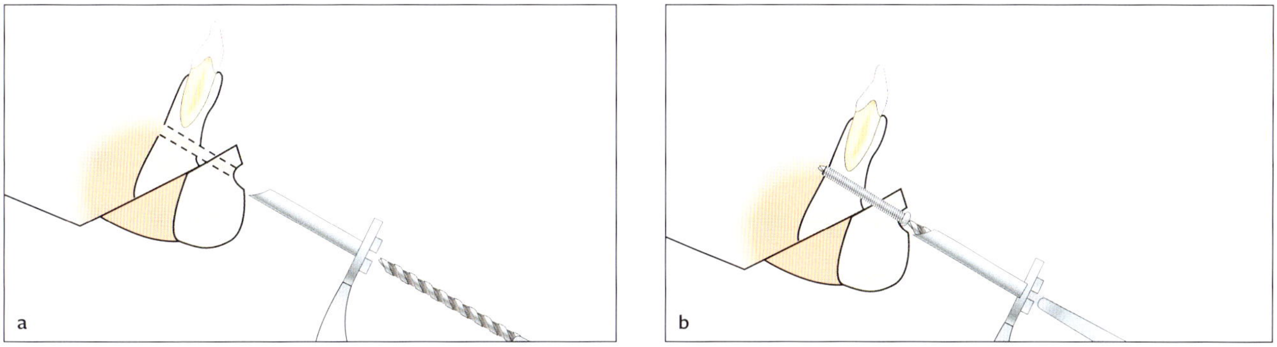

Fig 6-82 (*a*) A hole is drilled through all three cortices using a trocar to protect the soft tissue. (*b*) A trocar is used to place a tricortical screw to fixate the chin segment. At least two screws should be placed to secure the bone segment.

Step 15: Bone plate fixation as an alternative to screw fixation

Use a prefabricated chin fixation plate, an X- or H-shaped bone plate, or two straight bone plates with two screws on either side of the osteotomy. The positioning wire and digital pressure help stabilize the chin segment in its planned position (Fig 6-83) while the bone plates are bent to fit accurately and passively. Avoid damaging the roots of the incisors with the screws. It is recommended that fixation be placed on each side of the midline.

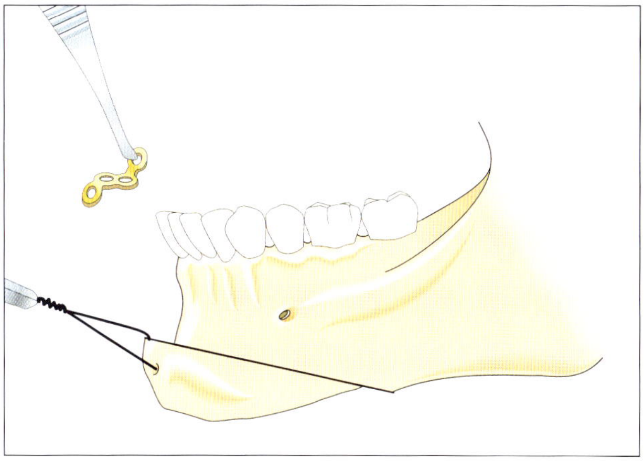

Fig 6-83 As an alternative to tricortical screw fixation, bone plates may be used as rigid fixation.

Step 16: Anteroposterior reduction of the chin

Position the chin using extraoral digital pressure, check the position of the bone using a caliper, and use a prefabricated chin fixation plate or bend the appropriate plate to fit accurately and passively (Fig 6-84a). Use a prefabricated chin fixation plate, an X- or H-shaped bone plate, or two straight plates. When the chin is set back, the posterolingual area often has a palpable step defect at the inferior border of the mandible, which may concern the patient. To contour this area, the osteotomized segment is pulled downward and forward, and the posterolingual aspect of the chin segment is contoured (Fig 6-84b). Protect the soft tissue at all times during this step.

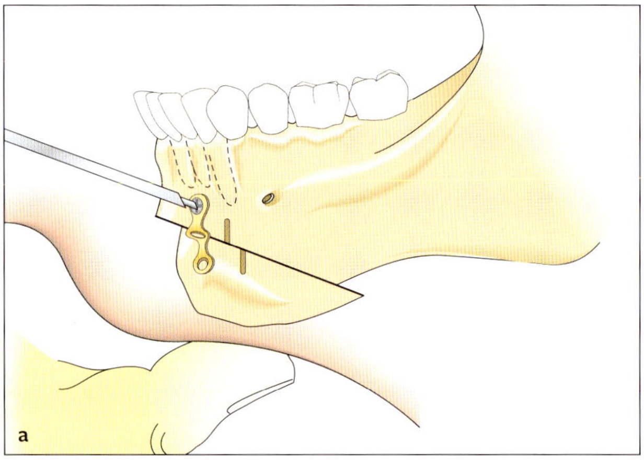

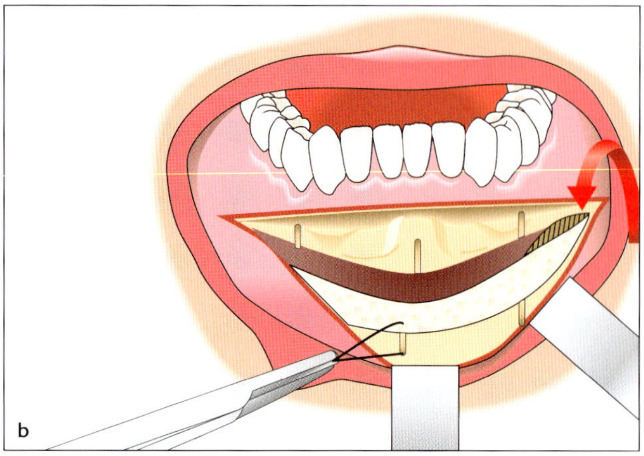

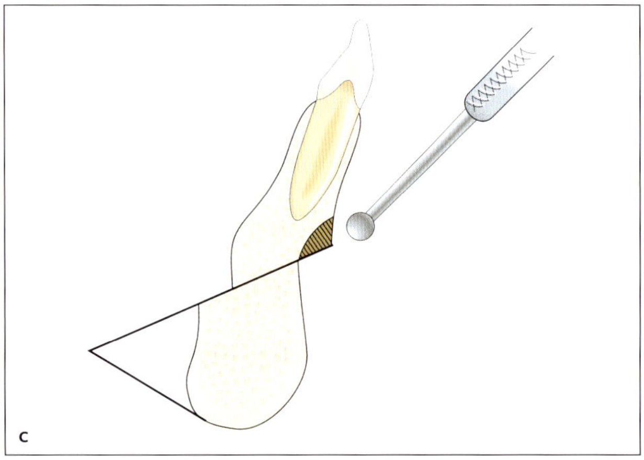

Fig 6-84 (*a*) For setback procedures of the chin, bone plate fixation is the method of choice. In setback procedures, the use of a positioning wire is impractical. (*b*) The medial aspect of the posterior area of the chin segment is removed to prevent a palpable step defect on the lower border of the mandible (*arrow*). (*c*) The labiomental fold is enhanced by contouring the anterior edge on the superior aspect of the mandible.

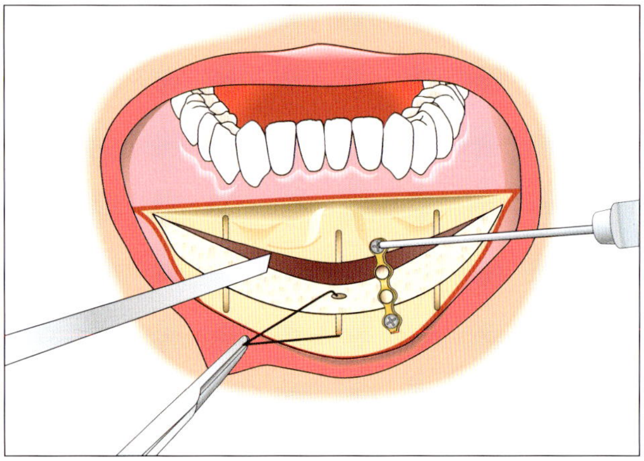

Fig 6-85 Vertical increase of the chin. The chin segment is held at the planned height with a positioning wire. Two bone plates are then placed to fixate the segment. Finally, the defect is grafted.

Anteroposterior reduction of the chin may result in flattening of the labiomental fold. The sharp anterior edge on the superior aspect may be contoured to counter this effect and enhance the depth of the labiomental fold and chin shape (Fig 6-84c).

Step 17: Vertical increase of the chin

Using a 701 fissure bur, drill reference holes recording the vertical dimensions of the chin. To maintain the symmetry of the chin, the reference marks should be made in the midline as well as approximately 15 mm lateral to the midline and the distances between them recorded. Place a bone plate while the assistant uses the positioning wire and an instrument wedged between the segments to maintain the required space between the bony segments (Fig 6-85). At least two screws should be placed superiorly and inferiorly to the osteotomy using an H- or X-shaped plate or two straight plates to secure the segment and maintain the vertical height. It is recommended that a bone graft be placed in the defect; however, do not force the bone graft into the defect because doing so might displace or mobilize the chin segment.

Step 18: Vertical reduction of the chin

Drill reference marks recording the vertical dimensions of the chin. To maintain symmetry of the chin, place the marks in the midline and approximately 15 mm lateral to the midline, and record the distances between them. Perform

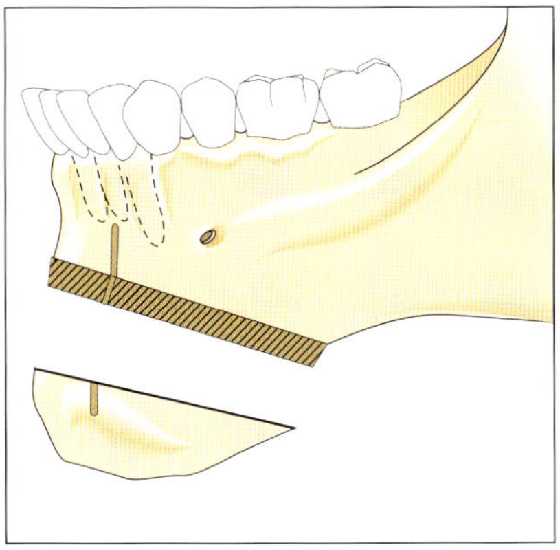

Fig 6-86 Vertical reduction of the chin. The lower osteotomy is performed first, and the planned amount of bone is then removed superiorly.

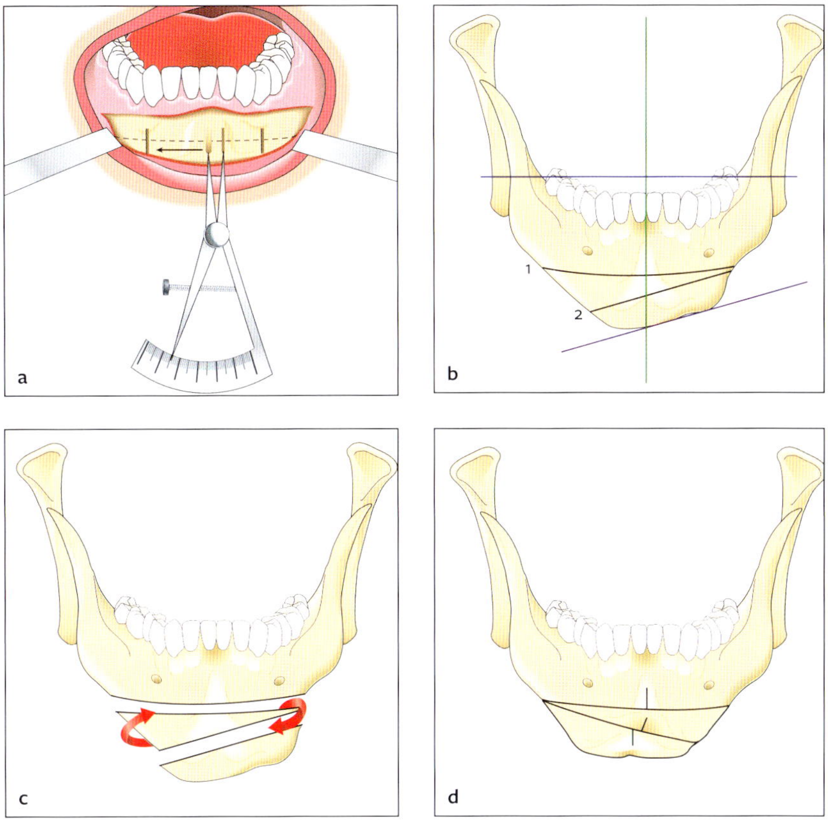

Fig 6-87 (*a*) Lateral movement of the chin. The midline of the chin is marked below the osteotomy line and the facial midline above the osteotomy line. After mobilization of the chin, the chin segment is moved laterally until the lines coincide. (*b*) Propeller osteotomy. A first osteotomy (1) is performed parallel to the interpupillary line. A second osteotomy (2) is then performed parallel to the lower border of the chin. (*c*) The triangular segment, pedicled to the hyoid muscles, is rotated 180 degrees. (*d*) The two segments are secured by rigid fixation.

the first osteotomy low enough to facilitate performing the second osteotomy from the superior aspect (Fig 6-86). Complete the lower osteotomy, and mobilize the chin. Mark the amount and shape of bone to be removed, and then complete the superior osteotomy. The shape of the ostectomized bone will influence the final anteroposterior position of the tip of the chin; that is, if the ostectomy is wider anteriorly, the chin will rotate anteriorly, whereas an ostectomy that is wider posteriorly will rotate the chin posteriorly. Maintain as much soft tissue attachment to the chin as possible to ensure good blood supply to the repositioned bone and to reduce dead space. This will also yield a more predictable esthetic result.

Step 19: Correction of asymmetry of the chin

Drill reference holes recording the dimensions of the chin. For lateral movement of the chin, the dental midline is marked on the superior aspect of the osteotomy line whereas the midline of the chin is marked on the inferior aspect (Fig 6-87a). When correction of asymmetry requires vertical change as well, marks are placed lateral to the midline to record vertical dimensions on both the left and right sides. Large cants in the chin contour (eg, in unilateral condylar hyperplasia or hypoplasia) may have to be corrected by a propeller osteotomy. The first osteotomy is performed superior and parallel to the occlusal plane or interpupillary plane. A second osteotomy is performed parallel to the lower border of the chin (Fig 6-87b). The small, triangular segment is rotated 180 degrees while its muscle attachment is maintained (Fig 6-87c). The inferior segment can now be secured by rigid fixation (Fig 6-87d).

Step 20: Altering the width of the chin

Using a 701 fissure bur, drill reference marks recording the presurgical chin dimensions.

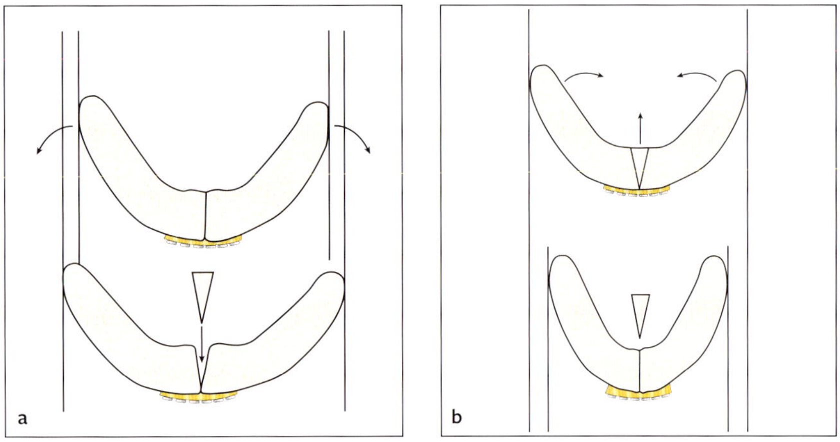

Fig 6-88 (*a*) Widening the posterior dimension of the chin. A midline osteotomy is performed through the chin segment after placement of a bone plate on the anterior surface. The plate is now used as a hinge, widening the posterior chin, and a small bone graft is placed in the midline defect. (*b*) Narrowing the posterior dimension of the chin. A bone plate is placed on the anterior surface of the chin and a triangular midline ostectomy performed. The segment is now bent medially to narrow the chin.

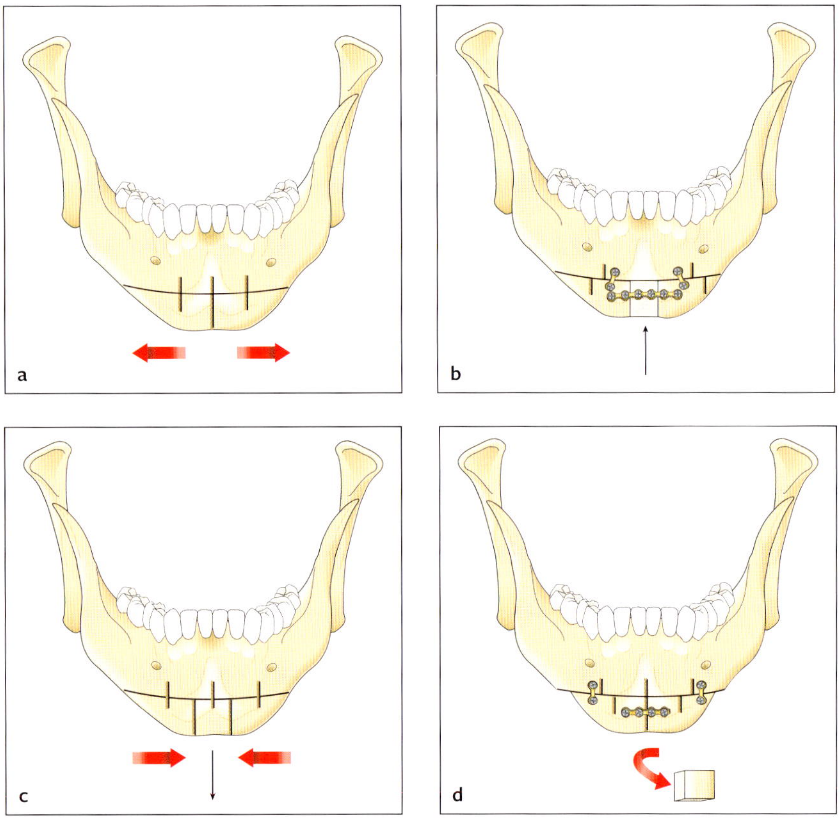

Fig 6-89 (*a*) Widening the anterior dimension of the chin. An osteotomy is performed in the center of the chin segment. (*b*) After increasing the anterior width of the chin, a bone graft is placed between the segments. (*c*) Narrowing the anterior dimension of the chin. A midline ostectomy is performed in the center part of the chin. (*d*) After removal of the ostectomized bone, the lateral segments are moved medially.

Widening or narrowing the posterior dimension of the chin

Before the chin is mobilized, a four-hole straight plate fixation is done horizontally across the midline to the labial cortex of the chin. To widen the chin, perform a midline osteotomy through the buccal and lingual cortex, and complete the osteotomy with a small osteotome. The chin can now be widened by using the bone plate as a hinge (Fig 6-88a). To narrow the chin, perform a triangular midline ostectomy on the lingual aspect of the chin segment, again using the bone plate as a hinge (Fig 6-88b).

Once the desired shape of the chin has been achieved, additional fixation can be placed. Fixation should be placed on both sides of the midline osteotomy.

Widening or narrowing the anterior dimension of the chin

In widening the chin, a predetermined width can be achieved by performing a midline osteotomy and increasing the anterior width by moving the segments laterally (Fig 6-89a). Secure the graft between the segments with a bone plate before fixation of the segments to the mandible (Fig 6-89b).

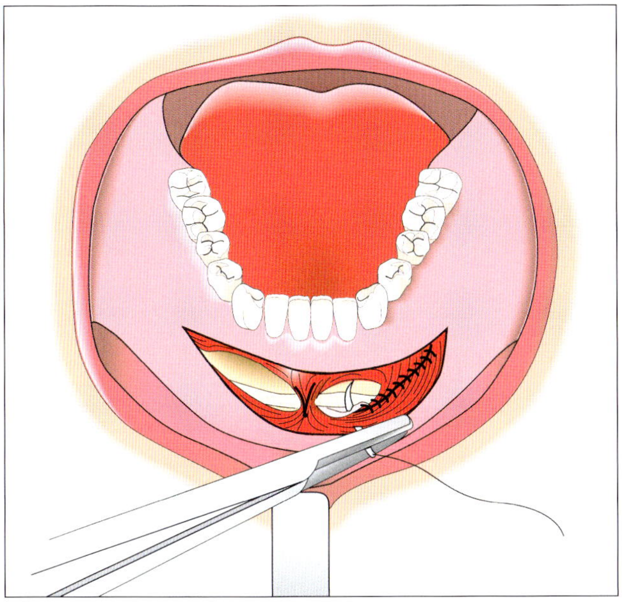

Fig 6-90 To achieve the best esthetic results, it is mandatory that the mentalis muscles be accurately reapproximated. Mucosal suturing should follow.

To narrow the chin, a predetermined amount of bone is ostectomized from the mobilized segment. To simplify the removal of the ostectomized bone from the center of the chin, complete all the osteotomies before mobilizing the segments (Figs 6-89c and 6-89d).

Step 21: Suturing the submucosal tissue

Place an interrupted midline suture to accurately reestablish midline soft tissue alignment. Then use a continuous 3-0 chromic suture to reapproximate the periosteum and muscle (Fig 6-90). Accurate reapproximation of the mentalis muscle is of the utmost importance in maintaining the soft tissue contour.

Step 22: Suturing the mucosa

Place a single midline 4-0 chromic suture to maintain lip symmetry. Use a continuous suture to secure the rest of the mucosa.

Step 23: Applying a pressure dressing

Vertical and horizontal pressure is applied to the chin via a pressure bandage. Postoperative hematoma formation and swelling is limited by keeping the bandage in place for approximately 3 days.

Complications

Although postoperative complications are infrequent, the following complications may occur:

- Damage to the mental nerve
- Damage to the roots of the canines and/or incisors
- Unexpected esthetic results due to excessive soft tissue stripping
- Postoperative hemorrhage and sublingual hematoma formation
- Wound dehiscence
- Unfavorable bone fracture

Recommended Reading

Acebal-Bionco F, Vuylstek PL, Mommaerts MY, De Clercq CA. Perioperative complications in corrective facial orthopedic surgery: A 5-year retrospective study. J Oral Maxillofac Surg 2000;58:754–760.

Axhauser G. Zur Behandlung veralteter distozierter gerheilter Oberkieferbrüche. Dtsch Zahn Mund Kieferheilkd 1934;1:334.

Bell WH. Correction of maxillary excess by anterior maxillary osteotomy. Oral Surg Oral Med Oral Pathol 1977;43:323–332.

Bell WH, Fonseca RJ, Kennedy JW, Levy BM. Bone healing and revascularization after total maxillary osteotomy. J Oral Surg 1975;33:253–260.

Betts NJ. Surgically assisted maxillary expansion. Atlas Oral Maxillofac Surg Clin North Am 2016;24:67–77.

Blair VP. Operations on the jaw bone of the face. Surg Gynecol Obstet 1907;4:67–78.

Blair VP. Treatment of deformities and malrelations of the jaws. In: Surgery and Diseases of the Mouth and Jaws. St Louis: Mosby, 1912.

Burch RJ, Bowden GW, Woodward HW. Intraoral one-stage ostectomy for correction of mandibular prognathism: Report of a case. J Oral Surg 1961;19:72–76.

Caldwell JB, Letterman GS. Vertical osteotomy in the mandibular rami for correction of prognathism. J Oral Surg 1954;12:185–202.

Collins P, Epker BN. The alar base cinch: A technique for prevention of alar base flaring secondary to maxillary surgery. Oral Surg Oral Med Oral Pathol 1982;53:549–553.

Dal Pont G. Retromolar osteotomy for the correction of prognathism. J Oral Surg Anesth Hosp Dent Serv 1961;19:42–47.

da Fontura RA, Vasconcellos HA, Campos AE. Morphologic basis for the intraoral vertical ramus osteotomy: Anatomic and radiographic localization of the mandibular foramen. J Oral Maxillofac Surg 2002;60:660–665.

De Clercq CA, Neyt LF, Mommaerts MY, Abeloos JV, De Mot BM. Condylar resorption in orthognathic surgery: A retrospective study. Int J Adult Orthodon Orthognath Surg 1994;9:233–240.

Dingman RO. Surgical correction of mandibular prognathism: An improved method. Am J Orthod Oral Surg 1944;30:683–692.

Edwards RC, Kiely KD. Resorbable fixation of Le Fort I osteotomies. J Craniofac Surg 1998;9:210–214.

Edwards RC, Kiely KD, Eppley BL. Resorbable PLLA-PGA screw fixation of mandibular sagittal split osteotomies. J Craniofac Surg 1999;10:230–236.

Epker BN. Modifications in the sagittal osteotomy of the mandible. J Oral Surg 1977;35:157–159.

Ferretti C, Reyneke JP. Genioplasty. Atlas Oral Maxillofac Surg Clin North Am 2016;24:79–85.

Guyman M, Crosby D, Wolford LM. The alar base cinch suture to control nasal width in maxillary osteotomies. Int J Adult Orthodon Orthognath Surg 1988;3:89–95.

Hall HD. Intraoral vertical ramus osteotomy. In: Bell WH (ed). Modern Practice in Orthognathic and Reconstructive Surgery: Mandibular Prognathism. Philadelphia: Saunders, 1992.

Hinds EC, Girotti WJ. Vertical subcondylar osteotomy: A reappraisal. Oral Surg Oral Med Oral Pathol 1967;24:164–170.

Hunsuck EE. A modified intraoral splitting technique for the correction of mandibular prognathism. J Oral Surg 1968;26:250–253.

Jones JK, Van Sickels JE. Facial nerve injuries associated with orthognathic surgery: A review of incidence and management. J Oral Maxillofac Surg 1991;49:740–744.

Le Fort R. Étude expérimentale sur les fractures de la machoire supérieure. Rev Chir 1901;23:208–227.

MacIntosh RB. Experience with the sagittal split osteotomy of the mandibular ramus: A 13-year review. J Maxillofac Surg 1981;9:151–165.

McKenna SJ, King EE. Intraoral vertical ramus osteotomy procedure and technique. Atlast Oral Maxillofac Surg Clin North Am 2016;24:37–43.

New GB, Erich JB. The surgical correction of mandibular prognathism. Am J Surg 1941;53:2–12.

Obwegeser H. Eingriffe am oberkiefer zur korrektur des progenen zustandsbildes. Schweiz Mschr Zahnheilk 1965;75:365–374.

Obwegeser H, Trauner R. Zur operationstechnik bei der progenie und anderen unterkieferanomalien. Dtsch Zahn Mund Kieferheilkd 1955;23:H1–H2.

O'Ryan F, Schendel S. Nasal anatomy and maxillary surgery. II. Unfavourable nasolabial esthetics following the Le Fort I osteotomy. Int J Adult Orthodon Orthognath Surg 1989;4:75–84.

Park HS. A clinical study on prognosis of intraoral vertical ramus osteotomy for mandibular setback in the mandibular prognathism. J Korean Assoc Oral Maxillofac Surg 1997;23:561–580.

Park HS. Transoral vertical ramus osteotomy (TOVRO). In: Fonseca RJ (ed). Oral and Maxillofacial Surgery, ed 2, vol III. Philadelphia: Saunders, 2009:119–136.

Precious DS, Goodday RH, Bourget L, Skulsky FG. Pterygoid plate fracture in Le Fort I osteotomy with and without pterygoid chisel: A computed tomography scan evaluation of 58 patients. J Oral Maxillofac Surg 1993;51:151–153.

Reyneke JP. The anterior maxillary osteotomy [in Afrikaans]. J Dent Assoc S Afr 1979;34:217–221.

Reyneke JP. The Art and Science of the Sliding Genioplasty. Gainesville: RAEduction, 2018.

Reyneke JP. Evaluation of the vitality of teeth following subapical osteotomy. J Dent Assoc S Afr 1981;36:19–22.

Reyneke JP. The Le Fort I Maxillary Osteotomy Surgical Manual. Jacksonville: Lorenz Surgical, 2000.

Reyneke JP. Johan P Reyneke's Techniques, Tips, Tricks and Traps. Vol 1: The Bilateral Sagittal Split Mandibular Ramus Osteotomy. Gainesville: RAEducation, 2018.

Reyneke JP. Johan P Reyneke's Techniques, Tips, Tricks and Traps. Vol 2: The Le Fort I Osteotomy. Gainesville: RAEduction, 2019.

Reyneke JP, Ferretti C. Intraoperative diagnosis of condylar sag after bilateral sagittal split ramus osteotomy. Br J Oral Maxillofac Surg 2002;40:285–292.

Reyneke JP, Ferretti C. The bilateral sagittal split mandibular ramus osteotomy. Atlas Oral Maxillofac Surg Clin North Am 2016;24:27–36.

Reyneke JP, Johnson T, van der Linden WJ. Screw osteosynthesis compared with wire advancement genioplasty: A restrospective study of skeletal stability. Br J Oral Maxillofac Surg 1997;35:352–356.

Reyneke JP, Masureik CJ. Condylar hyperplasia: An alternative method of treatment. J Dent Assoc S Afr 1979;34:335–339.

Reyneke JP, Masureik CJ. Treatment of maxillary deficiency by a Le Fort I downsliding technique. J Oral Maxillofac Surg 1985;43:914–916.

Reyneke JP, Tsakiris P, Becker P. Age as a factor in the complication rate after removal of unerupted/impacted third molars at the time of mandibular sagittal split osteotomy. J Oral Maxillofac Surg 2002;60:654–659.

Robinson M. Prognathism corrected by open vertical subcondylotomy. J Oral Surg 1958;16:215–219.

Schuchardt D. Ein beitrag zur chirurgeschen kieferorthopadie unter berucksichtigung ihrer bedeutung für die behandlung angeborener und erworbener kieferdeformitaten bei soldaten. Dtsch Zahn Mund Kieferheilkd 1942;9:73.

Sullivan SM. Le Fort I osteotomy. Atlas Oral Maxillofac Surg Clin North Am 2016;24:1–13.

Turvey TA. Intraoperative complications of sagittal osteotomy of the mandibular ramus: Incidence and management. J Oral Maxillofac Surg 1985;43:504–509.

Turvey TA, Scully JR, Waite PD, Costello BJ, Ruiz RL. Orthognathic surgery. In: Fonseca RJ (ed). Oral and Maxillofacial Surgery, ed 2, vol III. New York: Saunders, 2009:848–863.

Van de Perre JP, Stoelinga PJ, Blijdorp PA, Brouns JJ, Hoppenreijs TJ. Perioperative morbidity in maxillofacial orthopaedic surgery: A retrospective study. J Craniomaxillofac Surg 1996;24:263–270.

Van Sickels JE, Larsen AJ, Triplett RG. Predictability of maxillary surgery: A comparison of internal and external reference marks. Oral Surg Oral Med Oral Pathol 1986;61:542–545.

Wassmund M. Lehrbuch der probleschen chirurgie des mundes und der kiefer, vol 1. Leipzig: Meuser, 1935.

Willmar K. On Le Fort I osteotomy; A follow-up study of 106 operated patients with maxillo-facial deformity. Scand J Plast Reconstr Surg 1974;12(suppl 12):1–68.

Wolford LM. Computer-assisted surgical simulation for concomitant temporomandibular joint custom-fitted total joint reconstruction and orthognathic surgery. Atlas Oral Maxillofac Surg Clin North Am 2016;24:55–66.

Woford LM, Mercuri LG, Schneiderman ED, Movahed R, Allen W. Twenty-year follow-up on a patient-fitted temporomandibular joint prosthesis: The Techmedica/TMJ Concepts device. J Oral Maxillofac Surg 2015;73:952–60.

INDEX

Page numbers followed by "f" denote figures; those followed by "t" denote tables